John M. Graham

Glenis K. Scadding

Peter D. Bull

Editors

Pediatric ENT

John M. Graham
Glenis K. Scadding
Peter D. Bull

Editors

Pediatric ENT

With 355 Figures and 79 Tables

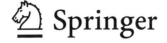
Springer

Mr. John M. Graham
Royal National Throat, Nose and Ear Hospital
330 Gray's Inn Road
London WC1X 8DA
United Kingdom

Dr. Glenis K. Scadding
Royal National Throat, Nose and Ear Hospital
330 Gray's Inn Road
London WC1X 8DA
United Kingdom

Mr. Peter D. Bull
Sheffield Children's Hospital
Western Bank
Sheffield S10 2TH
United Kingdom

2nd Printing 2008

ISBN   978-3-540-69930-9   e-ISBN   978-3-540-33039-4

Library of Congress Control Number: 2007923510

© 2007 Springer-Verlag Berlin Heidelberg

Cover design: Frido Steinen-Broo, EStudio, Calamar, Spain

Printed on acid-free paper

9 8 7 6 5 4

springer.com

Foreword

Children are special! This book is special!

Hospitals for sick children were founded in the first decade of the 20th century, and even before. Dedicated nurses and doctors with an interest in children were pioneers in those child-friendly hospitals, although diagnostic and therapeutic techniques were modest.

Currently, medical and surgical disciplines cooperate with paramedical professionals and specially trained nurses in the treatment of children. The contribution of professionals with an expertise in biochemistry and biophysics has also become essential, since routine procedures and research are dependent on advanced and advancing technology.

The scope of pathologists has broadened to the cellular and subcellular level. Molecular medicine is making progress. Information technology has contributed to the development of disciplines like epidemiology, clinical epidemiology and genetics. Modern imaging techniques produce data pertinent to the anatomy and metabolism of pathological processes.

Pediatric otorhinolaryngology has largely benefited from these new technologies and data produced by recent research. Moreover, interdisciplinary teamwork in audiology, vestibular pathology, neuro-otology, speech and hearing disorders, and allergy and genetics, together with the contributions of intensive care specialists, pediatricians and anesthetists have all contributed to raise the quality of patient care in pediatric otorhinolaryngology.

The biannual international congresses of the European Society of Pediatric Otorhinolaryngology (ESPO) have provided a prominent worldwide forum, presenting the latest research and evaluation of new and current practice, and acting as a meeting point for all colleagues with an interest in treating children with otorhinolaryngology-related pathology.

It is my great pleasure to welcome and recommend this book. We should be most grateful to John Graham, former president of the ESPO, Glenis Scadding, eminent in the field of allergy, and Peter Bull a distinguished pediatric laryngologist, and appreciate their great efforts to present a state of the art account of our specialty. They have brought together a group of eminent authors, presenting recent advances in all aspects of pediatric otorhinolaryngology. You will certainly appreciate their up-to-date information and critical evaluation of the field of pediatric otorhinolaryngology.

Carel Verwoerd
Secretary General
European Society of Pediatric
Otorhinolaryngology (ESPO)

Preface

This book has been written to fill a need for a basic but comprehensive text dealing with all aspects of paediatric ENT. It is aimed at trainees in our specialties who are developing an interest in the paediatric aspects of their work, at established ENT surgeons and audiologists who have decided to specialise in this most enjoyable subspecialty, or who wish to know more about paediatric ENT, and as a work of reference for those who encounter particular problems in their paediatric patients.

The scope of paediatric ENT has grown over recent years to the extent that doctors may now subspecialise in paediatric otology, laryngology or rhinology rather than dealing with all aspects of the field. It was therefore necessary to cover a large number of different topics in considerable depth.

We have been truly fortunate in our authors, who come from many parts of Europe, the USA and South Africa. All share our great enthusiasm for our specialty, as we hope the reader will recognise. We are grateful to them all for working to a short timescale. This has allowed us to put together a fairly large multi-author book in a relatively short time, with up to date contributions. Our authors are active in international academic work and meet each other regularly at the international gatherings of the European Society of Pediatric Otorhinolaryngology, American Society of Pediatric Otolaryngology and Society for Ear, Nose and Throat Advances in Children, as well as at the many national paediatric ENT societies that have been formed in the last 25 years.

Paediatric ENT has developed, during the careers of the editors, from being considered a relatively simple and minor part of our professional life into a broad, complex and often difficult subject. It no longer deals primarily with tonsillectomy, adenoidectomy and the insertion of ventilation tubes. However, these common procedures remain important and this book contains detailed analyses of these well-known aspects of paediatric ENT life, whose rôles are still being defined.

There are some variations in the depth of cover among the 47 chapters of this book. Some surgical topics are dealt with clearly but fairly briefly. In contrast, fields such as immunology, allergy and genetics, in which there continues to be quite rapid scientific progress, needed more detail.

It is a commonplace understanding that children are not small adults. Similarly, much of paediatric ENT is significantly different from the practice of ENT in adults. Children benefit from being looked after in dedicated clinics, able to accommodate the activities that children usually indulge in, and not threatening to them. Wards staffed by nurses trained in childcare as well as in ENT nursing are now considered essential, and need to include play areas and accommodation for parents. Many aspects of the care of children with ENT problems involve several different disciplines: a multidisciplinary team. The rôles of team members need both defining and acknowledging. The ENT doctor needs to accept and to encourage this. The book includes some general chapters dealing with these aspects of the specialty.

With contributors from many different countries, the use and the spelling of medical terms inevitably vary. In general we have accepted both standard US and standard British spellings, trying to keep to one or the other within the confines of separate chapters. Some medical terms appear to be interchangeable: tracheotomy and tracheostomy are an example; some authors hold strong views on this subject and we have encouraged them to use the term they prefer.

We end by acknowledging the support we have received from our publishers and the staff at Springer Verlag. We have also received considerable help from friends and colleagues, including those authors of chapters who have taken the time and trouble to review other chapters and offer advice. Kevin Gibbin and Will Hellier in particular have given much time and sound advice. Emily Graham has contributed great skill and some hours of work in manipulating tables, figures and all kinds of illustration to fit the requirements of several chapters.

Every text of this kind inevitably includes a sincere vote of heartfelt thanks to the spouses and family of the editors. We now understand why. Sharing one's marriage with a book is not necessarily something to be recommended. We, too, would like to thank Sandy Graham, Hilary Bull and Adam Pearson for their patience, forbearance, much sound advice and constructive criticism.

Letting a book loose on the public could be thought an irresponsible act. We hope this is not the case and that you, our readers, find its contents informative, useful and absorbing.

It is inevitable in a book of this nature that errors will have crept in. For these we apologise and crave your indulgence.

John M. Graham
Glenis K. Scadding
Peter D. Bull

Introduction

Each patient is a part of a society: successful care given to that patient adds value to that society. Pediatric otolaryngology encompasses the traditional purposes of medicine in the prevention and curing of illness. It also focuses especially on hearing, speech, gustation and the sense of smell, swallowing and respiration. Children able to express themselves will say "Thank you, I can hear better, smell and taste better, breathe better, sleep better, look better…". Pediatric otolaryngology has particular importance because it deals with communication by language, through the vehicles of hearing, voice and speech.

This is critically important in two ways. The first relates to the economic basis of our society – the way in which we make our livelihoods; this underwent fundamental change during the last half of the 20th century (Ruben 2000). In earlier periods we depended largely on manual labor. Today we depend upon communication skills, mediated through hearing, voice, speech and language, and directly linked to literacy. Pediatric otolaryngology contributes to the economic basis of society by facilitating the development of the skill of communication in individual children. Comparing three different countries (Ruben 2003): one very highly dependent upon communication skills (the Netherlands), one highly dependent upon communication skills (the USA), one a developing nation less dependent upon communication skills (the Philippines), reveals that all three nations are adversely affected economically and socially by communication disorders. It is estimated that the USA loses between 2.5 and 3% of its gross domestic product from the economic sequelae of communication disorders.

A second substantial impact related to pediatric otolaryngology is in the relationship between communication disorders and juvenile crime. The prevalence of communication disorders is many times greater in populations of juvenile delinquents than in the general population. Communication disorders appear to act synergistically with diminished economic and social resources in leading to violent behavior and crime.

The pediatric otolaryngologist's role in the prevention, cure and care of communication disorders is therefore one of the most important fields of medical care for the 21st century – the age of communication.

Robert J. Ruben, MD, FACS, FAAP
Distinguished University Professor
Albert Einstein College of Medicine
Department of Otolaryngology
Montefiore Medical Center

1. Ruben RJ (2000) Redefining the survival of the fittest: communication disorders in the 21st century. Laryngoscope 110:241–245
2. Ruben RJ (2003) Valedictory – why pediatric otorhinolaryngology is important. Int J Pediatr Otorhinolaryngol 67: S53–61

Contents

List of Contributors

David Albert FRCS
Consultant Otolaryngologist
Department of Paediatric Otolaryngology
Great Ormond Street Hospital for Children
Great Ormond Street
London WC1N 3JH
UK
Email: albert@easynet.co.uk

Sonia Ayari-Khalfallah MD
Department of Otorhinolaryngology
and Cervico-Facial Surgery
Edouard Herriot Hospital
5 place d'Arsonval
69437 Lyon cedex 03
France
Email: sonia.khalfallah@chu-lyon.fr

C. Martin Bailey BSc, FRCS
Consultant Otolaryngologist
Department of Paediatric Otolaryngology
Great Ormond Street Hospital for Children
Great Ormond Street
London WC1N 3JH
UK
Email: bailem@gosh.nhs.uk

Helen Bantock BSc, MB BS, FRCP, FRCPCH
Senior Lecturer in Paediatrics
and
Consultant Physician (Retired)
University College London
Gower Street
London WC1E 6BT

Ian Barker MB ChB, FRCA
Consultant Anesthetist
Sheffield Children's Hospital
Department of Anaesthesia
Western Bank
Sheffield S10 2TH
UK
Email: i.barker@sheffield.ac.uk

Timothy G. Barrett PhD, MB, BS, MRCP, MRCPCH, DCH
Professor of Paediatric Endocrinology
Paediatric Thyroid Service
Birmingham Children's Hospital
Steelhouse Lane
Birmingham B4 6NH
UK
Email: thyroid@bch.nhs.uk

Judith Barton BA (Hons) RGN, RSCN
Head of Nursing
Operating Theatres
Sheffield Children's Hospital
Western Bank
Sheffield S10 2TH
UK

Timothy Beale MB, BS, FRCS, FRCR
Department of Radiology
Royal National Throat Nose & Ear Hospital
330 Grays Inn Road
London WC1X 8DA
UK
Email: timothy.beale@royalfree.nhs.uk

Maria Bitner-Glindzicz BSc, MBBS, DCH, PhD, FRCP
Reader in Clinical and Molecular Genetics
Clinical and Molecular Genetics Unit
Institute of Child Health
30 Guilford St.
London WC1N 1EH
UK
Email: mbitnerg@ich.ucl.ac.uk

John Boorman BSc (Hons), MB, ChB, FRCS (Plast)
Queen Victoria Hospital
Holtye Road
East Grinstead
West Sussex RH19 3DZ
UK
Email: john.boorman@virgin.net

Mark Boseley MD, MS
Pediatric Otolaryngologist
Madigan Army Medical Center
9040 A Fitzsimmons Drive
Tacoma, WA 98431
USA
Email: mboseley@comcast.net

Mary Beth Brinson Au.D, FAAA CCC-C
Royal National Throat Nose & Ear Hospital
330 Grays Inn Road
London WC1X 8DA
UK
Email: mbbrinson@aol.com

Peter D. Bull FRCS
Sheffield Children's Hospital
Western Bank
Sheffield S10 2TH
UK
Email: peter.bull@sheffield.ac.uk

Andrew Bush MB, BS (Hons), MA, MD, FRCP, FRCPCH
Professor of Paediatric Respirology
Department of Paediatric Respiratory Medicine
Royal Brompton Hospital
Sydney Street
London SW3 6NP
UK
Email: a.bush@rbh.nthames.nhs.uk

Sean Carrie MB, ChB, FRCS (ORL)
Consultant Otolaryngologist
Department of Otolaryngology
Freeman Hospital
Newcastle upon Tyne NE7 7DN
UK
Email: sean.carrie@nuth.nhs.uk

Ray W. Clarke FRCS
Alder Hey Children's Hospital
ENT Department
Eaton Road
Liverpool L12 2AP
UK
Email: rayclarke@aol.com or raymond.clarke@rlc.nhs.uk

Peter A.R. Clement MD, PhD
Professor of Otorhinolaryngology
A.Z.-V.U.B. (Free University Brussels)
ENT-Department
Laarbeeklaan 101
1090 Brussels
BELGIUM
Email: knoctp@az.vub.ac.be or cknonsk@az.vub.ac.be

Fiona Connell MB, ChB, MRCPCH
Specialist Registrar in Clinical Genetics
NE Thames Regional Genetics Service
Great Ormond Street Hospital NHS Trust
Great Ormond Street
London WC1N 3JH
UK
fconnell@sgul.ac.uk

C.W.R.J. Cremers MD, PhD
Professor in Otology
University Medical Centre Nijmegen St. Radboud
P.O. Box 9101
6500 HB Nijmegen
The Netherlands

Frank Declau MD, PhD
Research Associate
University Hospital of Antwerp
ENT Department
Wilrijkstraat 10
B-2650 Eedegem
Belgium
Email: frank.declau@pandora.be

Ingeborg Dhooge MD, PhD
Department of Otorhinolaryngology, Ghent University
Belgium
Deputy Head, ENT-Clinic, Ghent University Hospital,
Belgium
De Pintelaan 185
B-9000 Ghent
Belgium
Email: ingeborg.dhooge@ugent.be

Milanka Drenovak MSc, Au.D
Audiological Scientist
Nuffield Centre for Speech and Hearing
Royal National Throat, Nose and Ear Hospital
330 Gray's Inn Road
London WC1X 8DA
UK
Email: milanka@compuserve.com

Adam Finn MA, PhD, FRCP, FRCPCH, DBPP
David Baum Professor of Paediatrics
University of Bristol
Institute of Child Life & Health
Department Clinical Sciences at South Bristol
Level 6, UBHT Education Centre
Upper Maudlin Street
Bristol BS2 8AE
UK
Email: adam.finn@bristol.ac.uk

Patrick Froehlich MD, PhD
Department of Otorhinolaryngology and Cervico-Facial
Surgery
Hôpital Edouard Herriot
Pavilion U
5 Place d'Arsonval
69437 Lyon cedex 03
France
Email: patrick.froehlich@chu-lyon.fr

Noel Garabédian MD
Service d'ORL Pédiatrique
Hôpital d'Enfants Armand-Trousseau
26 Ave du Dr Arnold Netter
75571 Paris Cedex 12
France
Email: noel.garabedian@trs.ap-hop-paris.fr

Kevin Patrick Gibbin FRCS
Consultant Paediatric Otolaryngologist
Department of Otorhinolaryngology, Head & Neck Surgery
Queen's Medical Centre
Nottingham NG7 2 UH
UK
Email: kevin.gibbin@qmc.nhs.uk

John M. Graham FRCS
Royal National Throat, Nose and Ear Hospital
330 Gray's Inn Road
London WC1X 8DA
UK
Email: john.graham10@virgin.net

Alexander N. Greiner MD
Assistant Clinical Professor
University of California
San Diego School of Medicine
Allergy & Asthma Medical Group & Research Center
A P.C.
9610 Granite Ridge Dr., Suite B
San Diego, CA 92123
Email: greineran@yahoo.com

John Hamilton FRCS
Consultant ENT Surgeon/Otologist
Gloucestershire Hospitals NHS Trust
Great Western Road
Gloucester
GL1 3EE.
UK
Email: ymg34@dial.pipex.com

Jonny Harcourt MBBS (Hons) MA (Oxon) FRCS
Consultant ENT Surgeon
Department of Paediatric Respiratory Medicine
Royal Brompton Hospital
Sydney Street
London SW3 6NP
UK
Email: jh@harco.demon.co.uk

Benjamin Hartley MB BS, BSc, FRCS (ORL-HNS)
Consultant Paediatric Otolaryngologist
Great Ormond Street Hospital for Children
London WC1N 3JH
UK
Email: hartlb1@gosh.nhs.uk

Christopher Hartnick MD
Department of Otolaryngology
Massachusetts Eye and Ear Infirmary
243 Charles Street
Boston, MA 02114
USA
Email: christopher_hartnick@meei.harvard.edu

William P.L. Hellier FRCS (ORL-HNS)
Consultant ENT Surgeon
Royal South Hants Hospital
Southampton
Hampshire
Email: whellier@hotmail.com

Werner J. Heppt MD
Professor and Director
Department of Otorhinolaryngology
Head and Neck Surgery
Klinikum Karlsruhe
Moltkestr. 90
76133 Karlsruhe
Germany
Email: hnoklinik@klinikum-karlsruhe.com

Hans L.J. Hoeve MD, PhD
Department of Otorhinolaryngology
Sophia Children's Hospital
Dr. Molewaterplein 60
3015 GJ Rotterdam
The Netherlands
Email: l.j.hoeve@erasmusmc.nl

Pekka Karma MD, PhD
Helsinki University Central Hospital (HUCH)
Eye and Ear Hospital
P.O. Box 220
FIN – 00029 HUS
Finland
Email: pekka.karma@hus.fi

Michael Kuo PhD, FRCS (ORL-HNS) DCH
Consultant Paediatric Otolaryngologist
Head and Neck Surgeon
Birmingham Children's Hospital
Steelhouse Lane
Birmingham B4 6NH
United Kingdom
Email: Michael.Kuo@mac.com

Mich Lajeunesse BSc, DM MRCPCH
Lecturer in Paediatrics and Infectious Diseases
University of Bristol
Institute of Child Life & Health
Department Clinical Sciences at South Bristol
Level 6, UBHT Education Centre
Upper Maudlin Street
Bristol BS2 8AE
UK
Email: mich.lajeunesse@bristol.ac.uk

Emmanuel Le Bret MD, PhD
Paediatric Cardiothoracic Department
Centre Cirurgical Marie Lannelongue
133 Avenue de la Résistance
92350 Le Plessis Robinson
France
Email: e.lebret@ccml.fr

Linda Luxon BSc, MB, BS, FRCP
Academic Unit of Audiological Medicine
Great Ormond Street Hospital
London WC1N 3JH
UK
Email: l.luxon@ich.ucl.ac.uk

Fiona B. MacGregor MB, ChB, FRCS, FRCS (ORL)
Consultant Otolaryngologist
Royal Hospital for Sick Children
Yorkhill
Glasgow G3 8SJ
Email: fiona.macgregor@northglasgow.scot.nhs.uk

Gitta Madani MBBS, FDSRCS, MRCS, FRCR
Specialist Registrar in Radiology
Royal National Throat Nose and Ear and University College
Hospitals London
330 Grays Inn Road
London WC1X 8DA
UK

Amy McConkey Robbins MS, CCC-SP
Speech-Language Pathologist
Communication Consulting Services
8512 Spring Mill Road
Indianapolis, IN 46260
USA
Email: amcrobbins@aol.com

Gavin Morrison MA, FRCS
Consultant Otolaryngologist
Guy's, & St Thomas' and The Evelina Children's Hospitals
Lambeth Wing
St Thomas' Hospital
Lambeth Palace Road
London SE1 7EH
Email: gajm@gavinmorrison.com

Richard Nicollas MD
La Timone University Children's Hospital
Department of Pediatric Otolaryngology
Head and Neck Surgery
Bd. Jean Moulin
13385 Marseille Cedex 5
France
Email: richard.nicollas@ap-hm.fr

Waheeda Pagarkar MRCPCH
Consultant in Audiovestibular Medicine
Donald Winnicott Centre
Coate Street
London E2 9AGH and,
Royal National Throat, Nose and Ear Hospital
330 Gray's Inn Road
London WC1X 8DA
UK
Email: apargarkar@nhs.net

Anne Pitkäranta MD
Docent, Head of Section
Helsinki University Central Hospital (HUCH)
Eye and Ear Hospital
P.O. Box 220
00290 Helsinki
Finland
Email: anne.pitkaranta@hus.fi

Chris Prescott MB, ChB FRCS (Eng)
ENT Department
Red Cross Children's Hospital
Klipfontein Road
Rondebosch, 7700
Cape Town
South Africa
Email: Christopher.Prescott@uct.ac.za

David Proops BDS (Hons), MB ChB, FRCS, FRCS (Ed) Hon
Consultant ENT Surgeon, Hon. Senior Lecturer
Department of Paediatrics, University of Birmingham
Department of Paediatrics and ENT
The Birmingham Children's Hospital
Steelhouse Lane
Birmingham B4 6NH
Email: david.proops@talk21.com

David Rawat MB, BAO, ChB, LRCP & SI (Irl), MRCP (Irl), MSc
Consultant Paediatric Gastroenterologist
Chelsea and Westminster Hospital
369 Fulham Road
London SW10 9NH
UK
Email: rawatdavid@hotmail.com

Chris Rittey MB, ChB, FRCP, FRCPCH
Consultant Paediatric Neurologist
Sheffield Children's Hospital
Western Bank
Sheffield S10 2TH
UK
Email: chris.rittey@sch.nhs.uk

Peter J. Robb BSc (Hons) FRCS FRCSEd
Honorary Senior Lecturer, Middlesex University
Consultant ENT Surgeon
Epsom and St. Helier University Hospitals NHS Trust
Epsom KT18 7EG
Surrey UK
Email: peter.robb@epsom-sthelier.nhs.uk

Stéphane Roman MD, PhD
La Timone University Children's Hospital
Department of Pediatric Otolaryngology
Head and Neck Surgery
Bd. Jean Moulin
13385 Marseille Cedex 5
France
Email: stephane.roman@mail.ap-hm.fr

Michael Rothera FRCS
Manchester Children's Hospital
Department of ENT Surgery
Hospital Road
Pendlebury
Manchester, M27 4HA
UK
Email: mprothera@aol.com

Robert J. Ruben MD, FAAP, FACS
Distinguished University Professor
Departments of Otorhinolaryngology
Head and Neck Surgery and Paediatrics
Albert Einstein College of Medicine
Montefiore Medical Center
Medical Arts Pavilion
3400 Bainbridge Avenue - 3rd Floor
Bronx, New York 10467-2490
USA
Email: ruben@aecomyu.edu

Michael J. Rutter FRACS
Cincinnati Children's Hospital Medical Center
Division of Pediatric Otolaryngology/ Head & Neck
Surgery
3333 Burnet Avenue
Cincinnati, OH 45229-3039
USA
Email: mike.rutter@cchmc.org

Glenis K. Scadding MA, MD, FRCP
Royal National Throat, Nose and Ear Hospital
330 Gray's Inn Road
London WC1X 8DA
UK
Email: g.scadding@ucl.ac.uk

Neville P. Shine MB, FRCS (ORL-HNS)
ENT Fellow
Royal Perth Hospital
Perth
Western Australia
Email: shiner1@gmail.com

John Stein FRCP
Lecturer in Neuroscience
University Laboratory of Physiology
Parks Rd.
Oxford OX1 3PT
UK
Email: jfs@physiol.ox.ac.uk

Michael Thomson MB, ChB, DCH, FRCP, FRCPCH, MD
Paediatric Gastroenterologist
Centre for Paediatric Gastroenterology
Sheffield Children's Hospital
Western Bank
Sheffield S10 2TH
UK
Email: mike.thomson@sheffch-tr.trent.nhs.uk

Jean-Michel Triglia, MD
La Timone University Children's Hospital
Department of Pediatric Otolaryngology
Head and Neck Surgery
Bd. Jean Moulin
13385 Marseille Cedex 5
France
Email: jean-michel.triglia@ap-hm.fr

Paul H. Van de Heyning MD, PhD
Professor and Chairman
University Department of Otorhinolaryngology
and Head and Neck Surgery
Antwerp University Hospital
University of Antwerp
Wilrijkstr 10
2650 Antwerp
Belgium
Email: paul.van.de.heyning@uza.be

Carel D.A. Verwoerd MD, PhD
Emeritus Professor Otorhinolaryngology
and Head -Neck Surgery
Erasmus University Medical Center Rotterdam
Secretary-general European Society of Pediatric
Otorhinolaryngology ESPO
Email: kroeskarper@hotmail.com

Brian J. Wiatrak MD
Pediatric ENT Associates
The Children's Hospital of Alabama
1940 Elmer J. Bissell Road
Birmingham, AL 35243
USA
Email: brian.wiatrak@chsys.org

Rosalind Wilson RGN, RSCN
Ward Sister
Dundas Grant Ward
Royal National Throat, Nose and Ear Hospital
330 Gray's Inn Rd.
London WC1X 8DA
UK
Email: rosalind.wilson@royalfree.nhs.uk

Chapter 1

A Paediatric Overview of Children Seen in the ENT Outpatient Department

Helen Bantock

1

Core Messages

- Special techniques are needed for a successful paediatric consultation.
- It is important for the clinician to be aware of the normal stages of a child's development, in order to identify delay in an individual child. In the field of paediatric ENT, this particularly applies to delays in speech and language.
- One child in five will have special needs, either minor or major, at some time during childhood.
- The paediatric ENT doctor needs to be aware of disorders such as autism, global delay, specific learning difficulty, Down and other syndromes, behavioural, social and cultural difficulties and the possibility of abuse.
- Liaison with other agencies is an integral part of the management of the child in an ENT clinic.

Contents

Introduction: Paediatric Consultation

Children are not small adults and their developmental status and metabolic needs must be considered carefully by those entrusted with their medical care. In a paediatric consultation, the history (anamnesis) is especially important, as it is essential to have a clear idea of the nature of the problem before examining the child. This is because children are often reluctant to be examined by strangers.

1. After discussing the reason for the referral with parents or carers, go over the child's developmental history and especially their communicative abilities.
2. Enquire about the family history, especially first-degree relatives: siblings and parents.
3. Observe how the child interacts with others and uses play materials.
4. Look for dysmorphic features, also physical signs, such as mouth breathing and dribbling.

5. Try to engage children in simple play by following their lead in the choice of play materials.

6. Only examine the children physically once you have gained their confidence, and leave possibly stressful things, such as tympanoscopy, till last.

7. Do not forget to ask older children about their own concerns.

8. At the end of the consultation explain what you feel the problem is and how you plan to proceed. Ask the accompanying adults or older children if they have any questions.

Development in the First Five Years of Life

In assessing a child's development, it is usual to look at gross and fine motor development, speech and language development, including social interaction, and visual and hearing capabilities. Older children are able to have a more formal assessment of their cognitive abilities, both verbal and non-verbal.

In terms of infant development, huge gains are made in terms of visual skills in the first few months. A key stage is the development of reciprocal social interaction at about 6 weeks of age. Not only do babies smile back at their caregivers at this stage and vocalise, they have begun to read facial expressions and will look distressed if people frown at them. Parents of children later diagnosed with autism often notice the lack of these early socialisation skills, especially if they have other children who are not autistic.

Motor development is a very obvious developmental parameter, and by the age of 7 months, children are sitting securely and able to transfer objects from one hand to another. Soon afterwards, they begin to crawl, although it is worth remembering that 10% of children are bottom shufflers, who may not walk till around 2 years of age, especially if they are lax jointed. In this situation there is often a family history of bottom shuffling. Most children are walking by 18 months, but it is worth emphasising that most children who walk later than this will have no long-term difficulties. On the other hand, children with global delay often have slow motor development as part of the picture. However, they may not and it is essential to look at the whole child, and especially at how he or she attempts to communicate (Hall et al. 1999).

Children with Special Needs

One child in five has special needs at some point in childhood. These range from major health and developmental problems to temporary and more minor ones, and include medical conditions such as epilepsy and diabetes mellitus, speech and language difficulties, conductive deafness ("glue ear"), visual acuity problems that require spectacle prescription, and mental health problems.

Speech and Language Delay or Disorder

Speech and language difficulties are very common, with children in the lowest 10th centile being more than 1 year behind the average with their expressive language, although their comprehension is age appropriate. If 100 children with the same birthday are considered, 10 of them will fall on or below the 10th centile in terms of speech and language development. These children do catch up, but even a temporary hearing impairment may slow down their development further. If children also have a delay in the understanding of language, the difficulties are greater and if they have both a receptive and expressive delay greater than 1 year, they have a speech and language disorder. About 0.5–1% of children have a language disorder.

Before they begin to talk, children develop their pre-verbal skills. For example, if you give a cup, especially a familiar one, to an 8-month-old child, he or she will look inside it. By 18 months definition by use has progressed so that when shown simple items, such as a cup, spoon, brush, ball or doll, a child should be able to play appropriately with them all, showing an understanding of what they are for. Many children at this age will hand over the items on request, even if they cannot name them, thus showing that they are beginning to understand verbal labels.

As a rule of thumb, by the age of 2 years, children will have a single word vocabulary of about 200 words and by then are beginning to link two words together. At 3 years, simple three-word sentences with subject, object and verb are achieved. For more details of developmental milestones in speech and language see Chapter 5.

Autistic Spectrum

As mentioned above, children on the autistic spectrum have difficulties with social communication. As a consequence, most have delayed speech and language development, although children with Asperger's syndrome, who often present later, in the early school years, may speak at the normal time but have difficulties with the use (pragmatics) and meaning (semantics) of words, as well as more subtle difficulties with social interaction. Because the more severely affected children appear to live "in a world of their own", a hearing loss is often suspected. Because they do not enjoy turn taking with another person, it is difficult to test an autistic child using behavioural testing, such as play audiometry.

The introduction of newborn hearing screening programmes means that these children have usually been shown to have the potential for normal hearing and there is less need to resort to auditory brainstem response testing. Of course, they may suffer from glue ear and conductive hearing difficulties, so a history of mouth breathing and snoring needs to be taken seriously. All children with developmental social and communication difficulties are at risk of incurring further delay in their development if they suffer from conductive hearing loss (see Table 5.2 for warning signs that assist in the differential diagnosis of communication disorders).

Global Delay

As with children with social and communication difficulties, children with global delay are disadvantaged by hearing loss. The causes of generalised delay include some syndromes (see below and Chapter 8), but in about one-third of children it is still not possible to find a cause.

Specific Learning Difficulties

Specific learning difficulties are common and can lead to educational failure if they are not recognised. Problems may occur with reading and spelling (often called dyslexia) and with coordination and fine motor difficulties (developmental coordination disorder or dyspraxia).

Syndromes

A syndrome is defined as a group of symptoms that collectively indicate or characterise a disease, a psychological disorder or other abnormal condition. There are many paediatric syndromes, several of which are associated with deafness (see Chapter 8). Many syndromes are associated with learning difficulties and because of this, conductive deafness, which affects as many as one in five under fives at some time, needs to be treated if it occurs.

Down Syndrome

Down syndrome, or trisomy 21, is the commonest syndrome encountered in paediatrics and affected individuals have a 30% risk of "glue ear" and a 30% risk of later sensorineural deafness. Regular hearing assessment is needed, and many children benefit from temporary hearing aids if the conductive deafness persists. Children with trisomy 21 have other physical difficulties. They are often very floppy at birth and may have abnormalities of the cardiovascular and digestive systems. For this reason they benefit from a multidisciplinary approach (see below under The Child Development Team).

Behaviour Difficulties

Child mental health problems are common and some, such as attention deficit hyperactivity disorder (ADHD), affect a child's educational progress, especially if specific learning difficulties are also present.

Attention Deficit Hyperactivity Disorder

Conservative estimates suggest that between 1 and 5% of children, mostly males, are affected by ADHD. The behavioural features are inattention, hyperactivity and impulsivity. The DSM-IV definition (Diagnostic and Statistical Manual of Mental Disorders, 1994) is the one most often used to classify the condition. Affected children are unable to concentrate on activities other than self-chosen ones, such as computer games. They fidget and are constantly on the move, interfering and butting in on the activities of others. Affected girls are more likely to have attention deficit disorder (ADD) and are not hyperactive. They are more placid and tend to daydream, and their difficulties are not easily apparent to their carers and teachers. Children with ADHD and ADD frequently fail screening hearing tests at school entry and form one of a group of children with non-organic hearing loss. Children who have been abused and neglected in early childhood develop behaviour that is very similar to ADHD, and care needs to be taken in separating these conditions. However, especially in children with associated learning difficulties, medication such as methylphenidate (Ritalin) can dramatically improve school progress (Guevera and Stein 2001). The exact mode of action is not fully understood, but Ritalin appears to stimulate inhibitory pathways, leading to improved concentration and short-term memory (UK National Institute for Clinical Excellence 2006).

Social Difficulties

Children who have been abused and neglected are frequently encountered in paediatric practice. Child Protection services are coordinated by the local Social Services in the United Kingdom and there are regular interagency meetings in all areas to discuss how to improve local services. Within each local authority area, a designated doctor and nurse take the strategic lead in all aspects of child protection, ensuring that the necessary policies and procedures are in place and that training and supervision are available for everyone who works in the local health services, including reception staff, managers, doctors and nurses, and members of all the professions allied to medicine. In addition, in the UK, local health services for children have both a named doctor and nurse who are responsible for ensuring that child protection strategies for the hospital or community are in place. Comparable systems exist in other developed countries.

Types of Abuse

Neglect is the commonest form of abuse, but is often accompanied by physical, emotional or sexual abuse. A more detailed description of the types and presentation of abuse can be found in Barker and Hodes (2004).

Child Abuse in the Context of an ENT Clinic

Most usually, the clinician will be aware of Social Services involvement, as this is likely to have been mentioned in the referral letter. However, it is useful to include a question about any other agencies working with the family as part of the history, just in case such details have been omitted. The aim of Social Services involvement is to improve conditions for children in the family and thus enable the childrens' names to be removed from the Child Protection Register. The intent is to work in partnership with parents, but many parents still find the process stigmatising and may be reluctant to mention involvement of the Social Services.

Alerting Signs of Non-Accidental Injury and Abuse in a Clinic Setting

Parents who neglect their children often fail to attend outpatient appointments. For this reason, a robust system should be in place whereby details of children who fail to attend are sent to the referrer and to Social Services, if they are known to be involved. Presenting signs of abuse in toddlers and young children include:

1. Emotional withdrawal and lack of a warm relationship with parents.
2. Bruises, especially on the face or behind the legs.
3. Delay in the notification of injuries and inconsistent explanations of how they were incurred.
4. Dirty clothing and lack of personal hygiene.
5. Aggressive parents.
6. Evidence of substance abuse in parents.

If any of the above features are present, the examining doctor needs to consider the possibility of child abuse. Most often, several factors coexist. It is possible for any toddler to accidentally hurt themselves and bruises on the forehead or shins are often seen. When they are clearly accidental and family relationships are secure, there is no cause for concern.

What to do if Abuse is Suspected

As mentioned above, local health services for children have to have a named doctor and nurse who can be consulted for advice. However, in the first instance, trainees should consult with their senior colleagues if they have Child Protection concerns. At the beginning of every clinical attachment, trainees should enquire about Child Protection policies and procedures and establish the correct means of communicating any concerns they may have.

If the consulting doctor feels that it is not safe for children to leave the clinic with their parents or caregivers, it is necessary to arrange for parents to wait while more senior staff are consulted. A child could be sent for a hearing test, for example, to allow time for this. It is possible to consult Social Services about whether there is or has been involvement with the family, but they will not be able to interview a family without the referring clinician explaining the nature of his or her concerns to the childrens' parents or carers.

Links with Local Services

Within the UK, a network of organisations is responsible for the delivery of Children's services, and a similar pattern occurs in all developed countries.

Primary Care Team

The primary care team is based around medical centres (general practices), but includes close cooperation with community initiatives, such as "Sure Start", where preventive services are available to help those thought most in need. Parents in Sure Start areas have access to drop-in centres where advice about health, education and social services is available in a user-friendly way.

The Child Development Team

Most districts will have a Child Development Team, which, although located in a local clinic or hospital, carries out a lot of work with parents and children in their homes or at nursery and in school. The staff include therapists (occupational, physiotherapy and speech and language therapy), psychologists, as well as medical staff and staff seconded from Education and Social Services. Each child with complex needs should have a package of care and objectives that are reviewed regularly.

The Education Service

The Education Services are involved very early on, especially in the case of children with complex needs who may attend nursery from the age of 2 years in the UK. The type of provision may be in a specialised nursery or in a mainstream nursery with additional support. By 5 years of age, all children with complex needs, such as cerebral palsy or autism, will have a formal Statement of their Special Educational Needs, and all professionals helping the child, including hospital practitioners, may have to contribute to this.

Child and Adolescent Mental Health Services

Because many children and families have associated mental health needs, the Child and Adolescent Mental Health Services play a major role in supporting families.

Social Services

Each Local Authority has its own department of Social Services. In most cases the social workers working with children form a department within the main social services organisation. Each hospital also has its own social work department and the people working there are able to liaise with their colleagues within the community.

Non-Statutory Organisations

The role of non-statutory organisations is ever increasing. Many are listed in "Contact a family" (www.cafamily.org.uk). Often, organisations have been started by parents of children with unusual conditions and they provide information and support to other people and often fund raise for the medical profession.

Summary for the Clinician

- Children are not small adults. Those treating children need to be aware of several important factors that should be borne in mind during a paediatric consultation, and to apply these in the assessment and management of the child under their care.

References

1. Barker J, Hodes D (2004) The Child in Mind: A Child Protection Handbook. Routledge, New York
2. Contact a Family – For Families with Disabled Children. www.cafamily.org.uk
3. Diagnostic and Statistical Manual of Mental Disorders (1994) 4th edition
4. Guevera JP, Stein M (2001) Evidence based management of attention deficit hyperactivity disorder. Br Med J 323:232–235
5. Hall D, Hill P, Elliman D (1999) The Child Surveillance Handbook. Blackwell, Oxford
6. UK National Institute for Clinical Excellence (2006) NICE guidelines on ADHD. www.nice.org.uk

Chapter 2

Nursing Aspects of Paediatric ENT

2

Rosalind Wilson and Judith Barton

Core Messages

- A child admitted to hospital needs to be nursed on a paediatric ward staffed by nurses with both paediatric and ENT training.
- Surgeons and anaesthetists responsible for the treatment of children should have appropriate training and have a paediatric workload sufficient to maintain their level of skill.
- Effective and sympathetic communication with the child, the child's family and the nursing staff is important for the ENT surgeon at all levels of seniority.
- Other professionals, including psychologists and play therapists, may play an important role in the management of the child in hospital, especially a child who may need a series of admissions and operations.
- Skill in managing tracheostomies is essential in an ENT ward and can be life-saving. The nursing staff have an essential role in the training of parents with children who have tracheostomies.
- Parents should be resident on the wards where their children are being nursed. It is also normal for parents to be with their children during anaesthetic induction and, when possible, during recovery from anaesthesia.
- Day surgery is increasingly common. Those responsible for the care of children undergoing day-case surgery should be clear about their duties, especially in informing parents of the risks of post-operative problems and the correct action to take if such problems arise. Written information should be provided.
- Pain control is now an important consideration in the care of children after surgery. Proper training for nurses and doctors is essential.

Contents

Introduction

ENT surgery accounts for nearly 40% of all paediatric surgery, as recorded in the report of the Childrens' Surgical Forum published by the Royal College of Surgeons of England (2000) "Childrens Surgery: a first class service". The UK National Service Framework for Children, together with this report, require that children should be nursed on dedicated paediatric wards, staffed by trained nurses with both paediatric and ENT training, and that ENT surgeons who operate on children, and anaesthetists who anaesthetise them, perform sufficient numbers of operations to keep their skills honed. Other countries will have similar principles and clinicians should be aware of them.

Communication

Good communication between healthcare professionals and the child and his or her family is essential if a trusting relationship is to be fostered. It is particularly important that children are always told the truth, within the bounds of their understanding of their condition and subsequent treatment.

Good communication is also needed between ward staff and the medical team: surgeons, anaesthetists and paediatricians. The ward staff should not hesitate to contact senior clinicians directly if circumstances demand urgent action, since where children are concerned, delay may be fatal.

Different surgeons may have different protocols for post-operative care and permitted activities. The nursing staff need to be aware of these and communicate with the medical team to agree what post-operative instructions the parents and child receive.

In the UK, to fulfil the requirements of the National Service Framework for Children, hospitals have to ensure that there are paediatric nurses in all areas where children are seen, including outpatient departments. Play therapists are invaluable in helping the medical staff with their interactions with the child by the use of distraction therapy at appropriate times, for example when blood or skin-prick tests are being undertaken.

There may be an advantage in the child's family visiting the ward (or even the operating department) prior to admission in order to allay some of the fear of the unknown. It will help parents and children to understand the system and alleviate some of the very understandable anxiety. Such visits may be conveniently arranged after the outpatient attendance and it can form a part of the play therapist's role to facilitate these visits. Children with conditions requiring many operations, for example those with laryngeal papillomas, may well become very frightened when the time comes for them to return to hospital. Play therapists and, if needed, paediatric clinical psychologists can be very helpful in this situation.

Consent for Surgery

At the time of booking for elective surgery, the proposed procedure should be explained carefully both to the parents and to the child in terms that they can understand. An explanatory leaflet may also be helpful. If necessary, a reliable interpreter should be used and a leaflet provided, if available, in the language of the parental home. It is not good practice to rely on children to interpret to parents who do not speak English, and this should be avoided except in an emergency.

On admission, the same explanation should be repeated and fully informed consent to undergo the planned procedure obtained. However, now that so many cases are dealt with as day cases, it is good practice to obtain consent to operation at the time of the outpatient attendance, to save delay at the time of admission and to ensure that a sufficiently experienced doctor is dealing with consent to surgery. In the UK it is also necessary to obtain the child's own consent, at a level appropriate to that child's age and intellectual development (British Medical Association 2003). The Student BMJ website (www.studentbmj.com/issues/06/03/education/94.php) also has a short paragraph summarising consent for children. Other countries will have similar principles and clinicians should be aware of them.

Staffing

It is considered to be best practice for nursing staff on a paediatric ENT ward to be fully trained in paediatric nursing. Specialist ENT nursing expertise is also required. Specific courses are not readily available in many countries, and this expertise has to be gained at ward level. Ideally, a senior member of the nursing staff should have a formal training role and time in which to perform this task.

The most important factor to be taken into consideration is the post-operative airway. At all times on the ward, there should be at least one member of staff capable of nursing a child with a compromised airway. That person should also be capable of guiding their colleagues in the swift recognition and treatment of children with respiratory difficulties.

The Physical Environment

A children's ENT ward should consist of areas where the children can be easily seen and heard at all times. Thought must be given to identifying cases that can be nursed safely in a side room and those for whom closer observation after surgery is required. For example, following tonsillectomy, which still carries a significant risk of bleeding, a child should be recovered in plain view since using side rooms can increase the risk of delay in the detection of post-operative haemorrhage, unless a nurse is assigned to that side room more or less full-time. Post-tonsillectomy bleeding may be occult initially and only recognised by a persistent tachycardia and moist pharyngeal sounds, relieved by swallowing the blood. Such cases need experienced observation if danger is to be avoided.

Tracheostomy

Many children and babies with tracheostomies live healthy lives at home with their parents who have been trained in their care, but when in hospital the parent should not be expected to be the sole carer, especially if the child is unwell; shared care should be negotiated between the child's named nurse and the resident parent.

Children with tracheostomies should be admitted only to units where staff experienced in the care of children with artificial airways will be available and who can both recognise and manage sudden respiratory difficulties. Children's tracheostomy tubes are often one-piece tubes without a separate inner tube, and any problems, such as tube blockage or displacement, must be dealt with instantly; there must therefore always be experienced staff nearby who are capable of recognising the situation and are able to replace the tube if necessary. All of the personnel who deal with such children, including the parents and play specialists, should be able to change or replace a tube in an emergency.

Student nurses should gain valuable supervised experience in changing tubes during their ENT placement. The operating theatre provides an ideal opportunity for staff at all grades to gain experience in changing tracheostomy tubes under (more or less) controlled conditions after routine airway endoscopy under general anaesthesia.

Children with tracheostomies should be nursed in side rooms only if there is someone experienced in their care in the room with them at all times. If that person is a parent, there should be a ward policy of covering for them when they need a break. It should be recorded how this is to be achieved and who will assume responsibility for the child's safety. If the ward cannot provide this level of staffing then the child should be nursed in the open ward where any respiratory distress can be quickly observed.

Children leaving the ward, for example to go to X-ray or Audiology, must be accompanied by a nurse or parent who is confident in changing tubes.

Suction is performed to clear the tube, not the lungs, and should be performed when it sounds as if the tube needs cleaning, not simply according to a timetable. If performed correctly, cleaning the tube while not irritating the mucosa should not provoke the production of bloodstained secretions. Suction catheters should never be used twice: re-use can introduce or spread infection.

Parents

Resident parents have been a feature of paediatric wards for over 20 years. Times have changed from the days when visiting by parents was forbidden on the day of operation and severely limited at other times. Parents now quite rightly share in the care of their children and participate in decisions. It would be unthinkable nowadays to prevent parents staying with their child while the child is going through unfamiliar and sometimes frightening or painful experiences. It took many years for hospital staff to believe that it was beneficial to themselves as well as to the children, even though research on the psychological damage of separation was published as long ago as 1952 (Robertson et al. 1952).

On admission to hospital, the child's main fear may not be the operation itself, as might be assumed, but the fear of being separated from their parents. When the child can be reassured that a parent will be able to stay with them at all times, they are much more likely to be cooperative with all the required procedures and have a better hospital experience.

It is now common practice for a parent to be present in the anaesthetic room during the induction of anaesthesia, helping the anaesthetist with reassurance and distraction. This may be traumatic for the parent, but significantly reduces the anxiety on the part of the child. In non-compliant children, especially young children, the presence of a well-prepared parent allows better control and reduces any risk of accusations of forced restraint. The ward nurse, who has built up a trusting relationship with the child and parent, should also be there to offer assistance and should be the one to lead the parent away at the appropriate moment and to provide reassurance as they return to the ward.

When the hospital has the appropriate environment, the post-anaesthetic recovery staff should accept a parent's presence as the child awakes from anaesthesia.

Provision of facilities for parents in hospital remains varied, but all paediatric wards should be providing fold-down beds and a means to make drinks at the very least. Plans for new children's wards should reflect a commitment to making parents both welcome and comfortable.

Day Surgery

Many ENT procedures performed on children are suitable for day-case or short-stay surgery. This can be safely undertaken only if children are skilfully prepared and recovered from surgery by nurses who fully understand the possible complications of such surgery and the speed at which they can occur.

At discharge from the day-surgery unit, clear discharge information must be given to the parent or the carer who will be supervising the recuperation in the home. Parents must understand that safe recovery after a child returns home is largely dependent on their actions.

Some areas can offer a visit the next day by a community paediatric nurse; this may allow larger numbers of children to be treated as day cases who would otherwise require a longer stay in hospital.

Some studies have looked at the stress day-case surgery puts on parents, highlighting the need for care and consideration in the selection of suitable candidates. Criteria such as a home or mobile telephone, availability of transport, especially at night, and the ability to communicate in the language of the country in which the hospital stands are essential. There should be two responsible adults in the home and the child should live within a reasonable distance (or access time) to the hospital.

There must be a clear policy of readmission without delay to the ward and beds must be available for such a contingency. The parents must have a contact telephone number so that they can ring without delay.

Many parents are keen for their child's tonsils to be removed, but remain unaware of the very real risk of the child bleeding 1 week later. Understanding the pain and dealing with it effectively will ease the reintroduction of meals after surgery, which will aid recovery. Adequate advice, preferably printed, should be given before discharge from hospital.

2

Pain Control

If the child's pain can be controlled effectively throughout the hospital stay, it will not only improve their remembered experience of hospital, but improve enormously their recovery after discharge. In the past, inadequate doses of analgesia were prescribed, largely on demand. Now in situations such as following tonsillectomy, where moderate to severe pain is expected, effective doses of analgesia are given at regular intervals, rather than waiting for pain scores to rise. This gives better control, allows the child to regain confidence in eating and drinking, and promotes safe recovery.

Successful pain control also allows the parents to gain confidence in their ability to supervise their child's recovery and may increase early discharge rates.

Summary for the Clinician

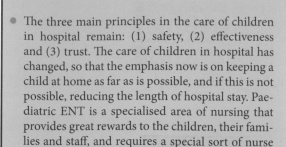

- The three main principles in the care of children in hospital remain: (1) safety, (2) effectiveness and (3) trust. The care of children in hospital has changed, so that the emphasis now is on keeping a child at home as far as is possible, and if this is not possible, reducing the length of hospital stay. Paediatric ENT is a specialised area of nursing that provides great rewards to the children, their families and staff, and requires a special sort of nurse who is able to accept the considerable responsibilities attached to the care of these children.

References

1. Bowlby J, Robertson J, Rosenbluth D (1952) A two-year-old goes to hospital. Psychoanal Study Child 7:82–94

2. British Medical Association (2003) Consent Toolkit. BMA, London

3. Children's Surgery – a First Class Service (2000) Report of the Paediatric Forum of the Royal College of Surgeons of England. www.rcseng.ac.uk

4. Student BMJ (2007) www.studentbmj.com/issues/06/03/education/94.php

Chapter 3

Anaesthesia for Paediatric ENT Surgery

3

Ian Barker

Core Messages

- The anaesthetist and surgeon should communicate and anticipate well.
- Intravenous fluids containing no sodium or concentrations of sodium less than 0.45% (less than 75 mmol.l^{-1}) are dangerous. The standard paediatric maintenance fluid is 5% dextrose with 0.45% saline.
- The three "Hs" of neonatal anaesthesia are hypoxia, hypothermia and hypoglycaemia.
- Beware the quiet child who is bleeding after tonsillectomy. The patient may be shocked to the point of unconsciousness.
- Hypotension is a very late sign of shock in the bleeding child.
- Anaesthetic induction can be longer than anticipated if the patient has a partially obstructed airway.
- Laser safety is everybody's responsibility.
- Severe obstructive sleep apnoea necessitates a thorough pre-operative assessment and sometimes post-operative high-dependency care.
- The pulse oximeter can give an incorrectly optimistic impression of the status of an anaemic patient.

Contents

Introduction

The paediatric anaesthetist works very closely with his ENT surgical colleague. Surgery may be undertaken on the airway, responsibility for which is, of necessity, shared by both practitioners, who must understand each other's requirements to ensure safe patient care. Good communication and understanding between surgeon and anaesthetist are essential for the safe management of the more challenging problems of paediatric ENT surgery.

This chapter deals with some of the relevant general considerations of paediatric and neonatal anaesthesia, reviews some specific conditions in which anaesthetist and surgeon interact significantly, and finally considers some items of anaesthetic equipment that the surgeon will encounter.

3

General Considerations

Anaesthesia for Children

The psychological aspects of paediatric anaesthesia should not be underestimated. Children are frightened of hospitals. The environment is unfamiliar, there are many strangers and the underlying reason for admission is often a terrifying mystery. Children (as ever) heighten the anxiety by relating melodramatic tales of operations to each other, stories that lose nothing in the telling. Above all is the fear of being "put to sleep" because that is what happens to pets at the end of their lives.

There is no easy answer. A welcoming, appropriate (for age) child-friendly environment helps a great deal. Familiarity with the hospital and ward also makes a big difference and many units run pre-admission groups at which children can look round the ward and theatre on a day unrelated to their admission. The greatest asset, however, is the calm reassurance of a loving parent. Modern paediatric practice encourages parental presence at all stages of admission (except the surgical procedure under general anaesthesia).

Pharmacological pre-medication is of use in managing the uncooperative younger child and can help to allay adolescent anxiety. This should be regarded as symptomatic relief rather than treatment of an underlying problem, which may require considerable psychological intervention particularly if the child is to undergo repeated procedures such as resection of laryngeal papillomatosis.

Healthy children, as opposed to the newborn, behave physiologically much like healthy small adults with the considerations that equipment needs to be smaller, physiological parameters differ according to age, veins are harder to find, drug doses and fluid requirements vary by weight, and the increased metabolic rate produces hypoxia rapidly in the apnoeic patient.

Anaesthesia for the Newborn

Textbooks have been written on the subject of neonatal anaesthesia. This chapter considers the three Hs: hypoxia, hypothermia and hypoglycaemia.

Hypoxia

Neonates have a very high metabolic rate; they use up oxygen extremely quickly and are therefore liable to become clinically hypoxic (cyanosed) following a period of apnoea lasting for no more than a few seconds. They compound this with a reflex bradycardia, a precursor to cardiac arrest. Anaesthesia for surgery on the neonatal airway is usually undertaken in 100% oxygen.

Hypothermia

Neonates and infants have a much higher surface area to volume ratio than older patients. They lose heat rapidly, cooling to dangerously low temperatures during some procedures. The head is a particularly good radiator of heat and it is most important that the patient is covered, a warm environment is provided and body temperature is monitored. Clear plastic drapes (and a hat) mean that the baby can be covered but observed, and the heated air blower can produce a warm environment for the patient whilst maintaining a comfortable temperature for staff in the operating theatre.

Hypoglycaemia

Newborns do not have good glycogen reserves. They need frequent feeds or can become severely hypoglycaemic, which can be as dangerous to the growing brain as hypoxia. A dextrose-containing infusion is usually administered during surgery and care must be taken that the fasting time prior to theatre is not prolonged. This time is much better controlled if the patient is first on the operating list.

Intravenous Fluid Therapy for Children

With a few simple guidelines, this is not difficult. All fluids containing no sodium or concentrations of sodium less than 0.45% (less than 75 mmol.l^{-1}) are dangerous and can produce hyponatraemia, leading to convulsions and possibly cerebral oedema.

For resuscitation, use normal saline, full-strength Hartmann's solution or a colloid. Do not use dextrose-containing fluids. Give boluses of 10 ml.kg^{-1}. Tell somebody that you are doing it and stop after two boluses until you have taken advice from a paediatrician or anaesthetist.

For maintenance, the best fluid to use in the first instance is 5% dextrose with 0.45% saline. You (or somebody else) can worry about more sugar and adding potassium later, stick to this in the first instance.

With regard to the rate of administration, fluids are prescribed by weight at an hourly rate. Lighter children need proportionally more fluid. So:

1. Up to 10 kg: 4 ml.kg^{-1}.h^{-1}, so that, for example a 5-kg baby gets 20 ml.h^{-1} and a 10 kg baby gets 40 ml.h^{-1}.
2. 10–20 kg: 40 ml.h^{-1} for the first 10 kg then 2 ml.h^{-1} for every 1 kg between 10 kg and 20 kg. A 15-kg toddler will thus get 50 ml.h^{-1} (10 kg = 40 ml.h^{-1} plus 5 kg = 10 ml.h^{-1}) and a 20-kg infant will get 60 ml.h^{-1}.
3. Above 20 kg: 60 ml.h^{-1} for the first 20 kg and then 1 ml.h^{-1} for every 1 kg above that. Therefore, a 30-kg

child will receive 70 ml.h^{-1} (that's 20 kg = 60 ml.h^{-1} plus 10 kg = 10 ml.h^{-1}).

This does not work in the first few days of life, so ask for help. This is basal maintenance only, more fluid is required in pyrexia and on hot days, so again ask for help. In any case, if the infusion has been running for more than a few hours ask for help from a paediatrician or your friendly anaesthetist.

Specific Conditions

Post-Tonsillectomy Bleeding

Assessment

Pain, fear and blood everywhere heighten the anxiety for all involved with the management of this problem. As with all anaesthesia, pre-operative assessment is undertaken first. This follows the usual lines of ABC: A (airway), B (breathing) and C (circulation). The child will usually have a clear airway and good breathing, letting the whole ward know about the problem! Beware the quiet withdrawn child who may have lost so much blood that hypovolaemic shock is setting in.

The management focuses on the circulatory system. It is impossible to assess blood loss from, for example, the sheets and vomit bowl, and a stomach full of blood must always be assumed. Assessment of blood loss concentrates on examination of the patient. A child who has lost a significant volume of blood will be pale, peripherally cold and have a tachycardia. Their capillary refill time will be prolonged to more than 3 s (press with one finger on the sternum for 5 s, let go and see how long the blanched skin takes to go pink). Substantial blood loss may lead to the absence of peripheral pulses such as the radial pulse, but more central ones such as the carotid and femoral pulses may still be palpable. A very shocked child may be drowsy because of reduced cerebral perfusion.

Blood pressure is not a good indicator of hypovolaemia in the unanaesthetised child. Normotension is not necessarily a reassuring sign; children vasoconstrict to maintain blood pressure and hypotension occurs very late as a pre-terminal sign.

Resuscitation

The management of this condition is to summon help, administer oxygen and correct the hypovolaemia. This last is done by the establishment of venous access, or intraosseous access if no veins can be found, sampling of blood for cross-match and the rapid administration of a fluid bolus. The first bolus will usually be 10 ml.kg^{-1} of a crystalloid solution such as normal saline or Hartmann's solution, or a colloid plasma substitute. This is followed by reassessment of ABC and usually a second similar bolus. In the absence of congenital heart disease, this volume of liquid (25% of the blood volume) will do no harm in the normovolaemic child and could be life saving in the shocked patient. By now the anaesthetist should have arrived.

Anaesthesia

The ongoing anaesthetic management is to complete the resuscitation to normovolaemia, which may require blood transfusion. This must be done prior to surgery as anaesthesia in the shocked patient is dangerous. There is little point in trying to empty the stomach with a gastric tube prior to surgery, the protestations of the patient will produce more bleeding. Anaesthesia usually follows the "rapid sequence induction" pattern of pre-oxygenation, intravenous induction, cricoid pressure (occlusively compressing the oesophagus), suxamethonium and intubation. An experienced senior anaesthetist should be present.

Airway Endoscopy

Indications

This procedure is performed for numerous indications in neonates and children. Congenital abnormalities, infections (croup, epiglottitis and papillomatosis) and foreign bodies are probably the most common. The principles of anaesthesia are similar for all.

Pre-operative assessment will consider the likely diagnosis, the degree of urgency of the procedure and the extent of airway compromise. As with every anaesthetic, questions must be asked about general health, personal and family history of problems with anaesthesia, and last oral intake.

Epiglottitis is an emergency requiring urgent endoscopy and intubation in order to secure the airway. Croup may be managed somewhat more conservatively, but these patients are still at imminent risk of obstruction. It is unusual for the child with an inhaled foreign body to require immediate endoscopy, time can normally be allowed for radiology and digestion of a recent meal. Congenital abnormalities producing stridor, and papillomatosis are usually managed urgently but electively. Any child with a partially obstructed airway, any child with stridor, can develop acute airway obstruction necessitating urgent intervention.

It is a basic tenet of anaesthesia that a patient should not be rendered apnoeic unless the anaesthetist knows that he can artificially ventilate. This is never more important than in children and babies with partial airway obstruction. Furthermore, paediatric airway endoscopy is a dynamic, physiological investigation looking at moving structures rather than a static anatomical diagnostic technique. The fundamental rule is to keep the patient breathing.

Induction

Anaesthesia is usually induced using 100% oxygen with a volatile anaesthetic agent added. Nowadays most practitioners induce anaesthesia with sevoflurane because it is non-irritant and the patient goes to sleep quickly. Having produced unconsciousness, but not apnoea, a vein is cannulated and an anticholinergic drug such as atropine is administered. Atropine is given to prevent the bradycardia resulting from the vagal stimulation produced when the laryngoscope or bronchoscope is inserted over the posterior surface of the epiglottis. Simultaneously, physiological monitoring is applied to the patient (electrocardiogram, pulse oximetry and capnography). The eyes should be protected.

Anaesthesia is now deepened to render the still breathing patient intubatable. Some anaesthetists continue with sevoflurane, whereas others may use halothane to achieve this state. When managing a patient with an obstructed airway, anaesthetic induction can take quite a long time simply because it takes longer to absorb sufficient "gas". When the child is judged to be "ready", an attempt is made to ventilate artificially using the bag and mask. If ventilation is not possible, one is very grateful for spontaneous breathing. Laryngoscopy is performed using the appropriate equipment and local anaesthetic spray (lidocaine) applied to the cords. The trachea may or may not be intubated by agreement between surgeon and anaesthetist, we shall assume that intubation is to be performed. Should it be impossible to visualise the larynx, an alternative approach such as fibre-optic endoscopy or rigid tracheoscopy with a rigid ventilating bronchoscope may be necessary.

Maintenance

The intubated, deeply anaesthetised, breathing patient is positioned with the neck extended over a pillow. If rigid bronchoscopy is to be performed the Storz bronchoscope is inserted with simultaneous removal of the endotracheal tube. Oxygen and anaesthetic vapour are administered through the side arm of the apparatus forming a conventional anaesthetic breathing system. Bronchoscopy is carried out in a controlled, unhurried fashion.

Should laryngoscopy be required, the preferred surgical laryngoscope is positioned and fixed with suspen-

sory apparatus. Supraglottic examination can now be performed, but examination below the cords requires an extubated patient. Extubation poses the questions of continuing oxygenation and anaesthesia. Both of these can be provided by some means of insufflation of gases either via the side arm of the laryngoscope or an appropriately positioned catheter in the pharynx. This produces pollution of the theatre atmosphere, and alternatively anaesthesia may be maintained by the infusion of intravenous agents. Oxygen should still be insufflated as described above.

The above technique is the author's personal choice, it is not recommended that you suggest a change to your anaesthetist!

Laser Surgery

The laser can be used for the resection of lesions of the paediatric airway and elsewhere on a child's head and neck. This piece of equipment poses significant dangers for patients and staff alike. In essence, an intense monochromatic, coherent, collimated light beam burns anything that gets in its way (including the surgeon's finger). Specific considerations for the anaesthetist are protection of the patient, maintenance of the airway and flammable gases.

Protection of the patient is everyone's responsibility, but the anaesthetist should ensure specifically that the patient's eyes and skin are suitably protected, usually with water soaked swabs and drapes.

The patient's airway needs to be maintained, but the endotracheal tubes in routine use are made from highly inflammable PVC and airway fires are usually fatal. There are several alternatives available. The first, for airway surgery, is to use a tubeless technique; as described above for other airway endoscopy, any insufflating catheter must not protrude posterior to the soft palate. The second is to protect a PVC tube with reflective metal tape or foil. Whilst effective, this is a home-made solution that carries with it considerations of product liability (if it catches fire there's only one person to blame!). The third are purpose-made laser-safe tubes. These are constructed from flexible metal or PVC covered with a fire-proof foam that can be soaked in water. They are excellent and 100% effective but are, at their smallest, too big for use in neonates and most infants and often obstruct the laser rather than facilitate the procedure.

Oxygen is the recommended anaesthetic gas for airway endoscopy, which at 21% in room air will support combustion well, while at 100% in the airway it can lead to the explosive ignition of flammable material. Some practitioners recommend never using 100% oxygen; all advocate extreme vigilance that the only flammable material in the line of the laser is the intended tissue for ablation. Nitrous oxide also supports combustion.

Obstructive Sleep Apnoea

What's all the fuss about? Obstructive sleep apnoea (OSA) in children ranges from snoring to episodes of apnoea resulting in significant hypoxia (see Chapter 15). In most cases (up to 95%), adenotonsillar hypertrophy is the cause and uneventful adenotonsillectomy the cure. The problem is that some children with severe OSA can develop post-operative respiratory complications. These are the younger patients (age <3 years), those with craniofacial or neuromuscular abnormalities, the morbidly obese and those with the cardiac complications of OSA. This last group have longstanding OSA, resulting in pulmonary hypertension and eventually cor pulmonale. Moreover, their normal respiratory drive becomes altered as they develop carbon dioxide (CO_2) insensitivity. These patients are also much more sensitive to the respiratory depressant effects of anaesthesia and opiate analgesia. A 20% incidence of post-operative respiratory complications has been reported in this severe group (Rosen et al. 1994).

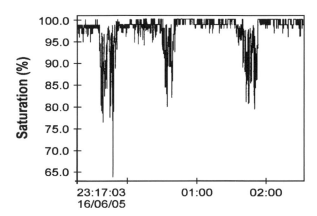

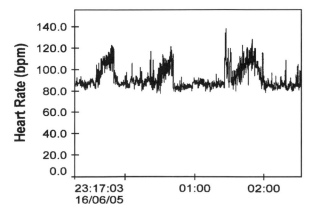

Fig. 3.1 A simple polysomnograph showing saturation and heart rate only. Note that in this child with obstructive sleep apnoea, the saturation falls profoundly each hour and the pulse rate increases simultaneously

How do we identify the at risk children? A full history and examination are of course essential, but the gold standard investigation is polysomnography (Fig. 3.1) in which the patient's respiratory pattern and pulse oximetry (amongst other parameters) are monitored during sleep (Subcommittee on Obstructive Sleep Apnea Syndrome 2002).

"What do I do, we haven't got polysomnography in our hospital?" Discuss the patient with the anaesthetist, well in advance, who may suggest that it is preferable to refer the child to a specialist centre for further management.

How is the anaesthetic managed? There is little concrete advice in the literature (Warwick and Mason 1998). Sedative pre-medication and sedation as an alternative to anaesthesia can have disastrous outcomes. A personal technique:

1. A full pre-operative assessment including polysomnography and possibly cardiac ultrasound are undertaken.
2. Sedative pre-medication is avoided; remember these children stop breathing when they fall asleep!
3. Anaesthesia is induced preferably intravenously and the child is intubated and ventilated for the procedure (ventilation with a relaxant reduces the requirement for a volatile anaesthetic agent). Opiates are avoided entirely and analgesia provided by local anaesthetic infiltration, paracetamol and non-steroidal analgesics such as diclofenac.
4. Children with severe OSA are admitted to a high-dependency environment for a period post-operatively until normal sleep has been proven.

Anaesthetic Equipment

Endotracheal Tubes

"The tube" is one of the major interfaces between the ENT surgeon and anaesthetist. These are almost always made from synthetic material; latex rubber has been replaced because of hypersensitivity and the requirement for a single-use product. Most commonly the material is PVC. The ENT surgeon will also encounter the reinforced endotracheal tube (ETT) usually made from silicone rubber with a steel or nylon spiral embedded into the wall to prevent kinking.

The length of the ETT is important because if too long the tube may enter one or other main bronchus, and if too short it may be pulled out of the airway. Extension of the neck by the surgeon will move the tube higher in the trachea. Flexion and placement of a tonsillectomy mouth gag will move it lower. Neck extension and placement of a mouth gag may therefore move the tube up or down, but removal of the gag always carries the risk of accidental removal of the ETT.

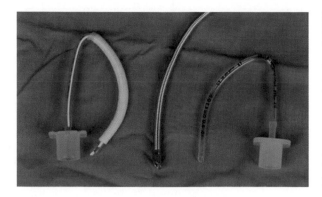

Fig. 3.2 Three endotracheal tubes: from the left, two tubes for use with the laser and a Ring-Adair-Elwyn (RAE) pattern tube for facial surgery. All of these tubes have the same 3-mm internal diameter but different external diameters

The diameter of the ETT is relevant for several reasons. First it should be noted that conventionally, historically, the internal diameter in millimetres is used when referring to tube size, taking no account of wall thickness (Fig. 3.2). Secondly, gas flow within an endotracheal tube is laminar (or streamlined) in nature, and therefore physics dictates that resistance to flow is inversely proportional to the radius (or diameter) of the tube to the power of four (R^4). A tube with an internal diameter of 4 mm will have more than twice the resistance to flow as one of 5 mm (i.e. $5^4 = 625$, $4^4 = 256$).

Cuffed ETTs are rarely used in children and a small leak around the tube is desirable in paediatric practice because a tightly fitting one risks the development of oedema in the tracheal mucosa. Using the power of four calculation described above it can be seen that a small amount of oedema can produce a surprisingly large increase in airway resistance.

Laryngeal Mask Airway

The laryngeal mask airway (LMA) device, which was invented in the 1980s, consists of a length of tubing welded to a shallow soft cup surrounded by an inflatable cuff. The cup fits in the pharynx over the glottic inlet and thus the airway is rendered patent. The LMA has been used in many circumstances. It is used when intubation is not necessary (e.g. for myringotomy), keeping the anaesthetist's hands free. It is used to maintain a patent airway when the larynx cannot be visualised. The LMA is a useful conduit for the fibreoptic laryngoscope or bronchoscope. Most interestingly, perhaps, is its use at tonsillectomy, where it has been demonstrated to result in very little airway soiling (Webster et al. 1993). At present, most LMAs are reused, sterilised by autoclave between patients.

Pulse Oximeter

This monitor gives two pieces of information: the pulse rate and the amount of oxygen in the patient's blood as a percentage of the total oxygen-carrying capacity. The transducer or "probe" has two light-emitting diodes and a receiving photocell. The diodes emit light alternately at a frequency of approximately 1 kHz, giving the appearance of a continuous red light. One emits visible red light at 660 nm, the other invisible infra red light at 940 nm. These two wavelengths are chosen because oxygenated haemoglobin absorbs the infrared light well but not the red light, and vice versa in the case of "blue" deoxygenated haemoglobin. By measuring the differences in absorption of the two wavelengths, the monitor is able to calculate the relative quantities of oxygenated and deoxygenated haemoglobin, giving a percentage oxygen saturation. The algorithm is sensitive to pulsatile flow and thus can use this to determine heart rate.

Limitations

Incident light and patient movement can produce false readings. Failure of circulation, whether caused by tourniquet or circulatory arrest, will inevitably produce no reading at all. Abnormal haemoglobin and artificial colouration such as nail varnish produce erroneous readings. Modern pulse oximeters can discount skin pigmentation. The monitor averages a reading over several heartbeats and so does not give an instant response.

The most dangerous limitation is that the pulse oximeter can give a reassuringly normal result in a profoundly anaemic patient. One gram of fully saturated haemoglobin carries 1.39 ml of oxygen. A patient with a normal haemoglobin concentration of 14 g.dl^{-1} who has a saturation of 100% will have 19.5 ml of oxygen in 100 ml (1 dl) of his arterial blood, whereas a profoundly anaemic patient with a haemoglobin concentration of 5 g.dl^{-1} and a saturation of 100% will only have 7 ml of oxygen in 100 ml of his arterial blood. Remember also that a patient needs 5 g.dl^{-1} of deoxygenated (blue) haemoglobin in order to appear cyanosed. Thus, the profoundly anaemic patient can never appear cyanosed. Within its limitations, the pulse oximeter is an excellent monitor but it doesn't tell everything.

Carbon Dioxide Monitor

The CO_2 monitor, or capnograph, measures the concentration of CO_2 in the gases the patient breathes. It works on the principle that CO_2 absorbs infrared light in direct proportion to its concentration in the gas mixture. The monitor usually determines the concentrations of oxygen and anaesthetic gases as well, but the advantages of the capnograph are several:

1. Tracheal intubation is confirmed by the presence of CO_2 in the expired gas. There may be a little CO_2 in the oesophagus and stomach, but positioning of the ETT in the airway is confirmed by regular, repeated detection of the gas.

2. Disconnection of the breathing circuit or accidental extubation is rapidly signalled by the failure of detection of CO_2.

3. A rapid decline in CO_2 concentration in the exhaled gas can be indicative of failure of pulmonary perfusion because of hypovolaemia, pulmonary embolus or cardiac arrest.

4. An increase in CO_2 concentration can have many causes. The anaesthetic system may be failing to remove the gas because the CO_2 absorber has expired or the patient may be being hypoventilated. Of greater concern is that the patient may be producing more CO_2 because of an increased metabolism. Most commonly this signifies a patient whose muscle tone is returning as the relaxant wears off, it might indicate an infected patient who is developing a raised temperature, but rarely, yet of great concern, is the rapidly rising expired CO_2 concentration pathognomic of malignant hyperpyrexia.

Summary for the Clinician

- It is hoped that this chapter has given a little insight into some of the techniques used and challenges faced by the paediatric ENT anaesthetist. The two "take home messages" are: (1) adequate communication and pre-operative planning between surgeon and anaesthetist are essential for safe patient care and (2) if the anaesthetist is taking a long time in the anaesthetic room he might appreciate a bit of help, he won't be having a cup of tea or doing the crossword.

References

1. Rosen GM, Muckle RP, Mahowald MW, et al. (1994) Postoperative respiratory compromise in children with obstructive sleep apnea syndrome: can it be anticipated? Pediatrics 93:784–788

2. Subcommittee on Obstructive Sleep Apnea Syndrome. American Academy of Pediatrics (2002) Clinical practice guideline: diagnosis and management of childhood obstructive sleep apnea syndrome. Pediatrics 109:704–712

3. Warwick JP, Mason DG (1998) Obstructive sleep apnoea syndrome in children. Anaesthesia 53:571–579

4. Webster AC, Morley-Forster PK, Dain S, et al. (1993) Anaesthesia for adenotonsillectomy: a comparison between tracheal intubation and the armoured laryngeal mask airway. Can J Anaesth 40:1171–1177

Chapter 4

The Evolution of Speech and Language

4

John F. Stein

Core Messages

- The specializations required for speech did not develop all at once, but over millions of years.
- Left-sided hemispheric specialization for precise timing was found in primitive mammals (i.e. 200 million years ago)
- Mirror neurones enabling imitation developed 45 million years ago.
- Descent of the larynx had occurred by 5 million years ago.
- The increase in the brain size and connectivity of *Homo sapiens* was complete by 100,000 years ago.
- Full speech had developed in *H. sapiens* only 50,000 years ago.

Contents

Introduction

Most people feel rather uneasy when reminded that we share 90% of our DNA with our ape ancestors. The idea that we evolved from monkeys was Darwin's most controversial claim in the Origin of the Species, much more unsettling than his hypothesis that the mechanism of evolution was by natural selection; "nature red in tooth and claw" actually fitted very easily with Victorian beliefs in unbridled capitalism. However, human descent from apes was embarrassing and seemed to denigrate our spirituality, so it was natural to seek ways of distancing ourselves from biology. The most quintessentially human attribute to emphasise was obviously the human ability to communicate by speech and language. Hence, until very recently it was believed that speech was uniquely human. Even chimpanzees, it was thought, could not be taught to communicate beyond rudimentary emotional calls. The power of speech had been bestowed on humans to make us human, all at once by a lucky mutation in the 1% of DNA we do not share with chimps. Chomsky and followers thought that this endowed us with an "encapsulated linguistic processing module" (Chomsky 1975) and a generative language "instinct" (Pinker and Jackendoff 2005).

However, this scenario has turned out to be thoroughly at odds with what we now know about the evolution of our capacity for language. Unfortunately, the organs of verbal communication do not turn to stone as bones do, so we are unlikely ever to know for certain from the fossil record how it did evolve. Nevertheless, we know from study of the evolution of other complex systems, such as the eye, that they never evolve all at once, but rather in small steps spread over millions of years. Each of those small steps must have had some adaptive value in the environment in which they evolved, but these may have had nothing to do with what we think of as their main purpose now. Thus we shall see that evolution of hemispheric specialisation, mirror cells and descent of the larynx preceded language by millions of years, and evolved for quite different purposes.

4

Is Language Innate or Learnt?

The first question we have to consider is whether speech is genetically endowed and innate or learnt via cultural experience. Although most people would now accept Chomsky's view that the "deep" structure of language is innate in the sense that all languages have grammatical rules consisting of similar basic elements, these probably derived from the sequential programming of limb gestures and were not evolved specifically for speech or language. Every element of explicit speech has to be learnt from others rather than being innate.

Our basic evidence for the importance of learning from others comes from brutal experiments bringing up children with little or no human contact. In 7000 BC, the Egyptian pharaoh Tsammtemichus had a child brought up in guarded isolation in a cage to find out whether he would learn to speak without any teaching. His first word turned out to be the Phrygian word for bread, which he had clearly learnt from his guards, so the experiment suggested that language is learnt, not innate. In Agra, in the 17th century AD, Mogul Akbar Khan ensured strict silence in his brutal version of the same experiment by employing dumb nurses to rear 12 children in isolation. He found, contrary to his religious conviction, that none of the children learned to speak at all, again implying that language had to be learnt by example. In the 1960s, a 10-year-old girl, Genie, was found in Los Angeles completely unable to talk. Her obsessionally religious parents had deprived her of almost all sensory input to protect her from any possibility of sin, by locking her up in a dark cupboard for the first 10 years of her life. No amount of teaching since then has managed to give her a full command of language. This again shows not only that children need exemplars to learn to speak, but also that these must be available before the age of 10 years.

Thus, there is a great deal of evidence that language has to be learnt. The English learn English from their parents; the French learn French; and chimps learn chimp. Johann, who was abandoned as a baby in Burundi, was brought up by chimpanzees for 5 years. When found, he was happily using chimpanzee vocalisations and gestures to communicate successfully. Interestingly he has now learnt to speak German quite well, but his hand and finger use remains very chimpanzee-like, suggesting that much of our fine finger control also has to be learnt, even earlier than speech, rather than being innate. Thus, our evolutionary past seems to equip us to learn languages but does not provide us with language itself; nor does it specify the language we learn. The capacity to learn to speak is innate but language itself is not; it is handed down to us culturally. The evolutionary prerequisites to be able to learn your language are genetically endowed, but their development took place over a very long period of time.

Human Evolution

To understand how this capacity to learn language evolved we need first briefly consider the controversial question of how *Homo sapiens* evolved from our ape ancestry (Bradshaw 1997). This story is highly controversial because the fossil record is incomplete and currently fails to explain many really obvious characteristics about humans, such as our lack of hair, our profligacy with water and our upright posture.

Mammals first appeared on the earth about 200 million years ago; primates around 65 million; the first anthropoids about 45 million and chimpanzees some 12 million years ago. The first hominoid, *Ankarapithecus*, split from the chimp line about 9 million years ago, *Australopithecus* appeared around 3 million years ago, *H. erectus* at 2 million, Neanderthals 250,000 years ago and *H. sapiens* maybe only 100,000 years ago.

From the point of view of language development, there are five important adaptations associated with this history. Some 200 million years ago the left side of the brain seems to have begun to become specialised for timing the order of sounds and movements; it is found in many birds and as low down in the mammalian line as rodents. Then "mirror cells" appeared as long as 65 million years ago and these enabled learning others' movements by imitation. Bipedalism developed in the first phase of hominoid evolution around 8 million years ago. This probably developed for quite different reasons but had the incidental effect of potentially freeing the arms and fingers for more efficient food gathering, tool use and gesturing. Descent of the larynx around the same time was also probably nothing to do with speech, but it subsequently, much later, made the voicing of phonemes possible, and greatly increased their potential number. It was only around 1 million years ago however that the very large increases in our brain size began. Actually, the brains of Neanderthals were somewhat larger than our own. Speech probably began only about 100,000 years ago and finally, in modern times, writing was invented only about 5000 years ago.

Left-Sided Specialisation

The origins of left-sided cerebral specialisation can actually be discerned from almost the very beginning of life in that the laevo-isomers of biological molecules are always favoured. This means that there is a non-genetic molecular bias towards favouring the left side. Although most invertebrates are bilaterally symmetrical, gastropods and crustaceans are asymmetrical, shells twisting either clockwise or anticlockwise, or one claw being much bigger than the other. There is no tendency to favour the left side.

Clear left-sided brain specialisation can, however, begin to be seen in birds and lower mammals. In most songbirds the left hyperstriatum, which is equivalent to the mammalian cerebral cortex, is specialised for controlling the vocal organ, the syrinx. Neurones in the left-sided nuclei crucial for song production divide in the breeding season, with each new division adding to the complexity of the song, and then die away in the autumn and winter.

It has been found that rodents can respond much more accurately to differences in sound order if the stimuli are delivered to their right ear (projecting to the left hemisphere) rather than to the left. At the same time, there is evidence that the right hemisphere of both rodents and chicks is somewhat better at large-scale visuospatial orientation than the left. Thus, it seems that as early as 200 million years ago in vertebrate evolution the left side of the brain began to become specialised for timing sensory and motor processes and the right side became specialised for visuospatial functions.

After birds, only humans have such a strong left hemisphere specialisation. In about 97% of humans (including 70% of left-handers), the left cerebral hemisphere is chosen to contain the network of areas that are specialised for mediating the perception and production of speech. How the left sidedness of L-amino acids translated in humans into this site in the left hemisphere of all the neural networks specialising in timing remains a mystery, but it is surely no accident that the two groups, birds and humans, that make the most use of acoustic communication, site their control systems on the left side.

Yet most features of animals are bilaterally symmetrical and perfectly satisfactorily controlled from both sides of a bilaterally symmetrical brain because there are good cross communications between the two sides. So what advantage does hemispheric specialisation on one side confer? Probably one side has to be favoured to prevent both trying to take control. Both hemispheres have the potential to control the vocal musculature. If they both attempted to, they would compete with each other and cause chaos. Hence the majority of the cross connections between the two hemispheres are inhibitory to prevent the two sides trying to do the same thing. Placing the control of vocalisations predominately in the same hemisphere thus simplified the control problem. Another contributory factor may be that joining sensory and motor language areas within the same hemisphere slightly shortens the length of the connections required, compared with linking the two hemispheres. Since precise timing of the vocal musculature requires millisecond accuracy, reducing these delays is crucial.

Emotional Vocalisations

In lower mammals, however, including monkeys, all of their vocalisations are controlled by a medially placed system of neurones that involves the cingulate cortex, basal ganglia and hypothalamus. This system seems to have evolved primarily to express emotions; and it is clear that in primates other than man, all vocalisations are completely automatic, driven by the emotions and not under voluntary control. Only Man has gained voluntary control of vocalisations using a separate lateral system, to express ideas other than emotions. It is therefore highly significant that the emotionally controlled medial system does not involve the monkey homologue of Broca's speech area in the left lateral frontal cortex. Therefore, lesions in this area do not at all affect the ability of monkeys to make their vocalisations.

Hence, all attempts to teach primates to actually talk have failed; it is almost impossible to harness primate vocalisations for other kinds of communication because they are simply not under the animals' voluntary control. It took 5 years to teach a chimpanzee to say just four words, "mum", "dad", "cup" and "up", and even then the words were not very intelligible. Yet it has been shown clearly that chimpanzees can be taught to communicate to the level of a 3-year-old human, by other means, such as gestures, sign language or using symbol boards. They are quite intelligent enough to learn to communicate to some extent; they simply cannot gain sufficient voluntary control over their vocalisations.

Mirror Neurones

The ability of chimps to communicate so successfully manually has been powerfully illuminated by the discovery of "mirror" neurones (Rizzolatti and Fadiga 1998). These seem to have evolved as long as 45 million years ago and they suggest strongly that human speaking and language evolved via gesture and facial expression rather than vocalisation. Mirror neurones are found in the ventrolateral frontal pre-motor cortex (ventrolateral Brodman area 6) just in front of the face and arm representation in the primary motor cortex. Note that Broca's speech production area is in precisely this location in the left hemisphere in humans.

The crucial characteristic of mirror neurones is that they fire not only when a monkey reaches out to grasp an object, but also when the monkey observes somebody else doing the same thing: that is why they were named "mirror" neurones. Further experiments have shown that in both humans and lower primates these neurones represent the "goal" of a movement. So their responses are not tied to its details; whether made by the hairy hand of a monkey or the very different hand of a human moving perhaps in the opposite direction, but they respond when the movement has a particular purpose, if this is understood by the monkey or human. In humans, the same area appears to be activated not only when the subject reaches out to grasp something or when he sees somebody else doing it, but also when he plans or imagines doing it himself. Thus, mirror neurones probably underlie how we learn to produce speech by enabling us to imitate our parents.

Bipedalism and the Aquatic Ape Hypothesis

Walking on only two legs seems not to have commenced with *H. erectus*, just 2 million years ago, but more likely 6–8 million years ago. There is great controversy as to why this happened at all, because it is a remarkably difficult feat to perch 70 kg over a footprint of only 30 cm and keep it stable, with no obvious selective advantage in doing so. Running on four legs is faster and more economical, and even though most of our close relatives live in trees, when on the ground they usually use all four legs. From the point of view of communication and speech, however, bipedalism had the advantage of leaving the hands free for tool use and manual gestures. Nevertheless, this is unlikely to have been its evolutionary drive because bipedalism probably preceded language communication by several million years.

There is also much controversy about several other features that distinguish us from apes. Why are we hairless, when hair is such a good insulator both from external heat in the summer and cold in the winter? Why are we so profligate with water, needing to drink at least 2 l/day and much more in hot environments? Our kidneys fail to concentrate urine very powerfully unlike, for example, the desert rat. The rest of our requirement for water is due to our sweating, which is a highly wasteful means of losing heat, far more wasteful of water than having a thick layer of hair and panting when necessary. Such conspicuous failure to preserve water probably rules out the theory that we evolved on the dry savannah. Further unsolved questions are why do we have so much subcutaneous fat where apes have none? And why do our nostrils point downwards rather than forwards.

Alistair Hardy put forward the aquatic ape hypothesis to answer these and many other questions, and Elaine Morgan has been a forceful resuscitant of it (Morgan 1997). But the theory is still met with profound scepticism, and needs much more evidence to be thoroughly accepted. Hardy suggested that hominids separated from the ape lineage 6–8 million years ago by becoming semi-aquatic, living around lakes or near the sea. This is supported by the fact that most of the fossils of hominids from around that time are found in the vicinity of areas that once were lakes; the most famous example is the Turkana basin in the Rift valley.

Furthermore, living in shallow water would have made the upright posture not only essential for breathing, but it would probably also have made the neural control required to accomplish it much simpler, since water will help to support standing on two legs. A watery environment might also explain why we are hairless; wet hair is useless as an insulator, and so almost all water-living animals are hairless. The ready availability of water would also explain why our kidneys have not evolved very long loops of Henlé to concentrate our urine more, and why wasting water as sweat was not a problem. Moreover, our profuse subcutaneous fat may be the answer to insulation in water. Heat conservation by subcutaneous fat is carried to much greater lengths in the blubber of whales and other sea-living mammals. And maybe our nostrils point downwards so that they do not fill with water when swimming.

The aquatic ape hypothesis may also answer another conundrum of which Alistair Hardy was not aware in the 1960s: 20% of the dry weight of our brains is made of very unusual long-chain unsaturated fatty acids such as docosahexanoic acid, a 22-carbon fatty acid with six double bonds between the carbons, the first at the third carbon from the terminal methyl group ("omega-3"). These fatty acids are only found in fish, although they can be very slowly synthesised from alpha linoleic acid, an 18-carbon fatty acid found in some nuts and seeds. But the very high proportion of long-chain omega-3 fatty acids found in our brains suggests strongly that during a crucial period in our evolution a major part of our diet came from fish and shellfish. These would have been readily available during our aquatic period, and piles of shellfish shells have been found alongside hominid remains from this period.

Larynx Descent

This aquatic ape hypothesis can also explain another very troublesome difference between us and the apes, namely the descent of the larynx. Although this was important for the development of speech, it probably pre-dated the development of language by several million years. True speech probably did not evolve until perhaps only 50,000 years ago, so the requirements of speech cannot have driven the descent of the larynx much earlier.

On the face of it, it seems a crazy development. Chimpanzees with a high larynx can keep the airway and oesophageal food path completely separate, so that the danger of inhaling food is almost completely eliminated, whereas a common cause of death in humans with a much lower larynx is just that, inhalation of water or food into the lungs because air and food share the same pathway in the pharynx.

Elaine Morgan, following Alistair Hardy, suggested that the descent of the larynx in hominids may actually have been driven by the requirements of being able to breath sufficiently deeply whilst swimming in water. The nose offers too high a resistance to airflow when the lungs have to be kept inflated during swimming, and mouth breathing is only possible with a lower larynx, so this might have been the evolutionary selective pressure to lower it in humans. But this also had the unforeseen benefit of enlarging the vocal cavities. Much later, this enlarged the number of phonetic distinctions that we can now produce.

Brain Enlargement

About 2.5 million years ago, the fossil record shows that hominids quite rapidly achieved an increase in brain size of about 50%, from about 600 cm³ to 900 cm³. This increase was accompanied by the first clear use of tools. Our ancestors had begun to learn how to split flint stones to make hand axes; these they used not only to kill animals (and maybe each other), but also to split open bones and skull to eat the fatty marrow and brain. This improved nutrition may well have helped to drive the increased brain size.

Then for about 1 million more years there appears to have been no further increase in brain size, nor any improvement in tool technology. However, about 1 million years ago another increase took place that enlarged our brains to their present size of about 1500 cm³. This increase was accompanied by a very noticeable improvement in tool technology and it coincided with a diaspora of hominid species out of Africa into Europe. Even then, however, there is no evidence that speech emerged; this required enlargement of the cervical spinal cord in order to control breathing precisely for the production of speech. There is no evidence that this occurred until much later.

Right-Handedness

From the point of view of language development, the most important change that these increases in brain size seem to have promoted is the development of right-handedness. Despite the evidence that in many animals left-brain structures are specialised for timing processes, no lower animal shows such strong right-handedness as humans do. Many animals choose to use either left or right hands for particular tasks, but not even chimpanzees choose the right so systematically. But the hand axes fashioned by hominids 1 million years ago show clear signs of having been made mainly for right-handers. This suggests strongly that left-brainedness had progressed far enough to cause specialisation of the right hand for accurate tasks.

Selective Advantages of Speech

So why did speech emerge at this point? Three interconnected explanations have been offered. The first is that speech was essential to improve collective use of tools. This development of technology encouraged speech communication to explain how tools should be used, to keep the hands free for using them and to discuss the best ways of employing them. It has been pointed out that chattering away would not lead to a very successful hunt; but, of course, the conversations would have taken place earlier in order to plan the hunt.

If these tools happened to be weapons, then they would have been used not only for hunting animals for food, but also for killing enemy Neanderthals. Sad to say, it seems that our ancestors simply annihilated their main competitors. Despite their larger brains, our Neanderthal cousins probably did not develop a sophisticated means of communication and this left them at a fundamental disadvantage in the face of the ability of H. sapiens to plan the means of killing them off.

The requirement for such planning gives rise to the second main suggestion about the pressure to develop language, namely that language enables you to discuss what is likely to happen by planning, predicting and representing it in abstract terms (i.e. language gives you the tools to think about things). This representation need not be confined to planning a hunt, but can also be used as the basis of thinking about all manner of things.

Perhaps the most important of these would be helping to determine what others are likely to be thinking about: developing a "theory of mind". Cynics believe this to be the basis of "Machiavellian intelligence", working out what people are likely to be thinking, thus putting yourself in a powerful position to deceive them and gain advantage. I prefer to emphasise how developing a theory of mind would naturally lead to the invention of the tools of thought: categorisation, quantification, abstraction, causality and logic.

The third kind of pressure that definitely contributed to the development of language capacities was the drive to find a mate. This sexual pressure is certainly the main driving force behind bird song. As we have seen, the left-sided brain structures that control song production by the syrinx actually increase in size during the breeding season; they grow new neurones under the influence of testosterone, and then during the winter, they lose these song neurones and the nuclei regress. In addition, because of the long childhood of humans, females have the need to retain their mate for several years to help bring up the children. This is, therefore, the only account that can explain why females are in general slightly better at communication than males.

These three suggestions are not mutually exclusive; probably all three contributed. But they are almost impossible to confirm or refute. Hence, they are to a certain extent like Kipling's Just So Stories: "how the rhinoceros got his skin" might have been as Kipling suggested, because the Parsee put itchy raisins into it when he'd taken it off to swim; but this seems very unlikely. Our stories about the selective advantage of communication by speech sound much more plausible, but since they are unproveable they might be just as totally off beam.

Gesture and Speech

The final steps leading to true speech probably evolved only about 200,000 years ago, and took the form of manual and facial gesturing and signing. Gaining control of vocalisations probably came even later (Corballis 2003). Our larger brains would contain more mirror neurones and greater connectivity between them. The "plasticity" of these connections means that they can be modified by experience. By learning to respond to the communicatory goal of a seen manual gesture, these mirror neurones would enable an observer to imitate it and thus to enable communication by means of these gestures, whose meaning is understood by both communicant and observer.

Liberman and colleagues at the Yale-Haskins laboratory of speech science long argued that the basic elements of speech are not, as generally assumed, consonants and vowels, but rather the vocal gestures that generate them, namely the movements of the lips, tongue and larynx (Liberman et al. 1967). Thus, mirror neurones in Broca's area probably came to represent lip, tongue and laryngeal gestures that would generate the different phonetic elements of speech. In fact, most of us still gesture with our hands when speaking and when we gesture, our vocal production is synchronised with our hand gestures. Moreover, the sign language gestures used by the completely deaf are controlled by the same left hemisphere centres, particularly Broca's area, that speech occupies in those who can hear.

These mirror neurones also established means of voluntary control over the vocal tract musculature. Even in monkeys, some of them project directly into the lateral corticospinal (pyramidal) tract that synapses monosynaptically on laryngeal motor neurones. More project back to the face and vocal tract area of the primary motor cortex, which lies just behind them, and the upper motor neurones here provide the major input to the pyramidal tract. Thus, evolution of the capacity for speech probably involved mirror neurones superimposing their voluntary control by the lateral corticospinal system on to the much older, medially descending, emotional system that controls automatic vocalisations. But the latter system probably does still supply important emotional components to speech such as the basic intonation and prosody of sentences.

This account of the development of speech from gesture has received further support from the study of sign language. In sign language, syntax, the grammatical ordering of ideas, is expressed in the trajectory of each gesture. The grammatical structure of a signed sentence is determined by the evolution of the gesture from shoulder to fingers. This is probably the basis of the "deep" grammar that all languages demonstrate, and this structure is enshrined in our genome. But language details, inflexions, the grammar of individual languages, word gender and pronunciation, for example, are handed down culturally and cannot be said to be hereditary.

Writing

The final step in this history is the invention of writing. This is even more of a cultural invention and even less enshrined in our genome than our capacity for language, because it was only invented about 5000 years ago; most of the population was illiterate until the last century. Learning to read and write has only become greatly advantageous very recently, so that only since the 20th century has it carried any particular selective advantage. The capacity to write is therefore much too recent to have entered our genome; it is most unlikely that we will ever find a gene specifically underlying reading, contrary to what is sometimes claimed. But, like speech before it, the invention of writing depended on prior adaptations developed for other purposes. Thus, for example, functional imaging has shown clearly that Broca's area, long thought to be exclusively involved in speaking, is highly activated during reading, even when the subjects are reading entirely silently.

The development of right-handedness was equally important for the invention of writing. Hieroglyphs and letters are very impoverished visual signals, but it matters greatly whether they are pointing to the left or to the right. It is easiest for us to agree which way round they should be if we all write from the same side. Ambidextrous animals and children therefore have extreme difficulty knowing which way round bs and ds should go, and children who fail to develop consistent handedness, whether on the left or the right, are the ones most likely to develop reading difficulties.

Because reading and writing are man-made inventions, they are much more difficult to learn than speaking. The written word does not map as easily onto articulatory gestures as speech does. The phonemes that are represented by letters are wholly artificial subdivisions of the articulatory gestures that generate them, and these subdivisions have to be taught and learnt. Hence, a very high proportion (some 10–20%) of humans never master this art properly; it is the most difficult thing that most of us ever have to learn.

Conclusion

The acquisition by *H. sapiens* of the capacity for language and literacy did not result from a single mutation that endowed us with a linguistic processor, all in one jump. Rather, the adaptations required for speech accumulated gradually over many millions of years, coat tailing on a series of developments that evolved for completely different purposes. Only when all were in place, including the necessary enlargement and interconnectivity of the brain, was speech possible. And even then we must not think of language has having evolved and being enshrined in our genome: all the details of whichever language you acquire are handed down culturally and you have to learn them explicitly. Admittedly, the adaptations that make this possible are innate and genetically endowed, but you have to learn your language from your parents or other carers.

The pre-eminence of phonology follows from the descent of the larynx and the specialisation of Broca's area for the voluntary control of articulatory gestures. Syntax and grammar can be viewed as a direct consequence of the evolution of sentences out of gestures that can involve the whole body from axial back muscles to distal finger-movers. In rather the same way that identical Chinese logographs represent the same idea, but totally different sounding words, in Chinese and Japanese, so the same deep structure, the same flow of ideas conveyed by a particular gesture, can be represented by different strings of articulatory gestures producing the thousands of different languages that have developed throughout the world.

What makes this whole enterprise more than just curiosity is that it can provide new insights into what can go wrong with language. Because ontogeny repeats phylogeny to some extent, elucidating how language gradually evolved from archaic gestures means that potentially we now have a new approach to understanding developmental disorders of language. Counterintuitively, both speech production and comprehension seem to depend on our mirror neurones being able to represent articulatory gestures. Hence, although comprehension clearly makes greater demands on the auditory system, and speech production makes greater demands on Broca's area and the voluntary motor vocalisation system, Broca's area is clearly engaged in both activities, as modern imaging methods have clearly shown. As expected, therefore, children with developmental dysphasia are significantly worse at lip-reading, which depends on deciphering articulatory gestures. Also, whereas a good speaker's hearing of a phoneme is greatly altered if the speaker's lips appear to be generating a different one (the McGurk effect), in developmental dysphasia this mishearing of the phonemes is much less apparent, because in them the mirror system is not working as well as it ought to be.

The bottom line of all this is that the capacity for learning to speak a language is endowed upon us by our evolution, but the language itself is handed down by our culture.

Summary for the Clinician

- The adaptations required to learn to speak took place over many millions of years. The first important one was left-sided specialisation of the neural apparatus controlling involuntary emotional vocalisations, which began more than 200 million years ago. The next was the development in primates of "mirror neurones" in the pre-motor cortex some 45 million years ago. These enabled us to control voluntarily and to imitate previously involuntary manual gestures and vocalisations. The third important adaptation was the descent of the larynx about 6 million years ago. Although this probably survived because it made diving and mouth breathing when swimming easier, much later, only about 100,000 years ago, when the human brain had increased greatly in size, it also permitted an increase in the phonological range of vocalisations that could be made. The capacity for speaking then emerged because it enormously improved communication between members of the group, facilitated learning how to use tools and weapons, enabled the planning of hunting, war and defence, helped us to imagine what other people are thinking, and so to develop a "theory of mind" and the tools of thought, and better communication improved our abilities to attract and keep a mate. Thus, our capacity for language did not develop all at once, but evolved gradually over millions of years, building upon adaptations originally meeting quite different needs.

References

1. Bradshaw JL (1997) Human Evolution. Psychology Press, Hove
2. Chomsky N (1975) Reflections on Language. Pantheon, New York
3. Corballis MC (2003) From mouth to hand: gesture, speech, and the evolution of right-handedness. Behav Brain Sci 26:199–208
4. Liberman AM, Cooper FS, Shankweiler DP, Studdert-Kennedy M (1967) Perception of the speech code. Psychol Rev 74:431–461
5. Morgan E (1997) The aquatic ape hypothesis. Condor Independent Voices, New York
6. Pinker S, Jackendoff R (2005) The faculty of language: what's special about it? Cognition 95:201–236
7. Rizzolatti G, Fadiga L (1998) Mirror neurones: grasping objects and grasping action meanings: the dual role of monkey rostroventral premotor cortex (area F5). Novartis Found Symp 218:81–95

Chapter 5

Evidence-Based Management of Speech and Language Delays

5

Amy McConkey Robbins

Core Messages

- Published data exist that allow us to construct valid milestones for communication development at frequent points in early childhood.
- Early speech and language intervention produces better outcomes than does late intervention; early identification and diagnosis is, therefore, critical.
- Hearing loss, a severe detriment to normal communication development, can be identified and treated as early as the newborn period.
- Through parent interview and observation of children, the doctor plays a critical role in making a differential diagnosis of several communication impairments, including: autism spectrum disorder, developmental delays, and hearing loss.
- The paediatrician, ENT or audiology specialist should be familiar with a cluster of speech/language characteristics that are often found with reading disability.
- An evidence-based approach to the management of children's speech and language development is possible for the paediatric, ENT and audiology specialist.

Contents

"Serious problems in speech and language development have major, negative consequences for children. As a result, professionals who work with young children need to know more about both the processes and the products of children's speech and language development. When professionals better understand why and how children learn language, and what it is that they learn as they progress from those first rude attempts at words at 1 year of age to thousands of well-structured sentences at 3 years of age, they will be better prepared to deal with children who have serious problems in speech and language. They also will be better prepared to call for and support the special efforts needed to help children better their skills in these crucial behavioural domains." (McLean and Snyder-McLean 1999, p. 5)

Introduction

One of the most remarkable things about human development is that within the span of approximately 5 years, babies progress from making only physiological noises, such as crying and coughing, to being fluent users of the language (or languages) spoken around them without receiving any direct instruction to do so. Mastery of such complex skills as knowing when to use the pluperfect tense, embedding dependent clauses and using thousands of different words productively occurs before children begin formal, academic schooling. This mastery occurs in children living all over the world, hearing thousands of different languages, under vastly different socioeconomic conditions.

For the purpose of this chapter, the word "doctor" will be used to describe medically qualified professionals. Where necessary, the word "specialist" will be used to refer to medically qualified specialists of various kinds. Doctors play a critical role in managing the speech and language development of young children due to their knowledge of the child's overall health status, the respect they command and parents' reliance on the doctor's assessment and advice. They are also "gatekeepers", in setting up the onward referral of children who need help with speech and language. Primary care physicians are well placed to identify all developmental problems in young children and to institute onward referral. ENT and audiology specialists have the expertise to identify or to confirm the presence of hearing and communication disorders or delay. Paediatricians and clinical geneticists will also be in a position to diagnose a wide range of developmental disorders. Access to developing children and expertise in these fields brings responsibility. Doctors must be prepared to use this access and these skills to identify developmental problems, to employ correct diagnostic tools and to make appropriate onward referrals for diagnosis and treatment.

Perhaps it is because the development of language does appear to be so natural and so inevitable in most children that doctors may be hesitant to call a child a "late talker", to suggest assessment by a communication specialist or to recommend intervention at an early age. In fact, two features of normal language development seem to work against late communicators from receiving the early attention they need: the apparent naturalness of language acquisition, and the variability that is seen across normally developing talkers. Other factors cited include lack of awareness of research-based speech and language milestones, a reluctance to over-refer for speech-language assessments for fear of burdening therapists, and clinical experience with other late-talking children who have "grown out of their problem" without intervention. Although some children who are late in communicating do catch up on their own, at least half have language problems that persist (Wetherby et al. 2004). Deficits in language have far-reaching and life-altering consequences, including decreased reading ability, lower academic achievement and limited career choices.

Reports of some parents' experiences show the negative consequences of a wait-and-see approach to delayed communication. In-depth interviews with parents were conducted by two local education authorities in Merseyside, in the UK (Rannard et al. 2005). In many cases, parents were the first to realise that there was something wrong with the speech and language development of their child. Parents reported that doctors tended to underestimate speech and language problems, and failed to take parental views into account. In some cases, parents found that even when children were attending a specialist unit or hospital they still were not referred to a speech and language therapist, resulting in the children reaching school age before referral for speech and language therapy. In other cases, health professionals appeared to rely on the hope of spontaneous recovery, and gave inappropriate advice to parents, which again resulted in delayed referral to speech and language therapists. The authors concluded that health professionals failed to use systematic, evidence-based approaches in responding to early parental concerns. For this group of parents, such an approach resulted in long delays in referral for specialist intervention.

In this chapter, we advocate a more active role by the ENT and audiology specialist in managing speech and language delays in children. Benchmarks of communication development are provided, based upon current, published studies. These benchmarks are presented in tabular form for easy referencing. Abnormal findings or red flags are listed that alert physicians to make referrals to speech-language or hearing specialists, allowing an evidence-based approach to the management of speech and language development.

Milestones for Communication Development

Normal Variation in Language Learning

Child language research has revealed fascinating variations in language learning styles in young children. For example, researchers have identified groups of babies whose early communication is referential (high proportion of object labels) versus others whose communication is expressive (high proportion of words to express feelings, needs and social functions). Some linguists have described "word babies", who produce many words in early speech, and "intonation babies" who use prosodic patterns more than words in early speech. A dichotomy proposed by Peters (1983) separated "analytic language learners", children who produced one-word utterances of one or two syllables that were quite distinct from "gestalt language learners", children who produced whole phrases or sentences rather than single words, without evidence of using individual words referentially. Gestalt babies were described as learning the tune before the words. These and other findings confirm that there are variations in language learning styles across normal babies and that there is more than one way to learn to talk.

Normal Variation versus Communication Delay

In spite of the variations in communication style observed across babies, the vast majority of children achieve language milestones within a circumscribed timeframe, allowing us to construct milestones for communication development throughout early childhood. There exists a sequence and scope of skills that develop over the first few years of life that are the foundations for normal speech and language development. Likewise, certain behaviours are not typical of children with normal communication, even allowing for variations in learning style. As an introduction to Table 5.1, let us review some of the significant milestones that occur in the first 12 months of life.

Communication Milestones in the First Year of Life

From birth to 2 months, babies show a definite response to voice and loud sounds and show an interest in the faces of people. Expressively, the baby is limited to crying. Between 2 and 4 months, though, a baby's crying already can be differentiated for such things as pain and hunger, and the baby engages in reciprocal cooing, an important foundation for establishing turn-taking in communication. Receptively, the 2- to 4-month-old baby calms and responds to a familiar voice and alerts to sound-making toys. The 4- to 9-month-old baby deliberately turns toward sound, recognises tones of voice (e.g. will cry to an angry voice or quiet to a soothing voice) and already responds to his or her name. By 9 months of age, babies begin to string consonant/vowel sequences together ("babababab") to produce babble, an important expressive landmark. By the end of the 1st year of life, babies respond appropriately to "no", comprehend verbal routines such as "Wave bye-bye" and smile and laugh as a reaction to others. The 12-month-old baby also points out inter- esting objects or people, uses gestures and vocalisation to get his or her needs met and produces "jargon", or complicated babbling and intonation patterns that resemble meaningful speech.

A noteworthy point about the milestones in the 1st year of life is how many of them involve auditory attention, social routines, and responsiveness to significant caregivers. These are the very behaviours that are often overlooked when professionals interview parents because such behaviours do not involve the sounds or words a child is using, but rather the social context within which communication occurs. It is, in fact, the establishment of these reciprocal social interactions that is the most important milestone of the 1st year of communication. Conversely, absence of reciprocal social interactions is a red flag for concern, and warrants referral to a specialist.

The findings listed in Table 5.1 (Moeller 2003) have been endorsed as a resource for physicians (American Academy of Pediatrics' continuing education website, PediaLink: www.pedialink.org). Note that for each chronological age range, the table lists the most salient milestones for a child's receptive and expressive lan-

Table 5.1 Developmental milestones in language (Moeller 2003). Used with permission M.P. Moeller and PediaLink, American Academy of Pediatrics *(see next page)*

Age of acquisition	Child's receptive skills	Child's expressive skills	Abnormal findings or "red flags" for full assessment
Birth to 2 months	- Responds to sound and voice - Shows social interest in faces and people - Awakens or stirs at loud sounds - Startles at loud noises	- Cries - Varies crying by state	- Lack of response to sound at any age - Lack of interest in interaction with people at any age
2–4 months	- Alternates vocalising and listening in face-to-face interaction - Calms at the sound of a familiar voice - Responds to voice (smiles or coos) - Notices rattle or other sound making toys	- Differentiates crying for pain, hunger and so on. - Coos (musical sounds) - Reciprocal cooing and turn-taking	- Lack of any drive to communicate after 4 months of age
4–9 months	- Deliberately turns head toward sound - Responds appropriately to tone of voice - Responds to name	- 4–6 months - explores vocal tract (squeals, growls, raspberries, mostly vowels) - Uses one or two consonants and sometimes strings consonant/vowel sequences together by 9 months (babble)	- Poor sound localisation or lack of responsiveness to sound - Limited amount of vocalisation - Limited or no use of babble; limited variety in sounds produced

5

Table 5.1 *(Continued)* Developmental milestones in language (Moeller 2003). Used with permission M.P. Moeller and PediaLink, American Academy of Pediatrics *(see next page)*

Age of acquisition	Child's receptive skills	Child's expressive skills	Abnormal findings or "red flags" for full assessment
9–12 months	– Comprehends verbal routines, such as "wave bye-bye" – Responds appropriately to "no" – Understands pointing – Smiles and laughs responsively and looks to see if parent is watching them play	– Points for needs and for interesting objects or actions – Lets family know he/she needs help or wants object out of reach with gestures and vocalisations – Creates complicated babbling called jargon which sounds like sentences – Uses six conventional gestures (12 months; i.e. wave, nod, point, reach, lift arms) – Uses voice to get help and attention	– Poor comprehension of verbal routines, such as wave bye-bye by 12 months – Reaching or pointing for wants or needs but no pointing at interesting objects or actions
10–16 months	– Points to body parts or objects to show comprehension – Understands more words than produces – Follows single step command – Responds to name – Understands familiar words and phrases like, "Where's mama?" and "Get your bottle."	– Produces at least three consonant sounds (by 12 months) – Produces single words – Has vocabulary that grows gradually to 30–50 words – Communicates needs or interests by giving, showing and pointing – Plays social games – Makes known what they want and do not want	– Failure to use words, add new words, or loss of most words previously learned – Slow progress in learning words receptively and expressively – Failure to point to body parts or follow single step commands – Limit variety of sounds and/or limited vocalisations
18–24 months	– Comprehends simple sentences – Points to pictures in response to words – Identifies objects when named – Listens to stories, songs and rhymes	– Experiences vocabulary spurt – Concurrently begins to use two-word phrases – Makes six or more different consonant sounds, like p, m, n, b, d and g – Imitates words spoken by others – Requests information (i.e. asks "what's that?") – Begins to provide information about things in the past	– Minimal comprehension and limited symbolic play, such as doll or truck play – Less than 50 words in expressive vocabulary at 24 months – Limited sound repertoire and limited imitation
24–30 months	– Understands personal pronouns – Understands negatives – Understands some prepositions such as in and on – Listens to 5- to 10-min story	– Uses two-word utterances – Produces simple sentences like "Mommy go outside" and "What's that?" – Shows good intelligibility for familiar people such as family members – Greater mastery of nouns and verbs than grammatical words or markers – Comments increasingly relevant to the remarks of others – Can express emotion verbally	– Less than 100 words at 30 months – No two-word utterances when vocabulary is >50 words – >Half of the utterances are unintelligible to family after age 2 years

Table 5.1 *(Continued)* Developmental milestones in language (Moeller 2003). Used with permission M.P. Moeller and PediaLink, American Academy of Pediatrics

Age of acquisition	Child's receptive skills	Child's expressive skills	Abnormal findings or "red flags" for full assessment
30–36 months	– Follows two-step commands – Identifies objects by use – Understands concepts like big/little, high/low	– Converses through asking and answering questions – Use pronouns I, you, mine, my, this, that – Can express emotion verbally	– Frequent immediate or delayed repetition of what others say ("echolalia") – Rote memorisation with failure to generate novel sentences
36–48 months	– Knows colours – Knows what to do if hungry, tired, thirsty – Answers yes/no, which, and what questions	– Shows good intelligibility for unfamiliar adults – Full, well-formed sentences – Shows some developmental dysfluency – Asks many questions – Begins to tease	– One-quarter of utterances are unintelligible to strangers after age 4 years – Consistent use of only short, simple sentences – Repetition of individual sounds of words or other signs of stuttering
4 years	– Understands same/different – Follows three-step command – Answers how much, how long, what if?	– Tells stories – Knows colours and numbers – Enjoys rhyming – Reasons with why and because – Talks about the imaginary – Asks what, where, who, why and yes/no?	– Persistent stuttering – Inability to express thoughts and ideas – Poor comprehension – Difficulty understanding or asking questions – Speech intelligibility <90%
5 years	– Comprehends most of what is said, limited only by conceptual development – Comprehends "what happens if"	– Pronounces all basic consonants correctly – Produces more logical personal stories – Adept at expressing ideas, wants, feelings and beliefs	– Errors in consonants such as b, p, d, t, p, k, m, n, l, r, w, s, by 5 years
7 years	– Participates in lengthy conversations	– Pronounces all speech sounds correctly – Begins to develop figurative language and slang – Knows some double meaning words	– Immature production blends such as st, sh, sp at 7 years

guage. The milestones are based upon current, published research about early communication development. The last column on the right lists red flags that signal a definite need to explore further communication assessment. Findings in the "Red Flags" column represent behaviours that are unlikely to go away on their own and that are not considered normal variations in communication development.

Clinical Use of Table 5.1 by Physicians

It is recommended that in the process of taking a history, physicians question parents about their child's communication development. The most fruitful opening question, based upon clinical experience and reports from Matkin (2005; personal communication) is likely to be "Do you have any concerns about your child's speech and lan-

5

guage?" Matkin found that, when examining the reliability of reports from a variety of informed adults in a child's life (mother, father, child's primary care physician, maternal grandparents, paternal grandparents), the mother's concern was the most reliable source for predicting communication delays. The maternal grandmother's concern was the second most reliable source. Thus, if parents (particularly mothers) express a concern about a child's communication development, further questioning is appropriate. In other words, healthcare professionals should take seriously the concern by a mother of delayed communication development in her child. Also helpful are open-ended question such as, "Tell me about Clarence's communication – how does he let you know what he wants?" or "Describe how Junior 'talks' to you and others". These sorts of open-ended questions set up scenarios and allow families to describe their child's communication in an open-ended way. Extensive research on the validity of parent reports demonstrates that such reports can be highly reliable if gathered in a non-biased manner. On the other hand, leading questions with yes/no answers have a tendency to over-credit the child, as insecure parents may assume that if the professional is asking, the child should be demonstrating that skill.

Because speech and language "explode" so rapidly in the first 3 years of life, an appropriate time to wait-and-see is 1 or 2 months, but not more than 3 months. In addition, for any child who shows delays in the use of or response to sounds and words, it is essential to have an audiological assessment to rule out hearing loss.

Speech and Language Intervention is Correlated with Young Age at Identification

A compelling reason for greater vigilance in identifying young children at risk for communication disorders is the published evidence regarding the superiority of early, rather than late, intervention. Numerous studies have shown the effectiveness of intervention when it is accomplished early. These studies have evaluated children with a wide range of communication impairments including developmental disabilities, specific language impairment, autism (Birnbrauer and Leach 1993; Harris and Handleman 2000), reading disability (Torgesen 1998) and hearing loss (Yoshinago-Itano et al. 1998; Moeller 2000). The latter investigation, a retrospective study, revealed the combined effects of two variables on the communication progress of children with hearing impairment. That is, there was an important interaction between: (1) age of enrolment in communication therapy and (2) family involvement. The negative impact of late intervention of services (some children had received intervention by age 3 years; others had not received services until aged 5 years) was particularly dramatic for children who had average to low-average family involvement ratings. Early enrolment in therapy was of benefit to language learning,

even with limited family involvement. Children who had the combined benefits of early intervention and strong family involvement were consistently the strongest communicators at age 5 years, whereas children enrolled late and with limited family involvement were at the greatest risk for poor communication at age 5 years. We summarise these findings clinically to mean that late intervention is undesirable for any child with communication delays, but disproportionately penalises children with lower family involvement.

Hearing Loss can be Identified and Treated as Early as the Newborn Period

Hearing loss is one of the most serious impediments to normal communication development, often leading to life-long deficits in achievement and career attainment. Hearing loss in adults is an annoyance – it interferes with the listener's ability to perceive all of the information cues in the spoken language "code" – but a hearing loss in babies impedes the code from being established in the first place. The presence of hearing loss alters dramatically a child's ability to extract linguistic cues from the auditory language models around them and deprives them of one of the primary sources of language information: the linguistic models that are available during "overhearing" language through various sources in the environment. Children with hearing loss have been shown to experience substantial delays in their mastery of all aspects of communication. Investigators have documented hearing-impaired children's deficiencies in vocabulary, grammar, concepts, pragmatics and speech intelligibility (Robbins 2000).

It is clear that identifying hearing loss as early as possible is critical. Several factors argue in favour of a Universal Newborn Hearing Screening (UNHS) as the preferred approach to for early identification. First, hearing loss is the most frequently occurring birth defect (approximately 3 in 1000 births). Second, as we have just noted, if hearing loss is not identified early, the consequences are negative and often irreparable. Conversely, if the loss is identified early, much can be done to restore a good developmental trajectory. Finally, a growing body of research has shown that the success of alternative means of identifying infant hearing loss pales in comparison to UNHS (Grill et al. 2005; Kennedy et al. 2005; Russ et al. 2002).

Professionals are well aware that severe-to-profound hearing loss has devastating consequences for the development of speech and language. However, more subtle forms of hearing loss, including minimal or mild hearing loss, unilateral hearing loss (with normal hearing in the contralateral ear), fluctuating hearing loss and conductive hearing loss have all been documented to put communication and academic success at risk.

Where UNHS has been implemented, it has lowered dramatically the average age at which paediatric hearing loss is identified. However, since it does not identify hearing loss that is acquired after the newborn period, UNHS does not eliminate the need for vigilance in auditory assessment throughout childhood. Recent data from White (2005) suggests that approximately 23% of all babies with permanent hearing loss at 9 months of age will have passed newborn auditory brainstem response screening. It is impossible to determine whether these are primarily congenital or late-onset hearing losses, although most will be mild sensorineural losses. The 2000 Position Statement from the Joint Committee on Infant Hearing notes that all infants who pass newborn hearing screening but who have risk indicators for other auditory disorders and/or speech and language delay should receive ongoing audiological and medical surveillance and monitoring for communication development. The position statement also recommends that infants with indicators associated with late-onset, progressive or fluctuating hearing loss as well as auditory neural conduction disorders and/or brainstem auditory pathway dysfunction should be monitored.

While ear and hearing specialists are aware that hearing aids may be fitted on children as young as newborns, there appears to be misunderstanding in the larger medical community regarding how early hearing aid fitting is possible. In a recent survey of 1375 general practice doctors in 21 states of the USA, approximately 50% erroneously thought that a baby had to be 6 months of age or older in order to be fitted with hearing aids and over 20% of those surveyed reported their impression that hearing aids were not able to be fitted until a child was 1 year of age or older. Such misinformation on the part of doctors could seriously compromise a deaf baby's chances of achieving a good outcome in auditory, speech and language acquisition.

Informal hearing screening in a doctor's office cannot be used to rule out hearing loss. Likewise, parents may report that their child "hears fine", unaware that hearing may be normal in certain frequencies and impaired in other frequencies, thereby decreasing speech understanding. Formal audiological assessment is the only way to verify normal hearing across all speech frequencies and to evaluate middle ear function (the reader is referred to the website, www.infanthearing.org for thorough and up-to-date information on many aspects of hearing health care in young children.)

Differential Diagnosis of Several Communication Disorders

A series of investigations has been invaluable in providing evidence-based information about children with various communication disorders. Wetherby and colleagues

Table 5.2 Developmental red flags supporting differential diagnosis

Identifying behaviours	Autism Spectrum disorder [a]	Developmental delays [a]	Deaf or hard of hearing [b]
Lack of appropriate eye gaze	X		
Lack of warm, joyful expressions with gaze	X		
Lack of sharing enjoyment or interest	X		
Lack of response to name	X		X
Lack of coordination of gaze, facial expression, gesture and sound	X		
Lack of showing	X		
Unusual prosody (e.g. vocal inflection)	X		X
Repetitive movements or posturing of the body, arms, hands or fingers	X		
Repetitive movements with objects	X		
Lack of response to contextual cues	X	X	
Lack of pointing	X	X	
Lack of vocalisations with consonants	X	X	X
Lack of playing with a variety of toys conventionally	X	X	

[a] Data from children ages 12–24 months of age (Wetherby et al. 2004)
[b] Moeller 2000

have studied over 3000 children using the Communication and Symbolic Behavior Scales Developmental Profile (Wetherby and Prizant 2002). Their work has generated a list of communication behaviours that differentiate reliably between three groups of children: those with autism spectrum disorders, developmental delay and normal development (Wetherby et al. 2004). Table 5.2 shows the 13 behaviours that were found to differentiate, with a high degree of statistical significance, between groups of children in the first two columns ages 12–24 months of age. In addition, a third column in Table 5.2 includes red flags for hearing impairment. Doctors are encouraged to utilise this differential diagnosis information in examining children and interviewing parents. Wetherby and colleagues have made a wide array of additional tools available for parents and professionals online at: http://firstwords.fsu.edu

Association Between Some Speech/Language Characteristics and Reading Disability

As children begin academic schooling, much of language development focuses on reading and writing. Reading and writing are extensions of oral language proficiency; and reading has its basis in spoken language. Evidence from the literature shows strong links between speech and language impairment in early life and reading difficulties in school. About one in three children in the United States entering kindergarten at age 5 years are poorly prepared to learn because they lack the oral vocabulary and sentence structures needed for school success (Whitehurst and Lonigan 1998). As reading proficiency is the strongest predictor of academic success, struggling readers are at high risk for academic failure. Sadly, some children struggle for years in school before professionals recognise their disability and make referrals for assessment and intervention. Shaywitz (2003) describes behaviours that may be indicative of struggling readers who require intervention (See Table 5.3). Some of these behaviours are related to traditional reading skills, whereas others are related to speech and language skills, emphasising the continuum of language proficiency in oral and written forms.

Recent reading research shows that children who get off to a poor start in reading rarely catch up. Several studies have documented that a child who is a poor reader in first grade almost invariably continues to be a poor reader (Francis et al. 1996; Torgesen and Burgess 1998). As with oral language delay, early intervention for reading delay is paramount and doctors are in a position to recommend assessment for a child whose reading is not up-to-par, sometimes before the school has intervened. Torgesen (1998) notes that the best solution to the problem of reading failure is to identify children who need extra help in reading before they experience serious failure.

Table 5.3. Findings in school-aged children that suggest the need for further assessment of reading, speech, language (compiled by Shaywitz 2003)

Use of imprecise language ("stuff", "that", "thing")

Confusion in finding the right words when speaking (e.g. "magician" for musician)

"Spoonerisms" (e.g. "grayplound" for playground; "toin coss" for coin toss)

Problems remembering rote information (e.g. phone number, months of year)

Latencies in responding to verbal queries; needs extra time to formulate answers

Disorganised verbal expression – description of a film or book plot is jumbled and poorly sequenced

Very slow progress in reading acquisition

Reading is choppy, dysfluent, monotone

Leaves out parts of words when reading; (e.g. "par-y" for particularly)

Inability to read small grammatical words (e.g. for, were, are, of, from)

Trouble sounding out new words; takes wild guesses

Strong dislike of reading; resistance to reading and homework

Struggles or guesses on longer words; may almost create a new story

Fear of reading aloud

Poor spelling; laboured and messy handwriting

A history of speech, language or reading problems in the family

Evidence-Based Approach to the Management of Children's Speech and Language Development

Collaboration between the doctor and the speech and language therapist is essential in the early diagnosis and treatment of communication disorders. The scope of practice of speech and language therapists grows broader over time as therapists incorporate research findings, new teaching approaches and technological advances into their work. We have touched on, but not in any way fully covered, the range of communication problems that may be successfully remedied by the speech and language clinician (See Table 5.4). Referral for speech

Table 5.4 Some paediatric communication impairments that are responsive to speech and language therapy

Communication impairment	Recommended therapy
Articulation errors; unintelligible speech	Phonological processes, articulation treatment
Delayed/disordered language; vocabulary, syntax, concepts, connected language; comprehension or production	Language intervention/parent–child training
Voice disorder; hoarseness, vocal abuse, abnormal resonance	Voice/resonance treatment
Dysfluencies, "blocking", repetitions that disrupt speech	Stuttering therapy
Disordered social language; poor conversational discourse	Pragmatic/social skills language training
Hearing impairment – language and speech delays; weak auditory skills	Auditory-oral rehabilitation; language intervention with parent involvement
Dysphagia; feeding/swallowing problems	Swallowing; oral motor therapy
Motor speech disorders; dysarthria, dyspraxia	Oral motor therapy
Limited oral or cognitive potential	Alternative/augmentative communication
Autism spectrum/ pervasive developmental disorder	Communication/social language; parent training
Dyslexia; weak reading, spelling, written language	Systematic reading instruction; phonological awareness/phonics training

and language therapy from informed doctors is the first critical step to restoring a normal developmental trajectory in many children with communication impairments.

Summary for the Clinician

- We have presented to paediatric ENT specialists a rationale for maintaining a vigilant approach to communication delays in children from the early, pre-linguistic period to reading and writing in the academic setting. We have presented tools that may be clinically useful in such an approach. We conclude that an evidence-based approach to the management of speech and language development is not only possible, but yields the best chance of successful outcome in childhood and beyond.

References

1. American Speech Language Hearing Association (2000) Position Statement of the Joint Committee on Infant Hearing. www.asha.org

2. Birnbrauer JS, Leach DJ (1993) The Murdoch early intervention program after 2 years. Behav Change 10:63–74

3. Francis DJ, Shaywitz, SE, Stuebing KK, et al (1996) Developmental lag versus deficit models of reading disability: a longitudinal, individual growth curves analysis. J Educ Psychol 88:3–17

4. Grill E, Hessel F, Siebert U, et al (2005) Comparing the clinical effectiveness of different newborn hearing screening strategies. A decision analysis. BMC Public Health 5:12, doi:10.1186/1471-2458-5-12

5. Harris S, Handleman J (2000) Age and IQ at intake as predictors of placement for young children with autism: a four- to six-year follow-up. J Autism Dev Disord 30:137–142

6. Kennedy C, McCann D, Campbell MJ, et al (2005) Universal newborn screening for permanent childhood hearing impairment: an 8-year follow-up of a controlled trial. Lancet 366:660–662

7. McLean J, Snyder-McLean L (1999) How Children Learn Language. Singular Publishing, San Diego

8. Moeller MP (2000) Early intervention and language development in children who are deaf and hard of hearing. Pediatrics 106:E43

9. Moeller MP (2003) Differential Diagnosis Table; Pedialink Program, Early Hearing Detection and Intervention module; American Academy of Pediatrics

10. Peters A (1983) The units of language acquisition. Cambridge University Press, Cambridge, UK

11. Rannard A, Lyons C, Glenn S (2005) Parent concerns and professional responses: the case of specific language impairment. Br J Gen Pract 55:710–714

12. Robbins AM (2000) Rehabilitation after cochlear implantation. In: Niparko JK (ed) Cochlear Implants: Principles and Practices. Lippincott Williams Wilkins, Baltimore, pp 323–363

13. Russ SA, Rickards F, Poulakis Z, et al (2002) Six year effectiveness of a population based two tier infant hearing screening programme. Arch Dis Child 86:245–250. doi:10.1136/adc.86.4.245

14. Shaywitz S (2003) Overcoming Dyslexia. Alfred A. Knopf, New York

15. Torgesen JK (1998) Catch them before they fall: identification and assessment to prevent reading failure in young children. Am Educator 22:32–39

16. Torgesen JK, Burgess SR (1998) Consistency of reading-related phonological processes throughout early childhood: evidence from longitudinal-correlational and instructional studies. In: Metsala J, Ehri L (eds) Word Recognition in Beginning Reading. Lawrence Erlbaum Associates, Hillsdale, NJ, pp 161–188

17. Wetherby A, Prizant B (2002) CSBS Developmental Profile. Paul Brookes Publishing, Baltimore

18. Wetherby A, Woods J, Allen L, et al (2004) Early Indicators of autism spectrum disorders in the second year of life. J Autism Dev Disord 34:473–490

19. White K (2005) Improving newborn hearing screening and follow-up. Paper presented at Early Hearing Detection and Intervention Symposium, April 3, 2005; Greensboro, NC. www.infanthearing.org

20. Whitehurst GJ, Lonigan CJ (1998) Child development and emergent literacy. Child Dev 69:848–872

21. Yoshinaga-Itano C, Sedey AL, Coulter D, et al (1998) Language of Early- and later-identified children with hearing loss. Pediatrics 102:1161–1171

Chapter 6

Paediatric Voice

Mark E. Boseley and Christopher J. Hartnick

6

Core Messages

- The vocalis process makes up 75% of the vocal fold length at birth. The length of the newborn true vocal fold is between 2.5 and 3.0 mm. The membranous portion of the vocal fold is dominant by 3 years of age.

- Hirano (1975) was the first person to describe the three-layered structure of the vocal fold, consisting of the superficial, intermediate and deep layers of the lamina propria. Hartnick et al. (2005) further characterized the timing of vocal fold maturation. He described a single layer at birth, which progressed to a fully mature trilaminar structure by age 12 or 13 years.

- New technologies in the office make examining paediatric patients with voice disorders less difficult than in the past.

- Outcome-based research is important if we want to adequately assess our treatment of these patients. There now are two paediatric validated voice surveys to objectively assess voice before and after therapy. These are the Paediatric Voice Outcomes Survey and the Paediatric Voice-Related Quality of Life Instrument.

- Vocal fold nodules are the most common cause of hoarseness in the paediatric population. Voice therapy is the first line of therapy. The role of gastroesophageal reflux has not been established definitively. Surgery is reserved for the most refractory cases and should only be considered if the child cannot make himself or herself understood.

- Voice following laryngotracheal reconstruction is often "functional," but is almost always abnormal. Many of these children had no voice prior to surgery and therefore it is difficult to assess the impact that airway expansion surgery has had on their voice.

- Unilateral vocal fold paresis often presents with a hoarse voice or weak cry. A history of birth trauma or cardiac surgery is important to obtain. If no trauma has occurred, it is important to image the entire course of the recurrent laryngeal nerve. Medialization procedures should be generally delayed until the child is greater than 4 years of age.

Contents

Introduction

Paediatric laryngology is a discipline that is in its infancy when compared to the practice of adult laryngology. One reason is that a young child is often more difficult to examine than an adult, which can impede our ability to make an accurate diagnosis. Another is the lack of knowledge that has existed about the fine structure and development of the vocal fold as a child grows. Furthermore, outcome-based results have not previously existed for our treatments of common paediatric vocal fold pathologies.

As the field of paediatric laryngology moves forward, there is a need to understand the particular issue of anatomic and structural development as it relates to evaluating a child's voice. Clinicians also have to keep in mind that children are not "small adults," taking into account where the child is developmentally and emotionally and realizing that their desires and motivations (as well as those of their parents) may well change as they mature and develop.

It is the goal of this chapter to shed some light on these issues. We will first discuss anatomic considerations, including histologic changes, in the vocal fold over time. This will be followed by a discussion of the current di-

6

agnostic techniques available to the paediatric laryngologist. The importance of outcome-based research will be emphasized and the use of paediatric voice outcome surveys. Finally, common paediatric voice pathologies and their surgical management will be discussed. We do not intend to extensively review the etiologies and treatments of distinct anomalies, but rather to discuss voice-related issues. Where paediatric outcome-based results do not exist, we will discuss and relate this to the known adult literature.

Anatomy

Gross

The larynx consists of the laryngeal framework (the laryngeal and cricoid cartilages) and the true vocal folds. The framework provides a buttress upon which the intrinsic and extrinsic laryngeal muscles can exert their effect. The larynx itself changes in position and structure throughout childhood. The larynx descends in the neck in relationship to the cervical vertebrae from infancy (where the inferior aspect of the cricoid is at the level of the fourth cervical vertebra) to the mature position (C6–C7) by mid-adolescence (Cummings et al. 1998).

Kahane (1988) compared specimens before and after puberty and showed that the laryngeal and cricoid cartilages undergo significant changes as a child grows. These changes included increase in length, height, width, and weight of both cartilages. As one might expect, these changes were greater in males than in females.

The growth of the true vocal folds has also been studied. Male vocal folds undergo over twice the growth of female true vocal folds (Kahane 1988). Hirano and colleagues expanded on this work by differentiating the length of the membranous and cartilaginous portions of the vocal fold (Hirano et al. 1983). His measurements comparing a newborn vocal fold with adult male and female vocal folds are presented in Table 6.1. Important to note is that the vocal process of the arytenoids comprises 75% of the vocal fold length at birth. The membranous aspect of the vocal fold is dominant by 3 years of age (Hirano et al. 1983).

Histology

The "modern" description of the microanatomy of the human vocal folds has been properly attributed to Dr. Hirano, which he described in his seminal work entitled "Phonosurgery. Basic and Clinical Investigations" (Hirano 1975). It was here that Hirano defined the trilaminar structure of the human vocal fold; the superficial, intermediate and deep layers of the lamina propria. He found that the superficial layer lacked elastic and collagenous fibers and that it appeared loose and pliant. This layer is also known as Reinke's space (Hirano 1975, 1977, 1981).

The intermediate layer is composed of primarily elastic fibers and is stiffer than the superficial layer. The deep layer is composed mostly of collagen fibers and is the stiffest of the layers. The intermediate and deep layers together make up the vocal ligament. The boundary between these two layers is sometimes difficult to distinguish (Hirano 1975, 1977, 1981).

The lamina propria is instrumental in producing voice. This is often explained by using the "cover-body" theory of phonation. Definitions of what layers of the vocal fold make up the cover and body vary. Perhaps the most common definition is that the cover consists of the superficial layer and superficial portion of the intermediate layer of the lamina propria. This cover moves over the relatively stationary body that is made up of the deep layer of the lamina propria and the vocalis muscle, allowing the vocal fold to vibrate with consistency and control (Hirano 1975, 1977, 1981).

Much of the histologic analysis of the vocal fold had been done on adult larynges, and not much was known about the histologic development of the true vocal folds as a child grows. Hartnick examined histologic specimens in order to elucidate when the human vocal fold develops into a bilaminar and later trilaminar structure. From this work, it appears that the vocal fold consists of just one layer at birth. The vocal fold then shows evidence of an immature trilaminar structure by age 7 or 8 years, and appears to reach its adult form by age 12 or 13 years. This could have important implications in the development of voice and also in the timing of paediatric phonosurgery (i.e., whether phonomicrosurgery should be withheld until the development of a trilaminar structure; Hartnick et al. 2005).

Table 6.1 True vocal fold lengths

Age	Overall vocal fold length	Membranous vocal fold length	Cartilaginous vocal fold length
Newborn	2.5–3.0 mm	1.3–2.0 mm	1.0–1.4 mm
Adult Males	17–21 mm	14.5–18 mm	2.5–3.5 mm
Adult Females	11–15 mm	8.5–12 mm	2.0–3.0 mm

Diagnostic Techniques

Physical Examination

The gold standard examination of an adult patient with a voice complaint has traditionally involved a video and stroboscopic examination with a 70° rigid endoscope. This provides the laryngologist with invaluable information regarding the anatomy and function of the true vocal folds. Unfortunately, peroral endoscopy has technical limitations in children due to the size of the telescope and patient compliance. Paediatric otolaryngologists have therefore relied on a 2.7-mm paediatric flexible fiber-optic laryngoscope for evaluating these children; the result is often a fleeting glimpse of the vocal folds that would, at best, give information only about gross anatomic abnormalities.

Fortunately, technology now exists to obtain a more useful examination of children with voice complaints. This evaluation begins with obtaining a thorough history from the child's caregiver. Particularly important are questions about voice quality (breathiness, hoarseness, pitch breaks, for example) and any related problems with swallowing (gastroesophageal reflux, coughing when eating, chronic cough). The clinician should also document any family history of voice disorders and any environmental factors such as exposure to smoke that may play a causative role.

A flexible fiber-optic laryngoscopy can then be performed. Digital fiber-optic scopes as small as 2.9 mm now allow for improved video and often stroboscopic evaluation of these patients. The flexible scope offers the advantage of improved patient tolerance, a more normal head position, and allows for more ease in speech during the examination. A significant disadvantage when compared to the rigid peroral technique is that only limited information regarding mucosal pliability can be seen using the flexible scope (Hartnick and Zeitels 2005).

Stroboscopic examination is reliable by the time a child reaches 6 years to 8 of age, since this is when the trilaminar development of the vocal fold begins to develop. However, the digital flexible fiber-optic scope also affords a much clearer view of the laryngeal anatomy than had previously been available in children less than aged 6 years. Videos can also be archived for pre- and post-treatment comparisons. This exam can usually be performed in the office on the youngest of patients.

There are still rare occasions when a child cannot be fully evaluated in the office. It is for these children that a direct laryngoscopy in the operating room with the aid of a microscope is necessary. The advantages of this technique are that the surgeon has a clear view of the larynx, the ability to palpate the lesion, and the opportunity to obtain a biopsy sample for diagnosis. The disadvantages are that the child requires a general anesthetic and there can be no dynamic evaluation of the vocal folds.

Voice Outcome Surveys

Despite our improved ability to document the anatomic changes of the vocal folds, this tell us little about the functional changes in voice. A complete evaluation by our voice therapy colleagues is extremely important. The aerodynamic profile allows for subjective measurement of voice changes following therapy. A second method of obtaining subjective measurements involves administering quality-of-life surveys. This was not possible until recently. We now have two validated paediatric voice quality-of-life instruments, the Paediatric Voice Outcomes Survey (PVOS; Hartnick 2002) and the Paediatric Voice-Related Quality of Life Instrument (PV-RQOL; Boseley et al. 2006).

The PVOS (Fig. 6.1) was validated by examining a specific population of children with and without tracheotomies. The survey was shown to be internally consistent as well as "to be able to support a proposed interpretation of scores based upon theoretical implications within the constructs" (a concept known as discriminant validity; Hartnick 2002). In order to broaden the applicability of the PVOS to children with a full spectrum of vocal disorders, normative scores were identified for a paediatric otolaryngologic population who presented without voice concerns (Hartnick et al. 2003). The PVOS was shown to be a brief, valid, and reliable instrument, simple to administer and to complete, and was responsive to changes in voice-related quality of life.

The brevity of the instrument, however, hindered the ability of the PVOS to reflect specific subdomains such as the socioemotional concerns associated with voice problems. To this end, the Voice-Related Quality of Life (V-RQOL) instrument was converted from its adult application to allow for parent proxy administration in order to measure two components of V-RQOL, namely the "physical-functioning" and "socioemotional" subdomains (Fig. 6.2; Boseley et al. 2005). The resulting PV-RQOL has now been validated for use in the general paediatric otolaryngology patient population. This is a 10-question survey that is scored on a scale of 0–100. Lower scores reflect less impact on quality of life than higher scores. Further validation studies are under way for use in specific voice disorders.

Common Voice Pathologies

Vocal Fold Nodules

True vocal fold nodules are the most common cause for prolonged hoarseness in the paediatric age group (Gray et al. 1996). They are considered to be the result of phonatory trauma and consist of subepithelial fibrovascular depositions (in the superficial layer of the lamina propria) along the membranous vocal fold (Hirano 1977, 1981;

6

1) In general, how would you say your child's speaking voice is:

☐ Excellent

☐ Good

☐ Adequate

☐ Poor or inadequate

☐ My child has no voice

The following items ask about activities that your child might do in a given day.

2) To what extent does your child's voice limit his or her ability to be understood in a noisy area?

☐ Limited a lot

☐ Limited a little

☐ Not limited at all

3) During the past 2 weeks, to what extent has your child's voice interfered with his or her normal social activities or with his or her school?

☐ Not at all

☐ Slightly

☐ Moderately

☐ Quite a bit

☐ Extremely

4) Do you find your child "straining" when he or she speaks because of his or her voice problem?

☐ Not at all

☐ A Little bit

☐ Moderately

☐ Quite a bit

☐ Extremely

Fig. 6.1 The Paediatric Voice Outcomes Survey (PVOS)

Please answer these questions based upon what your child's voice (your own voice if you are the teenage respondent) has been like over the past 2 weeks. Considering both how severe the problem is when you get, and how frequently it happens, please rate each item below on how "bad" it is (that is, the amount of each problem that you have). Use the following rating scale:

☐ 1 = none, not a problem

☐ 2 = a small amount

☐ 3 = A moderate amount

☐ 4 = A lot

☐ 5 = Problem is "as bad as it can be"

☐ 6 = Not applicable

Because of my child's voice, how much of a problem is this?

Q1)   My child has trouble speaking loudly or being heard in noisy situations.   1 2 3 4 5 6

Q2)   My child runs out of air and needs to take frequent breaths when talking.   1 2 3 4 5 6

Q3)   My child sometimes does not know what will come out when s/he begins speaking.   1 2 3 4 5 6

Q4)   My child is sometimes anxious or frustrated (because of his or her voice).   1 2 3 4 5 6

Q5)   My child sometimes gets depressed (because of his or her voice).   1 2 3 4 5 6

Q6)   My child has trouble using the telephone or speaking with friends in person.   1 2 3 4 5 6

Q7)   My child has trouble doing his or job schoolwork (because of his or her voice).   1 2 3 4 5 6

Q8)   My child avoids going out socially (because of his or her voice).   1 2 3 4 5 6

Q9)   My child has to repeat himself/herself to be understood.   1 2 3 4 5 6

Q10) My child has become less outgoing (because of his or her voice).   1 2 3 4 5 6

Fig. 6.2 The Paediatric Voice-Related Quality of Life Survey (PV-RQOL)

Gray et al. 1996). Generally they are symmetric and are located at junction of the anterior and middle one-third of the vocal fold; in other words at the midpoint of the membranous vocal fold (Fig. 6.3).The etiology of vocal fold nodules may well be multifactorial and include genetic predisposition, behavioral factors, as well as environmental factors such as exposure to laryngopharyngeal reflux (LPR; Gray et al. 1996).

Videostroboscopy can sometimes be used to differentiate nodules from intracordal polyps and cysts. The mucosal wave can be present or absent with nodules depending on their size. The wave is often present or increased when a polyp is present. Finally, the mucosal wave is usually absent or diminished with vocal fold cysts (Johns 2003).

LPR has not been studied extensively in the paediatric population as a potential causative factor. Kuhn and colleagues have been the only group to objectively measure the presence of reflux using a triple pH probe. They found in a group of 11 adult patients with nodules that pharyngeal reflux was more prevalent in these patients when compared to a group of control patients. They suggested a contributory role in the pathogenesis of nodules (Kuhn et al. 1998).

The largest published series of paediatric patients with vocal fold nodules involved 254 children over a 7-year period. This study revealed that the majority of nodules were found in boys (72%) and that the average age at presentation was 7.7 years. Hyperfunction was noted in 75% and laryngoesophageal reflux in only 25% (only a subjective assessment was made, based on endoscopic findings). Acoustic measurements seemed to correlate with the size of the nodules. Treatment options and outcomes were not evaluated (Shah et al. 2005).

Most would agree that children with nodules should first be treated with maximal medical management. This should include six to eight sessions of voice therapy. Improvement is expected within 4 weeks; if no improvement, further examination is required. In addition, good vocal hygiene should be stressed and gastroesophageal reflux treated if it is thought to exist. Vocal hygiene includes reducing vocal fold trauma by limiting abusive behaviors (e.g., talking in a loud environment, screaming, throat clearing), limiting risk factors for reflux, and keeping well hydrated.

Initial therapy typically consists of two, 1-h sessions per week, teaching both the child and parent techniques of breath control and muscle relaxation. The parents play an important role in continuing therapy in the home environment and must take an active role if the child is to get the maximum benefit. Improvement in voice is usually seen over a 2- to 3-month period. A plateau in the therapeutic benefit of speech therapy is often reached by 6 months. The end-point of therapy is patient and family satisfaction with voice and maintenance of good vocal hygiene (Wohl 2005).

If conservative therapy fails, surgical excision appears to be a viable treatment option, although only in a very small minority of cases before puberty. Only children or parents who complain about difficulty with being able to communicate should be considered for this treatment. Children should be over the age of 6 or 8 years since this is when the trilaminar structure of the vocal fold appears to begin to be developed (Hartnick et al. 2005). In addition, if surgery is considered, one should be relatively certain that the traumatic vocal pattern that produced the nodules has been corrected preoperatively. This fact also limits the role for surgery at a younger age since young children are often unable to comply with good vocal hygiene.

If surgery is performed, voice rest is usually recommended for 1 week afterwards. However, a survey of current practices amongst clinicians that perform this surgery revealed that there is no consensus and that the efficacy of voice rest has not been established (Behrman and Sulica 2003).

Currently, there are no published data on pre- and posttreatment voice outcomes for paediatric patients with vocal nodules. Zeitels has published the largest series on surgical outcomes in the adult population. His was a single-arm, non-controlled study that included 185 patients with 201 nodules that were excised. Four of these patients developed recurrent nodules and required a second operation. A subepithelial microdissection technique was employed in each case with the epithelial cordotomy being performed either immediately superior or lateral to the lesion. Overall, 182 out of 185 patients had a subjectively improved performing voice (of note is that not all of these patients had nodules, nodules made up 201 of the 365 benign vocal fold lesions removed from this population). All objective acoustic measurements for those patients that returned to the office were within normal limits (Zietels et al. 2002).

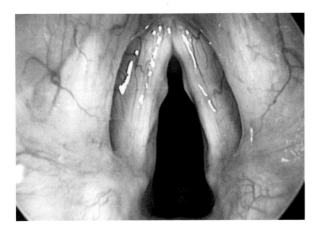

Fig. 6.3   True vocal fold nodules

Voice Results Following Laryngotracheal Reconstruction

The primary goal of laryngotracheal reconstruction (LTR) is to reestablish a patent laryngeal and subglottic airway. For those children who are tracheotomy dependent, this includes the ability to decannulate these patients. A secondary goal of surgical reconstruction is to improve the ability of these children to communicate. Unfortunately, it is often difficult to determine how successful we have been when it comes to postoperative voice results.

Many of these children have tracheotomies at a very young age prior to reconstructive surgery and therefore never had a "normal" preoperative voice. Therefore, it has been difficult to determine whether the voice is improved following surgery. In addition, most of the published data on post-LTR voice have included a heterogenous group of patients. Many have had prior open and endoscopic airway surgery, some included patients who had had stents placed, and the subjective results often have relied on nonvalidated caregiver questionnaires. Thus, it is difficult to form definitive conclusions. However, all of the published studies report a high incidence of abnormal voice following LTR.

Zalzal was the first to publish on post-LTR voice. He noted in a group of 16 patients that 12 had a functional voice postoperatively, as compared to only 6 preoperatively. However, 15 of the 16 patients had "abnormal" voices, as evidenced by low pitch, breathiness, and hoarseness (Zalzal et al. 1991). These findings were further substantiated by Smith et al. in 1993, who documented postoperative voice in a group of eight patients. Videostroboscopic findings revealed that two patients had glottal insufficiency, three had vocal fold asymmetry and stiffness, and three exhibited phonation with supraglottic structures (Smith et al. 1993). MacArthur et al. found similar results among a small sample of patients. They examined speech samples in six patients and found 100% had decreased vocal quality, 50% had decreased intelligibility, 100% had decreased volume, and 80% had a low fundamental frequency and increased jitter (MacArthur et al. 1994). Finally, in the largest reported series of 50 patients, Bailey reported that 52% had an "acceptable" voice following airway reconstruction. The assessment consisted of a parental questionnaire, voice analysis, video nasendoscopy and videostroboscopy, electrolaryngography, and pulmonary function tests (Bailey et al. 1995).

While it might be impossible to determine absolute change in voice after LTR since many children have no voice prior to surgery, there are several observations that can be made. The first is that when the anterior commissure is divided, it is more likely that the voice will be altered. The ability of the surgeon to reapproximate the true vocal folds in the correct anatomical position is crucial in determining how much voice will be affected (Fig. 6.4). A second important consideration is that use of stents that

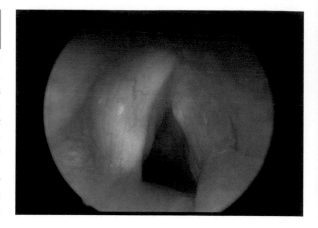

Fig. 6.4 Uneven true vocal folds following open-airway reconstruction with division of the anterior commissure

sit above the level of the true vocal folds can cause granulation tissue and scarring to form on the vocal folds. If this were to occur, there would obviously be an adverse affect on voice.

Future surgical considerations may include limiting the need to divide the anterior commissure. This may be a more practical consideration in older children since their larger airway may allow for better visualization to place the cartilage graft without the additional exposure that dividing the vocal folds affords. In addition, the development of new techniques to stabilize cartilage grafts without the need for stenting should prove helpful. Finally, it is important to continue to gather data on these children, particularly prior to them undergoing their first airway procedure. This should include gathering objective data from aerodynamic voice analysis and qualitative information using validated voice instruments.

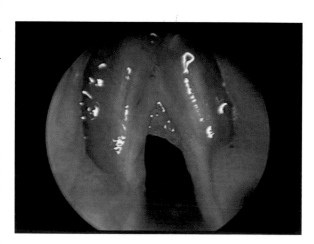

Fig. 6.5 Juvenile recurrent papilloma of the anterior commissure

Recurrent Respiratory Papillomatosis

Please also refer to Chapter 29. Most studies have not specifically addressed voice outcome following treatment of juvenile-onset recurrent respiratory papillomatosis (JORRP). Wiatrak has looked at quality of life in children with quiescent JORRP, but we still do not know which therapies offer the best posttreatment voice (Lindman et al. 2004). Future studies utilizing validated paediatric voice-outcome surveys should prove useful in this regard. The working premise is that techniques that preserve the vocal fold epithelium, such as the pulsed-dye laser, should produce the best voice.

Vocal Fold Paralysis

Vocal fold paralysis is the second most common cause of stridor in neonates. Airway obstruction is typically only seen in cases of bilateral true vocal fold paresis (BTVCP; Link et al. 1999). Since this chapter's primary focus is on voice, we have elected to focus our attention on unilateral true vocal fold paresis (UTVCP). The most common symptoms of UTVCP, when symptoms exist, are a hoarse or weak voice and aspiration of thin liquids.

The diagnosis of UTVCP involves first taking a thorough history, including questions regarding birth trauma or of cardiac surgery, which carries a risk of left-sided recurrent laryngeal nerve palsy. Neurologic disorders such as Arnold Chiari and Charcot-Marie Tooth can also present with vocal fold paresis (although these disorders more commonly present with BTVCP; Boseley et al. 2005). Indirect laryngoscopy should be performed, utilizing either a flexible fiber-optic or 70° rigid laryngoscope. Acoustic measurements should also be obtained in a cooperative child. The PVOS or PV-RQOL can also be administered to obtain information about quality-of-life issues. The role of laryngeal electromyography (EMG) in these patients continues to be defined. Perhaps as this test becomes less invasive, EMG will be more widely used in children. Certainly if one is to consider more permanent types of medialization procedures, a preoperative EMG would be useful. Finally, radiologic imaging should be used to evaluate the course of the vagus nerve from the skull base to the chest in order to search for anatomic causes.

The question then becomes how and when to treat the symptomatic child. Many of these children are able to compensate without surgical intervention. Certainly very young children (<6 months) should be followed for an extended period of time before considering a medialization procedure. If aspiration is a problem in these children, alternate means of giving nutrition should be sought, such as a thickened diet if proven safe on a modified swallow study. If this is not possible, a feeding tube or gastrostomy tube are other options. For children who are older (>4 years) and who have continued symptoms

from UTVCP for at least 9 months, surgical treatment is a viable option. Children between these ages should be managed on a case by case basis.

There are numerous surgical options to treat UTVCP. Each has advantages and disadvantages. The most common surgical treatment is injection thyroplasty. Many substances have been used in an attempt to medialize the vocal fold. Currently, autologous fat (Umeno et al. 2005), gelfoam (Coskun and Rosen 2003), and alloderm (Milstein et al. 2005) are probably the most commonly used. There is also a new product consisting of carboxymethylcellulose that has just been approved by the US Food and Drug Administration and may be useful (Kwon et al. 2005). The advantages and disadvantages of each are summarized in Table 6.2.

The next most common medialization procedure is the Ishikii thyroplasty. A carved silastic block is placed through a small window in the laryngeal cartilage. The amount of required medialization is typically determined by using a combination of direct visualization and, in adults, having the patient speak during the procedure.

This technique has been recently modified for use in the paediatric patient. One series of 12 type I thyroplasty procedures (children between the ages of 2 and 17 years) showed that the anterior commissure is often at a lower level than is found in the adult larynx. A technique was used whereby needles were passed through the laryngeal cartilage in order to localize the anterior commissure in the final four patients in their series. This allowed for more predictable placement of the implant (Link et al. 1999).

The other consideration when performing a medialization procedure in a child is the fact that most young children are under general anesthesia and so unable to speak during the procedure. We have found a helpful technique to better visualize the larynx when performing a thyroplasty. This involves using a laryngeal mask airway. A flexible fiber-optic laryngoscope is passed through the mask in order to visualize the vocal folds. Although not ideal, this at least allows the surgeon the ability to better approximate how much the vocal fold needs to be medialized.

There is still a lack of good data on voice outcome following medialization thyroplasty in children. One of the largest published series looked at results in a group of 45 adult patients. They utilized objective voice measurements, a global health quality-of-life survey, and two validated disease-specific quality-of-life surveys (Voice Outcomes Survey and the Voice Handicap Index). Patients appeared to have a significant improvement in scores on the disease-specific instruments as well as improved acoustic measurements. However, scores did not return to normal following surgery (Spector et al. 2001).

The best technique in treating paediatric patients with UTVCP remains to be determined. The assumption is that similar results will be found to those reported in the adult population. A prospective multi-institutional study would be helpful in this respect.

6

Table 6.2 Surgical options for treatment of paediatric unilateral vocal fold paresis. *FDA* Food and Drug Administration, *UTVCP* unilateral true vocal fold paresis

	Advantages	Disadvantages	Citation
Autologous fat	Effective for >2 years in most patients	Large needle required for injection, donor site morbidity	Umeno et al. 2005
Gelfoam	Effective for 4–6 weeks, FDA approved	Large needle required for injection, viscous substance	Coskum et al. 2003
Alloderm	May be effective for >12 months in select patients	Cost, theoretical risk of disease transmission	Milstein et al. 2005
Carboxymethyl-cellulose	Effective for 2–3 months, FDA approved, less viscous and can be injected through a small-gauge needle	New product, need further studies to document effectiveness	Kwon et al. 2005
Ishikii thyroplasty	Provides for permanent medialization of vocal fold	Children are often unable to cooperate by vocalizing during the procedure, the location of the anterior commissure is not as predictable in children	Link et al. 1999
Nerve reinnervation	May provide for improved tone and decrease atrophy of the paralyzed vocal fold, minimal morbidity associated when done in conjunction with medialization, long-term success seen in 88% of patients with UTVCP	Its role still unclear in light of study revealing no difference in voice between patients receiving arytenoid adduction alone and those having an arytenoid adduction with reinnervation	Tucker 1989; Chhetri et al. 1999
Arytenoid adduction	Provides for better closure of a posterior glottic chink, perhaps better option of foreshortened vocal fold with an anteriorly displaced arytenoid	Technically difficult operation, role has not been established in children	Chhetri et al. 1999

Summary for the Clinician

- The discipline of paediatric laryngology has come a long way in a relatively short period of time. Our knowledge of the microscopic anatomy and the development of the true vocal folds have been instrumental in guiding how we currently treat children with voice complaints. In addition, technologic advances in office equipment have made it much easier to examine these children. The ability to archive laryngeal images gives the clinician an opportunity to view anatomic changes over time. Finally, there are now validated voice outcome surveys that can be used to determine changes in voice quality of life after treatment. The net result is that our treatments will continue to be refined as more results become available.

References

1. Bailey CM, Clary RA, Pengilly A, et al (1995) Voice quality following laryngotracheal reconstruction. Int J Pediatr Otorhinolaryngol 32:S93–S95
2. Behrman A, Sulica L (2003) Voice rest after microlaryngoscopy: current opinion and practice. Laryngoscope 113:2182–2186
3. Boseley ME, Bloch I, Hartnick CJ (2005) Charcot-Marie-Tooth disease type 1 and paediatric true vocal fold paralysis. Int J Pediatr Otorhinolaryngol 70:345–347
4. Boseley ME, Cunningham MJ, Volk MS, Hartnick CJ (2006) Validation of the paediatric voice-related quality of life instrument. Arch Otolaryngol Head Neck Surg 132:717–720
5. Chhetri DK, Gerratt BR, Kreiman J, Berke GS (1999) Combined arytenoid adduction and laryngeal reinnervation in the treatment of vocal fold paralysis. Laryngoscope 109:1928–1936

6. Coskun HH, Rosen CA (2003) Gelfoam injection as a treatment for temporary vocal fold paralysis. Ear Nose Throat J 82:352–353

7. Cummings CW, Fredrickson JM, Harker LA, et al (1998) Otolaryngology – Head and Neck Surgery. Mosby, St. Louis, Missouri

8. Gray SD, Smith ME, Schneider H (1996) Voice disorders in children. Pediatr Clin North Am 43:1357–1384

9. Hartnick CJ (2002) Validation of a paediatric voice quality-of-life instrument: the paediatric voice outcome survey. Arch Otolaryngol Head Neck Surg 128:919–922

10. Hartnick CJ, Volk MS, Cunningham MJ (2003) Establishing normative voice-related quality of life scores within the paediatric otolaryngology population. Arch Otolaryngol Head Neck Surg 129:1090–1093

11. Hartnick CJ, Rehbar R, Prasad V (2005) Development and maturation of the paediatric human vocal fold lamina propria. Laryngoscope 115:4–15

12. Hartnick CJ, Zeitels SM (2005) Paediatric video laryngostroboscopy. Int J Pediatr Otorhinolaryngol 69:215–219

13. Hirano M (1975) Phonosurgery. Basic and clinical investigations. Otologia (Fukuoka) 21:239–260

14. Hirano M (1977) Structure and Vibratory behavior of the vocal folds. In: Sawashima M, Franklin S (eds) Dynamic Aspects of Speech Production. University of Tokyo Press, Tokyo, pp 13–30

15. Hirano M (1981) Structure of the vocal fold in normal and disease states: anatomical and physical studies. ASHA Rep 11:11–30

16. Hirano M, Kuriuta S, Nakashima T (1983) Growth, development, and aging of human vocal folds. In: Bless DM, Abbs JH (ed) Vocal Fold Physiology. College Hill Press, CA pp, 23–43

17. Kahane JC (1988) Histologic structure and properties of the human vocal folds. Ear Nose Throat J 67:322–330

18. Johns MM (2003) Update on the etiology, diagnosis, and treatment of vocal fold nodules, polyps, and cysts. Curr Opin Otolaryngol Head Neck Surg 11:456–461

19. Kuhn J, Toohill RJ, Ulualp SO, et al (1998) Pharyngeal acid reflux events in patients with vocal cord nodules. Laryngoscope 108:1146–1149

20. Kwon T, Rosen CA, Gartner-Schmidt J (2005) Preliminary results of a new temporary vocal fold injection material. J Voice 19:668–673

21. Lindman JP, Gibbons MD, Morlier R, Wiatrak BJ (2004) Voice quality of prepubescent children with quiescent recurrent respiratory papillomatosis. Int J Pediatr Otorhinolaryngol 68:529–536

22. Link DT, Rutter MJ, Liu JH, et al (1999) Paediatric type I thyroplasty: an evolving procedure. Ann Otol Rhinol Laryngol 108:1105–1110

23. MacArthur CJ, Kearns GH, Healy GB (1994) Voice quality after laryngotracheal reconstruction. Arch Otolaryngol Head Neck Surg 120:641–647

24. Milstein CF, Akst LM, Hicks D, et al (2005) Long-term effects of micronized alloderm injection for unilateral vocal fold paralysis. Laryngoscope 115:1691–1696

25. Shah RK, Woodnorth GH, Glynn A, et al (2005) Paediatric vocal nodules: correlation with perceptual voice analysis. Int J Pediatr Otorhinolaryngol 69:903–909

26. Smith ME, Marsh JH, Cotton RT, et al (1993) Voice problems after paediatric laryngotracheal reconstruction: videolaryngostroboscopic, acoustic, and perceptual assessment. Int J Pediatr Otorhinolaryngol 25:173–181

27. Spector BC, Netterville JL, Billante C, et al (2001) Quality-of-life assessment in patients with unilateral vocal cord paralysis. Otolaryngol Head Neck Surg 125:176–182

28. Tucker H (1989) Long-term results of nerve-muscle pedicle reinnervation for laryngeal paralysis. Ann Otol Rhinol Laryngol 98:674–676

29. Umeno H, Shirouzu H, Chitose S, et al (2005) Analysis of voice function following autologous fat injection for vocal fold paralysis. Otolaryngol Head Neck Surg 132:103–107

30. Wohl DL (2005) Nonsurgical management of paediatric vocal fold nodules. Arch Otolaryngol Head Neck Surg 131:68–70; discussion 71–72

31. Zalzal GH, Loomis SR, Derkay CS, et al (1991) Vocal quality of decannulated children following laryngeal reconstruction. Laryngoscope 101:425–429

32. Zeitels SM, Hillman RE, Mauri M, et al (2002) Phonomicrosurgery in singers and performing artists: treatment outcomes, management theories, and future directions. Ann Otol Rhinol Laryngol 111:21–40

Chapter 7

Genetics of Non-Syndromic Deafness

Maria Bitner-Glindzicz

7

Core Messages

- ENT surgeons who practice otology need to have a working knowledge of genetics relevant to their field.
- A large proportion of those with deafness of unknown aetiology have a genetic cause.
- *GJB2* testing should be offered to all those with bilateral permanent non-syndromic hearing loss.
- Many genes can cause non-syndromic deafness, and genetic testing is not yet available for a significant number.
- Some genetic causes of non-syndromic deafness may have distinct phenotypes that may be a clue to the underlying aetiology.
- It is likely that within a few years, a precise aetiological diagnosis of deafness will be necessary in order to determine appropriate medical and surgical management.
- Consent should always be sought before genetic testing, because of implications for other family members.
- The audiological/cochlear implant team may benefit from close liaison with their Regional Genetics Service, for difficult or rare syndrome diagnoses, for genetic counselling and for interpretation of genetic laboratory results.

Contents

Introduction

The prevalence of permanent sensorineural hearing loss in the UK has been shown to be approxmately 1:1000 children under 3 years and 2:1000 of children under 16 years (Fortnum et al. 2001). The late identification of congenital hearing impairment in particular may lead to delay in language development, significant educational underachievement and ultimately reduced employment opportunities. A Health Technology Assessment review conducted by Bamford and Davis in 1997 highlighted that large numbers of hearing-impaired children were being diagnosed late, and recommended the introduction of a universal neonatal hearing screening programme (Newborn Hearing Screening or NHS), which has since been established in the UK and which exists in other countries (Davis et al. 1997).

However, when hearing loss is diagnosed so early in an infant, the question of aetiology is particularly pertinent for parents who are often still in their reproductive years. Furthermore, it may be important for management (see below). The aetiology of hearing loss has long been known to be heterogeneous with both pre- and postnatal environmental factors implicated. In the last decade, however, genetic research into non-syndromic and syndromic deafness has proven that identifiable genetic causes account for a significant proportion of childhood and adult-onset deafness. Therefore, it is now important for the otologist and audiologist to have a working understanding of the genetics of non-syndromic hearing loss and its practical implications.

Investigation of the Aetiology of Hearing Loss

Reasons

Whilst many otologists and audiologists are concerned primarily with the management and rehabilitation of hearing loss, it is also important to discuss and investigate its aetiology for the following reasons:

1. Parents may want to know the aetiology if they are thinking of having further children (recurrence risk) and to obtain any prognostic information about their child's hearing loss (e.g. progression).
2. Young adults with hearing loss may wish to have information about having deaf or hearing-impaired children themselves (offspring risk).
3. To exclude syndromic forms of deafness that may initially present as non-syndromic deafness (prognostic information, career planning).
4. To follow-up long-term outcomes (e.g. cochlear implant, other therapeutic interventions).

Protocol

Guidelines exist that describe the aetiological investigation of hearing loss in children (see http://www.nhsp.info/cms.php?folder=22, and http://www.baap.org.uk/Audit___R_D/Guidelines/guidelines.html)

History

It is important to enquire about pregnancy and birth history as well as neonatal factors, since environmental causes of deafness, especially pre- and post-natal infections, are often suspected from this information. Perhaps the greatest exception to this is hearing impairment caused by congenital cytomegalovirus (CMV) infection. CMV is probably underdiagnosed and may be asymptomatic in the majority of cases, but may cause a progressive hearing impairment in childhood (Barbi et al. 2003). Exposure to ototoxic medications (e.g. aminoglycosides) should be noted as well as co-existing medical conditions (e.g. diabetes, renal disease in the individual and in the family). Record should be made of developmental milestones, since this may indicate global or specific language or motor delay (delay in motor milestones is an impor-

tant indicator of vestibular problems). A specific enquiry should be made about family history of hearing loss in first- and second-degree relatives, consanguinity and ethnic origin (because some forms of genetic hearing loss appear to be common among some ethnic groups).

Examination

The major aim of this is to exclude clinical features that may suggest a syndrome diagnosis (see Chapter 8). Often these are subtle. Additional physical features that should be particularly sought include: unusual pigmentation of the hair, skin or eyes (which may indicate an auditory pigmentary disorder), shape and position of the external ears (many syndromes), examination of the neck for cysts, sinuses and scars (branchio-oto-renal syndrome), swelling of the thyroid gland (may indicate Pendred syndrome) and abnormalities of stature. However, the overall appearance of the person is also important, and if in doubt about unusual features, advice should be sought from a clinical geneticist, since there are hundreds of genetic syndromes in which hearing loss is a feature.

Investigation

This will depend on findings from history and examination, but if there are no clues from these, the following tests should be requested:

1. Electrocardiogram in cases of profound hearing loss, especially where there is motor delay to look for long QT interval of Jervell and Lange-Nielsen syndrome (although a very rare syndromic diagnosis, the mortality of the condition is high).
2. Electroretinogram, especially if motor milestones are delayed and hearing loss is profound (to diagnose type 1 Usher syndrome).
3. Dipstick of urine (although associated undiagnosed nephritis and nephropathy are rare, this a cheap and non-invasive test).
4. Specific consent should be sought for *GJB2* (connexin26) testing in all types and severities of bilateral sensorineural hearing loss.
5. Temporal bone neuroimaging (computed tomography or magnetic resonance imaging) should be performed where the hearing loss is severe/profound or progressive or a syndrome diagnosis is suspected. Widened vestibular aqueducts, semi-circular canal aplasia/hypoplasia or Mondini malformation may be clues to particular genetic conditions and can only be found on imaging (see Chapter 40).
6. Ophthalmology: all children should be referred to an ophthalmologist for assessment of visual acuity and dilated fundoscopy as a minimum. Abnormal findings may prompt further examination by the ophthalmolo-

gist. Features of "syndromic" interest include cataracts, optic atrophy and retinal dystrophy. See also "Quality standards: vision care for deaf children and young people" at http://www.sense.org.uk/publications/all-pubs/professionals/deafblindness/.

7. There should be full characterization of the type of hearing loss, severity, audiometric configuration (some audiometric patterns may be a clue to aetiology), whether the hearing loss is conductive, mixed or sensorineural, and whether or not there is progression. Formal vestibular evaluation may be helpful in cases where the patient has prominent vestibular symptoms and in children in whom there is delay of motor milestones.

Genetic Hearing Loss

Once environmental factors have been excluded (as far as possible), a genetic aetiology becomes more likely. Although hearing impairment can be inherited as an autosomal recessive, dominant, X-linked or matrilineal (mitochondrial) trait, recessive causes account for about 80% of all cases of genetic deafness. The implication of this is that most children with genetic deafness will be born to normally hearing parents and will have no family history of deafness, yet their parents have a 25% chance of having a subsequent child with a similar hearing impairment. The difficulty is that in many cases, a genetic cause cannot be excluded as not all genes can be tested (see below), so the geneticist may have to rely on empirical data in order to provide recurrence risks. It may be a surprising fact that for children born with a severe/profound hearing impairment in whom no definite aetiology can be ascribed, that about 1:8 of their parents will go on to have a further deaf child. This is presumably because the group of children with "unknown causes" will include both recessive cases (with a 1:4 recurrence risk) and those with an undiagnosed environmental cause with a lower recurrence risk.

Many genes that cause autosomal recessive deafness have now been identified, and these encode a wide diversity of different types of molecules such as ion channels and ion transporters, gap junction proteins, cytoskeletal proteins, transcription factors and components of the hair cell stereocilia. They are summarized in Tables 7.1 and 7.2, adapted from the Hereditary Hearing Loss Homepage (http://webhost.ua.ac.be/hhh/). A disease locus merely describes a location on a chromosome where the gene is to be found, which may be approximate before the gene itself has been identified. For deafness, loci are designated by the letters DFN, followed by "A" if the gene is dominant and "B" if it is recessive. Loci are numbered according to the order in time in which they were first described. Thus, DFNB2 is the locus for the second autosomal recessive deafness gene described. X-linked genes are simply annotated as *DFN*, followed by a number (e.g.

DFN3). Of these however, the most prevalent in terms of aetiology is the gap junction beta 2 gene, *GJB2*, which encodes the gap junction protein, connexin26.

Table 7.1 Autosomal recessive genes identified to date (adapted from the Hereditary Hearing Loss Homepage, http://webhost.ua.ac.be/hhh/)

Locus	Gene	Protein
No locus assigned	*PRES*	Prestin
DFNB1	*GJB2(Cx26)*	Connexin26
DFNB1	*GJB6(Cx30)*	Connexin30
DFNB2	*MYO7A*	Myosin7A
DFNB3	*MYO15*	Myosin15
DFNB4	*SLC26A4*	Pendrin
DFNB6	*TMIE*	Transmembrane inner ear expressed gene
DFNB7/11	*TMC1*	Transmembrane cochlear expressed gene1
DFNB8/10	*TMPRSS3*	Transmembrane protease, serine 3
DFNB9	*OTOF*	Otoferlin
DFNB12	*CDH23*	Cadherin23
DFNB16	*STRC*	Stereocilin
DFNB18	*USH1C*	Harmonin
DFNB21	*TECTA*	Tectorin
DFNB22	*OTOA*	Otoancorin
DFNB23	*PCDH15*	Protocadherin15
DFNB28	*TRIOBP*	Trio and F-actin binding protein
DFNB29	*CLDN14*	Claudin14
DFNB30	*MYO3A*	Myosin3A
DFNB31	*WHRN*	Whirlin
DFNB36	*ESPN*	Espin
DFNB37	*MYO6*	Myosin6
DFNB67	*TMHS*	Tetraspan membrane protein of hair cell

Table. 7.2 Autosomal dominant genes identified to date (adapted from the Hereditary Hearing Loss Homepage, http://web-host.ua.ac.be/hhh/)

Locus	Gene	Protein
No locus assigned	*CRYM*	Cyratallin, Mu
DFNA1	*DIAPH1*	Diaphanous
DFNA2	*GJB3(Cx31)*	Connexin31
DFNA2	*KCNQ4*	Voltage-gated potassium channel
DFNA3	*GJB2(Cx26)*	Connexin26
DFNA3	*GJB6(Cx30)*	Connexin30
DFNA4	*MYH14*	Myosin heavy chain 14
DFNA5	*DFNA5*	DFNA5
DFNA6/14	*WFS1*	Wolframin
DFNA8/12	*TECTA*	Tectorin
DFNA9	*COCH*	Cochlin
DFNA10	*EYA4*	Eyes absent 4
DFNA11	*MYO7A*	Myosin7A
DFNA13	*COL11A2*	Collagen11alpha2
DFNA15	*POU4F3*	Pou4 factor3
DFNA17	*MYH9*	Myosin heavy chain 9
DFNA20/26	*ACTG1*	Actin, gamma-1
DFNA22	*MYO6*	Myosin6
DFNA28	*TFCP2L3*	Transcription factor CP2-like3
DFNA36	*TMC1*	Transmembrane cochlear expressed gene 1
DFNA48	*MYO1A*	Myosin1A

Recessive Genes: Common/ Recognizable Types of Non-Syndromic Genetic Hearing Loss

GJB2 (Connexin26)

GJB2 encodes the protein connexin26, a component of intercellular gap junctions. These allow the passage of ions and small molecules between neighbouring cells. Connexin26 aggregates into hexamers (a group of six connexin molecules) called connexons, which form a hemi-channel traversing the cell membrane; two connexons from adjacent cells then dock with each other to form a complete gap junction channel. Connexin26 is expressed in the supporting cells that surround the mechanosensory hair cells of the inner ear, but not in the hair cells themselves, and are likely to be important for the recycling of potassium and other small molecules within the endolymph.

Genetics

Mutations in the *GJB2* gene have now been shown to account for up to 30–50% of recessive deafness (i.e. families where there are affected siblings or there is known consanguinity) in Caucasians, and between 10 and 30% of "sporadic" cases (where there is no family history of deafness and no consanguinity) in some European countries. In other populations, prevalence varies, although in most reported ethnic groups prevalence is always significant (Kenneson et al. 2002). Mutations may be described according to the base that is changed in the DNA sequence, or according to the change to the amino acid in the predicted protein. In Caucasians, the most common mutation is 35delG (a deletion of a single G nucleotide at position 35 of the coding nucleotide sequence of the gene). This mutation accounts for nearly 70% of all mutations in Northern European and Mediterranean Caucasians, but other ethnic groups have different common mutations. Among the Ashkenazi Jews, 167delT (a deletion of a single T nucleotide at position 167 of the coding nucleotide sequence of the gene) is the commonest mutation and nearly 4% of this population carry it (Morell et al. 1998). The commonest mutation in Japan and China is 235delC, and R143W [substitution of the amino acid arginine (R) represented by codon CGG, to tryptophan (W) codon TGG, at position 143 of the polypeptide] is common among Africans. In the Indian subcontinent the commonest mutations are Q124X [mutation of the amino acid glutamine (Q), codon CAA, to a stop codon TAA (X) at position 124 of the polypeptide], W77X [mutation of the amino acid tryptophan (W) codon TGG to a stop codon, TGA, (X), at position 77 of the polypeptide], and W24X [tryptophan (W) TGG to a stop codon TGA (X), at position 24 of the polypeptide]. However, there are now over 80 deafness-causing mutations in *GJB2* listed on the connexin26 deafness homepage (http://davinci.crg.es/deafness/index.php).

Where a patient is found to have two pathogenic mutations in *GJB2* (e.g. 35delG/35delG), ascribing aetiology and subsequent genetic counselling is straightforward; the recurrence risk is 1 in 4 for subsequent children. However, if only a single mutation is found, it is unknown whether a second mutation could not be detected by laboratory screening methods or whether the patient happens to be a carrier by chance but whose deafness was caused by another factor or gene.

GJB2 is a small gene, with only one coding exon (genes are divided into exons, segments which are translated into RNA and generally encode protein, and intervening sequences called introns. Introns are spliced out of mature RNA by cellular machinery, which recognizes sequences at or close to intron–exon boundaries, and they do not encode the mature polypeptide). However there are some mutations that lie outside the coding region of the *GJB2* gene, often within introns, and cause abnormal splicing of RNA into mature mRNA. For example, the mutation IVS1+1 G>A, in which there is a G-to-A mutation at the very beginning of intron 1, abolishes the splice signal at the beginning of the intron. In addition there are mutations (large deletions) that lie some distance away from the gene, but that are likely to have an effect on gene transcription and therefore levels of protein expression (del Castillo et al. 2003; Lerer et al. 2001). Both of these mutations are quite common in some populations. Therefore, it is useful for requests for *GJB2* testing to be accompanied by information on the patient's ethnic origin and any family history of consanguinity, so that genetic testing may be tailored specifically to include these non-coding mutations.

Finally, there are some amino acid changes, which although they may alter the sequence of the polypeptide, may not be pathogenic, and the effect of these on the connexin26 protein may be difficult to interpret. Unfortunately, these latter variants are found commonly in some populations: M34T is present in 1–2% of Caucasians, and V37I is present in up to 11% of people from South East Asia, and so counselling can be difficult.

Genotype–Phenotype Correlations

Recent multi-centre studies have shown there to be correlation between type of mutation and severity of deafness (genotype–phenotype correlation). Mutations that are predicted to truncate or inactivate the protein (small frame-shifting mutations, for example 35delG, or nonsense mutations, for example W77X) cause a more severe deafness than those that alter a single amino acid (termed missense mutations, such as L90P) or affect splicing. Combinations of the two tend to cause deafness of intermediate severity. However, the correlation is not absolute, as even siblings with the same bi-allelic mutations can differ significantly in the severity of deafness. In addition, it is now clear that the severity of deafness caused by recessive mutations in *GJB2* can range from mild to profound. Most cases are, however, in the severe-to-profound range, because the commonest mutations are small frameshifts (35delG and 167delT). Hearing impairment is bilateral, usually stable, although documented cases of progression have certainly been reported, and usually congenital (although, again, cases of post-natal onset have been reported; Pagarkar et al. 2006). Thus, recent international guidelines now suggest that all children with bilateral permanent hearing impairment who are undergoing aetiological investigations for deafness should be tested for *GJB2* mutations regardless of the severity of their hearing loss (Mazzoli et al. 2004).

Management

Connexin26 and Cochlear Implantation

Several papers describe outcome after cochlear implantation in children whose deafness is caused by *GJB2* compared with those whose cause of deafness is unknown. The data have to be interpreted with caution. Sinnathuray and Fukushima described better speech intelligibility and speech discrimination (Fukushima et al. 2002; Sinnathuray et al. 2004a, b), and Bauer described better reading and cognitive outcomes, in those whose deafness was due to *GJB2*, whilst Cullen et al. (2004) and Taitelbaum-Swead et al. (2006) found no difference between the groups in terms of speech perception. Whilst *GJB2*-positive status may be an indicator of a "good" cochlear implant outcome, this may be a reflection of the fact that this type of deafness is truly non-syndromic, whereas a group of children whose deafness is of unknown aetiology may well include those with undiagnosed additional problems. Although all of these studies were small and the data perhaps currently inconclusive, there is no doubt that larger studies that correlate the aetiology of deafness (due to a variety of genetic or environmental factors) will be necessary in order to gain more accurate information about cochlear implant outcome.

Otologists and parents need to be aware that children whose deafness is due to *GJB2* and is of moderate severity may show some progression over time. These children need to be monitored. Siblings of children with *GJB2*-related deafness should have their hearing tested at birth and can be offered genetic testing, especially in cases where the older sibling did not have deafness at birth. Genetic testing of children to determine carrier status alone is not performed.

Connexin26 and Dominant or Syndromic Deafness

The recessive mutations discussed above are likely to result in complete absence of protein production, may prevent mutant connexin molecules from aggregating into the normal hexameric structure, or result in non-functional gap junctions. Thus, carriers of recessive mutations (parents of children with *GJB2*-related deafness) are likely to have fewer normally functioning remaining gap junctions (presumably 50%), but enough for them to be able to hear. However, there are some mutations in the protein, (in particular some mutations that change just a single critical amino acid) that may allow assembly of mu-

7

tant connexin molecules into connexons, but which cause the whole gap junction to function abnormally. Carriers of these mutations may therefore have very few gap junctions in which all 12 connexin molecules are encoded by the individual's normal copy of the gene and function normally. Carriers of these mutations would be predicted to have hearing impairment. Such mutations are said to have a "dominant-negative" effect because they interfere with the normal connexin molecules (Table. 7.3). There are also some dominant mutations that cause syndromic forms of deafness, usually involving the skin, as *GJB2* is also known to be expressed in the skin (e.g. palmoplantar keratoderma and deafness, keratitis ichthyosis deafness syndrome – KID – or Vohwinkel's mutilating keratoderma). The mutations that cause these two latter diseases are distinct and affect specific residues of the protein (e.g. D66H, which causes Vohwinkel syndrome, and D50N, G45E and S17F, which cause KID). It is not fully understood why these mutations have such a specific and severe effect.

SLC26A4 (Pendred and Non-Syndromic Enlarged Vestibular Aqueduct)

Pendred syndrome is the name given to the combination of thyroid dyshormonogenesis and congenital deafness and it is inherited in an autosomal recessive manner. The dyshormonogenesis often causes thyroid hyperplasia, which may not be apparent until the teenage years, and Pendred syndrome therefore often presents in childhood as non-syndromic deafness. Pendred syndrome cannot be excluded by normal routine thyroid function tests in childhood. Later, the failure of thyroid tissue to produce enough thyroxine leads to an increase in TSH, and hyperplasia, in order to raise thyroxine levels to normal. The patient then has "euthyroid goitre". This may progress to hypothyroidism if hyperplasia cannot maintain normal thyroid hormone levels. Other than the thyroid enlargement, which may not be apparent, the other clinical clue to this condition is the presence of dilated (enlarged) vestibular aqueducts (EVA) on computed tomography scan and of enlarged endolymphatic sacs on magnetic resonance imaging. About 80–90% of people who have Pendred syndrome have EVAs (Luxon et al. 2003; Reardon et al. 2000). Thus, someone who presents with deafness and EVA should be investigated for Pendred syndrome using molecular tests and the perchlorate discharge test (PDT). The latter is difficult to perform in young children as they need to sit still for some time.

Genetics

The gene that causes Pendred syndrome has been identified as *SLC26A4* and encodes an anion transporter protein called pendrin (Coyle et al. 1998; Tsukamoto et al.

2003). The precise function of this protein has not been clarified, but in the thyroid it is thought to transport iodide across the apical membrane of thyrocytes. In the inner ear it is expressed in a highly localized manner at the inner sulcus of the scala media, and may be important for the regulation of chloride in the endolymph. Abnormalities of function of the protein may cause a form of endolymphatic hydrops causing dilation of the endolymphatic sac. There are several "common" mutations in the gene, with four mutations accounting for almost 70% of alleles in the UK, and diagnostic testing is available (Coyle et al. 1998).

Genotype–Phenotype Correlations

Current thinking is that bi-allelic mutations in this gene give rise to full-blown Pendred syndrome with a deafness that is congenital, rapidly progressive, and which may be associated with abnormalities of vestibular function. Most often, vestibular dysfunction is asymptomatic, but some individuals present with florid vestibular symptoms. Individuals with Pendred syndrome may develop a goitre and will have an abnormal PDT.

However there are also clearly individuals with similar patterns of hearing loss and EVA but whose PDTs are normal. A recent publication suggests that there is a clear distinction between these two groups (Pendred syndrome and non-syndromic EVA) in that the group with normal thyroid hormonogenesis on PDT have only a single mutation or no mutation in the *SLC26A4* gene, whereas those with abnormal thyroid hormonogenesis have two (bi-allelic) mutations (Pryor et al. 2005). Such individuals are said to have non-syn-

Table 7.3 Dominant non-syndromic mutations of *GJB2* described to date (adapted from The Connexin-Deafness homepage, http://davinci.crg.es/deafness/index.php)

Mutation
delE42
W44S
W44C
R75Q
R143Q
M163L
D179N
R184Q
C202F

dromic EVA. The conclusion is that non-syndromic EVA is a "complex" condition (i.e. it requires more than one genetic or environmental factor to become manifest), and that a single mutation in *SLC26A4* is a predisposing factor to the development of EVA but that another genetic or environmental factor is likely to contribute to the condition. The rationale underlying this is that a single mutation is unlikely to cause deafness, otherwise the parents of children with Pendred syndrome would be deaf (which is not the case), but it is a fact that the prevalence of *SLC26A4* single mutations is much higher in those with EVA than in those with normal vestibular aqueducts.

Genetic testing for Pendred syndrome is now available on a diagnostic basis.

Management

As a result of the dilated vestibular aqueducts, patients should be told of the dangers of sudden deterioration in hearing following minor head trauma (Cremers et al. 1998; Luxon et al. 2003; Stinckens et al. 2001). Progression has been reported in about one-third of patients. The finding of EVA in a patient should always prompt investigation for Pendred syndrome.

There are no evidence-based guidelines for the monitoring of thyroid status in those with Pendred syndrome; however, individuals with Pendred syndrome need to be told that hypothyroidism is common after puberty, and it would seem sensible to monitor thyroid function annually until further clarification is obtained.

OTOF (Auditory Neuropathy)

Mutations in *OTOF*, the gene encoding the protein otoferlin, were shown to cause autosomal recessive non-syndromic deafness in Lebanese, Indian and Druze families. The gene is highly expressed in inner hair cells and is involved in synaptic transmission. This results in the presence of otoacoustic emissions (generated by outer hair cells), but in absent or abnormal auditory brainstem responses and a patient with severe or profound hearing loss. It is thus one of the causes of "auditory neuropathy", others being a more widespread neuropathic process (Charcot-Marie-Tooth Disease or Friedreich's ataxia), nerve hypoplasia or aplasia, a result of severe perinatal injury or hyperbilirubinaemia.

Auditory neuropathy is an important diagnosis to make, not only because of possible associations with more widespread neuropathies, and because of genetic implications if the cause is recessive as in this case, but also for reasons of management; such individuals tend to have variable hearing losses and speech perception that is out of proportion to the degree of measured hearing loss.

They tend to respond poorly to hearing aids and results from cochlear implant are variable.

Genetics

Several publications have now described mutations in *OTOF* that underlie auditory neuropathy in a significant proportion of non-syndromic patients (Rodriguez-Ballesteros et al. 2003; Tekin et al. 2005; Varga et al. 2006). In Spanish families, a single mutation Q829X, has been shown to cause deafness in about 4% of families with deafness, and this finding has been replicated in a second study (Migliosi et al. 2002; Rodriguez-Ballesteros et al. 2003). In some cases these patients have received cochlear implants and appear to have benefited, although follow-up data is limited at the present time (Rouillon et al. 2006). Interestingly, there has been a report of a specific "temperature-sensitive" mutation in which the patients' hearing was documented to worsen when they were pyrexial (Varga et al. 2006).

Genotype–Phenotype Correlation

The deafness is described as severe-profound in most cases and probably congenital in origin. Otoacoustic emissions are often preserved.

Management

If preliminary reports of successful cochlear implantation in patients with *OTOF* mutations are confirmed, then genetic testing of suitable cases would have important implications for management.

Dominant Genes: Common/Recognizable Types of Non-Syndromic Genetic Hearing Loss

WFS1 (Dominant Low-Frequency Sensorineural Hearing Loss)

This is an unusual type of hearing loss in which the frequencies below 2000 Hz are predominantly affected. This may be either genetic or non-genetic, but there are clearly specific genes that underlie the familial cases. Three loci have been identified – DFNA1 (*DIA1*, which encodes diaphanous protein, DFNA6/14/38; *WFS1*, which encodes wolframin), as well as an unknown gene at locus DFNA54. In the mouse, a specific mutation in *Myo7a* (encoding Myosin7a) also causes low-frequency sensorineural hearing loss (Rhodes et al. 2004). Of these genes, the *WFS1* accounts for a significant proportion of famil-

7

ial low-frequency hearing loss cases (probably 50%) and so it is worth screening the gene where a low-frequency hearing loss is familial (Cryns et al. 2002; Lesperance et al. 2003).

Genotype–Phenotype Correlations

Interestingly, the phenotypes associated with mutations in the gene appear to be expanding. Initially, the gene was shown to underlie the autosomal recessive condition, Wolfram syndrome or DIDMOAD (diabetes mellitus, diabetes insipidus, optic atrophy and deafness) with bi-allelic mutations resulting in this condition, but with asymptomatic carrier parents. The mutations that cause Wolfram syndrome are thought to be null mutations (i.e. mutations that result in the absence of protein production), and clearly the presence of 50% normal protein levels in carrier parents causes no symptoms. However, mutations that are localized to a specific amino acid substitution in the protein (missense mutations) are likely to result in near normal or normal protein levels, and yet give rise to low-frequency hearing impairment. It is likely that these mutations may act in a "dominant-negative" manner (see section on "Connexin26 and Dominant or Syndromic Mutations") or confer an abnormal gain-of-function on the mutant protein. More recently, however, families with a more intermediate phenotype have been described in which there is optic atrophy, hearing loss and impaired glucose regulation (again caused by missense mutation of a single copy of the gene; Eiberg et al. 2006).

Management

It seems that most individuals with mutations in *WFS1*, ascertained because of low-frequency hearing loss, will have non-syndromic deafness. However, individuals should have an ophthalmological review to exclude optic atrophy, and enquiries should be made about family associations of psychiatric disease.

COCH (Menière-Like Symptoms)

Deafness caused by mutations in *COCH*, the gene encoding a protein called cochlin, was mapped using a single large family, to the DFNA9 locus. The clinical picture in this type of deafness appears to be distinctive, and consists of adult-onset, progressive, high-frequency sensorineural hearing loss (onset in the 4th–5th decade of life, although onset in 3rd decade has also been reported) accompanied in several individuals by prominent vestibular symptoms. These include vertigo, aural fullness and tinnitus, giving

a rather "Menière-like" picture. The vestibular symptoms are of lower penetrance than the hearing loss and may not be present in every affected member of a family (de Kok et al. 1999; Fransen et al. 1999; Kamarinos et al. 2001).

Genetics

The protein cochlin is a secreted extracellular protein of unknown function, which is present in high abundance in the inner ear. Cochlin comprises about 70% of all protein in the inner ear and may be the target of autoantibodies in autoimmune hearing loss. In families with mutations in *COCH*, temporal bone studies have shown prominent acellular acidophilic mucopolysaccharide deposits in the inner ear in the structures in which the normal protein is usually expressed. These are the fibrocytes of the spiral ligament and limbus, and fibrocytes of connective tissue stroma underlying the sensory epithelia of the maculae of the otoliths and the cristae of the semicircular canals. The protein has an LCCL domain, important for normal folding of this protein, and two vWFA domains, involved in protein–protein interactions. All mutations described to date, bar one, occur in the LCCL domain. The exception, a deletion of a single amino acid, is a single missense change that has been shown to cause abnormal protein folding: all of the mutations have a localized effect on the protein. Mutant protein is secreted and forms insoluble aggregates in the normal sites of expression. This, together with the finding that the knockout mouse model (a mouse that has been engineered to have no copies of the *COCH* gene) has completely normal hearing and inner ear histology, has led to the hypothesis that the deafness is not due to haplo-insufficiency (a shortage of normal protein), but to a toxic gain-of-function mechanism. Thus, the abnormal protein is thought to cause strangulation and progressive degeneration of dendrites and progressive loss of cochlear and vestibular neurones.

Genotype–Phenotype Correlation

The clinical picture is one of adult-onset, progressive, high-frequency sensorineural hearing loss, accompanied by an associated family history of prominent vestibular symptoms.

Management

The course appears to be one of inevitable progression. There is a single report of cochlear implantation in several members of a large family with *COCH* mutation in whom outcome was reported as successful (Vermeire et al. 2006).

Summary for the Clinician

- Rapid progress in genetic research during the last decade has allowed the identification of the genetic aetiology in a significant proportion of deaf children. Those trusted with the care of children with hearing loss need to be aware of this work and to make available to a child's family the current methods of aetiological investigation. This should include referral to a genetics unit with the appropriate expertise in dealing with hearing loss in children. This chapter has covered the currently identifiable recessive and dominant non-syndromic genetic causes of hearing loss, with some explanation of the basics of genetics for the non-specialist.

References

1. Barbi M, Binda S, Caroppo S, et al (2003) A wider role for congenital cytomegalovirus infection in sensorineural hearing loss. Pediatr Infect Dis J 22:39–42

2. Bauer PW, Geers AE, Brenner C, et al (2003) The effect of GJB2 allele variants on performance after cochlear implantation. Laryngoscope 113:2135–2140

3. Coyle B, Reardon W, Herbrick JA, et al (1998) Molecular analysis of the PDS gene in Pendred syndrome. Hum Mol Genet 7:1105–1112

4. Cremers CW, Admiraal RJ, Huygen PL, et al (1998) Progressive hearing loss, hypoplasia of the cochlea and widened vestibular aqueducts are very common features in Pendred's syndrome. Int J Pediatr Otorhinolaryngol 45:113–123

5. Cryns K, Pfister M, Pennings RJ, et al (2002) Mutations in the WFS1 gene that cause low-frequency sensorineural hearing loss are small non-inactivating mutations. Hum Genet 110:389–394

6. Cullen RD, Buchman CA, Brown CJ, et al (2004) Cochlear implantation for children with GJB2-related deafness. Laryngoscope 114:1415–1419

7. Davis A, Bamford J, Wilson I, et al (1997) A critical review of the role of neonatal hearing screening in the detection of congenital hearing impairment. Health Technol Assess 1:i–iv, 1–176

8. de Kok YJ, Bom SJ, Brunt TM, et al (1999) A Pro51Ser mutation in the COCH gene is associated with late onset autosomal dominant progressive sensorineural hearing loss with vestibular defects. Hum Mol Genet 8:361–366

9. del Castillo, I, Moreno-Pelayo MA, del Castillo FJ, et al (2003) Prevalence and evolutionary origins of the del(GJB6-D13S1830) mutation in the DFNB1 locus in hearing-impaired subjects: a multicenter study. Am J Hum Genet 73:1452–1458

10. Eiberg H, Hansen L, Kjer B, et al (2006) Autosomal dominant optic atrophy associated with hearing impairment and impaired glucose regulation caused by a missense mutation in the WFS1 gene. J Med Genet 43:435–440

11. Fortnum HM, Summerfield AQ, Marshall DH, et al (2001) Prevalence of permanent childhood hearing impairment in the United Kingdom and implications for universal neonatal hearing screening: questionnaire based ascertainment study. BMJ 323:536–540

12. Fransen E, Verstreken M, Verhagen WI, et al (1999) High prevalence of symptoms of Meniere's disease in three families with a mutation in the COCH gene. Hum Mol Genet 8:1425–1429

13. Fukushima K, Sugata K, Kasai N, et al (2002) Better speech performance in cochlear implant patients with GJB2-related deafness. Int J Pediatr Otorhinolaryngol 62:151–157

14. Kamarinos M, McGill J, Lynch M, et al (2001) Identification of a novel COCH mutation, I109N, highlights the similar clinical features observed in DFNA9 families. Hum Mutat 17:351

15. Kenneson A, Van Naarden BK, Boyle C (2002) GJB2 (connexin 26) variants and nonsyndromic sensorineural hearing loss: a HuGE review. Genet Med 4:258–274

16. Lerer I, Sagi M, Ben-Neriah Z, et al (2001) A deletion mutation in GJB6 cooperating with a GJB2 mutation in trans in non-syndromic deafness: a novel founder mutation in Ashkenazi Jews. Hum Mutat 18:460

17. Lesperance MM, Hall JW, III, San Agustin TB, et al (2003) Mutations in the Wolfram syndrome type 1 gene (WFS1) define a clinical entity of dominant low-frequency sensorineural hearing loss. Arch Otolaryngol Head Neck Surg 129:411–420

18. Luxon LM, Cohen M, Coffey RA, et al (2003) Neuro-otological findings in Pendred syndrome. Int J Audiol 42:82–88

19. Mazzoli M, Newton V, Murgia A, et al (2004) Guidelines and recommendations for testing of Cx26 mutations and interpretation of results. Int J Pediatr Otorhinolaryngol 68:1397–1398

20. Migliosi V, Modamio-Hoybjor S, Moreno-Pelayo, et al (2002) Q829X, a novel mutation in the gene encoding otoferlin (OTOF), is frequently found in Spanish patients with prelingual non-syndromic hearing loss. J Med Genet 39:502–506

21. Morell RJ, Kim HJ, Hood LJ, et al (1998) Mutations in the connexin 26 gene (GJB2) among Ashkenazi Jews with nonsyndromic recessive deafness. N Engl J Med 339:1500–1505

7

22. Pagarkar W, Bitner-Glindzicz M, Knight J, et al (2006) Late postnatal onset of hearing loss due to GJB2 mutations. Int J Pediatr Otorhinolaryngol 70:1119–1124

23. Pryor SP, Madeo AC, Reynolds JC, et al (2005) SLC26A4/PDS genotype–phenotype correlation in hearing loss with enlargement of the vestibular aqueduct (EVA): evidence that Pendred syndrome and non-syndromic EVA are distinct clinical and genetic entities. J Med Genet 42:159–165

24. Reardon W, OMahoney CF, Trembath R, et al (2000) Enlarged vestibular aqueduct: a radiological marker of Pendred syndrome, and mutation of the PDS gene. QJM 93:99–104

25. Rhodes CR, Hertzano R, Fuchs H, et al. (2004) A Myo7a mutation cosegregates with stereocilia defects and low-frequency hearing impairment. Mamm Genome 15:686–697

26. Rodriguez-Ballesteros M, del Castillo FJ, Martin Y, et al (2003) Auditory neuropathy in patients carrying mutations in the otoferlin gene (OTOF). Hum Mutat 22:451–456

27. Rouillon I, Marcolla A, Roux I, et al (2006) Results of cochlear implantation in two children with mutations in the OTOF gene. Int J Pediatr Otorhinolaryngol 70:689–696

28. Sinnathuray AR, Toner JG, Clarke-Lyttle J, et al (2004a) Connexin 26 (GJB2) gene-related deafness and speech intelligibility after cochlear implantation. Otol Neurotol 25:935–942

29. Sinnathuray AR, Toner JG, Geddis A, et al (2004b) Auditory perception and speech discrimination after cochlear implantation in patients with connexin 26 (GJB2) gene-related deafness. Otol Neurotol 25:930–934

30. Stinckens C, Huygen PL, Joosten FB, et al (2001) Fluctuant, progressive hearing loss associated with Meniere like vertigo in three patients with the Pendred syndrome. Int J Pediatr Otorhinolaryngol 61:207–215

31. Taitelbaum-Swead R, Brownstein Z, Muchnik C, et al (2006) Connexin-associated deafness and speech perception outcome of cochlear implantation. Arch Otolaryngol Head Neck Surg 132:495–500

32. Tekin M, Akcayoz D, Incesulu A (2005) A novel missense mutation in a C2 domain of OTOF results in autosomal recessive auditory neuropathy. Am J Med Genet A 138:6–10

33. Tsukamoto K, Suzuki H, Harada D, et al (2003) Distribution and frequencies of PDS (SLC26A4) mutations in Pendred syndrome and nonsyndromic hearing loss associated with enlarged vestibular aqueduct: a unique spectrum of mutations in Japanese. Eur J Hum Genet 11:916–922

34. Varga R, Avenarius MR, Kelley PM, et al (2006) OTOF mutations revealed by genetic analysis of hearing loss families including a potential temperature sensitive auditory neuropathy allele. J Med Genet 43:576–581

35. Vermeire K, Brokx JP, Wuyts FL, et al (2006) Good speech recognition and quality-of-life scores after cochlear implantation in patients with DFNA9. Otol Neurotol 27:44–49

Chapter 8

ENT-Related Syndromes

David Albert and Fiona Connell

8

Core Messages

- Whenever a syndromic diagnosis is suspected the clinician should look for other diagnostic clues.
- Referral to a geneticist is important for diagnostic purposes, family counselling, and discussion of recurrence risk.
- Molecular testing is useful in some syndromes and should be requested when the diagnosis is in doubt and a diagnosis will make a difference, for example in counselling, pre-natal diagnosis or management.
- Just because a gene is known does not mean that molecular testing is available on a diagnostic basis.

Contents

8

Definition

A syndrome can be defined as a group of symptoms that collectively indicate or characterise a disease, psychological or congenital disorder. The derivation is from Συν-δρομη (Syn-drome), which means "running together".

Introduction

ENT surgeons dealing with children need to know the ENT features of a few common syndromes, for example Down syndrome, Treacher Collins syndrome and Goldenhar syndrome, as they are likely to meet children with these conditions in their paediatric practice. The ENT surgeon may be presented with two distinct clinical scenarios. In the first, a patient with a known syndrome presents with an ENT problem. In this instance, the ENT surgeon needs to be aware of the ENT features of the syndrome so that the appropriate investigations and management can be instigated. The second and less common situation is when the ENT surgeon suspects that a child may have a syndrome that has not yet been diagnosed. This is rightly the province of the geneticist and, while it is intellectually stimulating to try to piece together a syndrome, it is best to avoid mentioning any suspicions at this stage. Much anxiety can otherwise result from ready access to the Internet. Nevertheless, they should know how to find out about these less common syndromes. This chapter provides a brief list of the more common ENT-related syndromes. Referral to a geneticist is appropriate not only for children with undiagnosed conditions, but also for those with the common syndromes so that genetic counselling and genetic testing can be offered both to the immediate family and to those in the extended family. It may be surprising how many children with known genetic diagnoses who are under multiple hospital specialties, have never seen a geneticist.

Resources

A useful book to have in the ENT department is Smith's Recognizable Patterns of Human Malformation (Jones 2005). The book contains pictures of children with genetic syndromes and a brief description of the main clinical features. Gorlin's Hereditary Hearing Loss and its Syndromes (Gorlin et al. 2001) and Oxford Desk Reference. Clinical Genetics (Firth et al. 2005) are also useful reference sources, the former with a particular emphasis on syndromes incorporating deafness. The London Dysmorphology Database (Winter and Baraitser 2004) is a computerised database that is searchable using clinical features, and contains pictures, a brief summary of clinical features, and an abstract as well as lists of useful published papers. Two other useful websites are www.genetests.org and www.orpha.net.

Syndromes of Particular Relevance to the ENT Clinician

Down Syndrome

Genetics

Down syndrome is the most common chromosome disorder, and ENT sequelae occur frequently. Most cases of Down syndrome arise from free trisomy of chromosome 21, although a small proportion are caused by translocations in which there is a high recurrence risk. The overall population incidence is between 1 in 650 and 1 in 800 live births. There is a well-recognised relationship between increased risk of trisomy 21 conceptions and maternal age. The risk of Down syndrome in women aged 35 years is 1

in 385, compared to 1 in 28 in women aged 45 years. Antenatal diagnosis is available. There are, of course, more Down syndrome babies born to younger mothers because of their higher fertility compared with older women.

ENT Features

1. Small ears.
2. Narrow external ear canals: can make it difficult to view the tympanic membrane or insert grommets.
3. Increased incidence of glue ear: age related.
4. Otoacoustic emissions often non-reproducible, even in patients with normal hearing ability.
5. Abnormal ossicles.
6. Mixed deafness (7%).
7. Sensorineural deafness (8%).
8. Airway obstruction from small posterior nasal spine with large tonsils and adenoids.
9. Macroglossia.
10. Subglottis: usually require one anaesthetic tube size smaller than expected.
11. Unstable neck, with a risk of atlanto-occipital joint subluxation in 15%, especially during general anaesthetic.

General Features

1. Typical facial features include:
   - Brachycephaly.
   - Upslanting palpebral fissures.
   - Epicanthic folds and Brushfield spots (speckling of iris).
   - Flat facial profile.
   - Small nose with depressed nasal bridge.
2. Mental retardation: variable IQ – can range from 20 to 85.
3. Hypotonia: contributes to delayed motor milestones.
4. Joint laxity.
5. Congenital heart disease.
6. Single palmar crease.
7. Wide sandal gap (gap between first and second toes).
8. Other medical problems (e.g. hypothyroidism, leukaemia).
9. Other congenital problems (e.g. duodenal atresia, Hirschsprung disease).

Pierre Robin Sequence

Genetics

This condition is a disorder of embryological developmental characterised by a cleft palate and a small jaw. The primary anomaly is one of intrauterine mandibular hypoplasia, which results in the features listed below.

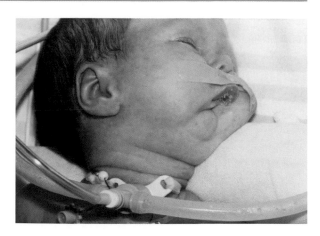

Fig. 8.1 Pierre-Robin syndrome, showing severe retrognathia, which in this case required a tracheostomy

ENT Features

1. Cleft palate.
2. Retrognathia/micrognathia (Fig. 8.1).
3. Airway obstruction, difficult intubation.
4. Small open mouth.
5. Prominent nose with squared-off nasal tip.

Treacher Collins Syndrome

Genetics

Treacher Collins syndrome (TCS) is a disorder of branchial arch development and individuals have a characteristic facial appearance. It is inherited in an autosomal dominant manner and the only gene currently known to be associated is *TCOF1*. A high proportion of cases are caused by new mutations, but significant clinical variability is common and so genetic testing may be extremely useful for recurrence risks. Classically, features are bilateral, symmetrical and congenital.

ENT Features

See Chapter 44, Fig. 44.1.

1. Microtia, dysplastic ears (bilateral ear anomalies).
2. Auricular pits/fistula/tags.
3. Deafness: usually conductive due to external auditory canal atresia and malformations of the ossicles.
4. Cleft palate.
5. Micrognathia: cleft palate and micrognathia together may result in significant airway problems in neonates.
6. Mandibular hypoplasia: occipitomental projection of skull and orthopantogram radiographs can assist in diagnosis.

7. Flat malar region.
8. Prominent nose.
9. Broad mouth.
10. Narrow nasopharynx.
11. Choanal atresia (rare).

General Features

Typical facial features include downslanting palpebral fissures, coloboma of inferior eyelid, sparse eyelashes.

Goldenhar Syndrome

Goldenhar syndrome is also known as oculo-auriculo-vertebral spectrum, hemifacial microsomia and first and second arch syndrome.

CHARGE Syndrome

The term "CHARGE" is taken from its main features: Coloboma, Heart defect, Atresia choanae, Retardation of growth and development, Genital defect and Ear anomalies and/or deafness.

Genetics

Unilateral or bilateral, asymmetrical congenital defects involving the first and second branchial arches are seen in this condition. Involvement of other systems is common. The aetiology of the condition is unknown and most cases are a single occurrence (i.e. only one family member affected), although cases with dominant and recessive inheritance are reported in the literature. Various chromosome anomalies have been reported in Goldenhar cases.

Reported risk factors include: maternal diabetes, bleeding in early pregnancy, twinning and teratogens (thalidomide, retinoic acid derivatives); it is also commoner in populations living at high altitude.

ENT Features

1. Microtia (Fig. 8.2a): variable severity ranging from partial to complete atresia of the auditory canal and from minor degrees of microtia to complete absence of the external ear. Although the condition is almost usually unilateral, it may occasionally be bilateral but is almost always asymmetrical.
2. Pre-auricular skin tags.
3. Skin tags: in line between the tragus and the corner of the mouth.
4. Deafness: sensorineural and/or conductive.

5. Macrostomia: occasionally with lateral facial clefting.

General Features

1. Facial asymmetry (Fig. 8.2b).
2. Epibulbar dermoid (Fig. 8.2c).
3. Vertebral defects.
4. Cardiac defects.
5. Renal anomalies.
6. Mental retardation: uncommon and chromosome analysis should be performed when this is present.

Genetics

CHARGE syndrome has a reported prevalence of 1 in 12,000. Diagnosis of CHARGE syndrome is made on the basis of clinical findings and temporal bone imaging. Mutations in the gene *CHD7* can be identified in approximately 65% of cases, mostly due to new mutations. In these cases, the inheritance pattern is autosomal dominant.

Patients with choanal atresia (unilateral and bilateral) need to be assessed to exclude features of CHARGE syndrome. Cardiology, ophthalmology and endocrine opinions should be sought, as well as audiology and temporal bone imaging.

ENT Features

1. Choanal atresia/stenosis (unilateral or bilateral).
2. Outer ear: short, wide ear with deficient lobe, often protruding, asymmetric.
3. Middle ear: ossicular malformations.
4. Temporal bone abnormalities; absent or hypoplastic semicircular canals.
5. Sensorineural deafness (mild to profound).

General Features

1. Coloboma – iris, retina, choroids, disc.
2. Microphthalmia.
3. Cranial nerve dysfunction: anosmia, facial palsy, swallowing problems.
4. Genital hypoplasia.
5. Developmental delay (ranges from mild to severe; those with absent semicircular canals will have significant motor delay).

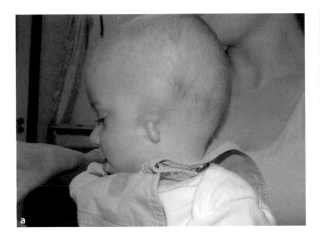
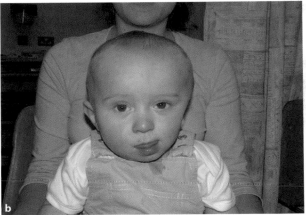
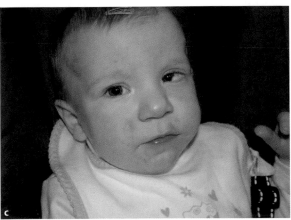

Fig. 8.2a–c Goldenhar syndrome. **a** Left-sided microtia. **b** Facial asymmetry, with left sided hemifacial microsomia. **c** Epibulbar dermoid over the sclera of the left eye

6. Congenital heart disease.
7. Cleft lip/palate.
8. Facial features: prominent forehead and nasal bridge, flat midface.
9. Growth deficiency.

Branchio-oto-renal Syndrome

Please also refer to Chapter 19.

Genetics

This autosomal dominant disorder is characterised by external, middle and inner ear anomalies, branchial sinuses and renal dysplasia. It is caused by mutations in the *EYA1* gene, and less commonly in the *SIX-1* gene. Extreme clinical variability can be observed within the same family. Patients with ear pits (with or without hearing loss) and branchial defects warrant a renal ultrasound scan.

ENT Features

1. Ear anomalies: pits in the pre-helical region and dysplastic pinnae (Fig. 8.3a).
2. Conductive (due to ossicular malformations), sensorineural, or mixed hearing impairment. Inner ear malformations may include Mondini dysplasia of the cochlea, and occasionally, dilated vestibular aqueducts (see Chapter 40). Hearing impairment is not always present, but the pre-helical ear pits are a very highly penetrant feature.
3. Branchial fistulae and/or cysts (Fig. 8.3b).

General Features

Renal malformations: duplex collecting system, hydronephrosis, dysplasia, unilateral or bilateral renal agenesis.

22q11.2 Deletion Syndrome

22q11.2 Deletion syndrome is also known as velocardiofacial syndrome, DiGeorge syndrome and Shprintzen syndrome.

Genetics

22q11.2 deletion syndrome is microdeletion syndrome which is inherited in an autosomal dominat pattern. The phenotype can be very variable. About 90% of probands

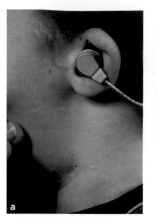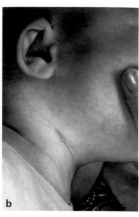

Fig. 8.3a,b Branchio-oto-renal syndrome. **a** Dysplastic pinna of left ear. Note the typical pre-helical pit and hearing aid. **b** Branchial fistula, right side of neck

have a *de novo* deletion of chromosome 22q11.2, but the remaining 10% have inherited it from either parent.

ENT Features

Palate

1. Overt or submucous cleft palate.
2. Velopharyngeal incompetence.
3. Hypernasal speech.

Ears

1. Small, low-set ears.
2. Prominent/overfolded helices.
3. Absent or hypoplastic ear lobules.
4. Pre-auricular tags.
5. Otitis media.
6. Sensorineural hearing loss.
7. Narrow external auditory canals.

Tracheal/laryngeal

1. Upper airway obstruction.
2. Laryngeal web.
3. Vascular ring.
4. Laryngomalacia.

General Features

1. Characteristic facial appearance: prominent nasal bridge, bulbous nose and long face.
2. Congenital heart abnormalities.

3. Mental retardation/developmental delay (variable).
4. Short stature.
5. Feeding difficulties.
6. Psychiatric illness.
7. Immune deficiency
8. Parathyroid dysfunction: hypocalcaemia

Craniosynostosis Syndromes

Genetics

Crouzon (see Fig. 8.4), Apert, Muenke and Pfeiffer syndromes are part or the *FGFR*-gene-related craniosynostosis syndromes (Hayward et al. 2004). They follow an autosomal dominant inheritance pattern, but new mutations are common. Saethre-Chotzen is a craniosynostosis syndrome that is caused by mutations in the *TWIST* gene.

ENT Features

1. Airway obstruction.
2. Pinna abnormalities: low-set, small or posteriorly rotated ears.
3. External canal atresia.
4. Middle ear abnormalities: both congenital ossicular fixation and Eustachian tube dysfunction.
5. Sensorineural deafness.

General Features

1. Craniosynostosis.
2. Hypertelorism.
3. Proptosis.
4. Syndactyly – Apert syndrome.
5. Broad, short thumbs/toes – Pfeiffer syndrome.

Alport Syndrome

Genetics

Condition characterised by nephropathy (proteinuria and haematuria) and sensorineural deafness. It is caused by mutations in genes that code for collagen IV. X-linked Alport syndrome is the most common form, affecting males more severely, but autosomal recessive and dominant forms also exist and therefore it is vital that a thorough family history is obtained.

ENT Features

Hearing loss: high-tone sensorineural (mild to moderately severe) affecting 83% males and 57% females.

Usually presents in school-age boys and exhibits a progressive deterioration. Adults tend to retain some hearing capacity and the impairment is more or less stable with time.

General Features

1. Renal impairment (onset in childhood; progression to end-stage renal failure in 100% of males, 15% of females)
2. Ocular lesions: lenticonus (most commonly anterior lenticonus) and macular flecks.

Pendred Syndrome

Combination of congenital deafness and thyroid dyshormonogenesis. As this often presents as non-syndromic deafness it is covered in Chapter 7.

Usher Syndrome

Genetics

Usher syndrome is characterised by sensorineural hearing loss and progressive retinitis pigmentosa (RP). It is one of the most common types of autosomal recessive syndromic hearing loss and there are three, usually distinct types recognised, based on the degree of hearing impairment and vestibular involvement. It presents initially as non-syndromic hearing loss until the RP is diagnosed.

Type 1

1. Profound congenital sensorineural deafness.
2. Absent vestibular function (resulting in delayed motor milestones). Such a presentation should prompt investigation for Usher syndrome. Children should have the option of cochlear implant assessment in view of the fact that they will ultimately develop severe visual handicap in addition to their deafness.
3. RP: asymptomatic at first (but may be diagnosed presymptomatically by electroretinogram), but symptoms of night blindness and tunnel vision become apparent around late childhood/early puberty.

Type 2

1. Congenital sensorineal hearing loss, severe in the high frequencies
2. Normal vestibular function

8

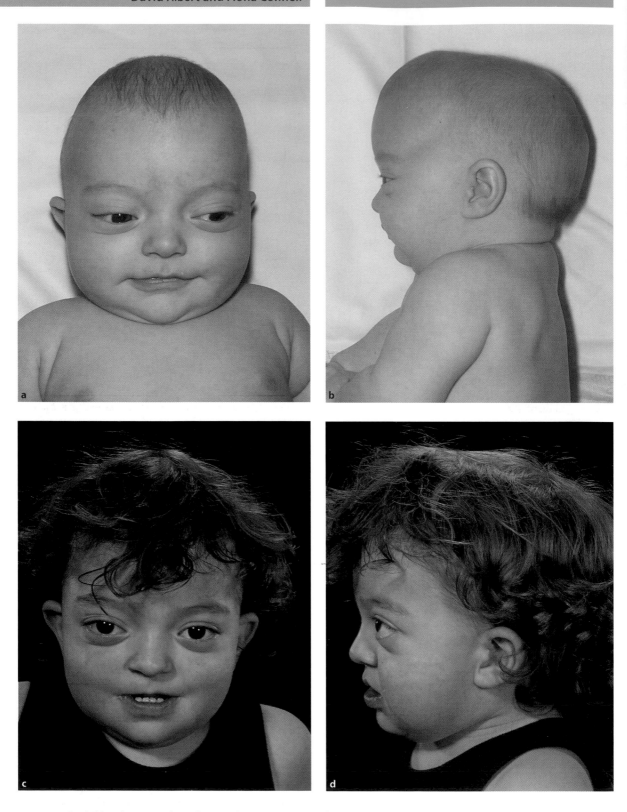

Fig. 8.4a–d Child with Crouzon's syndrome **a–b** age 4 months. **c–d** age 2 years

3. RP: onset is around puberty (slightly later than type 1 on average)

Type 3

1. Progressive hearing loss, may be post-lingual onset.
2. Normal or absent vestibular function.
3. RP: later and more variable age of onset.

Alstrom Syndrome

Genetics

Alstrom syndrome is a rare, autosomal recessive disorder caused by mutations in the *ALMS1* gene. It is characterised by retinal dystrophy, obesity and deafness. There is considerable clinical variability, even within sibships.

ENT Features

Progressive hearing impairment: tends to develop in the second decade of life.

General Features

1. Progressive retinal degeneration: beginning in infancy, no light perception by 20 years.
2. Photophobia and nystagmus.
3. Cone-rod dystrophy in which cones are predominantly affected.
4. Obesity.
5. Non-insulin-dependent diabetes mellitus: develops in the second/third decade of life.
6. Renal complications: progressive chronic nephropathy.
7. Cardiomyopathy.
8. Other endocrine involvement.

Syndromes Less Commonly Seen by ENT Surgeons

Achondroplasia

Genetics

Achondroplasia is the most common cause of disproportionate short stature and affected individuals have a characteristic appearance. It is an autosomal dominant disorder that is caused by activating mutations in the *FGFR3*

gene. Incidence is related to increasing paternal age. 80% of patients have *de novo* mutations.

ENT Features

1. Obstructive sleep apnoea (OSA) or central apnoea.
2. Adenotonsillar hypertrophy.
3. Narrow nasopharynx.
4. Frequent otitis media and glue ear.
5. Sensorineural and conductive hearing loss.
6. Midface hypoplasia.

General Features

1. Short stature.
2. Rhizomelic (proximal) shortening of the limbs.
3. Tibial bowing.
4. Thoracolumbar kyphosis in infancy.
5. Exaggerated lumbar lordosis, which develops when walking begins.
6. Large head with frontal bossing.
7. Small chest leading to respiratory compromise in infants.
8. Neurological involvement: cervical spine stenosis can lead to apnoea/sudden death (anaesthetic risk), spinal stenosis/nerve root compression.

Beckwith-Wiedemann Syndrome

Genetics

Beckwith-Wiedemann syndrome (BWS) is an overgrowth disorder caused by changes in the activity of growth-promoting and -suppressing genes, many of which are imprinted, found at 11p15.

ENT Features

1. Macroglossia (Fig. 8.5), which may constitute an anaesthetic risk and may occasionally require surgical reduction.
2. Ear lobe creases and/or posterior helical ear pits.

General Features

1. Overgrowth: large birth weight, macrosomia, visceromegaly, hemi-hypertrophy. Growth rate slows around age of about 7/8 years.
2. Neonatal hypoglycaemia.
3. Omphalocoele.

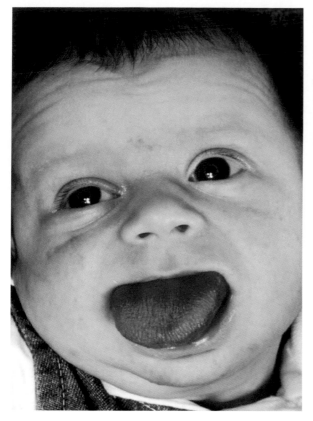

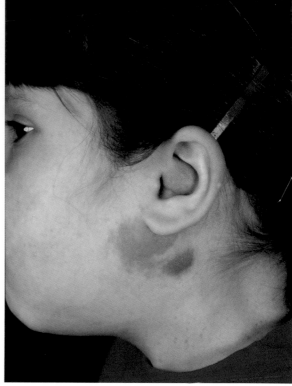

Fig. 8.5 Beckwith-Wiedemann syndrome, showing macroglossia

Fig. 8.6 Café au lait spot below left ear

4. Embryonal tumour risk increased: Wilm's tumour, hepatoblastoma, neuroblastoma, rhabdomyosarcoma.
5. Renal anomalies.

Neurofibromatosis Type 2

Genetics

Clinically and molecularly distinct condition from neurofibromatosis type 1 (NF1), neurofibromatosis type 2 (NF2) is inherited in an autosomal dominant pattern and is characterised by the presence of vestibular schwannomas. New mutations in the *NF2* gene arise in approximately half of cases.

Diagnostic criteria include one of the following:
1. Bilateral vestibular schwannomas.
2. First-degree relative with NF2 AND unilateral vestibular schwannoma OR any two of: meningioma, schwannoma, glioma, neurofibroma and posterior subcapsular lenticular opacities.
3. Unilateral vestibular schwannoma AND any two of: meningioma, schwannoma, glioma, neurofibroma and posterior subcapsular lenticular opacities.

4. Multiple meningiomas AND unilateral vestibular schwannoma OR any two of: schwannoma, glioma, neurofibroma and cataract.

All patients should be referred for genetic counselling as other family members may need to be monitored for the condition or tested to exclude it. Radiation therapy in NF2 patients should be considered carefully as radiation exposure, especially in childhood, can induce/accelerate tumour growth.

ENT Features

Hearing loss, tinnitus or vertigo caused by Schwannoma of the cranial nerves: typically unilateral or bilateral vestibular (acoustic) neuromas. Can cause facial paralysis depending on nerve involvement.

General Features

1. Other central nervous system tumours: meningiomas, ependymomas, spinal tumours, astrocytomas.

2. Peripheral nervous system manifestations: peripheral/subcutaneous schwannomas, cutaneous neurofibromas, NF2 plaques.
3. Café au lait patches (Fig. 8.6): these are less common than in NF1.
4. Ocular manifestations: cataracts, retinal hamartomas.

Noonan Syndrome

Genetics

Noonan syndrome is a relatively common autosomal dominant disorder. Mutations in *PTPN11* have been identified in 50% of patients. More recently, other genes have been implicated in causing Noonan syndrome (e.g. *KRAS* gene found in 5–10% of Noonan patients). Noonan syndrome has a clinically heterogeneous phenotype, even within families.

ENT Features

1. Low-set, posteriorly rotated ears.
2. Webbing of the neck, low posterior hairline.
3. Variable hearing loss.
4. Micrognathia.

General Features

1. Congenital heart disease; typically pulmonary stenosis. Hypertrophic cardiomyopathy is also characteristic.
2. Mild mental retardation.
3. Short stature.
4. Sternal abnormalities.
5. Widely spaced nipples.
6. Cryptorchidism.
7. Epicanthal folds.
8. Ptosis.

Osteogenesis Imperfecta

Genetics

Osteogenesis imperfecta (OI) comprises a group of inherited disorders, and is otherwise known as "brittle bone disease". The *COL1A1* and *COL1A2* genes code for collagen type 1 and mutations in these genes are responsible for causing OI. Trivial trauma can result in fractures due to the skeletal fragility. The severity of the disease and deformities depends on the type of OI.

Type I is the commonest form and shows autosomal dominant inheritance. It is a relatively mild form, which is non-deforming.

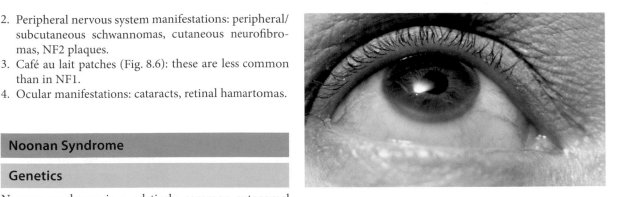

Fig. 8.7 Blue sclera in a case of osteogenesis imperfecta

ENT Features (Type 1)

Hearing loss.

General Features (Type 1)

1. Blue sclerae (see Fig. 8.7).
2. Fractures.
3. Mildly short stature.
4. Wormian bones visible on skull X-ray.

Prader-Willi Syndrome

Genetics

Prader-Willi syndrome is one of the more common genetic conditions and is characterised by poor neonatal feeding and childhood-onset obesity as a result of hyperphagia. It is caused by the absence of the paternally derived Prader-Willi syndrome region on chromosome 15.

ENT Features

Obstructive sleep apnoea (OSA): secondary to obesity, a cardinal feature of the disorder. The role of growth hormone (GH) in exacerbating OSA in Prader-Willi syndrome has been postulated following a series of fatalities of children with Prader-Willi syndrome on GH treatment. This is currently unproven but it has been suggested that GH leads to increased growth of lymphoid tissue in the airway, thus worsening already existing hypoventilation or OSA.

General Features

1. Overeating leading to obesity.
2. Hypogonadism.

3. Mental retardation.
4. Difficult behaviour.
5. Growth failure/short stature.
6. Hypotonia: particularly in neonatal period.

Stickler Syndrome

Genetics

Stickler syndrome is a hereditary arthro-ophthalmopathy. Children have a characteristic facial appearance. It is inherited in an autosomal dominant manner and the clinical phenotype can be very heterogeneous, even within families. It is a collagen disorder and the responsible mutations are found in *COL2A1* and *COL11A1*.

ENT Features

1. Flat faces with depressed nasal bridge and anteverted nares: facial features most evident in childhood.
2. Pierre Robin sequence.
3. Sensorineural deafness, may be progressive.
4. Glossoptosis.
5. Dental anomalies.

General Features

1. Severe myopia resulting from a congenital vitreous anomaly. Risk from retinal detachment.
2. Joint problems, especially joint hypermobility and premature arthritis.

Turner Syndrome

Genetics

Turner syndrome is caused by partial or complete absence of an X chromosome in some (Mosaic Turner syndrome) or all cells (Classical Turner syndrome) of the body. It has a frequency of about 1 in 1800 girls.

ENT Features

1. Increased incidence of glue ear.
2. Sensorineural deafness.
3. Webbed neck.
4. Low posterior hairline.

General Features

1. Short stature.

2. Ovarian dysgenesis.
3. Coarctation of aorta, bicuspid aortic valve.
4. Renal anomalies.
5. Mild learning difficulties.
6. Broad chest, widely spaced nipples.
7. Increased carrying angle.
8. Increased incidence of autoimmune conditions: hypothyroidism, coeliac disease, inflammatory bowel disease, diabetes mellitus.

Waardenburg Syndrome

Genetics

Waardenburg sydrome is the most common type of syndromic autosomal dominant syndromic hearing loss, characterised by hearing loss and pigmentary anomalies. There are four different types. Types 1 and 3 are characterised by subtle craniofacial anomalies (below). In type 2 the appearance is normal, as in type 4, which is characterised in addition by the association with Hirschprung's disease. Mutations in the *PAX3* gene are responsible for types 1 and 3. Mutation in the *MITF* gene causes some cases of type 2; the genes implicated in type 4 include, *EDNRB*, *EDN3* and *SOX10*.

ENT Features

1. Congenital sensorineural hearing loss.
2. Hypoplastic nasal alae (type 1).
3. High nasal bridge (type 1).
4. Synophrys (fused eyebrows) and medial eyebrow flare (type 1).

General Features

1. Pigmentary disturbances: heterochromia iridium, white forelock and eyelashes, with premature greying of the hair (these may be concealed with the use of hair dyes in adults), hypopigmentation of skin.
2. Dystopia canthorum (lateral displacement of inner canthus of eye) (type 1).
3. Limb anomalies (type 3).
4. Hirschprung's disease (type 4).

Jervell and Lange-Nielsen Syndrome

Genetics

Homozygous form of long-QT syndrome with profound congenital deafness. Inherited in an autosomal recessive manner. Disease-causing mutations in the potassium channel gene *KCNQ1* and its accessory subunit *KCNE1*, are responsible for both the cochlear and cardiac abnormalities. This is an important diagnosis to make because of its high mortality if left untreated, and children with severe/profound congenital hearing loss should be screened routinely with electrocardiogram.

ENT Features

Congenital profound sensorineural deafness with absent vestibular function.

General Features

1. Prolonged QTc interval on 12-lead electrocardiogram.
2. Risk of *torsade des pointes* ventricular tachycardia.
3. Risk of ventricular fibrillation, which can culminate in syncope or sudden death. Can be precipitated by general anaesthesia, fright/stress, exercise (particularly dangerous if swimming).

Gorlin Syndrome

Genetics

Gorlin syndrome is an autosomal dominant syndrome that is otherwise known as naevoid basal cell carcinoma syndrome. It is caused by mutations in *PTCH*, a tumour suppressor gene.

ENT Features

1. Jaw cysts.
2. Cleft lip and palate.

General Features

1. Basal cell naevi/basal cell carcinoma.
2. Macrocephaly.
3. Frontal and biparietal bossing.
4. Palmar/plantar pits.
5. Ocular anomalies: cataracts, developmental defects.
6. Calcification of falx cerebri.
7. Rib or vertebral anomalies.

Holoprosencephaly

Genetics

Holoprosencephaly is a genetically heterogeneous disorder. Chromosomal abnormalities are responsible for the majority of cases (e.g. trisomy 13, microdeletion of 7q36). Syndromic causes, familial autosomal dominant and *de novo* cases have all been described. There are five known genes implicated in the pathogenesis of holoprosencephaly to date: *SHH*, *SIX3*, *TG1F*, *ZIC2* and *PTCH*.

ENT Features

1. Oral defects: ranging from midline cleft upper lip to single central incisor/absent frenulum.
2. Pre-maxillary agenesis.
3. Midface hypoplasia.
4. Airway obstruction.
5. Nasal defects ranging from "proboscis" nose to single nostril.

General Features

1. Eye anomalies ranging from cyclopia or ocular hypotelorism.
2. Mental retardation.
3. Other midline anomalies: congenital heart defects, anal anomalies.

Mucopolysaccharidoses

Genetics

Within this group of storage disorders, each type has a distinct phenotype but they share many features. Mucopolysaccharidoses are inherited in an autosomal recessive manner with the exception of type II (Hunter syndrome), which is X-linked. For the purposes of this chapter the different types are not described individually, but awareness of the ENT complications is advised.

Please note that the features listed below are not universal to every type of mucopolysaccharidoses.

ENT Features

1. Obstructive airway disease and OSA.
2. Diffuse infiltration around the airway.
3. Hearing loss.
4. Atlanto-axial instability in types IV and VI.
5. Coarse or rough facial features with thick lips and enlarged mouth and tongue.

General Features

1. Short stature.
2. Skeletal irregularities.
3. Visceromegaly particularly hepatosplenomegaly.

4. Progressive joint stiffness.
5. Heart disease.
6. Corneal involvement in some types.
7. Mental retardation in some types.

Foetal Alcohol Syndrome

Genetics

Heavy alcohol exposure *in utero* can have multiple effects on the developing foetus. The resulting phenotype is variable.

ENT Features

1. Sensorineural hearing loss.
2. Cleft lip +/– palate (uncommon).

General Features

1. Low birth weight.
2. Growth retardation with disproportionately low weight to height relationship.
3. Developmental delay especially impaired fine motor skills and cognition.
4. Attention deficit disorder/behavioural difficulties.
5. Flat malar region.
6. Short palpebral fissures.
7. Smooth philtrum with thin upper lip.
8. Mild to moderate microcephaly.

Foetal Cytomegalovirus Syndrome

The severity of the syndrome depends on gestation at the time of intrauterine infection. Consequences of first trimester infection are relatively severe, whereas third-trimester infection can be asymptomatic in the foetus.

Features

1. Sensorineural deafness.
2. Microcephaly.
3. Learning difficulties and developmental delay.
4. Chorioretinitis.

Congenital rubella syndrome

Maternal infection prior to 16 weeks gestation can result in severe consequences for the foetus.

Features

1. Sensorineural deafness.
2. Growth retardation.
3. Mental retardation.
4. Ophthalmic defects such as cataracts, pigmentary retinopathy.
5. Congenital heart disease: patent ductus arteriosus, peripheral pulmonary artery stenosis, septal defects.

Summary for the Clinician

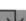

- This chapter has covered some of the more common genetic syndromes that may be seen in the ENT clinic, with emphasis on ENT-related complications and features. With the advent of Newborn Hearing Screening, hearing loss is diagnosed early, and it is likely that the ENT surgeon may be one of the first health professionals to see a child with a syndrome. It is recommended that patients with features of a syndrome and their families are offered genetic counselling. The genetic review aims to offer a diagnostic service but in addition to this, it is important that genetic testing is performed appropriately on the patient and necessary family members. It is also necessary for the family to receive counselling regarding inheritance patterns, recurrence risks and available pre-natal diagnosis options.

Acknowledgements

Maria Bitner-Glindzicz, Reader in Clinical and Molecular Genetics, Institute of Child Health and Great Ormond Street Hospital, London.

References

1. Firth HV, Hurst JA, Hall J (eds) (2005) Oxford Desk Reference. Clinical Genetics. Oxford University Press, Oxford

2. Jones KL (2005) Smith's Recognizable Patterns of Human Malformation, 6th edn. WB Saunders Company, Philadelphia

3. Gorlin RJ, Cohen MM Jr, Hennekam RCM (2001) Syndromes of Head and Neck, 4th edn. Oxford University Press, Oxford

4. Hayward R, Jones B, Dunaway D, et al. (eds) (2004) The Clinical Management of Craniosynostosis. Mac Keith Press, London

5. Winter R, Baraitser M (2004) London Dysmorphology Database. Version 1.0.7 2004. Oxford University Press (info. at www.lmdatabases.com)

EXIT – Antenatal (Pre-natal) Diagnoses and Management

9

Gavin Morrison

Core Messages

- 1. Ultrasound features of pre-natal airway disease include:
  - a. Polyhydramnios – non-specific.
  - b. Obstructive airway mass seen in relation to the airway.
  - c. Gross anomaly of the upper airway.
  - d. Tracheal dilatation and increased echogenicity of lungs in congenital high airway obstruction syndrome (CHAOS).
  - e. Incomplete laryngeal stenosis – may be a normal scan.
- 2. Sequence of ex-utero intrapartum treatment (EXIT) procedure. Caesarian section approach:
  - a. Deep general anaesthesia to relax uterus.
  - b. Deliver head and upper torso only.
  - c. Foetal scalp monitoring.
  - d. Intramuscular foetal paralysis.
  - e. Establish foetal airway endoscopically or by in-situ tracheotomy.
  - f. Clamp and divide umbilical cord and deliver baby.

Contents

Introduction

Over recent decades, antenatal diagnosis has been greatly enhanced by high-resolution ultrasonography, enabling the identification of potential airway anomalies in utero. The development of rapid-sequence magnetic resonance imaging (MRI) scanning of the foetus further enhances our diagnostic capabilities pre-natally. The role of the paediatric otolaryngologist in the management of these problems has become increasingly important, because the development of minimally invasive endoscopic techniques and advancements in intrauterine surgery and in endoscopic equipment now make the pre-natal surgical correction of airway conditions a possibility. Thus, airway obstruction in the unborn baby can be diagnosed early, and with a multidisciplinary approach, planned management of the possible neonatal airway compromise has become routine. The paediatric ENT surgeon's principal remit in this team is to secure the airway at the time of an ex-utero intrapartum treatment (EXIT) procedure. EXIT describes the technique of undertaking a Caesarian section approach, but delivering only the head and upper torso through the uterine incision, while maintaining the maternal foeto-placental circulation. This allows time for the otolaryngologist to secure the neonatal airway by intubation, tracheostomy, or other neck surgery. Once achieved, the Caesarian section delivery is completed. Subsequently, the congenital airway problem can be definitively corrected at the appropriate time by the paediatric airway surgeons. The management of these conditions is greatly enhanced by the support of a full multidisciplinary team. This chapter will describe the common antenatal diagnoses of potential airway problems, the indications for the EXIT procedure, techniques and pitfalls, and will touch on newer applications and foetal surgery. Counselling and ethical issues are also important.

Pre-natal Diagnosis

High-resolution ultrasonography and subspecialisation in this area has brought substantial advances in pre-natal diagnoses in recent decades. This has increased the chance of survival in patients with neonatal airway obstruction, because where the airway obstruction is anticipated, a management plan for ensuring oxygenation of the neonate can be developed. Ultrasonography enables the foetal airway to be viewed from the pharynx to the carina, and the presence, type and severity of most of the anatomical foetal abnormalities in these areas can be diagnosed. The airway conditions most commonly diagnosed by foetal ultrasound are listed in Table 9.1.

Table 9.1 Airway conditions diagnosed antenatally. *CHAOS* Congenital high airway obstruction syndrome

Cervical lymphangioma (cystic hygroma)
Lingual/pharyngolaryngeal lymphangioma
Cervical/thoracic teratoma
Epignathus (developed fetal organs arising from basi-sphenoid)
Laryngeal and tracheal atresia/stenosis (CHAOS)
Congenital thyroid goitre
Tongue tumour
Severe micrognathia
Conjoined twins
Embryonic rhabdomyosarcoma
Cervical neuroblastoma
Plunging ranula

It has been estimated that 4.8% of patients have one or more congenital anomalies diagnosed antenatally by ultrasound, and of these, 2.5% involve the head and neck region. Congenital teratomas affect 1 in 20,000–40,000 live births. Five percent of these occur in the head and neck and may cause airway compromise (Azizkhan et al. 1995) and 95% of congenital teratomas are benign (Kerner et al. 1998). Prior to the development of the EXIT procedure, 35% of babies born with cervico-facial teratomas had life-threatening airway obstruction, and prior to routine ultrasound scanning, the mortality rate was 30% at birth (Azizkhan et al. 1995).

Probably the most common antenatal diagnosis in the head and neck region is cervical lymphangioma. It is estimated to occur in 1 in 6,000 pregnancies, although when diagnosed before the 30th week of gestation, it carries a poorer prognosis, being associated with other congenital anomalies. Approximately 1 in 12,000 therefore, proceed to live birth. First-trimester diagnosis of cystic hygroma has the strongest pre-natal association with aneuploidy, with the major structural foetal malformations being primarily cardiac and skeletal. In one study, overall, two-thirds (89 of 132, 67.4%) of all cases of septated cystic hygroma were diagnosed with either chromosomal or major structural foetal abnormalities (Malone et al. 2005).

Complete congenital laryngeal atresia is rare, and before the advent of the EXIT procedure, was always fatal. It is associated with other major congenital anomalies in up to 50% of cases. All 48 cases that were reported in the world literature between 1826 and 1993 died; 16 cases reported in more recent years, between 1988 and 1994, also failed to survive (Hendrick et al. 1994). Since that time, with the use of the EXIT procedure, there have been several long-term survivors.

Diagnostic Ultrasound Features

Many congenital abnormalities, including those in the head and neck, are associated with polyhydramnios. Polyhydramnios is noted in 0.41% of pregnancies, and 20% of these will have a congenital abnormality in the head and neck (Stocks et al. 1997). Antenatal ultrasonography will be expected to identify an obstructive lesion seen in relation to the upper airway. Thus, a giant mass in the region of the head and neck, be it solid or cystic, will be observed directly, and its relative compression of the pharynx, larynx or nose should be apparent. Figure 9.1 shows such an example. Teratomas may also be associated with a raised maternal alphafetoprotein as well as elevated alphafeto-protein and acetylcholinesterase in the amniotic fluid. Cleft lip and palate is frequently diagnosed pre-natally, but choanal atresia would not be routinely seen. Recently, three-dimensional ultrasound has shown clefting well (Campbell et al. 2005).

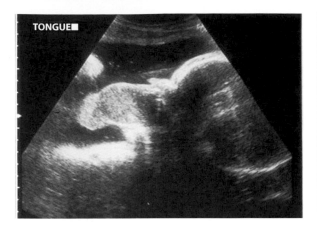

Fig. 9.1 Ultrasound of foetal tongue tumour

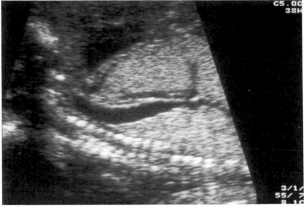

Fig. 9.2 Ultrasound at 18 weeks of congenital high airway obstruction syndrome (laryngeal atresia)

Congenital High Airway Obstruction Syndrome

If there is a complete atresia of the laryngeal airway, such that no liquor from the lungs can pass out through the pharynx, then this fluid progressively builds up, causing a secondarily widely dilated trachea and increased echogenicity of the lungs. These features are characteristic on ultrasound, and comprise the congenital high airway obstructive syndrome (CHAOS). The laryngeal atresia itself might be more difficult to visualise, but the tracheal dilatation is characteristic. The ultrasound findings in CHAOS can be summarised as polyhydramnios, increased echogenicity of the lungs, dilated trachea, flattened or inverted diaphragm, secondary abdominal ascites, and in severe cases cardiac compression (Fig. 9.2). Laryngeal atresia develops when the airway fails to recanalise at 9–10 weeks. There are various subclassifications. Up to 50% of cases will have other associated congenital anomalies.

Unfortunately, not all life-threatening airway problems are pre-natally diagnosable with a high degree of certainty. A particular difficulty arises if there is congenital laryngeal or subglottic stenosis, but a small airway exists to allow the passage of the liquor from the lungs, or perhaps more commonly where there is a complete laryngeal atresia but a coexistent tracheo-oesophageal fistula. In either of these circumstances the lung fluid can pass freely in and out through a small lumen to the pharynx and the amniotic sac. This means that there will be no dilatation of the trachea and no increased echogenicity of the lung structures antenatally. Unless the stenosis or atresia itself can be identified, the baby may be born with no antenatal diagnosis of an airway problem, with potentially fatal consequences. Hartnick et al. (2002) highlighted this problem and proposed the following working definition for paediatric cases of CHAOS: any neonate who needs a surgical airway within 1 h of birth owing to high upper airway (i.e. glottic, subglottic or upper tracheal) obstruction and who cannot be intubated tracheally other than through a persistent tracheo-oesophageal fistula. Therefore, CHAOS has three possible presentations: (1) complete laryngeal atresia without an oesophageal fistula, (2) complete laryngeal atresia with a tracheo-oesophageal fistula and (3) near-complete high upper airway obstruction.

Foetal MRI Scanning

Ultrasound scanning will usually identify a potential congenital airway problem, but the advent of foetal MRI scanning has further enhanced the diagnostic capabilities. Rapid-sequence MRI scanning using techniques such as the half-Fourier, single-shot, turbo spin echo (HASTE), or single-shot fast spin-echo (SSFSE) imaging sequences, allow the rapid acquisition of high-quality images in the transverse, coronal and sagittal planes, with movement artefact minimised. Fast MRI is therefore increasingly being used as a correlative imaging modality in pregnancy because it uses no ionising radiation, provides excellent soft-tissue contrast and has multiple planes for reconstruction and a large field of view. However, for sonographic evaluation of the foetus, it is still important to select the appropriate foetuses for MRI examination, (Glastonbury and Franzcr 2002). Such scanning is indicated for all conditions in which the nature and extent of the pathology cannot be ascertained accurately by ultrasound alone. Figure 9.3 shows an example of a foetal MRI scan demonstrating a large obstructive thyroid teratoma in the neck. Foetal MRI scanning has been reported as helpful in planning the EXIT procedure (Schwindt et al. 2003) and is now widely employed (Zaretsky and Twickler 2003).

9

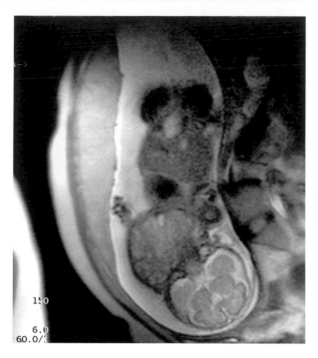

Fig. 9.3 Foetal magnetic resonance imaging scan of thyroid teratoma

The EXIT Procedure

The EXIT procedure was first described by Harrison's group (Mychaliska et al. 1997) in studies that attempted to treat congenital diaphragmatic hernias by clipping the trachea in the neck to promote lung growth, firstly in primates and then in humans. The principle of the treatment is to deliver the head and upper torso of the baby through a hysterotomy incision only (Fig. 9.4), thus maintaining the materno-placental and placento-foetal blood flow and utero-foetal gas exchange, while the airway surgeon

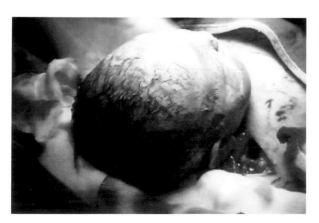

Fig. 9.4 Baby's head delivered at ex-utero intrapartum treatment (EXIT) procedure

secures the baby's natural airway. This will usually involve endoscopically assisted endotracheal intubation through the larynx, but might require the undertaking of an immediate tracheostomy to bypass an airway obstruction that precludes intubation. Occasionally, some excisional procedure will be required at the EXIT procedure before a tracheostomy becomes possible. Once the airway is safely established, the rest of the Caesarian section delivery can proceed, with clamping and ligation of the umbilical cord and initially elective ventilation of the neonate.

Indications for the EXIT Procedure

The indications for planning an EXIT procedure are when there is antenatal diagnosis of: (1) a mass considered likely to be compressing and/or obstructing the upper airway, (2) a grossly abnormal upper airway in which spontaneous respiration or neonatal intubation might prove unsuccessful and (3) where there is antenatal evidence for the CHAOS syndrome with a complete upper airway obstruction, typically from laryngeal atresia. Recently, a further indication has been developed: the planned EXIT procedure to retrieve an iatrogenic pre-natally placed tracheal balloon, in the treatment of congenital diaphragmatic hernias (CDH).

As a note of caution, it is worth stressing that the most common neonatal neck mass is a lymphangioma (cystic hygroma) and the EXIT procedure is not frequently indicated for this condition. When the hygroma comprises macrocysts in the soft tissues of the neck, the pharyngeal and laryngotracheal airway is not usually compromised very much. It the majority of babies with cystic hygroma, therefore, a planned EXIT procedure is not strongly indicated. Where the lymphangiomas involves the tongue, floor of mouth and luminal structures of the pharynx and larynx, however, the airway may be seen on ultrasound to be compromised and EXIT should be planned.

Techniques of the EXIT Procedure

The multidisciplinary team who may be involved in the mother and baby's care should draw together the relevant subspecialists (Table 9.2) and will include: a foetal medicine consultant, a specialist radiologist, an obstetrician, an obstetric anaesthetist, the paediatric otolaryngologist, neonatal intensivists, a paediatric anaesthetist and sometimes a paediatric surgeon, as well as the neonatal nurses, operating theatre nurses and operating department assistants.

Typically, a date for EXIT is planned at about 37–38 weeks, allowing for sufficient maturity but before the spontaneous onset of labour. A large operating theatre is selected, stocked with all of the equipment and staff for a standard Caesarian section delivery, including the neona-

Table 9.2 The Multidisciplinary ex-utero intrapartum treatment (EXIT) team

Foetal Medicine Consultant
Specialist Radiologist
Obstetrician
Obstetric Anaesthetist
Paediatric Otolaryngologist
Paediatric Surgeon
Paediatric Anaesthetist
Neonatal Intensivists
Theatre Nurses & Neonatal Nurses
Operating Department Assistants

tal team and ventilator, as well as the ENT surgeon and his full set of neonatal microlaryngoscopy and bronchoscopy equipment and tracheostomy instruments. The theatre is kept very warm to accommodate the baby and hopefully reduce the likelihood of stimulating an early change of foetal to infant circulation.

The mother is anaesthetised with a rapid-sequence induction and given a deep general anaesthetic to relax the uterus and maintain the foeto-placental circulation. Maternal hypotension should, however, be avoided. Typically, nitrous oxide and isofluorane might be used. The nitrous oxide is then discontinued before the hysterotomy incision is undertaken and an intravenous muscle relaxant such as vecuronium is given to the mother to maintain muscle relaxation. The position of the hysterotomy is determined by mapping the borders of the placenta, using sterile intraoperative ultrasonography. A transverse lower-uterine-segment hysterotomy is employed. The hysterotomy incision is best kept small, just large enough to allow careful delivery of the foetal head and shoulders without loss of much amniotic fluid, if possible. Haemostasis at this incision is important and some authors recommend use of uterine staples (Leichty et al. 1997).

The maternal legs will have been supported in the abducted position, allowing the ENT surgeon to access the baby from between the mother's legs. Obtaining adequate foetal neck extension is difficult and it helps to tilt the operating table somewhat foot-down (reverse Trendelenburg). The ENT surgeon should sit on a stool.

Once the foetal head has been delivered, foetal scalp monitoring including pH is routine and pulse oximetry can be applied to the baby's finger or ear. Foetal anaesthesia and paralysis can be administered intramuscularly (fentanyl and vecuronium, to supplement the inhalational anaesthetic that crosses the placenta). Warmed lactated Ringer's solution may be infused into the amniotic cavity to avoid hypothermia and oligohydramnios, and continuous echocardiography is used to monitor the foetal heart rate and cardiac function. An intravenous catheter may be placed in the foetus to administer fluid, medications or blood, as needed.

This technique will often allow up to 1 h, during which the placento-foetal circulation is maintained successfully. The ENT airway surgeon or the neonatal intensivist can then establish a safe airway, if possible by peroral endotracheal intubation. When the anatomy is obscure, it is very helpful to visualise the larynx and pharynx using a folding anaesthetic laryngoscope, held by an assistant, together with a zero-degree Storz rigid endoscope and camera system. The appropriately sized endotracheal tube can then be passed, with the use of a nearly straight stilette passed through it to provide additional rigidity. Another possible strategy, with the baby lying supine, is simply to lift the mass upwards, so that it no longer compresses the larynx and trachea; this may allow better visualisation of the larynx and easier intubation.

If this standard intubation is not possible, then a neonatal 2.5-Storz ventilating bronchoscope may be employed instead, with an endotracheal tube "railroaded" over its barrel. If even this proves impossible, then a tracheostomy, undertaken on the foetal neck, while the baby is placed over the maternal pelvis, is recommended, before further delivery. If necessary, surfactant is delivered at this stage through the tube to the foetal lungs.

As soon as the foetal airway is established, the rest of the Caesarian section delivery is completed, with clamping and ligation of the cord and transfer of the baby to the neonatal cot and ventilator.

Maternal as well as neonatal care remains paramount. There is a risk of significant maternal bleeding from the uterine incision, but more seriously from the placental bed. As soon as the baby is delivered, therefore, oxytocin is administered, and the maternal muscle relaxant can be reversed.

Tips and Pitfalls of EXIT

Spontaneous Onset of Labour

The EXIT procedure is usually planned at about 38 weeks gestation so long as the foetus is still viable and when it is as mature as possible but before the likelihood of spontaneous onset of labour. Much earlier premature or threatened labour might be reversed medically by the antenatal team, however, not infrequently, the mother may go into labour before the planned EXIT date. The success of the procedure depends on the expertise of a large team. It may be possible to muster most of them urgently at short notice, but if this is not possible, the choice will be to proceed with a more standard emergency Caesarean section delivery and rely on the neonatal team to attempt immediate resuscitation of the baby or to attempt an EXIT with the personnel available. In this regard, it has been our practice to educate the neonatologists as well as on-call residents and interested paediatric surgeons in specialist intubation and bronchoscopic techniques.

Cystic Hygroma

For cystic hygroma in the neck, puncture and drainage of large external macrocysts by ultrasound guided transuterine needling just prior to the EXIT procedure can be advantageous. This allows easier delivery of the head and shoulders and may secondarily decompress the airway obstruction.

Maintaining Placento-Foetal Circulation

Any excessive change in foetal conditions during the EXIT procedure could adversely influence the placento-foetal circulation and precipitate infantile circulatory changes, with loss of cord blood flow. Thus, changes in temperature and pressure may be important. The author has empirically undertaken EXIT in a very warm operating theatre, and we have employed a small lower-segment hysterotomy in an attempt to avoid loss of much amniotic fluid, until full delivery is undertaken. This precaution may maintain the intrauterine pressure. If necessary warmed Ringer's solution can be instilled to replace lost amniotic fluid. Maintenance of uterine relaxation is important to prevent placental separation and intravenous nitroglycerin to the mother has been recommended (Clark et al. 2004).

Loss of Placento-Foetal Circulation

Optimally, the EXIT procedure will allow up to 60 min of normal foetal oxygenation, giving plenty of time to establish the neonatal airway. Sometimes, however, for reasons that may remain unclear, the placeto-foetal circulation is lost and the neonate becomes hypoxic and acidotic. In this situation, the airway surgeon must rely on good preparation, having the full range of instruments to hand, and undertake an emergency intubation, if necessary using the Storz ventilating bronchoscope, or undertake an emergency tracheostomy, prior to delivery. Techniques such as transtracheal needle jet ventilation are not suitable in this situation.

Risks to Mother

Uterine atony can result in serious uterine blood loss. This should be minimised by administration of oxytocin before the cord is clamped. Uterine rupture following a subsequent pregnancy is always a small risk.

Outcomes of EXIT

EXIT is now well established, is a safe procedure for the mother and is a means of improving neonatal survival in cases of upper airway compromise. MacKenzie et al. (2002) successfully achieved either intubation or tracheostomy in 30 of 31 EXIT procedures. In another large series from the University of California (Noah et al. 2002), EXIT was compared with normal Caesarean section delivery. Post-partum wound complications were more common in mothers who underwent EXIT. The rate of chorioamnionitis and of endometritis was similar between the groups. There was no difference between groups in hematocrit level change or post-partum hospital stay.

This chapter's author reported his early experience of EXIT procedures (Ward et al. 2000), which now extends to a dozen cases, while the group's experience is over 20 (Morrison 2004). The airway was successfully established in all planned EXIT procedures, although in a few there was loss of placento-foetal oxygenation earlier than desired. Typically, however, up to 60 min of neonatal operating time is achievable. The procedure has proved reliable. Not all the births have subsequently survived without significant long-term morbidity, however.

Counselling and Ethical Issues

As soon as the antenatal team identify any potential anomaly in relation to the head and neck, a collaborative approach should be instigated with referral to the paediatric airway surgeon and multidisciplinary counselling. The foetal medicine team will advise if the pregnancy is likely to safely go to term, the otolaryngologist's role will be to advise about the potential neonatal problems and the likely success rate in terms of survival for the foetus. It is then important to give a clear picture to the parents of what the baby's prognosis and disabilities are likely to be. Parents may believe that the intervention will result either in the death of the foetus or complete correction of the problem. This is seldom the case; in congenital laryngeal atresia, for example, the expectation would be for a tracheostomy to remain in situ for several years and for multiple laryngotracheal reconstruction operations to be required. The eventual outcome in terms of airway and voice quality can not be predicted accurately. Similarly, teratomas and lymphangiomas can lead to the need for multiple operations for functional or cosmetic problems in future years, and do not guarantee the avoidance of long-term tracheostomy. Large obstructive masses can prove to be malignant, such as embryonal rhabdomyosarcomas, and will require further oncologic therapy.

Termination of Pregnancy

If the predicated morbidity for the neonate is considered too great, then elective termination of the pregnancy can be the correct choice. It should always be presented as a possibility, but a balanced view is required from the professionals.

Two Acts of Parliament, the Abortion Act of 1967 and the Human Fertilisation and Embryology Act of 1990, regulate the provision of abortion in England, Wales and Scotland. Section 37 of the Human Fertilisation and Embryology Act governs the time limits for abortion requiring that pregnancy has not exceeded 24 weeks. There is no time limit, however, if there is a substantial risk that if the child were born it would suffer from such physical or mental abnormalities as to be seriously handicapped.

The Abortion Act and Section 37 of the Human Fertilisation and Embryology Act do not apply to Northern Ireland. In the rest of Europe, abortions on demand are available up to 12 or 13 weeks into pregnancy. After that, they are allowed for medical reasons. In the United States, the legal limit for an abortion ranges from 14 to 28 weeks, depending on the state or territory. In most states, abortions after 20 weeks are considered late and can require the support of an ethics panel. If the foetus is mature and viable then a very late termination of pregnancy may raise ethical dilemmas for the medical staff, however. If possible, therefore, it would seem best to proceed with a planned termination before 23–24 weeks.

The physician's responsibility is for both the mother's health and that of the foetus. Increasingly, they are viewed as two separate, treatable patients. The first consideration will be to ensure that the mother's health is likely to be secure, and if not, the termination approach might be advised. Assuming the mother's health risk is low, however, then the counselling must focus on the risks to the foetus and the post-natal morbidity. The pregnant mother's choice should be respected and voluntary informed consent obtained. If the risk to the mother is considered negligible, non-intervention is dangerous to the foetus and EXIT is likely to result in survival with the ability to completely correct the anomaly, then it is reasonable to express this and if the parents still wish termination, to explain that this presents a relative conflict of interest for the team of professionals caring for the mother and foetus (Nelson et al. 1999).

Foetal Surgery

As antenatal diagnosis of head and neck pathologies becomes more sophisticated, and with advances in fibre-optic endoscopy and lasers, the prospect of successfully undertaking intrauterine foetal surgery to the airway has now been realised.

In the author's own series, the earliest attempt at a life-saving intrauterine foetal tracheostomy was undertaken. The foetus was diagnosed before 18 weeks gestation with CHAOS from complete laryngeal atresia. Initially, EXIT was planned at maturity, but the following week cardiac compression from lung expansion became life threatening and an endoscopic transuterine procedure to puncture the trachea and release the liquor was undertaken (Ward et al. 2000). This was not successful, but led to the development of more specialised instrumentation.

Procedures such as diagnostic foetoscopy, laser coagulation of intertwin placental vascular connections in twin–twin transfusion syndrome, foetal tracheal balloon occlusion in diaphragmatic hernia, laser perforation of posterior urethral valves, vocal cord division in CHAOS and, most recently, even coverage of spina bifida aperta, can be performed entirely percutaneously using minimally invasive foetoscopic techniques (Kohl 2004).

Such foetal surgery would only be indicated, currently, in rare situations. The risks to the mother should be small and the mortality risk to the foetus of non-intervention should be very high. Ethical consent and careful counselling must be undertaken. When the foetal intervention discussed is of unproven efficacy, parents must not be made to feel obliged to participate and the surgery should only be undertaken with full informed consent and as part of a clearly defined research protocol, already approved by an appropriate ethics board (Nelson et al. 1999).

Intrauterine Treatment of CHD and EXIT

Harrison (Mychaliska et al. 1997) first attempted to encourage lung development antenatally in CDH by clipping the trachea in utero, thereby obstructing the outflow of foetal lung liquor and expanding the lung volume. An EXIT birth was then required to release the clip at delivery. Iatrogenic tracheomalacia was one problem. He subsequently used a detachable balloon placed in the trachea (Harrison et al. 2001) and more recently, a collaborative group (the Fetal Endoscopic Tracheal Occlusion, FETO, task group), from the Catholic University of Leuven in Belgium and King's College Hospital in London, UK, under Professors Jan Deprest and Kypros Nicoaides, as well as Spanish, French and Californian colleagues, subsequently developed experience in the technique of intrauterine balloon placement within the foetal trachea (Deprest et al. 2004). The balloon obstruction promotes lung expansion and maturation and compresses the herniated abdominal contents downwards. A flexible Teflon cannula containing a pyramidal trocar is placed in the amniotic cavity through the abdominal and uterine walls and directed toward the foetal mouth. The trocar is withdrawn and the foetoscopic instruments are inserted: a sheath loaded with a fibre-optic endoscope and a catheter loaded with a detachable gold valve balloon. A side connector permits amnioinfusion with Hartmann's solution. After passing the endoscope through the vocal cords to the trachea, the catheter delivers the balloon into the trachea. The balloon is inflated with isotonic Omniscan, an MRI contrast agent.

The intratracheal balloon can subsequently be removed endoscopically at an EXIT procedure. The neonate is then stabilised in the Neonatal Intensive Care Unit and, if the foetal lung function and gases are compatible with survival, then the diaphragmatic hernia is repaired within the first few days of life (Jani et al. 2005b). This prospective study allowed long-term survival of approximately 50% of the neonates and survival of a greater percentage (64%), in the last 11 treated, towards the end of this series, when more experience had been gained. For comparison, of a group of CDH patients with similar severity of disease, whose parents declined the intervention, all but one died. Lung to head ratio and liver position allowed prediction of the outcome in this multicentre innovative research and confirmed control-matched study subjects. As the ratio of lung size to head size on ultrasound decreases, the prognosis worsens (Jani et al. 2005a).

Adequate balloon inflation is essential to achieve long-term tracheal occlusion. Experience has also been gained concerning the optimal time for the placement and removal of the balloon. Earlier balloon placement at 26 weeks allowed more successful lung maturation. EXIT balloon removal at about 36 weeks, involves needling and bursting the balloon and then retrieving it at EXIT tracheoscopy. The technique proved successful, unless there was early spontaneous onset of labour.

Newer Applications and the Future

There has been further evolution in the management of CDH. The Kings College Hospital and University of Leuven Group recently avoided the need for EXIT balloon retrieval by undertaking two transuterine foetal procedures: the first to endoscopically place the intratracheal balloon at 26 weeks, the second to burst it by transuterine needling at about 34 weeks. (without subsequent balloon retrieval). This allows a standard Caesarian section delivery later (Deprest et al. 2004, Jani et al. 2005b).

Foetal surgery can be undertaken entirely endoscopically or via a maternal hysterotomy, depending upon the condition. Apart from airway surgery, it has been shown to be possible in obstructive uropathy, congenital cystic adenomatous malformation of the lungs, sacrococcygeal teratomas, twin–twin transfusion syndrome and myelomeningocele (Farmer 2003). It seems likely that further advances in foetal surgery in the ENT regions will follow.

Summary for the Clinician

- The management of the neonatal airway is a multidisciplinary process. Antenatal diagnosis of potential airway obstruction is identified by ultrasound and MRI scanning in selected cases. Careful consideration of the risks to the mother and to the foetus should be made, and counselling the parents about these risks is important. The likely subsequent morbidity to the baby with congenital anomalies, if born successfully, must be discussed. The presence of coexisting non-airway anomalies will be a factor. Ethics require the foetus and the mother to be considered as two patients, in the best interests of both. Elective termination of pregnancy before 24 weeks gestation is one option. The EXIT procedure is indicated, however, when pre-natal diagnosis suggests that the upper airway is sufficiently compromised to lead to perinatal airway obstruction after natural or Caesarian birth. In such cases, at about 37–38 weeks, EXIT allows for safe and successful securing of the neonatal airway, by delivering the head and upper torso only, through a lower-uterine hysterotomy, while maintaining the placento-foetal blood flow and foetal oxygenation. The techniques described herein have proved reliable and successful. This procedure has greatly improved survival for babies with severe upper airway problems such as neck and thorax teratomas, laryngeal atresia and lymphangioma deeply involving the airway. Other applications have included the treatment of congenital diaphragmatic hernias by pre-natal balloon occlusion of the foetal trachea, with subsequent EXIT balloon retrieval.

References

1. Azizkhan RG, Haase GM, Applebaum H, et al. (1995) Diagnosis, management, and outcome of cervicofacial teratomas in neonates: a Childrens Cancer Group study. J Pediatr Surg 30:312–316

2. Campbell S, Lees C, Moscoso G, et al.(2005) Ultrasound antenatal diagnosis of cleft palate by a new technique: the 3D "reverse face" view. Ultrasound Obstet Gynecol 25:12–18

3. Clark KD, Viscomi CM, Lowell J, et al (2004) Nitroglycerin for relaxation to establish a fetal airway (EXIT procedure). Obstetrics Gynecol 103:1113–1115

4. Deprest J, Gratacos E, Nicolaides KH; FETO Task Group (2004) Fetoscopic tracheal occlusion (FETO) for severe congenital diaphragmatic hernia: evolution of a technique and preliminary results. Obstet Gynecol Surv 60:85–86

5. Farmer D (2003) Fetal surgery. BMJ 326:461–462

6. Glastonbury CM, Franzcr KA, (2002) Ultrafast MRI of the fetus. Australas Radiol 46:22–32

7. Harrison MR, Albanese CT, Hawgood SB, et al (2001) Fetoscopic temporary tracheal occlusion by means of detachable balloon for congenital diaphragmatic hernia. Am J Obstet Gynecol 185:730–733

8. Hartnick CJ, Rutter M, Lang F, et al (2002) Congenital high airway obstruction syndrome and airway reconstruction: an evolving paradigm. Arch Otolaryngol Head Neck Surg 128:567–570

9. Hendrick MH, Ferro M, Filly RM, et al (1994) Congenital high airway obstruction syndrome (CHAOS). J Pediatr Surg 29:271–274

10. Jani J, Benachi A, Keller R, et al (2005a) Lung-to-head ratio and liver position to predict outcome in early diagnosed isolated left sided diaphragmatic hernia fetuses: a multicenter study. Pediatr Res 58:386

11. Jani J, Gratacos E, Greenough A, et al; FETO Task Group (2005b) Percutaneous fetal endoscopic tracheal occlusion (FETO) for severe left-sided congenital diaphragmatic hernia. Clin Obstet Gynecol 48:910–922

12. Kerner B, Flaum E, Mathews H, et al (1998) Cervical teratoma: prenatal diagnosis and long-term follow-up. Prenat Diagn 18:51–59

13. Kohl T (2004) Fetoscopic surgery: where are we today? Curr Opin Anaesthesiol 17:315–321

14. Leichty KW, Crombleholme TM, Flake AW, et al (1997) Intrapartum airway management for giant fetal neck masses: the EXIT (ex-utero intrapartum treatment) procedure. Am J Obstet Gynaecol 177:870–874

15. MacKenzie, TC, Crombleholme TM, Flake AW (2002) The ex-utero intrapartum treatment. Curr Opin Pediatr 14:453–458

16. Malone FD, Ball RH, Nyberg DA, et al (2005) First-trimester septated cystic hygroma: prevalence, natural history, and pediatric outcome. Obstet Gynecol 106:288–294

17. Morrison G (2004) Antenatal balloon obstruction of the trachea for congenital diaphragmatic hernia and EXIT. Abstracts, 6th International Conference on Pediatric Otorhinolaryngology. Int J Pediatr Otorhinolaryngol 68:723–724

18. Mychaliska GB, Bealer JL, Graft NS, et al (1997) Operating on placental support: the ex-utero intrapartum treatment (EXIT) procedure. J Pediatr Surg 32:227–230

19. Nelson RM, Botkin JR, Levetown M, et al (1999) Fetal therapy – ethical considerations, American Academy of Paediatrics, Committee on bioethics. Paediatrics 103:1061–1063

20. Noah MMS, Norton ME, Sandberg P, et al (2002) Short-term maternal outcomes that are associated with the exit procedure, as compared with Cesarean delivery. Am J Obstet Gynecol 186:773–777

21. Schwindt J, Mittermayer C, Brugger PC, et al (2003) Planning EXIT-procedure with fetal magnetic resonance imaging. Ultrasound Obstet Gynecol 22:117

22. Stocks RMS, Egerman RS, Woodson GE, et al (1997) Airway management of neonates with antenatally detected head and neck anomalies. Arch Otolaryngol Head Neck Surg 123:641–644

23. Ward VMM, Langford K, Morrison G (2000) Prenatal diagnosis of airway compromise: EXIT (ex utero intra-partum treatment) and foetal airway surgery. Int J Ped Otorhinolaryngol 53:137–141

24. Zaretsky MV, Twickler DM (2003) Magnetic resonance imaging in obstetrics. Clin Obstet Gynecol 46:868–877

Chapter 10

The Immunocompromised Child

10

Mich Lajeunesse and Adam Finn

Core Messages

- Primary immunodeficiencies are under-diagnosed and can present to ENT practice.
- The type of infection may provide a clue to the type of underlying disease.
- A history of severe, prolonged, unusual or recurrent infections should alert to the diagnosis.
- Treatment will reduce morbidity and mortality from these conditions.
- Human immunodeficiency virus (HIV) is increasingly common amongst children.
- HIV infection can cause chronic upper respiratory tract symptoms and signs in its early stages.

Contents

Scope of Chapter

Many adults and children with an underlying immunodeficiency can present to the ENT surgeon. This chapter deals with the presentation, investigation and management of immunocompromised children in ENT practice. The reader should also consider the chapter on cystic fibrosis and primary ciliary dyskinesia. Both primary immunodeficiency (PID) and human immunodeficiency virus (HIV) infection are discussed, as PID is under-diagnosed and retroviral infection is an increasingly common problem in the UK. Immunodeficiency is a complex area of medicine and this chapter is not meant to be exhaustive, but instead we aim to outline basic principles to guide clinical practice.

Primary Immunodeficiency

The first PID was described over 50 years ago, and since then a profusion of different disorders has been identified. Novel immunodeficiencies continue to be discovered and with them, our knowledge of the immune system has grown (Primary Immunodeficiency Diseases. Report of an IUIS Scientific Committee 1999). Recent examples of novel immunodeficiency are the disorders of the gamma interferon (γIFN)/interleukin 12 (IL-12) signalling pathway that are associated with disseminated non-tuberculous mycobacterial infections (Picard and Casanova 2005). Some immunodeficiencies lead to a broad deficit in immunity, such as the T-cell deficiency associated with severe combined immunodeficiency (SCID), whilst others are quite specific and only permit opportunism by specific infections such as the γIFN/IL-12 pathway disorders. Because of this, even "big" holes in immunity can result in fairly specific spectra of infections, so that the clinical picture can be very informative even before any immunological tests have been performed.

Although severe immunodeficiencies are rare, at least half of children who present with histories that convince the specialist that an underlying problem is present, or at least that some form of management is warranted, do not have any demonstrable abnormality of immune function. These children clearly have an individual susceptibility to specific infections, which will vary according to polymorphisms in genes important for immune function and regulation (Sanders et al. 1994) as well as the "tissue typing" human leukocyte antigen (HLA) formation. In fact, such variation in susceptibility is normal within species as a "deliberate" evolutionary way of preserving diversity and defence against microorganisms. With advances in immunological understanding, the functional implications of more of these polymorphisms may be elucidated in the next few years. An interesting recent example is the association of respiratory papillomatosis with the HLA DRB1 haplotype (Gelder et al. 2003).

Natural History if Untreated

If undiagnosed, some immunodeficiencies will lead to repeated invasive infections and death. Others cause chronic infection, local tissue damage and long-term morbidity. There can be a wide spectrum of severity even among children with the same disorder. Many children will have significant problems, with recurrent infection leading to multiple hospital admissions and repeat courses of antibiotics, causing missed school and loss of parents' working time because of infection (Chapel 1994). They may also be seen in several different clinics for complications of infection such as sinusitis and bronchiectasis. We know of one case of X-linked agammaglobulinaemia (XLA) diagnosed by an astute ENT house officer at the time of admission clerking for grommet reinsertion. The child was 8 years old at the time of diagnosis and had been chronically and severely ill for 5 years. The potential complications of PIDs are legion and are outlined in Table 10.1.

Table 10.1 Complications of primary immunodeficiencies

General
Poor growth/failure to thrive
Recurrent fevers
Protracted infections
Respiratory
Bronchiectasis
Complicated pneumonias (i.e. pneumatocoele)
ENT
Recurrent and chronic rhinitis and sinusitis
Recurrent otitis media often with perforation
Gastrointestinal
Chronic diarrhoea (e.g. viral, *Giardia* and *Cryptosporidium*)
Malabsorption and failure to thrive
Hepatitis, biliary cirrhosis and cholangitis
Splenomegaly
Granuloma formation and atypical mycobacterial infection
Bones and joints
Septic arthritis and osteomyelitis – especially relapsing, unusual organisms
Chronic sterile arthritis
Blood/Bone marrow/Lymphoid system
Iron deficiency anaemia
Anaemia of chronic illness (normocytic)
Autoimmune haemolytic anaemia
Aplastic anaemia
Idiopathic thrombocytopaenic purpura
Lymphoma
Central Nervous System/Eyes
Chronic meningoencephalitis (e.g. enteroviral)
Uveitis and keratoconjunctivitis
Skin
Recurrent abscesses
Cold abscess formation
Severe eczema and other chronic rashes

10

Prevalence and Incidence

As a group, the PIDs remain under-diagnosed and this is especially true among ethnic minorities where the diagnosis is often overlooked. A common misconception is that PID is a rare condition. Individually, some forms are extremely rare; however, selective IgA deficiency (sIgAD) is relatively common, with around 1 in 600 individuals in the UK affected. Fortunately, sIgAD often causes only mild symptoms, but its consequences can be significant for some people and it should not be ignored.

Another reason for under-diagnosis is that many antibody deficiencies, and especially those caused by common variable immunodeficiency (CVID), do not develop and manifest until early adulthood. As such, it is not surprising that many people with PID already have chronic complications arising from multiple infections by the time of diagnosis.

PIDs are more common than you would think and can be diagnosed in adults as well as children.

Table 10.2 Ten warning signs of primary immunodeficiency (http://www.info4pi.org)

1. Eight or more new ear infections within 1 year.
2. Recurrent, deep skin or organ abscesses.
3. Two or more serious sinus infections within 1 year.
4. Persistent thrush in mouth or elsewhere on skin, after age of 1 year.
5. Two or more months on antibiotics with little effect.
6. Need for intravenous antibiotics to clear infections.
7. Two or more pneumonias within 1 year.
8. Two or more deep-seated infections.
9. Failure of an infant to gain weight or grow normally.
10. A family history of primary immunodeficiency.

Aetiology and Genetics

Many immunodeficiencies are inherited in an autosomal recessive or X-linked manner. An example is XLA, the first PID to be described and a severe antibody deficiency. The defect is in the Bruton's tyrosine kinase (*btk*) gene on the X chromosome. Absence of BTK protein leads to a defect in B-cell maturation so that the child has no functioning B cells able to synthesise antibody (Conley et al. 2005).

When PID is suspected, clues can be gained from a careful family history, and in particular, a family history of consanguinity should be sought. This is much more socially acceptable in certain communities than in others. Other pointers suggestive of immunodeficiency include siblings or relatives who have died, often in infancy from infection. An exception to the recessive rule is the complement deficiencies, which are often co-dominantly inherited. In these disorders, parents will be carriers and will have half the normal levels of circulating components and be asymptomatic, whilst the affected child has none. Similarly, mothers who are carriers of X-linked chronic granulomatous disease (CGD) may also have a significant proportion of neutrophils with low oxidative burst function. Although they do not usually exhibit the classic features of the immunodeficiency, they may have characteristic symptoms, such as a characteristic facial lupus-like rash.

Assessment and Diagnosis

Diagnosing children with immunodeficiency can be a difficult business and all children with suspected significant immunodeficiency should be referred to a paediatric immunologist for assessment, regardless of any prior immune work up that has been undertaken. Many paediatric ENT consultants have good working relationships with local immunologists, and some even run joint clinics together.

Children with immunodeficiency present with severe, prolonged, unusual or recurrent (SPUR) infections. Other common signposts to PID are given in Table 10.2. The nature of the infections will often provide a clue as to the type of immunodeficiency. This typical infection pattern is discussed in more detail below. There is often more than one clue to an immunodeficiency within the history.

Severe

The severity of infection is often out of proportion to the nature of the disease. For instance, a 4-year-old boy who required intravenous antibiotics to treat a sinusitis can be considered as a severe event because most cases of sinusitis are mild in this age group and improve with oral antibiotics. Severe infections will often spread to other local structures such as underlying bone or meninges, to distant sites such as joints and liver, or cause invasive infection and sepsis.

Prolonged

Prolonged infections should similarly be of concern, as should those that relapse off therapy and require several courses of antibiotics to cure. An example would be a child with hypogammaglobulinaemia presenting with prolonged or relapsing, bilateral discharging otitis media.

Unusual

Unusual infections are those not normally seen in that patient population (e.g. the boy with sinusitis) and those caused by opportunistic infections. Opportunistic organisms only rarely cause disease in the immune-competent host. The best known example is that of *Pneumocystis* pneumonia in patients with T-cell deficiencies. However, chronic ENT infections are frequently caused by polymicrobial infections including anaerobes and *Pseudomonas*, which makes the identification of an opportunist organism all the more difficult. Unusual infections also relate to those that do not often occur in that age group: for instance – a 6-week-old boy with mastoiditis caused by *Escherichia coli* infection.

Recurrent

Children with immunodeficiency experience episodes of recurrent infection. These include reactivation of infections such a herpes zoster, where a multidermatomal pattern is classical. For immunodeficiency, what constitutes a recurrent upper respiratory tract (URT) infection is difficult to define and requires experience and judgement. Most pre-school children have on average six to eight URT infections per year and this will be modulated by attendance at day care or pre-school, and elder siblings bringing home infections. Many children will have recurrent perforation of a damaged tympanic membrane over the course of a winter without time for healing in between, and this in itself is not suggestive of immunodeficiency. It is rather those children who present with recurrent perforating bilateral middle ear disease, or those with recurrent symptoms not explained by temporal or anatomic factors that should be considered. The severity of such recurrent infection can be further assessed in two ways, by its impact on schooling, and by its affect upon the child's growth. A history of an additional separate episode of invasive infection such as a pneumonia, meningitis or orbital cellulitis in this setting should also arouse suspicion.

Examination

Children with suspected immunodeficiency should be examined fully for evidence of chronic infection. Growth parameters should be plotted on centile charts. Pointers to the diagnosis include the presence of clubbing and chest signs, whilst absence of lymphoid tissue, or the converse situation of organomegaly may also be seen. Children may have signs associated with a congenital syndrome associated with PID such as severe eczema in Wiskott Aldrich and hyper-IgE syndromes, and conjunctival telangiectasia seen in older children with ataxia telangiectasia.

Classification

The PIDs are classified according to the defective part of the immune system affected by the condition or, where this is not yet known, the associated syndrome. We will discuss only the major types of PID that could present to ENT practice. The immune deficiencies that lead to ENT infection include antibody deficiency, neutrophil disorders and complement deficiency. A list of the potential commoner PIDs presenting to ENT are given in Table 10.3.

Table 10.3 Immunodeficiency presenting to ENT practice

Antibody deficiency
X-Linked agammaglobulinaemia (Bruton)
Common variable immunodeficiency
Selective IgA deficiency[a]
Hyper IgM syndrome (CD40 ligand deficiency)[b]
Immunoglobulin G subclass deficiencies (maturational defect)
Complement disorders
C3 deficiency (the most common)
Mannan binding lectin deficiency[a]
Neutropaenias and neutrophil disorders
Autoimmune neutropenia of infancy
Cyclic neutropenia
Kostmann syndrome (severe primary neutropenia)
Chronic granulomatous disease
Other Syndromes
di George syndrome (22q11 deletion, velocardiofacial; T-cell deficiency)
Down's syndrome[a] (associated immunodeficiencies often poorly defined)
Heterotaxy (asplenism)
Ataxia telangiectasia (antibody deficiencies, lymphomas)
Wiskott Aldrich syndrome (antibody deficiencies, low small platelets, lymphomas)
Hyper IgE (Job) syndrome (rashes and abscesses)

[a]Common
[b]Also involves T-cell function – may present with *Pneumocystis*

10

Antibody Deficiencies

Children with antibody deficiencies are prone to infection with encapsulated bacteria. These organisms are common causes of URT infections and include pneumococcus, *Haemophilus* and *Moraxella*. For this reason, children with antibody deficiencies frequently have URT problems. Encapsulated bacteria pose a particular problem to the antibody-deficient child because the B-cell antibody response against the polysaccharide antigens of the bacterial capsule is independent of T-cell help. The defective B cell is left to fend for itself and is unable to mount an adequate protective response. This T-independent response is immature in normal children, thus reducing their response to polysaccharide vaccines, and does not reach adult levels until at least the fourth birthday. For this reason, the majority of respiratory tract and invasive infections caused by encapsulated bacteria occur in children with no demonstrable immunodeficiency. However, antibody-deficient children are particularly prone to frequent, recurrent, persistent and relapsing infections, which may single them out from the rest.

Antibody deficiencies often become symptomatic at between 3 and 9 months of age as the levels of transplacentally acquired maternal antibody wane. This period of life is associated with low immunoglobulin concentrations in normal children (Fig. 10.1), but they soon recover and attain adult levels. Thus, when interpreting immunoglobulin concentrations, it is important to consider the age of the child and use age-specific normal ranges. Some children may lack a single antibody class, as in IgA deficiency, whilst in others all classes may be absent (XLA) or there may be combinations of low isotypes, for example IgA and IgG subclass 2 as commonly seen in CVID. Some children have less marked deficiency involving the four subclasses of IgG. Interpretation of these tests can be difficult and can require specialist input. A child should not be labelled as abnormal unless levels at least two standard deviations below mean levels for age are present on two or more successive occasions in the presence of significant clinical concerns.

Complement Deficiencies

The complement cascade is part of the innate immune system and is involved in the inflammatory process and the clearance of foreign antigens. The classical, alternate and lectin activation pathways channel through the C3 component and can trigger the cascade. Children with C2 and C3 deficiency can present in a manner similar to those with antibody deficiency. Deficiencies of the later complement components (C6–C9) predispose to infection with meningococcus. Any single component deficiency will lead to a decrease in the total haemolytic complement (CH_{50} and $APCH_{50}$), which is thus a good screening test. Deficiencies can also predispose to autoimmune disease.

Mannose-Binding Lectin Deficiency

Mannose-binding lectin (MBL) is an acute-phase plasma protein that binds to bacterial carbohydrates in the cell wall and capsule (Petersen et al. 2001). Bound MBL is capable of triggering the complement cascade via the lectin pathway. MBL is part of the innate immune system. Partial deficiencies are common. MBL deficiency has been associated with an increased risk of infection, post-operative infection, infection following chemotherapy, intensive therapy unit morbidity and systemic lupus erythematosus. MBL-deficiency-associated infection is seen when associated with minor humoral immunodeficiencies such as those of the IgG subclasses (Fevang et al. 2005). Whilst

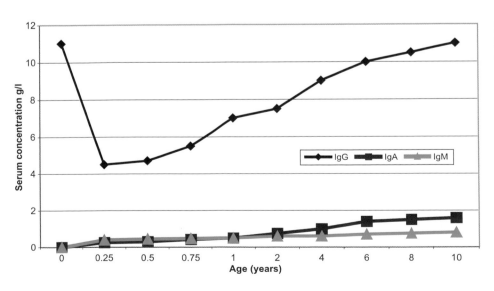

Fig. 10.1 Immunoglobulin levels in children vary with age

MBL has been associated with increased risk of infection, over 90% of those with low MBL concentrations have no such predisposition. Thus, the significance of MBL in the predisposition to infection has not been fully elucidated and remains an emerging area of immunology.

Neutrophil Disorders

Neutrophil disorders can be classified as abnormalities either in numbers or of function (Lakshman and Finn 2001). Children should have a full blood count and film to exclude congenital neutropaenias; a count should also be performed when the child is acutely unwell, as some neutropaenias are cyclical in nature. Even these tests may miss some cases, necessitating regular blood counts three times weekly for 6 weeks when concerns are high.

Children with disorders of neutrophil function such as CGD present with abscess formation, often deep-seated, and infection with catalase-positive organisms such as *Staphylococcus aureus*, *Nocardia*, *Serratia* and *Burkholderia* (Rosenzweig and Holland 2004). Invasive fungal infection with *Aspergillus* may also cause problems.

Laboratory Tests

Any child having a work up for immunodeficiency should be discussed with a paediatric immunologist. This is because the results are often difficult to interpret and absence of abnormal results does not exclude the diagnosis (Wahn 1995). A basic screen is shown in Table 10.4. Other tests may be required depending upon the clinical presentation. These second-line investigations are best dealt with in a specialist clinic and in liaison with a clinical immunology laboratory.

In all children with suspected immunodeficiency, early use of prophylactic antibiotics should be considered. This may best be done in discussion with a paediatric immunologist. Those who have had severe invasive infection or are chronically unwell should be referred for specialist opinion as a matter of urgency.

Treatment

Treatment will depend upon the nature of the immunodeficiency, but for antibody deficiencies there are two main avenues of treatment: prophylactic antibiotics and replacement immunoglobulin therapy.

Prophylactic Antibiotics

Agents that have been used for prophylaxis include amoxicillin, cotrimoxazole, and macrolides such as clarithomicin and azithromicin. Use should be weighed against local resistance patterns and side effects of therapy. We use cotrimoxazole as a first-line prophylaxis (Smith and Finn 1999). Children with suspected hyposplenism should be commenced on penicillin V or amoxicillin (Castagnola and Fioredda 2003).

Immunoglobulin Replacement Therapy

Human normal immunoglobulin is a blood product taken from pooled donors. It is screened during production for blood-borne viruses such as HIV and hepatitis B and C virus. Some of these viruses are also denatured during the manufacturing process. The risk of viral transmission is extremely low, but there remains a theoretical and unquantifiable risk, as with all blood products, for transmission of unknown agents or spongiform encephalopathies. Children with antibody deficiency can receive replacement infusions either intravenously or subcutaneously. Intravenous immunoglobulin is administered every 3 weeks or so and requires a venous cannula and often day ward admission for infusion. Some families are able to manage this at home. Subcutaneous therapy is given once a week and many parents are able to give these at home to their children with appropriate training. Subcutaneous therapy has fewer side effects during and after infusion and is generally preferred by parents (Gaspar et al. 1998).

Immunisation

Live vaccines are best avoided whilst an immunodeficiency is being investigated. However, on the whole we consider that immunisation may be beneficial, even in children with antibody deficiency (who may not make adequate antibody responses to vaccines) because of the cellular priming aspects of the immunisation. In addition to the routine schedule, we advocate an annual influenza vaccine and pneumococcal conjugate vaccine (PCV-7).

Table 10.4 First-line investigation of suspected immunodeficiency. *ESR* Erythrocyte sedimentation rate, *CRP* C-reactive protein

Full blood count, differential and film for Howell-Jolly and Heinz bodies (review previous blood counts for neutro- and lymphopaenia)
Liver function tests – to exclude low albumin protein losing states
Immunoglobulin classes G, A, M
ESR and CRP

This vaccine is different to the standard polysaccharide vaccine for adults (Lajeunesse 2004). Its conjugate technology enables good immune responses in pre-school children. In theory, PCV-7 should also protect against recurrent otitis media. To date this has been shown when it is added to the infant primary schedule (Black et al. 2000). However, the only study to address its use in children with recurrent acute otitis media did not demonstrate protection (Veenhoven et al. 2003) and so at present we would not recommend it PCV-7 for use in recurrent acute otitis media until further data are available.

Bone Marrow Transplantation

Bone marrow transplant is effective for those with SCID and some other forms of PID. Its use is limited to two quaternary centres in the UK. Depending on the transplant match, children may experience graft versus host disease and require long-term immunosuppression. Equally, failure of engraftment may lead to chronic cytopaenias and their attendant problems. Thus, some children may experience long-term problems with immunosuppression despite transplantation.

Gene Therapy

This is a novel and rapidly expanding area of clinical expertise (Chinen and Puck 2004). To date, trials have been conducted on several SCID variants including adenosine deaminase deficiency, although only a handful of children have been treated in this way. Whilst there have been some early successes, there have also been reports of haematologic malignancy following gene therapy, and the technique remains highly experimental.

Secondary Immunodeficiency

The majority of causes of acquired immunodeficiency in childhood are iatrogenic, due to immunosuppressive drug therapy. Children with inflammatory conditions are increasingly being treated with immunosuppression such as azathiprone, tacrolimus and cyclosporin. There are the thousands of children who receive regular inhaled steroid as nasal sprays for rhinitis or for asthma. In sufficient doses, these may lead to immunosuppression as well as suppression of the adrenal axis leading to poor growth and Addisonian crisis if therapy is abruptly withdrawn (Sim et al. 2003). Other causes of secondary immunodeficiency include protein-losing states such as nephrotic syndrome or a protein-losing enteropathy, and acquired hyposplenism following surgical excision after trauma or due to sickle cell disease. A list of causes of secondary immunodeficiency is given in Table 10.5.

Table 10.5 Causes of acquired immunodeficiency in children. *HIV* Human immunodeficiency virus

Physiological
Preterm neonates
Infection
HIV infection
Chronic disease
Diabetes mellitus – types I and II
Burns
Cirrhosis
Chronic renal failure
Juvenile idiopathic arthritis
Malnutrition (may itself be secondary to underlying gut pathology)
Following solid organ and bone marrow transplant
Haematological
Sickle cell anaemia
Leukaemia and lymphoma
Disseminated malignancy (neuroblastoma)
Hyposplenism
Iatrogenic
Glucocorticoid steroids (oral, topical or inhaled)
Immunosuppressants (cyclosporin, azathioprine, tacrolimus)
Following chemo- and radiotherapy

Human Immunodeficiency Virus

HIV infection amongst children is an increasingly common problem in the developed world. Almost all HIV infection in childhood is acquired through mother-to-child transmission (Sharland et al. 2002). This can occur at several stages either during pregnancy, labour and delivery, or from breastfeeding. If the mother's infection is identified during pregnancy, effective strategies are available to prevent mother-to-child transmission. However, children born outside the UK or those whose mothers have not been screened during pregnancy are still at risk of infection and the condition should not be overlooked.

Description

HIV is a retrovirus that first infected humans some time in the last century, probably evolving from an African monkey retrovirus. It is commonly transmitted through blood and body fluids – breast milk, semen and vaginal secretions, but not saliva. Thus, the infection is spread through both vaginal and anal sexual intercourse, oral sex, blood products (before routine screening occurred in the developed world) and by sharing needles amongst recreational drug users. The virus infects cells bearing the CD4, CCR5 and CXCR4 co-receptors. Such cells include T helper cells, and dendritic and glial cells. Once infected, the virus cannot be eradicated. The viral polymerase responsible for replication (reverse transcriptase) is prone to error. Thus, HIV has a high spontaneous mutation rate that allows selection of mutants resistant to environmental pressures such as antiretroviral drugs and immunisation. Continued viral replication leads to immune compromise with exhaustion of the pool of CD4 cells produced by the bone marrow. An immunodeficiency ensues that leads to opportunistic infection and malignancy and eventually death of the host. The time to progression varies between individuals and many remain asymptomatic for several years.

Natural History if Untreated and Complications

Two broad groups of children with HIV infection are seen. Rapid progressors develop severe disease in the 1st year of life. These children have life-threatening opportunistic infections such as cytomegalovirus pneumonitis or *Pneumocystis jiroveci* pneumonia. They have signs of neurodevelopmental delay or loss of developmental milestones and failure to thrive. Once they have presented to medical services, the diagnosis is usually in

little doubt. Left untreated they will die, although the use of antiretroviral therapy (ART) does not provide relief for all. Roughly 10% will still die of acquired immune deficiency syndrome in the first few years of life. In contrast, slow progressors will have few if any symptoms and will not have had an opportunistic infection. Left untreated, these children may remain asymptomatic until their teens. However, eventually they will succumb to opportunistic or recurrent infection or malignancy as their immune system fails. It is these slow-progressing children who are more likely to present to an ENT clinic.

Prevalence

HIV infection amongst children in the UK remains rare. To date, around 3000 children are known to be infected in the UK. This figure has increased since the early 1990s. The geographic distribution of children has also changed with the dispersal of asylum seekers and their families from London to most areas of the UK. Although the majority of children will have some parental link to sub-Saharan Africa or South East Asia, this is not always the case. HIV cannot reliably be inferred or excluded by a child's race or travel history.

Classification

HIV disease is categorised according to symptoms and signs (Caldwell et al. 1994) (summarised in Table 10.6), although in practice the child's CD4 cell count and retroviral load have replaced the slow deterioration to end-stage disease seen prior to effective treatment (Table 10.7). Table 10.6 shows that many of the first signs of HIV infection involve the ENT system, and early recognition at this stage will permit treatment to be started before immunodeficiency occurs.

Table. 10.6 Clinical categories for children with human immunodeficiency virus (HIV) infection. Summarised from Caldwell et al (1994) and modified to show main systemic and ENT features only. *HSV* Herpes simplex virus, *TB* tuberculosis, *PCP Pneumocystis jiroveci* pneumonia, *CNS* central nervous system

Category	Symptoms and signs
N: Not symptomatic	Children who have no signs or symptoms
A: Mildly symptomatic	Cervical lymphadenopathy and parotitis (+/– parotid swelling) with no systemic symptoms
B: Moderately symptomatic	Chronic oropharyngeal candidiasis, HSV stomatitis, zoster, and invasive bacterial infections, lymphocytic interstitial pneumonitis
C: Severely symptomatic	Recurrent serious bacterial infections, TB, opportunistic infections such as PCP, disseminated non-tuberculous mycobacteria, lymphoma (often primary CNS), encephalopathy and developmental regression, wasting syndrome with chronic diarrhoea (e.g. *Cryptosporidium*).

Table 10.7 Immunologic categories based on age-specific CD4+ T-lymphocyte counts and percent of total lymphocytes

Immune category		Age of child		
		<12 months cells/μL (%)	1–5 years cells/μL (%)	6–12 years cells/μL (%)
No suppression	1	≥1500 (≥25)	≥1000 (≥25)	≥500 (≥25)
Moderate	2	750–1499 (15–24)	500–999 (15–24)	200–499 (15–24)
Severe	3	<750 (<15)	<500 (<15)	<200 (<15)

Clinical Assessment

Some of the first signs of symptomatic HIV infection in children are chronic URT infections, cervical or axillary lymphadenopathy and chronic or perforated otitis media. Infected children may also have bilaterally enlarged parotid glands, sometimes markedly so, with a raised serum amylase. Dental caries is a frequent finding and often requires multiple extractions. They may have recurrent or persistent oral candidiasis, which outside the newborn period, is strongly suggestive of a T-cell disorder.

Children with suspected HIV infection should have a thorough history and examination, including details of pregnancy, delivery and mode of feeding for the 1st year. Any infections should be documented and risk factors for co-infection with tuberculosis considered. A full immunisation history should be taken. The child's height and weight should be plotted on a growth chart.

Diagnosis

Testing for HIV should be undertaken carefully. This is because the diagnosis of HIV in a child will also reveal the mother's diagnosis. Such inadvertent breach of confidentiality can lead to social pillory and has forced families in our practice to relocate schools and homes. This is an almost unique situation in medicine. The implications of testing the child should be made clear to the mother prior to testing. Some parents will not wish other members of the family to be involved initially, even their own partners. This is because HIV infection carries an enormous social stigma, especially in cultures where it is highly prevalent. Confidentiality should be respected. For this reason pre-pubertal children tend to not know that they are HIV positive, as they are unable to understand the full social implications of their diagnosis, and may inadvertently breach their own confidentiality and that of other family members. In contrast, it is important that teenagers know their diagnosis.

Consideration should be made as to how the test results are given. We arrange for the mother and child to be seen in clinic 1 week after testing to receive the results.

This prevents the diagnosis being given over the phone, and the stress to the family of a hastily arranged appointment when the child turns out to be infected. HIV testing is a delicate business and for these reasons we feel that paediatric HIV tests should be performed by trained staff wherever possible.

Following appropriate discussion, an HIV test should be taken along with the standard investigations outlined in Table 10.4. We would advise commencing the child on a prophylactic dose of cotrimoxazole to reduce the risk of pneumocystis and bacterial infections whilst the diagnosis is being established. An urgent referral should be made to a paediatrician experienced in the care of children with HIV infection even before the diagnosis has been established, to assist with investigation and acute management.

The virology tests required for diagnosis vary according to the age of the child. Children over 18 months old can be diagnosed by HIV serology. Less than this age the situation may be complicated by the presence of passively transferred maternal HIV antibodies. Thus, the child may be antibody positive but not infected. Test results may be difficult to interpret and should be discussed with a virologist or paediatric immunologist. HIV infection in this age group ideally should be undertaken using polymerase chain reaction (PCR) for pro-viral DNA, although more widely available RNA PCR tests ("viral load") may also be useful.

Other routine investigations can suggest undiagnosed HIV infection. These include raised serum amylase, globulin fraction and IgG. Blood counts may show thrombocytopaenia and lymphopaenia. Children may also have low CD4 counts, but these should never be taken as a surrogate for HIV testing for the reasons that we have just indicated and because they lack specificity.

Treatment

Over the last 10 years, the advent of ART has revolutionised the management of HIV infection (Sharland et al. 2004). There are now four licensed drug classes of ART; each acts upon a different aspect of the viral replication cycle. The use of three or more antiretroviral agents in combination can arrest viral replication and allow immune reconstitution. This is known as highly active ART (HAART). Many HIV-infected children live healthy lives and are progressing on to adulthood.

Despite these advances, problems remain. Adherence to therapy must be absolute (>95%) to ensure success. Rigid adherence to treatment is vital because viral resistance may emerge rapidly when drug levels are below the threshold of viral replication (Mullen et al. 2002). Because of the nature of the virus, drug resistance is selected almost automatically. The medicines are often not formulated for children; tablets are large and syrups foultasting, and most of the medicines have unpleasant side effects.

In spite of advances in therapy, it is extremely difficult for children to adhere to current HAART regimens. ART has multiple drug interactions as well as side effects, such that careful monitoring and support of the family is required.

10

Summary for the Clinician

- PIDs are more common than expected. They should be considered in any child presenting with a SPUR infection or organ damage following infection. Children should be commenced on antibiotic prophylaxis prior to referral to a paediatric immunologist. Baseline investigations may be normal in some immunodeficiencies. HIV infection can also present with ENT problems. Children may be otherwise asymptomatic. Diagnosis of a child also discloses the mother's status and this should be borne in mind when considering testing. For all forms of immunodeficiency, ENT surgeons should work in partnership with their colleagues in paediatrics and immunology.

References

1. Black S, Shinefield H, Fireman B, et al (2000) Efficacy, safety and immunogenicity of heptavalent pneumococcal conjugate vaccine in children. Northern California Kaiser Permanente Vaccine Study Center Group. Pediatr Infect Dis J 19:187–195

2. Caldwell MB, Oxtoby MJ, Simonds RJ, et al (1994) Revised classification system for human immunodeficiency virus infection in children less than 13 years of age. MMWR Morb Mortal Wkly Rep 43:1–10

3. Castagnola E, Fioredda F (2003) Prevention of life-threatening infections due to encapsulated bacteria in children with hyposplenia or asplenia: a brief review of current recommendations for practical purposes. Eur J Haematol 71:319–326

4. Chapel HM (1994) Consensus on diagnosis and management of primary antibody deficiencies. Consensus Panel for the Diagnosis and Management of Primary Antibody Deficiencies. BMJ 308:581–585

5. Chinen J, Puck JM (2004) Perspectives of gene therapy for primary immunodeficiencies. Curr Opin Allergy Clin Immunol 4:523–527

6. Conley ME, Broides A, Hernandez-Trujillo V, et al (2005) Genetic analysis of patients with defects in early B-cell development. Immunol Rev 203:216–234

7. Fevang B, Mollnes TE, Holm AM, et al.(2005) Common variable immunodeficiency and the complement system; low mannose-binding lectin levels are associated with bronchiectasis. Clin Exp Immunol 142:576–584

8. Gaspar J, Gerritsen B, Jones A (1998) Immunoglobulin replacement treatment by rapid subcutaneous infusion. Arch Dis Child 79:48–51

9. Gelder CM, Williams OM, Hart KW, et al (2003) HLA class II polymorphisms and susceptibility to recurrent respiratory papillomatosis. J Virol 77:1927–1939

10. Lajeunesse M (2004) Pneumococcal vaccines: the issues for primary care. Airways J 2:152–155

11. Lakshman R, Finn A (2001) Neutrophil disorders and their management. J Clin Pathol 54:7–19

12. Mullen J, Leech S, O'Shea S, et al (2002) Antiretroviral drug resistance among HIV-1 infected children failing treatment. J Med Virol 68:299–304

13. Petersen SV, Thiel S, Jensenius JC (2001) The mannanbinding lectin pathway of complement activation: biology and disease association. Mol Immunol 38:133–149

14. Picard C, Casanova JL (2005) Novel primary immunodeficiencies. Adv Exp Med Biol 568:89–99

15. Primary immunodeficiency diseases. Report of an IUIS Scientific Committee. International Union of Immunological Societies (1999) Clin Exp Immunol 118 1:1–28

16. Rosenzweig SD, Holland SM (2004) Phagocyte immunodeficiencies and their infections. J Allergy Clin Immunol 113:620–626

17. Sanders LA, van de Winkel JG, Rijkers GT (1994) Fc gamma receptor IIa (CD32) heterogeneity in patients with recurrent bacterial respiratory tract infections. J Infect Dis 170:854–861

18. Sharland M, Blanche S, Castelli G (2004) PENTA guidelines for the use of antiretroviral therapy, 2004. HIV Med 5:61–86

19. Sharland M, Gibb DM, Tudor-Williams G (2002) Advances in the prevention and treatment of paediatric HIV infection in the United Kingdom. Arch Dis Child 87:178–180

20. Sim D, Griffiths A, Armstrong D (2003) Adrenal suppression from high-dose inhaled fluticasone propionate in children with asthma. Eur Respir J 21:633–636

21. Smith J, Finn A (1999) Antimicrobial prophylaxis. Arch Dis Child 80:388–392

22. Veenhoven R, Bogaert D, Uiterwaal C, et al (2003) Effect of conjugate pneumococcal vaccine followed by polysaccharide pneumococcal vaccine on recurrent acute otitis media: a randomised study. Lancet 361:2189–2195

23. Wahn U (1995) Evaluation of the child with suspected primary immunodeficiency. Pediatr Allergy Immunol 6:71–79

Cystic Fibrosis and Primary Ciliary Dyskinesia

11

Andrew Bush and Jonny Harcourt

Core Messages

- Efficient mucociliary clearance is vital to the health of the respiratory tract.
- Defects may present to the ENT surgeon as chronic rhinosinusitis, nasal polyps or otitis media with effusion.
- A child with nasal polyps should have a sweat test, and if negative, tests for primary ciliary dyskinesia (PCD).
- Also consider specialist unit referral for severe unresponsive rhinosinusitis prior to surgery.
- A history of rhinitis and wet cough since birth suggests PCD, in which condition nearly 50% have situs inversus (mirror-image arrangement of the organs).
- Grommets are contraindicated in PCD since they lead to chronic discharging ears.
- ENT operations in children with mucociliary problems need collaboration with experienced anaesthetists and medical staff plus physiotherapists.

Contents

Introduction

Cystic fibrosis (CF) and primary ciliary dyskinesia (PCD) are inflammatory airway diseases that may impinge on ENT practice in one of two ways. Firstly, a child thought previously to be healthy may present to the ENT surgeon with features that are suggestive of one of these conditions. Such a child should be referred for a diagnostic work up to a specialist unit. Secondly, a child known to have one of these conditions may be referred for treatment, either of a known complication, or of an unrelated condition.

Cystic Fibrosis – The Disease

Molecular Defect

The gene for CF was localised to the long arm of chromosome 7 in 1989. It encodes for a multifunctional protein of 168,138 Daltons, coded by 27 exons, the CF transmembrane regulator, CFTR. The gene product undergoes complex post-translational processing, leading to different classes of mutation, which have prognostic significance (Table 11.1). The severe mutations, usually with pancreatic insufficiency, are classes 1–3, and these patients as a group have significantly poorer survival. These classes are of more than mere academic interest; they are the basis of the exploration of class-specific therapies. For example, gentamicin nose drops have been shown to bypass the premature stop codons in the class 1 mutation such as W1282X (Wilschanski et al. 2003), whereas molecular chaperones such as the class V phosphodiesterase inhibitor sildenafil may promote the transfer of the class 2 mutation ΔF_{508} CFTR to the apical cell membrane from the endoplasmic reticulum, where it would otherwise be ubiquitinated and destroyed (Dormer et al. 2005).

Pathophysiology

Lung Disease

The CF baby is born with essentially normal lungs. The link between CFTR dysfunction and the cycles of infection and inflammation that lead to bronchiectasis and eventually result in death is not completely clear (below). The current likeliest mechanisms are proposed by the so-called "low volume" hypothesis (Boucher et al. 2004). This proposes that the fundamental abnormality is the hyperabsorption of sodium by the sodium channel ENaC. Normally, the activity of airway ENaC is inhibited by CFTR. It is proposed in CF that uncontrolled ENaC activity results in a secondary hyperabsorption of water, with dehydration of the airway surface and a loss in height of the airway surface liquid. The consequence of this is that cilia are unable to function normally, lacking the necessary height of the periciliary fluid for the recovery stroke, and the mucociliary escalator function is lost. The most compelling evidence for this hypothesis is that the CF mouse is in general a very poor model of human CF lung disease, but a much better model is a CF mouse with normal CFTR function, but which has been genetically manipulated to over-express the β-subunit of the ENaC gene (Mall et al. 2004). The issue is still debated, and the interested reader is referred to a recent monograph (Bush et al. 2006).

Table 11.1 Classes of cystic fibrosis (CF) transmembrane conductance regulator (CFTR) mutation

Mutation class	Nature of defect	Example of genotype
Class 1	No synthesis of CFTR mRNA	Nonsense, G542X Frame shift, 394delTT
Class 2	Block in intracellular processing of CFTR protein, leading to destruction before reaching the apical membrane	ΔF_{508}
Class 3	Block in regulation of CFTR on arrival at the apical cell membrane	G551D
Class 4	Altered conductance of the ion channel function of CFTR at the apical cell membrane	R117H
Class 5	Reduced synthesis of CFTR	A455E Alternative splicing, 3849+10 kbC → T

Gastrointestinal and Other Disease Manifestations

By contrast with the lungs, babies with two severe mutations are usually pancreatic insufficient from birth, due to destruction of the exocrine pancreas. The pathophysiology is complex, but thought to include blockage of the pancreatic duct and autodigestion of exocrine cells. In later life, the islets of Langerhans atrophy, causing initially an insulin deficiency, and subsequently frank diabetes. The liver may be affected by a focal biliary cirrhosis, in part due to the effects of inspissated secretions. The loss of electrolytes in sweat, the basis of the most useful diagnostic test for CF (below) may also lead to heat exhaustion and dehydration.

Prevalence

In the UK, 1 in 25 of the white population is a carrier, giving a disease frequency of 1 in 2500 live births and making CF the commonest inherited disease of white races. The prevalence shows enormous variation between races, partly likely due to incomplete ascertainment in some developing countries, but in general, CF can be found in virtually every ethnic group. It would certainly be an error to fail to consider CF as a diagnosis because the child is not white.

Diagnostic Tests

Clinical Suspicion

There are many different, age-related presentations of CF. These are summarised in Table 11.2. Once considered, the diagnosis is usually easy to confirm; the usual cause of diagnostic delay is failing to think of the diagnosis. It should be noted that even in populations in which there is a newborn screening program, some children will slip through the diagnostic net, and being screened does not exclude the diagnosis.

Table 11.2 Presentation of CF by age group

Age group	Presenting complaint
Antenatal	• Chorionic villus sampling • Ultrasound diagnosis of bowel perforation • Foetal hyperechogenic bowel [1]
At or soon after birth	• Bowel obstruction (meconium ileus [2], bowel atresia) • Haemorrhagic disease of the newborn • Prolonged jaundice • Screening (population based or previous affected sibling) • Delayed passage of meconium
Infancy and childhood	• Recurrent respiratory infections • Diarrhoea and failure to thrive • Rectal prolapse • Nasal polyps (almost pathognomonic) • Acute pancreatitis • Portal hypertension and variceal haemorrhage • Pseudo-Bartter's syndrome, electrolyte abnormality • Hypoproteinaemia and oedema • Screening as a result of CF diagnosis in a sibling/relative
Adolescence and adult life	• Recurrent respiratory infections • Atypical asthma • Bronchiectasis • Nasal polyps (aspirin-sensitive asthma a commoner cause) • Male infertility (congenital bilateral absence of the vas deferens) • Electrolyte disturbance/heat exhaustion • Screening as a result of diagnosis in affected relative • Portal hypertension and variceal haemorrhage

[1] Most foetuses with hyperechogenic bowel are normal; around 6% have a trisomy, and 4% CF

[2] Note that meconium ileus may be seen in pancreatic-sufficient infants with CF, as well as rarely in those without CF

The Sweat Test

Virtually all CF patients can be diagnosed by a properly performed sweat test. It is essential that this test be carried out only in experienced centres, to prevent false negative and false positive diagnoses. Detailed guidelines have been published at www.acb.org.uk/Guidelines/sweat. htm. Techniques include the classical pilocarpine iontophoresis of Gibson and Cooke, and more recently the Macroduct collection. For the diagnosis to be established, tests should be performed in duplicate; an unequivocally abnormal result is sweat [chloride]>60 mmol, and sweat [sodium]<sweat [chloride]. Sweat [sodium], or even worse, sweat conductivity, on its own should not be relied on as a diagnostic test. A sweat [chloride] of <40 mmol is normal, and intermediate concentrations are equivocal. However, it should be noted that newborns have a much lower mean sweat [chloride], and a [chloride] of 39 mmol/ l is 6 standard deviations from the mean, so should not be uncritically accepted as normal. There are also undoubted cases of CF with normal sweat electrolytes, and the sweat test should always be interpreted in the light of the entire clinical picture. There are a few rare conditions that also cause elevation in sweat electrolyte concentration, but these are not usually a serious diagnostic consideration in practice; the most important causes of confusion are sweat testing by an inexperienced operator, and eczematous skin, which can make sweat collection difficult. False negative sweat tests have been reported in severely malnourished children with CF. The golden rule is, if anyone is in any doubt at all, perform a sweat test.

Genetic Testing

More than 1000 different CFTR mutations have been discovered, many of them extremely rare (www.genet. sickkids.on.ca/cftr/). Although highly specialised laboratories offer complete sequencing of the CF gene, in practice, most will identify around 30 of the commonest mutations, accounting for more than 90% of CF chromosomes. The commonest UK mutation (approximately 70%) is ΔF_{508}, in which a 3-base-pair deletion leads to a loss of the phenylalanine residue at position 508. The prevalence of mutations shows ethnic variation, and laboratories will test for specific panels, dependent on the ethnic group. It is essential to distinguish harmless polymorphisms from disease-producing mutations. It must be noted that failure to detect one or two mutations does not exclude the diagnosis.

Ancillary Testing

The abnormal potential difference across mucosal surfaces can be measured by passing a soft catheter under the inferior turbinate, referencing it to an electrode placed on the abraded skin of the forearm. Normal values are 0 to −30 mV, the CF range less than −34 mV. The test is unreliable if the patient has an upper respiratory tract infection or has chronic rhinitis. The diagnosis can be further refined by perfusing the nose with solutions of amiloride to block sodium transport, and isoprenaline/low chloride to stimulate CFTR (Middleton et al. 1994). Nasal potentials require extensive experience if results are to be accurate. This test is rarely necessary in clinical practice.

Tests of target-organ function may elicit features suggestive of CF. The status of exocrine pancreatic function is probably the most useful test, most easily achieved by measuring stool human faecal elastase-1. Other investigations such as high-resolution computed tomography of the chest or sinuses, and bronchoscopy, are part of the work-up of the difficult diagnosis in the older child. Faecal immunoreactive trypsin, which is useful as part of screening programs, is far too unreliable to be used as a diagnostic test in an individual child.

Features of the Disease

Upper Airway Disease

Perhaps surprisingly, middle ear disease is no commoner in CF than in the general population. Nasal polyps are common (Fig. 11.1); **The finding of nasal polyps in a child mandates referral for exclusion of CF, and if this has been done, PCD.** Evidence of sinus disease is almost invariably found if sought. Severe sinusitis (Fig. 11.2), including mucocoeles, are another important part of lower-airway pathology. Rarely, allergic fungal (usually *Aspergillus fumigatus*) sinusitis is seen.

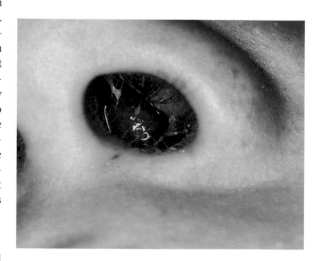

Fig. 11.1 Nasal polyposis in a child with cystic fibrosis (CF). The finding of nasal polyps in childhood mandates diagnostic testing for CF

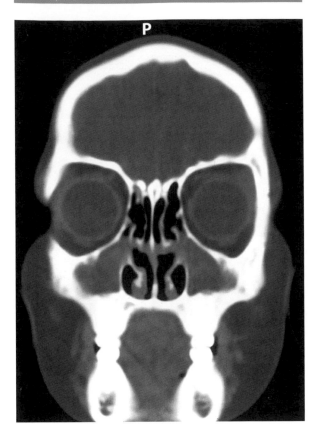

Fig. 11.2 Computed tomography (CT) scan showing severe maxillary sinus disease and mucosal thickening in a child with CF

than MRSA, these organisms do not pose a threat to non-CF patients. However, there is increasing evidence of cross-infection between CF patients, and segregation of these patients from each other is increasingly practiced.

Other Organ Disease

As CF patients live longer, new complications in almost every system of the body are being appreciated. The major ones are summarised in Table 11.3, and the interested reader is referred elsewhere for more detailed recent descriptions (Bush et al. 2006).

Medical Treatment

Upper Airway Disease

Asymptomatic sinus abnormalities rarely, if ever, merit treatment. If the child is symptomatic, prolonged courses of saline douching, oral antibiotics, topical steroids and decongestants are prescribed. Surgery may rarely be needed for troublesome disease. Nasal polyps are usually treated medically with topical steroids (Hadfield et al. 2000), but these are less effective than in eosinophilic allergic-type polyps. It should be remembered that prolonged use of potent topical steroids, such as betamethasone drops, may cause adrenal suppression and growth failure. An alternative is fluticasone drops, available as nasules containing 400 µg, which are minimally absorbed. If topical steroids fail to control symptoms, then surgery is required (see below).

Lower Airway Disease

The commonest cause of death from CF is respiratory failure secondary to bronchiectasis. The lungs are essentially normal at birth, but rapidly chronic infection and inflammation develop. There is controversy about whether the CF airway is pro-inflammatory in the absence of infection, but there is no doubt that chronic infection leads to an intense neutrophilic inflammation, which is itself damaging to the airway. The eventual result is bronchiectasis (Fig. 11.3), respiratory failure and death. Early on, common pathogens include *Staphylococcus aureus* and *Haemophilus influenza*. By the teenage years, around 80% of patients have chronic infection with mucoid *Pseudomonas aeruginosa*. Other important Gram-negative organisms include *Burkholderia cepacia*, *Stenotrophomonas maltophilia* and *Achromobacter (Alcaligenes) xylosoxidans*. Infection with methicillin-resistant *S. aureus* (MRSA) is also increasingly common. Other pathogens include *A. fumigatus*, which may set up a devastatingly destructive allergic reaction (allergic bronchopulmonary aspergillosis) requiring prolonged courses of oral prednisolone, and the non-tuberculous mycobacteria. Other

Lower Airway Disease

Aggressive treatment of infection, and airway clearance techniques, are mandatory. Typically, the child will be doing two sessions of chest physiotherapy per day. There are several techniques, including active cycle of breathing and autogenic drainage, and devices such as the flutter valve, positive-pressure mask and the cornet. Physical exercise is also encouraged. Mucus clearance may be enhanced by inhalation of rhDNase, which cleaves the DNA released from necrotic airway neutrophils and causes increased mucus viscosity, and hypertonic saline.

Antibiotics are given orally prophylactically in some centres, and for any positive respiratory culture of *S. aureus* and *H. influenza*. Infection with *P. aeruginosa* is treated energetically with oral ciprofloxacin, nebulised antibiotics, and when necessary, 2-week courses of intravenous antibiotics. Macrolide antibiotics have an extended range of anti-inflammatory and immunomodulatory properties, and have been shown to be beneficial in CF. They are increasingly used as part of routine treatment.

11

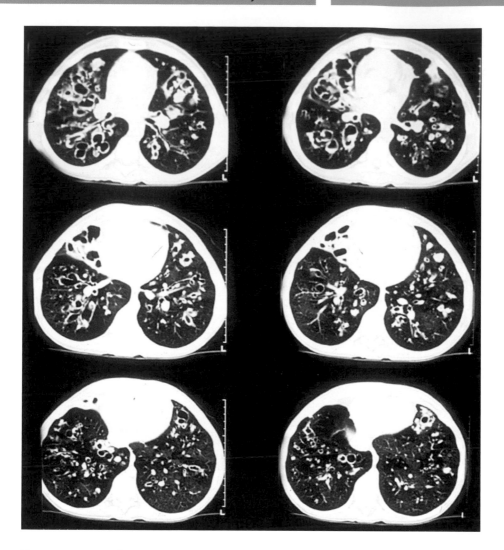

Fig. 11.3 CT scans showing severe bronchiectasis in a patient with CF

It may seem paradoxical to try to suppress inflammation in a child with chronic infection, but this approach may bear dividends in CF. The theoretical basis is that the huge burden of necrotic neutrophils releases neutrophil elastase and other mediators, which are themselves tissue damaging. Suppression of this response with oral prednisolone improves lung function, but at an unacceptable cost of side effects (Eigen et al. 1995). The hunt is on for anti-inflammatory agents with a more favourable profile. The non-steroidal anti-inflammatory ibuprofen has been the subject of clinical trials, but as yet has not found widespread use in the UK. However, there may be implications in terms of bleeding and interactions with other medications, for example intravenous aminoglycosides causing renal failure.

CF patients may be prescribed inhaled corticosteroids and bronchodilators; in general, these are over-prescribed, and should be discontinued unless there is clear evidence of benefit. An annual influenza immunisation is recommended for child and parents.

Other Systems

Pancreatic insufficient patients will be prescribed pancreatic enzyme replacement therapy with enteric coated microspheres. They are taken before and sometimes during meals and snacks, and the dose is adjusted to the ingested fat content. Fat-soluble vitamins are prescribed routinely. CF patients are particularly prone to gastro-oesophageal reflux, and may be prescribed proton pump inhibitors and prokinetic agents. Other therapies may include insulin for endocrine pancreatic failure, ursodeoxycholic acid and taurine for liver disease, and biphosphonates for CF bone disease. Important treatments are summarised in Table 11.3.

Table 11.3 A summary of the more important non-respiratory complications of CF, with their principal treatments. *DIOS* Distal intestinal obstruction syndrome, *PPIs* proton pump inhibitors, *GFR* glomerular filtration rate

Organ system	Disease Manifestation	Treatment
Exocrine pancreas	Malabsorption, steatorrhoea	Pancreatic enzyme replacement therapy; fat-soluble vitamin supplementation
Endocrine pancreas	Diabetes	Insulin (Rarely oral hypoglycaemics)
Gastrointestinal tract	Bowel obstruction (DIOS) Simple constipation Gastro-oesophageal reflux Rectal prolapse Intussuception Associated coeliac and Crohn's disease Increased risk of cancer	Oral Klean-prep, gastrograffin Lactulose, other laxatives PPIs, prokinetics
Hepatobiliary tree	Macronodular cirrhosis Portal hypertension and varices Gall stones	Ursodeoxycholic acid, Taurine Endoscopic variceal banding Care with medication doses necessary
Bones	Osteopaenia, pathological fracture	Biphosphonates
Male genital tract	Azoospermia Hypogonadism	Epididymal aspiration allows in vitro fertilisation; testosterone supplementation
Female genital tract	Reduced fertility Stress incontinence	Therapy for vaginal candidiasis if present
Sweat glands	Electrolyte depletion Heat stroke Failure to thrive	Electrolyte supplementation
Kidneys	Tubular damage, reduced GFR from repeated courses of aminoglycosides	Care with medication dosages

When Should an Apparently Healthy Child be Suspected of Having CF?

Traditionally, CF was thought of as an illness presenting in the early pre-school years with recurrent chest infections, and diarrhoea and failure to thrive. However, mild atypical phenotypes may present very late; 10% of CF diagnoses are made in adult life (Cystic Fibrosis Foundation patient registry, 1997). Undiagnosed children with mild CF may look perfectly healthy, be pancreatic sufficient, and have no chest problems at all.

The child with undiagnosed CF may present to the ENT clinic in one of two ways:

1. Nasal polyps: unlike in adult life, where polyps are most commonly related to aspirin-sensitive asthma, in children nasal polyposis should always prompt referral for exclusion of CF, and, if CF is excluded, PCD.

2. Severe sinusitis and its complications (mucocoele): sinus disease to some degree is almost always a feature of CF, but this diagnosis should be considered if sinusitis is severe, and in particular if surgery for sinusitis is being considered in a child. Mucocoele is a very rare feature of CF.

It is not expected that the ENT surgeon will have time to take a detailed general history if CF is suspected. The six key features to try to elicit include:

1. Does the child have a chronic productive cough, or atypical "asthma"? Sputum production or a moist cough when the child does not have a viral cold is suspicious of bronchiectasis of any cause, including CF and PCD.

2. Is there a history of diarrhoea or poor weight gain? About 15% CF patients are pancreatic sufficient and thrive, so the absence of these symptoms does not ex-

clude CF (Cystic Fibrosis Foundation patient registry, 1997).

3. Has the child had a rectal prolapse? All such children should have a sweat test
4. Is there abnormal sweat: does the child taste salty or has he suffered from significant dehydration (for example, requiring intravenous rehydration, or with significant electrolyte abnormalities), or an episode of heatstroke?
5. Is there a family history of CF?
6. Is there digital clubbing? This sign is often not sought in children, and if not sought, will not be found.

If there is any doubt – refer for testing, BEFORE performing surgery, unless in an acute emergency.

PCD – The Disease

Molecular Defect

PCD is the result of a congenital defect of ciliary function, often with an obvious structural defect on electron microscopy, which results in chronic upper and lower airway infection and inflammation, and in nearly 50% cases, mirror-image arrangement. PCD must be distinguished from states of secondary ciliary dysfunction, due for example to acute viral infection (Bush et al. 1998). The cilium is a complex structure (Fig. 11.4) and is constructed of more than 200 proteins. Only a very few genes have been described, and currently, except for a few families, genetic testing is not feasible.

Pathophysiology

The mucociliary escalator is one of the early and important defence mechanisms, trapping inhaled bacteria, and removing them from the normally sterile lower respiratory tract. Failure of this escalator due to immotile or dyskinetic cilia results in chronic infection and inflammation in the

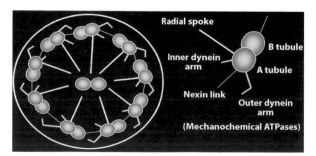

Fig. 11.4 Diagram of the components of respiratory cilia

lower respiratory tract. There is also a failure of clearance of upper airway secretions (middle ear fluid, nasal mucus). Sperm tails are structurally and functionally similar to cilia, and sperm may be immotile, but only in around 50% of males (Munro et al. 1994). There are ependymal cilia, but other than rare cases of hydrocephalus, central nervous system disease is not seen in PCD.

Prevalence

This is only an estimate, based on the proportion of people who have mirror-image arrangement, the number of these who have PCD, and anticipating a prevalence of twice that to account for PCD with normal organ arrangement. This gives a figure of 1 in 15,000. From the known diagnostic rate, it would appear that many patients are undiagnosed (Bush et al. 1998). Indeed, late diagnosis is even more common in PCD than in CF (Coren et al. 2002).

Diagnostic Tests

Diagnostic testing is usually a staged procedure (Table 11.4), in a specialist centre (Bush et al. 1998). Except in the most obvious cases, other conditions such as CF and agammaglobulinaemia will be excluded first. It must be noted that secondary ciliary dysfunction must be excluded; a heavily infected and inflamed epithelium may have cilia that are static or dyskinetic, with structural changes. These are reversible and must not be confused with PCD.

In Vivo Tests of Ciliary Function

The saccharine test is the simplest way of screening for PCD, A 1- to 2-mm pellet of saccharine is placed on the inferior turbinate, and the patient is asked to lean forward and remain still, without sneezing or sniffing. If the taste of saccharine is noted within 60 min, the patient is unlikely to have PCD. If no taste is noted, check that the patient actually can taste saccharine, and refer for further testing. Variants on this test include the use of albumen particles labelled with Evans Blue, detected by direct inspection of the pharynx. These tests are not useful in young children. If the patient sniffs back the pellet, the test is of course unreliable.

Nitric Oxide Studies

Nasal nitric oxide (NO) is usually <100 ppb in patients with PCD, and rarely if ever >500 ppb. A level above

Table 11.4 Staged diagnostic testing for primary ciliary dyskinesia (PCD). *nNo* Nasal nitric oxide

	Tests performed	Comments
Stage 1: Eliminate common disease	Immunoglobulins, specific antibody tests Sweat test Oesophageal pH probe	Bypassed if obvious suspicion (e.g. mirror image arrangement and neonatal onset rhinitis)
Stage 2: Screen for ciliary dysmotility	Saccharine test or variant	Not useful in small children Normal test excludes PCD, abnormal requires further testing
Stage 3: Nitric oxide studies	Nasal nitric oxide	In most centres, not useful in small children nNO>250 ppb; 95% sensitive and specific for PCD Low nNO also in CF, diffuse panbronchiolitis, so not diagnostic of PCD nNO>250 ppb, low probability clinical history, consider stopping testing
Stage 4: Direct assessment of ciliary motility	Nasal brush biopsy	Beware of secondary ciliary dyskinesia due to viral infections
Stage 5: Ciliary ultrastructure	Transmission electron microscopy	Beware of secondary ciliary structural changes due to viral infections
Stage 6: Culture of ciliated cells	Nasal brush biopsy or biopsy of inferior turbinates	Only needed if doubt still remains

250 ppb is 95% sensitive and specific for the disease. Exhaled NO is also low, but there is more overlap between disease groups (Narang et al. 2002). A high nasal NO can usually be taken to exclude PCD, but since a blocked nose, CF and diffuse panbronchiolitis are also causes of a low nasal NO, this test should not be used in isolation to diagnose PCD. Furthermore, active co-operation is required, and so in most centres NO studies can only be offered to older children and adults.

Measurement of Ciliary Beat Frequency and Pattern

Brushing the inferior turbinate with a cytology brush can detach strips of epithelium, which can be studied on a heated microscope stage. The beating cilia can be recorded using a video camera (Chilvers et al. 2003), and the beat pattern studied. Particular structural changes may be associated with recognisable patterns of abnormality. If the child has had a recent viral cold, it may be impossible to harvest healthy cilia. Likewise, chronic rhinosinusitis must be treated before attempting a brushing.

Electron Microscopy

The morphology of cilia can be studied by transmission electron microscopy of the epithelial strips. At least 100 cilia should be studied (Bush et al. 1998), and abnormalities may be seen in up to 10% of healthy cilia. Several different patterns have been described (Table 11.5, Fig. 11.5). There may be no structural abnormality visible in some undoubted cases of PCD, so electron microscopy should not be performed without also doing functional studies. It is true that if a classical abnormality such as absent dynein arms is seen, the diagnosis of PCD is secure, but performing electron microscopy alone will result in cases being missed.

A controversial variant of PCD is a primary orientation defect, in which normal cilia are not properly aligned with each other and therefore cannot beat in a coordinated fashion. Disorientation is also secondary to chronic infection, so such cases should always have a repeat biopsy to check the findings, after treatment of local inflammation or infection; alternatively, the findings should be confirmed by biopsy from another site, for example the lower airway.

Table 11.5 Common ultrastructural features seen on electron microscopy in PCD patients

Dynein arm defects	Absent or reduced number of inner, outer or both dynein arms
Tubular defects	Transposition, extra microtubules (these are particularly likely to be secondary abnormalities); absent central microtubule pair
Radial spoke defects	Absent spokes
Ciliary disorientation	Mean standard deviation of angles >20°, not reducing after treatment and present in two sites (nose, bronchus) (do not confuse with secondary ciliary dyskinesia)
Miscellaneous	Abnormal basal apparatus, ciliary aplasia, abnormally long cilia
Normal ultrastructure	Review of diagnosis mandatory

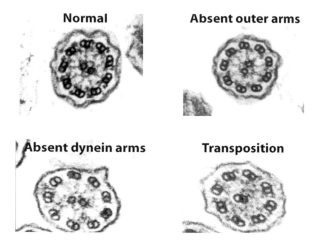

Fig. 11.5 Scanning electron micrographs of respiratory cilia (courtesy of Dr. Ann Dewar)

Electron microscopy is most conveniently performed on epithelial strips. A larger piece of tissue, such as parts of the turbinate, can be studied. However, before sending such tissue from an operation, it is essential to discuss the matter with the electron microscopist first.

Culture of Cilia

This technique is particularly useful when it is proving impossible to collect healthy cilia. Either a forceps or brush biopsy can be used to provide tissue culture material. Cilia will then re-grow, and can be studied functionally and structurally as above (Jorissen et al. 2000).

Features of the Disease

Upper Airway Disease

Characteristically, the child has persistent and unremitting rhinitis, often from the very first day of life. Inspection of the nose often reveals pooled, static mucopurulent secretions. No treatment has much effect. Nasal polyps have been described as common in some series; in our clinic, they are a very unusual manifestation of PCD. Other features include otitis media with effusion and rhinosinusitis. If the child has had tympanostomy tubes inserted, characteristically there is prolonged, foully offensive otorrhoea, with an obvious smelly discharge running down the side of the face from the ears. The usual pathogen cultured is *P. aeruginosa*.

Lower Airway Disease

Typically the child has a chronic productive ("wet") cough, every day. Although the parent may say the child wheezes, usually this is due to bronchial secretions rather than true bronchospasm. If untreated, the child will suffer from recurrent infection and ultimately severe bronchiectasis. Early on, the usual pathogens are *H. influenza* and *S. aureus*; in adult life, *P. aeruginosa* and non-tuberculous mycobacterial infection is seen (Noone et al. 2004).

Other Organ Disease

Mirror-image organ arrangement is observed in nearly 50% of patients with PCD, due to dysfunction of nodal cilia during embryonic development (Fig. 11.6). In addition, 50% of males with PCD have immotile sperm and need to resort to assisted conception techniques in order to father children. There is a higher prevalence of ectopic pregnancy amongst women with PCD, because of loss

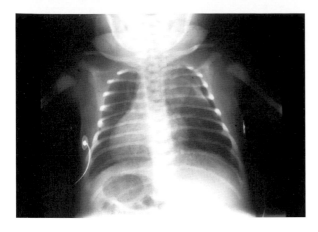

Fig. 11.6 A newborn with respiratory distress and mirror-image arrangement. This combination is a typical presentation of primary ciliary dyskinesia

of ciliary function in the oviduct. Complex congenital heart disease with disorders of laterality are seen in some children (Gemou-Engesaeth et al. 1993). Other rare associations include severe oesophageal disease (major reflux, oesophageal atresia), hydrocephalus and biliary atresia. Rare kindreds with retinitis pigmentosa and PCD have been described.

Medical Treatment

Upper Airway Disease

Rhinitis is treated medically with saline drops or sprays. Regular, age-appropriate hearing tests are essential. If there is a significant hearing deficit affecting speech, then hearing aids are the preferred treatment. Often however, if the teacher is sensitive to the child's hearing, and the child is placed in the front row of the class, no further action is needed. Hearing can be anticipated to be satisfactory by 12 years of age. If the child has a chronically discharging ear at presentation, then treatment with fluoroquinolones (ciprofloxacin) eardrops is needed. If these are not available, in our experience aminoglycoside drops can also safely be used.

Lower Airway Disease

The bedrock of treatment is regular chest physiotherapy, liberal use of antibiotics for any respiratory deterioration, and the encouragement of physical exercise. If oral antibiotics do not control infection, then intravenous treatment is prescribed. Nebulised antibiotics are used for chronic infection with *P. aeruginosa*. Bronchodilators and inhaled steroids are prescribed only if there is clear evidence of

benefit. Anti-pneumococcal immunisation and annual influenza immunisation is recommended.

Other Organ Disease

This is treated along standard lines. Severe reflux may mandate a Nissan's fundoplication. A referral to an infertility clinic may be necessary.

When Should an Apparently Healthy Child be Suspected of Having PCD?

The child with undiagnosed CF may present to the ENT clinic in one of five ways:

1. Chronic rhinitis; this usually commences at or soon after birth, and is present every day without remission. It has usually failed to respond to medical management.
2. Severe chronic suppurative otitis media.
3. Perforated eardrum with prolonged otorrhoea, usually after one or several attempts at insertion of tympanostomy tubes.
4. Severe sinusitis, sometimes despite multiple previous surgical procedures.
5. Nasal polyps; in paediatric practice, these should first prompt diagnostic testing for CF.

If PCD is suspected, the six key pieces of information to seek are:

1. Was there neonatal onset of rhinitis or unexplained respiratory distress soon after birth?
2. Does the child have a chronic productive cough, or been diagnosed with "asthma"; and if "asthma" has been diagnosed, what has been the response to therapy?
3. Is there rhinorrhoea that has persisted from early in life, with no response to treatment or remission over time?
4. Are the ears normal? If so, PCD is less likely, but cannot be excluded.
5. Has the child had previous ENT surgery, and how beneficial was it? In particular, prolonged offensive otorrhoea after tympanostomy tube insertion should prompt consideration of PCD BEFORE another set is inserted.
6. Has the child got mirror-image arrangement? Almost unbelievably, even children with such an obvious physical sign may suffer diagnostic delay.

The Child Referred for Surgery for an Unrelated Condition

Neither CF nor PCD is protective against, for example, adenotonsillar hypertrophy and obstructive sleep apnoea, which might lead to an ENT referral. Close liaison with the team that is responsible for the usual care of the child is essential, particularly if surgery is contemplated. Depending on the clinical situation, the centre may wish to give pre-operative oral or even intravenous antibiotics, even before a very short procedure. The antibiotics may need to be continued for a variable period after the operation. Extra chest physiotherapy may be prescribed; the parents will usually administer this, but occasionally one of the hospital physiotherapists may need to be involved.

It is essential that the anaesthetist is experienced in paediatrics and is aware of the problems that may arise during anaesthesia (Table 11.6). A detailed pre-operative assessment is essential, including disease-specific and generic anaesthetic issues. During the course of the anaesthetic, the opportunity may be taken to carry out other disease-related procedures. This may include a blind or bronchoscopic bronchoalveolar lavage to obtain material for culture, especially in children who find it difficult to produce sputum; if surgery is performed away from the CF centre, it is essential that the sample is cultured in the microbiology laboratory using appropriate media. Diagnostic testing may need to be performed if the underlying diagnosis is in doubt. Tests might include nasal or bronchial biopsy for ciliary studies; and the performance of nasal or bronchial potential difference measurements in a young child with an equivocal diagnosis of CF. In all cases, this should be discussed with the centre that is undertaking the routine care of the child.

ENT Surgery for CF

The majority of children with CF will have some degree of rhinosinusitis as an inevitable consequence of the disease process, although differential diagnoses of allergic rhinitis and adenoidal hypertrophy should be considered. Low-level symptoms of nasal obstruction, hyposmia, rhinorrhoea and post-nasal drip are common. Complicating infection may produce complaints of facial pain and headache. Worsening symptoms of blockage and discharge are likely to herald the onset of extensive polypoid rhinosinopathy, which is common in CF if screened for with nasal endoscopy. Typical endoscopic appearances are shown in Fig. 11.7. The polyps form a huge gelatinous mass filling most of the nasal cavity (Fig. 11.8).

Table 11.6 Potential anaesthetic complications in the child with CF or PCD

Disease (CF, PCD)	Timing	Organ system	Potential complication
CF, PCD	Peri- and post-operative	Lower respiratory tract	Atelectasis, blockage of endotracheal tube, and V:Q mismatch due to sputum retention, especially if the patient is in pain, inspired gases have been inadequately humidified or cough suppressing drugs have been prescribed
CF, PCD	Peri- and post-operative	Gastrointestinal tract, lungs	Gastro-oesophageal reflux and aspiration
CF, PCD	Pre-, peri- and post-operative	Any	Anaesthetic drug interactions with previously prescribed treatments
CF	Pre-, peri- and post-operative	Liver	Bleeding (deficiency of K-dependant clotting factors, thrombocytopaenia due to hypersplenism), drug toxicity
CF	Pre-, peri- and post-operative	Kidney	Drug toxicity due to iatrogenic renal impairment
CF	Peri- and post-operative	Endocrine pancreas	Hyperglycaemia due to known diabetes, or diabetes precipitated by surgery
CF, PCD	Per- and post-operative	Adrenal	Crisis due to current or prior oral steroid therapy
CF	Peri- and post-operative	Sweat gland	Sodium and potassium depletion, metabolic alkalosis, dehydration due to excessive loss
CF	Post-operative	Gastrointestinal tract	Constipation, especially if opiates prescribed, or dehydration

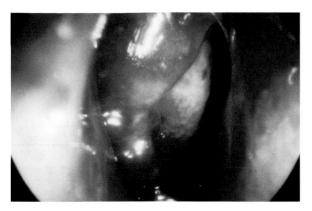

Fig. 11.7 Typical endoscopic appearances of nasal polyps

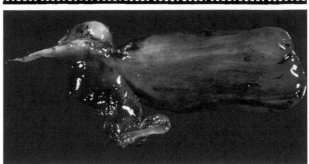

Fig. 11.8 Large polypoid mass post-excision, previously filling the nasal cavity

Endoscopic sinus surgery (ESS) has replaced external approaches as the surgical modality of choice. The potential advantages of surgery are symptomatic control of the majority of obstructive and infective symptoms. However there are potential risks in the procedure. A prolonged general anaesthetic or sedation may precipitate a lower respiratory tract infection and all precautions should be taken to protect the patient, including peri-operative antibiotics and pre- and post-surgical chest physiotherapy. The surgery could involve: (1) a simple nasal polypectomy, just removing the intranasal parts of the polyps, (2) an ethmoidectomy, middle meatal antrostomy, sphenoidotomy and fronto-nasal approach (although this is rarely required as the frontal sinuses are rudimentary in the majority) or (3) extensive removal of the lateral nasal wall including the middle turbinate and exteriorising the paranasal sinuses up to the anterior skull base. With more extensive procedures there is an increasing risk of local complications including primary haemorrhage, orbital damage and a cerebrospinal fluid leak. Some of the problems of bleeding and visualisation may be overcome with use of powered instrumentation such as a micro-debrider.

The benefits of surgery need to be weighed against the duration of control of symptoms. The onset of facial pain on the background of nasal obstruction that persists despite topical steroid treatment and systemic antibiotic therapy is a good indication for surgery with a high chance of symptomatic control. Symptoms of obstruction alone tend to fare less well with surgery. There is an inevitable recurrence of symptoms, and this may be prolonged by more extensive surgery. With surgery involving limited endoscopic resection there is a 50% chance of symptom control at 2 years post-operatively (Rowe-Jones and Mackay 1996). Although this is a much poorer outcome than with conventional rhinosinusitis, this may be a considerable period of time for children who have limited life expectancy. Typical post-operative appearances are shown in Fig. 11.9.

Chronic rhinosinusitis in children with CF may be complicated by the formation of paranasal sinus mucocoeles (DiCocco et al. 2005), which are secretory cysts that enlarge by concentric expansion. These affect predominantly the ethmoid sinuses and often present with proptosis and/or hyperteleorism in addition to the typical symptoms of rhinosinusitis. They can have local, orbital or even intracranial complications. Mucocoeles may be successfully managed with an endoscopic approach, as shown in Fig. 11.10.

Nasal polyposis can be a considerable challenge in patients who have undergone heart–lung transplanta-

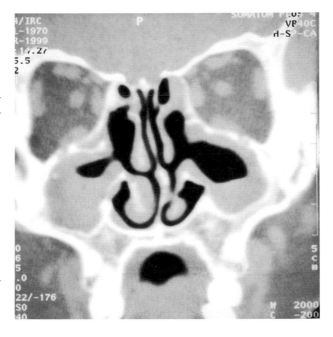

Fig. 11.9 Typical post-endoscopic sinus surgery CT appearance. Persistent mucosal thickening within the paranasal sinuses, though well aerated

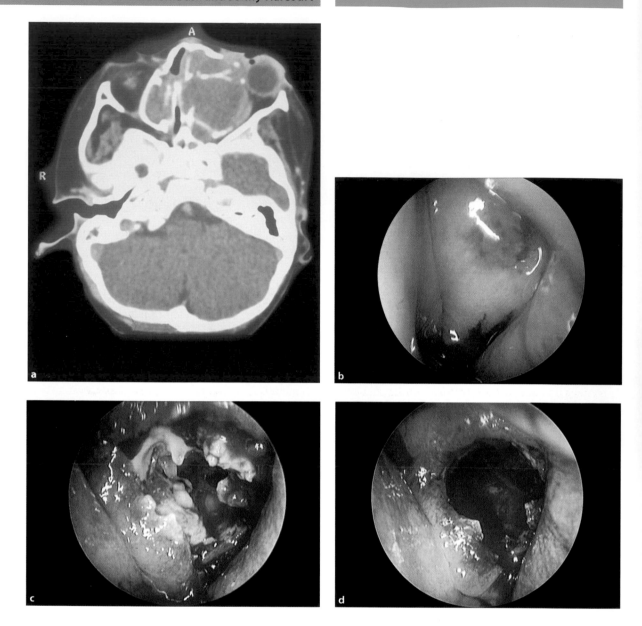

Fig. 11.10 a CT scan showing large left ethmoid mucocoele. **b** Endoscopic appearance of left ethmoid mucocoele. **c** Initial opening of mucocoele. **d** Post-operative endoscopy

tion for end-stage CF (Holzmann et al. 2004). The post-operative long-term immunosuppression often seems to precipitate a very aggressive form of nasal polyposis that involves a gross inflammation of the sinus mucosa, which will often lead to polyps extruding from the anterior nares and which rapidly recur after excision. These patients may suffer from severe airway obstruction and may require frequent nasal surgery, which is often quite bloody as the polyps are firm and vascular. Successful control of the polyps, however, may control post-transplant lower airway colonisation and infection.

Despite the frequency and severity of rhinosinusitis in CF, middle ear problems are relatively rare and indeed there seems to be a low level of otitis media compared with normal children (Haddad et al. 1994). This may be due to the protective effect of systemic antibiotic and anti-inflammatories that children with CF may be prescribed. If present, it should be treated on its own merits depending on the hearing levels in the better ear and the frequency of complicating episodes of acute otitis media.

ENT Surgery for PCD

The ENT clinical features of PCD are quite different from those of CF. Chronic rhinosinusitis without polyp

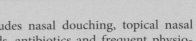

formation is the characteristic nasal finding in this condition. Due to the lack of effective ciliary action within the nose, mucus collects within the nasal cavity and paranasal sinuses leading to a low level nasal obstruction, rhinorrhoea and post-nasal drip. Nasal cleaning can be optimised by use of regular nasal saline douches. Complicating episodes of acute sinusitis are rare, but if patients present with additional symptoms of recurrent or chronic facial pain combined with endoscopic evidence of muco-purulent discharge form the lateral nasal wall, and are resistant to long-term systemic antibiotics, ESS can be considered (Parsons and Greene 1993). This should involve only a limited endoscopic resection to remove chronic infected material and improve drainage from dependant sinuses.

Otitis media with effusion is an almost universal finding in PCD. The gold standard treatment of ventilation tube insertion is, however, strongly contraindicated in this condition (Hadfield et al. 1997). Apart from the increased peri-operative risk of chest infection, there is an unacceptably high incidence of post-ventilation tube-insertion otorrhoea and subsequent tympanic membrane perforation. The conductive hearing loss resolves by the age of 13 years in more than 90% of patients, and so auditory rehabilitation is achieved with hearing aids until the spontaneous resolution of the condition (Majitha et al. 2005).

Complicating episodes of acute otitis media in infants are not uncommon. It occurs quite often in association with an increased frequency of lower respiratory tract infections and as such will usually respond to the long-term systemic antibiotics that are given to control the associated respiratory problems.

Summary for the Clinician

- Therapy includes nasal douching, topical nasal corticosteroids, antibiotics and frequent physiotherapy for the chest.
- Surgery may be needed for CRS/polyps; endoscopic sinus surgery results are inferior to those in non-CF CRS, with 50% of patients still reporting improvement at 2 years. Close liaison with the medical team, an experienced anaesthetist and very intensive physiotherapy are necessary.
- PCD with decreased ciliary function probably occurs in 1 in 15,000 individuals. There are usually abnormalities of cilia on electron microscopy. In 50% of cases there is a mirror-image arrangement of organs. There is a history of rhinitis from birth, unresponsive to treatment, associated with a chronic wet cough. Otitis media with effusion is common; grommet insertion results in a chronic discharge and should be avoided since hearing problems usually resolve with age.
- Diagnosis is made by examination of ciliary beating and electron microscopy; however, screening tests such as properly performed saccharine clearance and nasal NO can reduce the need for referral for these expensive procedures. Secondary ciliary dysfunction needs to be excluded.
- Therapy for PCD includes saline douching, liberal use of antibiotics when needed and physiotherapy. If ENT surgery becomes necessary, then conditions similar to those for CF apply.

Summary for the Clinician

- Innate immune defects in mucociliary clearance present to the ENT surgeon as nasal polyposis, chronic rhinosinusitis and otitis media with effusion, often resistant to therapy.
- CF has a prevalence of 1 in 2500 and occurs in every ethnic group. Nasal polyps and severe chronic rhinosinusitis (CRS), sometimes with mucocoele formation, are the usual ENT presentations, otitis media with effusion is rare. Nasal polyps or CRS with a history of chronic productive cough, diarrhoea, poor weight gain, rectal prolapse, dehydration or heat stroke or family history of CF should suggest investigation in a specialist unit, as should finger clubbing. A sweat test properly performed is often diagnostic, genetic tests can reveal the nature of the abnormality and counselling is needed.

References

1. Boucher RC (2004) New concepts of cystic fibrosis lung disease. Eur Respir J 23:146–158
2. Bush A, Alton EWFW, Davies JC, et al (eds) (2006) Cystic Fibrosis in the 21st Century. Progress in Respiratory Research, volume 34. Karger, Basel
3. Bush A, Cole P, Hariri M, et al (1998) Primary ciliary dyskinesia: diagnosis and standards of care. Eur Respir J 12:982–988
4. Chilvers M, Rutman A, O'Callaghan C (2003) Ciliary beat pattern is associated with specific ultrastructural defects in primary ciliary dyskinesia. J Allergy Clin Immunol 112:518–524
5. Coren ME, Meeks M, Buchdahl RM, et al (2002) Primary ciliary dyskinesia (PCD) in children – age at diagnosis and symptom history. Acta Paediatr 91:667–669
6. Cystic Fibrosis Foundation, Patient Registry 1996 Annual Data Report, Bethesda, Maryland, August 1997

7. Di Cocco M, Constantinou D, Palon R (2005) Paranasal mucoceles in children with cystic fibrosis. Int J Ped Otorhinolaryngol 69:1407–1413

8. Dormer RL, Harris CM, Clark Z, et al (2005) Sildenafil (Viagra) corrects DeltaF508-CFTR location in nasal epithelial cells from patients with cystic fibrosis. Thorax 60:55–59

9. Eigen H, Rosenstein B, FitzSimmons S, et al (1995) A multi-center study of alternate day prednisone therapy in patients with cystic fibrosis. J Pediatr 126:515–523

10. Gemou-Engesaeth V, Warner JO, Bush A (1993) New associations of primary ciliary dyskinesia syndrome. Pediatr Pulmonol 16:9–12

11. Haddad J Jr, Gonzalez C, Kurland G, et al (1994) Ear disease in children with cystic fibrosis. Arch Otolaryngol Head Neck Surg 120:491–493

12. Hadfield PJ, Rowe-Jones J, Bush A, et al (1997) Treatment of otitis media with effusion in children with primary ciliary dyskinesia. Clin Otolaryngol 22:302–306

13. Hadfield PJ, Rowe-Jones JM, Mackay IS (2000) A prospective treatment trial of nasal polyps in adults with cystic fibrosis. Rhinology 38:63–65

14. Holzmann D, Speich R, Kaufmann T, et al (2004) Effects of sinus surgery in patients with cystic fibrosis after lung transplantation: a 10-year experience. Transplantation 77:134–136

15. Jorissen M, Willems T, Van der Schueren B (2000) Ciliary function analysis for the diagnosis of primary ciliary dyskinesia: advantages of ciliogenesis in culture. Acta Otolaryngol 120:291–295

16. Majitha A, Fong J, Hariri M, et al (2005) Hearing outcomes in children with primary ciliary dyskinesia – a longitudinal study. Int J Ped Otorhinolaryngol 69:1061–1064

17. Mall M, Grubb BR, Harkema JR, et al (2004) Increased airway epithelial Na+ absorption produces cystic fibrosis-like lung disease in mice. Nat Med 10:487–493

18. Middleton PG, Geddes DM, Alton EWFW (1994) Protocols for in vivo measurement of the ion transport defects in cystic fibrosis nasal epithelium. Eur Respir J 7:2050–2056

19. Munro NC, Currie DC, Lindsay KS, et al (1994) Fertility in males with primary ciliary dyskinesia presenting with respiratory infection. Thorax 49:684–687

20. Narang I, Ersu R, Wilson NM, et al (2002) Nitric oxide in chronic airway inflammation in children: diagnostic use and pathophysiological significance. Thorax 57:586–589

21. Noone PG, Leigh MW, Sannuti A, et al (2004) Primary ciliary dyskinesia: diagnostic and phenotypic features. Am J Respir Crit Care Med 169:459–467

22. Parsons DS, Greene BA (1993) A treatment for primary ciliary dyskinesia: efficacy of functional endoscopic sinus surgery. Laryngoscope 103:1269–1272

23. Rowe-Jones J, Mackay, I (1996) Endoscopic sinus surgery in the treatment of nasal polyposis. Laryngoscope 106:1540–1544

24. Wilschanski M, Yahav Y, Yaacov Y, et al (2003) Gentamicin-induced correction of CFTR function in patients with cystic fibrosis and CFTR stop mutations. N Engl J Med 349:1433–1441

11

Chapter 12

Head and Neck Masses

Ben Hartley

12

Core Messages

- Paediatric head and neck masses are common and mostly benign.
- Cancer is the second commonest cause of death in children, and 25% of cases ultimately involve the head and neck.
- A systematic approach is required to clinically evaluate head and neck masses and biopsy-suspicious lesions.
- Haemangiomas are distinct biological entities and this term should not be sued for vascular malformations.
- Complete surgical excision of non-tuberculous mycobacterial neck lesions has several advantages over conservative management if the lesion is anatomically suitable.
- The spectrum of diseases that constitute paediatric head and neck malignancies are different from adults and a different approach is required.
- Epithelial carcinomas (e.g. squamous cell carcimomas) are extremely rare in children.

Contents

Introduction

Neck swellings in children are common. The majority are due to reactive lymphadenopathy associated with tonsillitis and other common upper-respiratory infections. These are usually self-limiting but may progress to cellulitis, suppuration and abscess formation. Chronic infections are less common but need to be considered if the swelling persists.

Congenital mass lesions may be present at birth, but not infrequently appear in older children, when the onset of the swelling may be precipitated by an acute inflammatory episode. These are best considered in two groups: midline neck abnormalities (which are most commonly associated with the thyroglossal duct) and lateral branchial anomalies. The congenital vascular lesions are subdivided into two groups: first, haemangiomas, with a distinctive growth pattern of proliferation and involution, and second, vascular malformations, which grow with the child.

Amongst those with common neck swellings are a small number of children with an underlying malignancy. These are most commonly lymphomas or sarcomas. Squamous cell carcinoma is rare in children and accounts for only a very small proportion of paediatric head and neck malignancies. For this reason, a child with a neck mass requires a different approach to an adult. It is very important to maintain an index of suspicion for malignancy in all persistent neck swellings in children and pursue a tissue diagnosis by biopsy sampling (or less often by fine-needle aspiration for cytology) when appropriate.

Part 1. Clinical Assessment of Neck Swelling in Children

History

1. Duration: This is important. Swellings that have been present for a few days are likely to represent acute inflammation. After 6 weeks, a swelling is generally regarded as chronic and further investigation should be considered. Investigation should be considered earlier than 6 weeks if there are suspicious clinical features (e.g. rapid enlargement or associated nerve palsies).
2. Size: Very large swellings or swellings that progressively enlarge despite antimicrobial treatment should be considered for further investigation.
3. Age: Most acute lymphadenitis occurs in children older than 6 months. Swellings occurring at or shortly after birth are likely to be congenital in origin, although congenital swellings also frequently present in older children.
4. Associated symptoms: A preceding upper-respiratory infection is often a feature of inflammatory lymphadenitis. Fever, rhinorrhoea, sore throat and malaise are common. With chronic swellings, enquiries should be made about weight loss, night sweats and swellings elsewhere in the body.
5. Contacts: Enquire about tuberculosis, other infections and exposure to cats, farm animals and ticks.
6. Medical History: Identify any known illnesses.
7. Family and social history: Identify any familial disease or congenital anomalies and any social factors. If a diagnosis of human immunodeficiency virus (HIV) infection is suspected then involve a paediatrician with a special interest in infectious diseases.

Examination of the Neck

Site of the Swelling

The site of the swelling within the neck gives important information about the possible aetiology.

Lateral Neck Swellings

Lymph nodes are distributed throughout the neck, but the commonest site is along the superficial and deep cervical chains. The deep cervical chain lies deep to the sternomastoid muscle in the upper neck and along its anterior border in the lower neck. Enlarged lymph nodes are the commonest cause of lateral neck swellings. The principle differential diagnosis includes congenital anomalies such as branchial cysts, which may also become acutely inflamed. The differential diagnosis of a lateral neck swelling in a child also includes congenital vascular lesions (haemangiomas and vascular malformations, including lymphatic malformations), benign and malignant neoplasia arising from the neural or connective tissue elements present, and rare secondary metastases.

Central Neck Swellings

The principal causes of a neck swelling in the central area of the neck around the midline are: (1) thyroglossal duct cyst, (2) lymph node and (3) dermoid cyst. It is not uncommon for thyroglossal duct cysts to become acutely inflamed. Less commonly, children can develop thyroid disease. Lymphatic malformations can occasionally involve this region.

Parotid Swellings

Please also refer to Chapter 17. Acute parotitis (mumps) is due to a self-limiting viral infection. Vaccination for measles mumps and rubella is now reducing the frequency of mumps. Bacterial parotitis may occur in children and may be recurrent. It is usually distinguished for other conditions by its acute painful presentation followed by resolution on antibiotics. Occasionally chronic inflammatory swelling persists and must be distinguished from neoplasia. Vascular malformations and haemangiomas are some of the commonest persistent swellings in the parotid region in children. Magnetic resonance imaging (MRI) can be very helpful with this differential diagnosis. Occasionally, fine-needle aspiration or biopsy sampling is required to exclude neoplasia. This may be lymphoid or salivary gland in origin (see also Chapter 17). Rhabdomyosarcoma or other connective tissue tumours occasionally present with a mass in this region.

Submandibular Swellings

Enlarged lymph nodes, floor of mouth infections, acute sialadenitis and occasionally lymphatic vascular malformations or congenital "plunging" ranula all cause swelling in this region.

Posterior Triangle Swellings

Most commonly these are lymph nodes, but branchial anomalies, vascular malformations and, rarely, neoplasia should be considered.

Nature of the Swelling

Classical signs of acute inflammation may be present, for example redness, tenderness and heat. Chronic swellings usually do not show these signs. If abscess formation has occurred, the clinical sign of fluctuance may be present and the mass may feel cystic. A classical tuberculous abscess lacks the clinical features of acute inflammation ("cold abscess").

Head and Neck Examination

A careful examination for a source of primary infection should be made. This should include examination of the pharynx, oral cavity, teeth, nose and ears as well as looking for any cutaneous lesion.

General Examination

Fever, tachycardia or rash should be identified. A general examination should include a search for any associated lymphadenopathy and hepatosplenomegaly.

Investigation

The investigation of neck swellings in children is dependent on the clinical assessment. In many cases no investigation is required. Simple observation of presumed viral infection or antibiotic treatment of bacterial infection, with careful clinical follow up, will often result in resolution.

Laboratory Tests

If the child is systemically unwell, a full blood count may demonstrate a neutrophilia consistent with bacterial infection. Occasionally, haematological malignancy may be detected. A Monospot test for infectious mononucleosis should be considered. Other serological tests for toxoplasmosis, *Bartonella* (cat scratch), or cytomegalovirus should be considered for persistent lymphadenopathy. Mantoux or Heaf tests for tuberculosis may be helpful, particularly in the non-immunised. If the thyroid gland is enlarged, then thyroid function tests and autoantibody titres should be performed (Table 12.1).

Radiology

There is only a limited place for plain radiographs. Plain films of the chest may be helpful, particularly if tuberculosis is a possibility. Lateral neck films may demonstrate a retropharyngeal mass but are not recommended routinely (Table 12.2).

Ultrasound examination of a neck mass is a very useful test. It may provide valuable information without sedation or anaesthesia. Ultrasound will help determine if this is a cystic lesion or whether it is solid. If an abscess is identified it will help with the anatomical relationships of the abscess and help with surgical planning. An experienced ultrasonographer can comment on the internal architecture of lymph nodes and may raise the suspicion of

Table 12.1 Laboratory investigations. *CMV* Cytomegalovirus, *HIV* human immunodeficiency virus

Full blood count
Monospot
Serology: toxoplasmosis, *Bartonella*, CMV and HIV
Mantoux or Heaf test
Biopsy procedure or, occasionally, fine-needle aspiration cytology

Table 12.2 Radiology. *TB* Tuberculosis, *CT* computed tomography, *MRI* magnetic resonance imaging

Plain films:	Not routinely performed but occasionally helpful for TB (chest x-ray) or retropharyngeal abscess (soft tissue neck x-ray).
Ultrasound:	Non-invasive, distinguishes cystic versus solid masses and provides information regarding lymph node architecture and size.
CT:	May require sedation or anaesthesia in children; distinguishes cystic versus solid masses, gives information regarding architecture of mass and surgical relationships; good information for bony structures.
MRI:	Usually reserved for persistent soft-tissue masses.

malignancy. Computed tomography (CT) scanning may require sedation or even general anaesthesia in small children. Good anatomical detail is, however, provided and it is helpful in surgical planning. MRI scanning rarely adds useful information in the case of acute inflammatory lesions, but is very useful for vascular malformations, salivary gland and soft-tissue masses.

Biopsy Sampling versus Fine-Needle Aspiration for Cytology

Persistent or rapidly enlarging masses raise the possibility of malignancy and a tissue diagnosis is required. The principle pathologies in the paediatric population (principally lymphomas and sarcomas – see below) are less easily diagnosed by fine-needle aspiration cytology, and biopsy remains the gold standard for the diagnosis and treatment of paediatric head and neck malignancy.

Fine-needle aspiration cytology following topical local anaesthesia can be helpful in the diagnosis of salivary and thyroid masses and also lymph node hyperplasia on older children (e.g. over age 4 years) who can tolerate the procedure under topical anaesthesia. An experienced cytopathologist is essential for interpretation of these samples and often the cytologist will recommend biopsy if lesions persist.

Part 2. Inflammatory Disorders of the Neck and Lymphadenopathy

Please refer to Table 12.3

Table 12.3 Inflammatory neck nodes in children

Infective Aetiologies
Viral
Upper respiratory: rhinovirus, adenovirus, enterovirus
Common childhood illnesses: measles, mumps, rubella, *Varicella*
Infectious mononucleosis
CMV
HIV
Bacterial
Acute lymphadenitis: *Streptococcus*, *Staphylococcus*, less commonly Gram-negative organisms
Suppurative lymphadenitis with deep or superficial neck abscess: usually pyogenic organisms (*Streptococcus* and *Staphylococcus*)
Mycobacteria : tuberculosis or 'atypical' mycobacteria
Other granulomatous bacterial infections: Cat scratch disease, actinomycosis, brucellosis, tularaemia, Bubonic plague, syphilis
Fungal
Histoplasmosis
Uncommon fungal infections (immunocompromised host) *Candida* and *Aspergillus*
Parasitic
Toxoplasmosis
Filariasis
Non-Infective Adenopathy
Kawasaki syndrome
Sarcoidosis
Sinus histiocytosis with massive lymphadenopathy
Kikuchi-Fujimoto disease

Viral Infections

Viral Upper Respiratory Tract Infections

Adenovirus, rhinovirus or enterovirus (Coxsackie A and B) may cause reactive lymphadenopathy. These are generally self-limiting.

Infectious Mononucleosis

This is an acute infection caused by Epstein-Barr virus. It occurs mainly in adolescence and is spread by close contact. Fever, fatigue, malaise and an exudative, "membranous" tonsillitis are characteristic. Cervical lymphadenopathy may be massive. Other lymphoid tissues including liver and spleen may be enlarged. There is a characteristic picture on the blood film with the presence of atypical lymphocytes. Serological tests such as Monospot or Paul Bunnell will usually confirm the diagnosis. Although the aetiology is viral, antibiotics may be needed to treat any co-existent bacterial infection. In cases where the acute tonsillitis is associated with airway obstruction, steroids may be considered. On occasion, endotracheal intubation may be required to protect the airway until the swelling subsides.

Cases with hepatosplenomegaly should be managed in co-operation with a paediatrician.

Human Immunodeficiency Virus

Please also refer to Chapter 10. Infection is associated with repeated opportunistic infections. Most cases of paediatric HIV infection are acquired from the mother by vertical transmission. Acute infection may mimic infectious mononucleosis. Persistent generalised lymphadenopathy including the cervical nodes becomes a feature as the disease progresses. Weight loss and recurrent fevers occur. Following HIV infection, it may be years or decades before the full acquired immune deficiency syndrome (AIDS) develops. There is increasing evidence of increased life expectancy with early antiretroviral treatment.

Bacterial Infections

Acute Lymphadenopathy with Suppuration

Cervical Abscesses

Bacterial infection within a cervical lymph node may progress to cause local cellulitis and abscess. Occasionally, a solid mass of inflammatory tissue forms, due to coalescence of a group of lymph nodes: this is clinically referred to as a phlegmon. The distinction between phlegmon and abscess is important, as abscesses usually require surgical drainage, whereas phlegmon settle with intravenous antibiotics. The most important assessment is clinical. Abscesses are tender, usually reddened and exhibit the clinical sign of fluctuance, confirming their cystic nature. Imaging is helpful. Neck abscesses require surgical drainage. This may be performed by a neck incision or transorally. There are advocates of each approach.

The author prefers to use a cervical approach for lesions with a palpable neck mass, but a transoral approach when the problem is principally a pharyngeal mass. A wide-bore needle aspiration may be adequate if the pus has coalesced and liquefied, although a proportion of these will recur and need formal surgical drainage.

Dental Abscess

An infected molar or pre-molar tooth may cause extensive swelling extending into the face and neck and should be considered in the differential diagnosis of a neck abscess.

Retropharyngeal Abscess

This occurs typically in the young child (under 2 years) and is due to suppuration in the loose aggregate of lymph nodes between the pharynx and the pre-vertebral fascia. It is now uncommon but should be recognised because of its potential to cause fatal airway obstruction. The child is febrile, drooling and may adopt a characteristic posture with the neck flexed and the head extended. Transoral drainage is usually preferred.

Mycobacterial Neck Infections

Tuberculosis is now uncommon in the Western world, but there is an increasing incidence of infection with non-tuberculous mycobacterial organisms, frequently referred to as atypical mycobacteria. There is a wide variation in practice in the management of children with cervical lymphadenopathy caused by atypical mycobacterial infection. There is also confusion about the relative roles of surgery and antimicrobial treatment.

To manage this condition it helps to understand the natural history of the disease process if left untreated. The mycobacteria infect the cervical lymph nodes of small children causing a cervical, submandibular or less commonly parotid swelling. In the early stages there are no skin changes and concern may be raised about the possibility of an underlying lymphoma. Left untreated, the lesions usually progress and characteristic redness develops in the overlying skin. A significant proportion then progress to formation of an abscess, which, if untreated, discharges and forms a fistula. The fistula may continue to discharge for weeks or months before gradually "burning out". Natural resolution with significant scarring and puckering of the skin is the ultimate conclusion for untreated disease, but this may take 2 years or longer.

The aims of treatment are firstly to confirm the diagnosis and exclude the two main differentials, which are lymphoma in the early stages and tuberculosis later on.

Secondly, the aim is to limit the severity and duration of the disease, preventing or controlling discharge and reducing scarring.

Mycobacteria are encapsulated organisms and are highly resistant to medical treatment with antibiotics. Antituberculous medication and clarithromycin have been used in treatment. The nature of the infection often means that long-term antibiotic treatment for several months is considered. Unfortunately, there is great controversy as to whether this long-term antibiotic treatment reduces the duration or severity of this disease, compared to no treatment. Despite this, medical treatment has its advocates.

Surgical treatment offers several advantages. Ideally, complete excision of infected lymph nodes at an early stage will both eradicate the disease and confirm the diagnosis. A neat surgical scar can be obtained and fistula formation can be prevented. If surgery is performed later in the disease, after suppuration has formed, then it may not be possible to eradicate the disease completely. Surgery at this stage is still of benefit in reducing duration, severity, fistula formation and ultimate scarring. It also provides material for histopathology and microbiology. The risks to the marginal mandibular nerve for submandibular lesions are small. In the parotid region, surgery should also be considered and superficial parotidectomy can eradicate early disease. Because of the facial nerve, a conservative management is more commonly chosen in more advanced parotid lesions; however, significant facial scarring can result.

If lesions are treated non-surgically, then needle aspiration should be performed to confirm the diagnosis. Unfortunately, this frequently itself leads to discharge, which may become chronic. Chest x-ray and Mantoux test should be performed as part of the work up to exclude tuberculosis. A negative Mantoux test is reassuring, but a positive test is not diagnostic for tuberculosis, as atypical mycobacterial infection may cause false positive results.

Non-Infectious Inflammatory Lymphadenopathy

Kawasaki Syndrome

This is an acute multisystem vasculitis of unknown aetiology. It tends to affect children under 5 years of age and the clinical presentation is similar to many childhood infectious diseases. The diagnosis is clinical and children should have four of the five criteria

1. Acute non-purulent lymphadenopathy, usually unilateral.
2. Erythema, oedema and desquamation of the hands and feet.
3. Polymorphous exanthema.
4. Painless bilateral conjunctival infection.
5. Erythema and injection of the lips and oral cavity.

There may be a thrombocytosis and pericardial effusion. In the subacute stage, coronary artery aneurysms develop in 15–20% of cases. The goal of management is to reduce inflammatory responses with anti-inflammatory or gamma globulin therapy. The vasculitis is self-limiting, but unfortunately causes permanent cardiac damage in around 20% of untreated patients. All patients should have an initial echocardiogram and cardiac follow up. A mortality of 1–2% is associated with this disease due to the cardiac sequelae.

Sinus Histiocytosis (Rosai Dorfman Disease)

Children present with massive cervical lymphadenopathy that is similar to infectious mononucleosis or lymphoma. This disease is thought to represent an abnormal histiocytic response to some precipitating cause, possibly a herpes virus or Epstein-Barr virus. Fever and skin nodules may be present. Treatment is expectant, but biopsy sampling is usually required to rule out malignancy. Histopathologic examination reveals dilated sinuses, many plasma cells and marked proliferation of histiocytes.

Kikuchi-Fujimoto Disease

This is an idiopathic disorder. It is characterised by lymph gland enlargement, which may occur anywhere in the body but is typically cervical. Fever, chills and weight loss are common. Women are more commonly affected, typically young adults. The disease is self-limiting, but biopsy sampling is often performed to rule out malignancy. Histology shows a characteristic necrotising lymphadenitis.

Part 3. Haemangiomas and Vascular Malformations

Terminology

Historically, a wide range of terms has been used to describe this group of lesions (e.g. strawberry naevus, port wine stain, capillary haemangioma). Unfortunately the same word was often used for a wide range of vascular pathologies and this caused confusion. The tendency to use the term haemangioma to encompass all congenital vascular lesions should be avoided. Greater understanding of the biology of the commonest lesion the "strawberry" haemangioma has enabled a simple and more accurate classification to be developed by Mulliken and Glowacki (1982), which is now widely adopted. They demonstrated that there are two major types of vascular abnormality

1. Haemangioma. This is a distinct biologic tumorous entity characterised by rapid endothelial proliferation shortly after birth. The lesion is flat or absent at birth and then undergoes rapid, growth in early infancy followed by spontaneous resolution in childhood.
2. Vascular malformation. These lesions are structural anomalies that have a normal growth rate and normal rates of endothelial turnover.

Vascular malformations can be subdivided according to the morphology of the vessels and the flow rate. Slow-flow lesions include capillary, venous and lymphatic malformations. Fast-flow lesions include arterial and arteriovenous malformations.

Haemangiomas

Incidence

These are extremely common lesions, with one in ten (10–12%) full-term white infants being born with a haemangioma pleural line. For premature babies under 1000 g birth weight the incidence is even higher (Amir et al. 1986).

Clinical Features

Although most haemangioma are absent at birth, there may be a red macule. Rapid growth follows in the first 6 weeks of life and continues for the first 8–12 months. The lesion then enters an involutive phase followed by regression. Regression occurs slowly over the course of 3–8 years. Lesions that involve the dermis will be red in colour, but deeper lesions may be pale or bluish in colour. Haemangiomas in the subglottic region of the larynx present with increasing stridor and are considered in Chapter 24.

Complications associated with haemangiomas include Kasabach-Merrit syndrome, where platelet trapping within the haemangioma causes a thrombocytopenia and associated purpura and haemorrhagic tendency. Bleeding into the pharynx, gastrointestinal tract and brain may result, and this condition has a 30–40% mortality despite therapy. In massive haemangiomas, the high blood flow may result in cardiac failure.

Treatment

For the majority of haemangiomas no intervention is required and the lesions regress spontaneously. The overlying skin may exhibit mild atrophy, pallor or telangiectatic vessels after resolution.

High-dose corticosteroids remain the mainstay of treatment for endangering haemangiomas. Oral prednisolone 2–3 mg/day can control proliferation. The dose can be gradually lowered over several weeks. Children will require careful monitoring during this period, including blood pressure monitoring and urinalysis. Intralesional steroid injections have been used with some success, particularly for lesions around the eye and on the nasal tip. Up to 40 mg triamcinolone can be injected, dependent on body weight, and several injections (up to five) can be used 4–6 weeks apart.

Interferon therapy (2–3 million units interferon alpha 2A subcutaneously) has been used extensively, particularly in association with Kasabach-Merrit syndrome. Side effects include fever and neutropenia. Increasing concern about neurologic side effects including spastic diplegia, has led to less wide use of interferon therapy for haemangiomas.

Surgery to excise a haemangioma should be considered in some situations. Orbital haemangiomas that are encroaching on vision, and airway haemangiomas are two examples. Surgery is occasionally advocated for the psychological problems associated with having a large and visible haemangioma.

Pathologic Features

Haemangiomas during the proliferative phase are composed of rapidly dividing endothelial cells that form syncytial masses with and without lumina. Growth factors are produced, including basic fibroblast growth factor, which can be detected in the serum and urine of children with proliferating haemangiomas. There is potential to develop this into a clinical test for the presence of a proliferating haemangioma, since levels of these peptides are normal in patients with vascular malformations.

Vascular Malformations

These lesions grow commensurately with the child. They are divided into low-flow and high-flow lesions and can be further divided according to the dominant type of blood vessel. Slow-flow lesions include capillary, venous and lymphatic malformations. Not uncommonly, they may be mixed, as in venolymphatic malformations.

Capillary Malformations

The term "port-wine stain" is so widely used for these lesions that this term is unlikely to disappear. Port-wine stains are, however, capillary malformations. The skin or mucosa contains abnormally dilated capillaries in the superficial dermis. The lesion is present at birth and slowly changes to a more deep purple colour in adulthood. When these abnormalities occur in the area of the trigeminal nerve there is an associated risk of choroidal and intracranial vascular anomalies. This is known as the "Sturge Weber Syndrome". There may be hypertrophy of the soft tissue of the face and bony overgrowth of the maxilla. CT and MRI may show focal cerebral atrophy, cortical calcification, leptomeningeal enhancement of the affected area and enlargement of the choroid plexus.

The mainstay for treatment of capillary malformations is the pulsed-dye laser, which can achieve significant lightening in 80% of patients. In some cases, surgical excision with skin grafting or advancement flaps has been employed with variable cosmetic success.

Venous Malformations

These lesions may occur in isolation or be part of a capillary venous malformation. They have often been inappropriately termed haemangiomas in the past. They present as a soft, often bluish swelling with varying degrees of varicosity. They are common in the skin and subcutaneous tissue, but may also occur in skeletal muscle. They grow with the child and may expand at puberty, and after trauma or subtotal excision. Treatment may be complex and for most lesions no treatment is indicated. Sclerotherapy with an agent such as 95% ethanol or sodium tetradecyl sulphate can cause occlusion and significant reduction in the anomaly. Complications include local necrosis, oedema and nephrotoxicity. Surgical resection may be required for large or symptomatic lesions. This is rarely straightforward and bleeding may be profuse. In many cases complete excision is impossible and subtotal resection to debulk the lesion is the primary aim.

Lymphatic Malformations

In the head and neck the term cystic hygroma is commonly used for these lesions. The term lymphangioma is also used, but lymphatic malformation is more accurate. A typical lesion consists of several dilated lymphatic channels lined by a single layer of epithelium. These channels form cystic swellings of variable size. There are commonly associated venous malformations.

Common presentations are with cystic masses in the head and neck, which are present at birth or develop during childhood. Sudden swelling may be associated with an upper respiratory tract infection, when the fluid content increases. Swelling may also occur following minor trauma, which leads to internal haemorrhage. Involvement of the tongue may cause macroglossia and the tongue may be covered in vesicles. Tongue-base involvement frequently causes airway obstruction and may necessitate a tracheostomy. There may be associated bone hypertrophy and progressive distortion of the mandible, leading to prognathism. There are various classifications based on location. Type 1 lesions are located below the mylohyoid muscle, and involve the anterior and posterior triangles of the neck. These are often macrocystic lesions and carry a more favourable prognosis. Type 2 lesions are found above the level of the mylohyoid and may involve tongue, cheek, parotid and lip. These lesions are often microcystic and may be impossible to excise completely. They also respond less well to sclerotherapy.

Treatment options include conservative management, surgery and sclerotherapy. Without intervention, the vast majority of lesions progressively enlarge and may become massive. Rare cases of spontaneous involution have, however, been reported. In these cases there is presumably an inflammatory episode, possibly associated with a viral upper respiratory tract infection, and the lesion undergoes an "autosclerotherapy" process. For type 1 lesions there is a choice between excisional surgery and sclerotherapy. If the lesion is amenable to complete excision then surgery is preferred (Fig. 12.1). In experienced hands, surgery carries a relatively low risk of nerve damage. Depending on the location, the marginal mandibular, hypoglossal, recurrent laryngeal and accessory nerves may be at risk. Complete surgical excision does, however, offer a one-stop, short-term curative approach. Sclero-

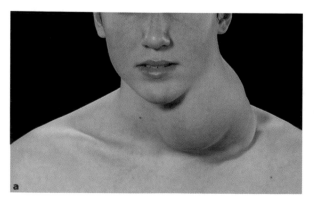 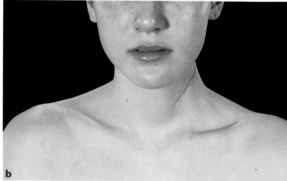

Fig. 12.1a,b Pre- (**a**) and post-operative (**b**) views of extensive lymphatic malformation (cystic hygroma)

therapy has a variable response, but is usually followed by dramatic swelling and then slow involution over several months. It may need to be repeated and the risk of late recurrence remains, as the lesion is still present. If there is airway compromise or dysphagia then sclerotherapy is usually best avoided as the subsequent enlargement will exacerbate the problem.

Type 2 lesions are usually treated with subtotal excision and sclerotherapy to any macrocystic areas. Partial glossectomy may be required for macroglossia, and surface lasering of tongue vesicles may be helpful. For children with facial disfigurement, psychological support for the children and their families is important.

Arteriovenous Malformations

These fast-flow lesions are relatively uncommon in the head and neck, compared to slow-flow lesions. The exception is the cranial cavity, where they are 20 times more common. They generally present in childhood or adolescence. A swelling appears that may be warm and pulsatile. A thrill may be palpable and Doppler ultrasound may confirm the presence of arteriovenous shunting. They may remain stable for years and then suddenly enlarge following trauma, infection or hormonal changes. Skin necrosis and destruction of the facial bones may occur.

No treatment is required for asymptomatic arteriovenous malformations. If pain, ulceration, bleeding or heart failure occurs, treatment may be required. MRI and angiography are essential. Selective embolisation may be helpful pre-operatively. Embolisation may have a role in palliation of surgically inaccessible lesions. Recurrence is likely after subtotal excision as new vascular channels form. Total resection is the only treatment that offers cure, and this may involve very extensive surgery.

Part 4. Head and Neck Malignancy in Children

Cancer is the second commonest cause of death in children (after accidents) and one in four paediatric malignancies will involve the head at some stage. An estimated 5% originate in the head and neck area (Boring et al. 1993).

There is a striking difference between the pathologies seen in children compared to those observed in adults. Squamous cell carcinoma is exceptionally rare and lymphomas and sarcomas are the predominant lesions, followed by thyroid carcinoma, nasopharyngeal carcinoma (predominantly affecting adolescents), salivary malignancy, neuroblastoma (especially under 1 year) and teratomas (newborn infants; Table 12.4).

A detailed account of the management of these diseases is beyond the scope of this text, but an overview will be given. Cases should be managed in co-operation with a paediatric oncologist.

Table 12.4 Histopathology of paediatric head and neck malignancy

Malignancy	Relative incidence
Hodgkin's lymphoma	32%
Non-Hodgkin lymphoma	29%
Rhabdomyosarcoma	13%
Other sarcoma	5%
Thyroid carcinoma	9%
Nasopharyngeal carcinoma	4%
Neuroblastoma	5%
Salivary malignancy	2%
Teratoma	1%
Other uncommon tumours	1%

Hodgkin's Disease

This is a malignant neoplasm of the lymphoreticular system that occurs predominantly in adolescents and young adults. It is distinguished pathologically from non-Hodgkin lymphoma (NHL) by the presence of Reed-Sternberg cells. It arises within lymph nodes in the vast majority of cases, and extra-nodal sites are rare (unlike NHL). Typical presentation is progressive enlargement of cervical or supraclavicular lymph nodes. Axillary and inguinal lymphadenopathy are less common. Enlargement of the liver, spleen and abdominal lymph nodes occurs as the disease spreads. The bone marrow may become involved, with neutropenia, thrombocytopenia and anaemia in the peripheral blood film as the disease progresses. Constitutional symptoms of fever, night sweats and weight loss may be present. Diagnosis is by lymph-node biopsy analysis. Staging is then performed and treatment is with chemotherapy or radiotherapy according to stage.

Non-Hodgkin Lymphoma

NHL is a mixed group of solid malignant neoplasms of the lymphoreticular system that usually affects a younger age group (2–12 years) than Hodgkin's disease. NHL may present as cervical or other lymphadenopathy, but not infrequently affects extra-nodal sites. Lesions may occur in the head and neck, oropharynx (enlarged tonsil), nasopharynx, orbit and skull base. Classification is confusing and controversial. Biopsy staging and treatment with chemotherapy or radiotherapy is required. As in Hodgkin's disease, surgery plays little role after initial biopsy analysis.

Rhabdomyosarcoma

After lymphoma, this is the commonest malignancy in the paediatric age group, and 35% occur in the head and neck. The commonest sites are the orbit, nasopharynx, middle ear and mastoid and sinonasal cavities. A typical presentation is a rapidly enlarging mass in one of these sites, most frequently the orbit, in a child under 12 years of age. In the nasopharynx, a delayed diagnosis is common due to the presentation with rhinorrhoea and nasal obstruction in school-age children. Similarly with tympanomastoid disease, a diagnosis of otitis media is usually made until a haemorrhagic mass in the external ear canal is identified or there are neurological sequelae due to skull-base involvement. Biopsy and detailed imaging (usually CT and MRI) are required.

Staging is performed with chest CT, abdominal ultrasound, bone marrow aspiration and trephine and, in selected cases, lumbar puncture to look for cerebrospinal fluid involvement.

Treatment is according to Intergroup Rhabdomyosarcoma Studies (IRS) 1 and 2 guidelines. Localised disease may be completely resected, but, because of the location and frequently delayed diagnosis, primary surgical treatment is rarely possible. There remains an important role for surgery in the management of residual or recurrent disease. Multimodality treatment involving chemotherapy, radiotherapy and surgery according to the IRS guidelines have significantly improved the morbidity and mortality associated with rhabdomyosarcoma.

Non-Rhabdomyosarcoma Sarcomas

Fibrosarcomas, synovial sarcomas and neurofibrosarcomas may occur in the head and neck region in children presenting with an enlarging mass. Biopsy, staging and treatment with chemotherapy or radiotherapy is usually the management of choice. Surgery remains an option for soft-tissue sarcomas and, if they can be excised completely with a margin of normal tissue, this can be curative. In reality, this is often not possible and may carry significant morbidity.

Thyroid Carcinoma in Children

This is considered separately in Chapter 31.

Salivary Gland Malignancy

Fortunately, salivary gland malignancies these remain rare in children (see also Chapter 17). The spectrum of pathology is similar to that in adult salivary malignancy, although children have a slightly higher proportion of malignant compared to benign disease. Mucoepidermoid carcinoma is the commonest salivary gland malignancy in childhood, and parotid malignancy is more common than submandibular. Adenocarcinoma, acinic cell carcinoma, adenoid cystic carcinoma and malignant mixed tumours are less common. Lymphomas and sarcomas may rarely present as salivary swellings.

Neuroblastoma

This is the commonest malignancy in children under 1 year of age, and 90% present before the age of 10 years. They arise from undifferentiated sympathetic nervous system cells of neural crest origin. The predominant sites are the adrenal and sympathetic chain. A small number present as a primary neck mass arising from the cervical sympathetic trunk and may have an associated Horner's syndrome. Metastasis is commonly observed at the time of presentation. After biopsy, imaging and staging, a treatment plan is made. Surgery may be curative for localised lesions. Radiation therapy and chemotherapy are considered for unresectable or metastatic lesions. For young patients with resectable disease, surgery offers a 90% survival.

Nasopharyngeal Carcinoma

This is one of the few epithelial malignancies affecting the head and neck in children and predominantly affects adolescents. There is an association with raised Epstein-Barr virus antibody titres, suggesting a possible infectious aetiology between undifferentiated and non-keratinising nasopharyngeal carcinoma. Most children presenting with nasopharyngeal carcinoma will have metastatic disease in the neck. Unilateral otitis media, rhinorrhoea and nasal obstruction are commonly present. Cranial nerve palsies and facial pain suggest skull-base involvement. Delayed diagnosis is frequent, with an average of 18 weeks between onset of symptoms and diagnosis of carcinoma. Biopsy, imaging with CT and MRI, and staging are performed. Treatment is based on type, location and extent of spread. Traditionally, the disease has been frequently considered non-resectable and chemotherapy and radiotherapy have been the mainstay treatments. However, advances in craniofacial and skull-base surgery makes surgery an important option both in primary and recurrent disease.

Teratoma

These occur in 1 in 4000 births and are thought to be derived form pluripotent cells; 7–9% are localised to the head and neck. The majority occur in the sacrococcygeal region, ovaries, testes, anterior mediastinum and retro-peritoneum. Overall malignant change occurs in 20% of teratomas, but it is rare in the head and neck. The typical head and neck presentation is a huge neck mass present at birth (see also Chapter 9). Although these are benign, the associated morbidity and mortality is significant. Treatment is by surgical resection (Fig. 12.2). Careful follow up with monitoring of tumour markers (alpha fetoprotein and beta human chorionic gonadotrophin) in the blood is recommended.

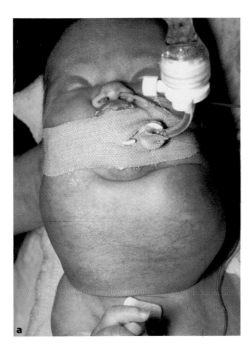

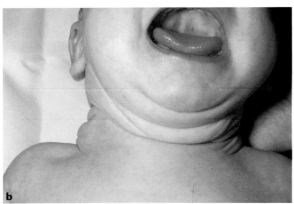

Fig. 12.2a,b Pre- (**a**) and post-operative (**b**) views of cervical teratoma

Juvenile Nasopharyngeal Angiofibroma

This is a benign tumour with potentially severe morbidity and a small associated mortality and is included in this section for completeness. It is a highly vascular lesion that originates in the region of the sphenopalatine foramen in adolescent males. The median age of presentation is 14 years, although lesions are often extensive at the time of diagnosis. Typical clinical features are nasal obstruction and epistaxis. This may progress to upper airway obstruction, facial mass or proptosis. If undetected, the lesion will progress to intracranial involvement affecting the anterior or middle cranial fossae or pituitary. The tumour also tends to spread laterally through the pterygo-maxillary fissure into the infratemporal fossa. CT scanning demonstrates the mass and a characteristic bowing of the posterior wall of the maxillary sinus due to progressive enlargment of the tumour. It also demonstrates the bony erosion that may involve sphenoid, ethmoids and pterygoid plates. MRI scanning gives good soft-tissue detail and information with regard to intracranial spread. In extensive cases, both forms of imaging are performed, as they are complementary.

Most authorities agree that primary surgery is the preferred treatment. This has been achieved successfully using endoscopic techniques for small lesions. The principle approach is an anterior approach, which may be performed by a midfacial degloving incision, to avoid facial scarring. More extensive lesions may require lateral skull-base approaches or collaboration with a neurosurgeon.

There is controversy as to the management of very extensive lesions with widespread intracranial extension. Complete surgical excision may be impossible and may carry significant morbidity and potential mortality. Primary radiotherapy has been used for some of these cases with control of growth in the majority.

Subtotal surgery with post-operative radiotherapy of the residual tumour is often preferred as it will substantially reduce the radiation exposure.

Summary for the Clinician

- Most of the head and neck masses the ENT surgeon will encounter in children are benign; however, cancer is the second commonest cause of death in children in developed countries and a quarter of these involve the head and neck. The spectrum of head and neck malignancies in children is different from that in adults and requires a different approach. In particular, epithelial malignancies are very uncommon in children.

References

1. Amir J, Metzker A, Krikler R, et al (1986) Strawberry hemangioma in preterm infants. Pediatr Dermatol 3:331–332

2. Boring CC, Squires TS, Tong T (1993) Cancer Statistics, 1993. CA Cancer J Clin 43:7

3. Mulliken JB, Glowacki J (1982) Hemangiomas and vascular malformations in children: a classification based on endothelial characteristics. Plast Reconstr Surg 69:412–422

12

Chapter 13

Paediatric ENT in Developing Countries

13

Neville P. Shine and Christopher A. J. Prescott

Core Messages

- In so-called developing countries, poverty and poor access to limited healthcare facilities are the predominant features of the less advantaged.
- Ear disease:
  - a. Acute infection often presents with complications.
  - b. Acute infection is commonly neglected or inadequately treated and progresses to a state of chronic or recurrent suppuration.
  - c. The lack of trained ENT specialists in these countries to undertake definitive surgery means that for the majority of affected children this will remain a life-long problem with consequences for hearing impairment and the risk of complications.
- The expense associated with hearing aids and the lack of audiological rehabilitation services condemns children with both conductive and sensorineural hearing impairment to developmental impairment and a lifetime of social isolation.
- Even relatively simple surgery such as adenotonsillectomy is not readily available, thus condemning children with recurrent infection to prolonged periods of ill health, and those with hypertrophy to the potentially fatal consequences of chronic upper-airway obstruction.

- The expense of antiretroviral therapy means that children infected with human immunodeficiency virus usually progress to acquired immune deficiency syndrome and die within a few years, often contracting associated tuberculosis.
- Tracheotomy for severe airway obstruction is often a death sentence for affected children due to lack of facilities for appropriate management of either the cause or the subsequent care.
- Head and neck trauma is a common problem: largely a consequence of poor driving and children playing in the streets of overcrowded settlements.
- Internal trauma to the pharynx and larynx from ingestion of small objects or corrosives is also a common problem.
- Developing countries present a challenging clinical environment: specialists from developed countries can provide a huge beneficial input by assisting and training local healthcare practitioners.

Contents

Introduction

The term "developing country" essentially refers to a country with low levels of economic development generally accompanied by poor social and infrastructural development. The United Nations compares countries in terms of the Human Development Index, a relative measure of wealth. This is assessed by: (1) gross domestic product, (2) health (life expectancy at birth) and (3) education (literacy levels).

While the nomenclature relating to poorer countries has moved on from "Third World" to "Developing World", the reality is that many inhabitants of this planet live in abject poverty, with little or no access to healthcare or education. The world population is now in excess of 5 billion and of them, an estimated 1.2 billion people live on less than US$1 per day and 800 million go to bed hungry every night. Obviously in such a context, it is the children who suffer most and even now, in the third millennium, 6 million children die every year from malnutrition.

Ill health and poverty are inextricably linked. The presence of one often determines the other and they cannot be dealt with in isolation. On an individual level, particularly in developing countries, the onset of illness often precipitates a spiral into poverty, draining meagre savings to pay for treatment while the patient is not able to earn. The poor are more prone to illness, which further limits the opportunities to escape from the poverty trap. On a national scale, developing countries have less money available to spend on healthcare, with the result that many of these countries lack the appropriate infrastructure and personnel to administer an effective healthcare programme for their citizens. Such challenges are being addressed on the world stage by the Millennium Development Goals and The Commission of Macroeconomics and Health, under the auspices of the World Health Organisation (WHO) and the United Nations.

For many poor people living in developing countries the reality is that when they are sick (and they are sick more frequently than the wealthy), they may not have a healthcare practitioner to attend locally, a public transport/ambulance system to transport them to an appropriate facility or the funds to pay for necessary investigations or treatment.

Children are the most vulnerable in society, and poor children in developing countries are the subjects of some appalling statistics. Of the total of 11 million children who die every year before their fifth birthday, 4 million are under 1 month old; 54% of deaths are related to malnutrition, and 99% of deaths occur in low- and middle-income countries (i.e. sub-Saharan Africa and South Asia). The majority of deaths are due to a handful of diseases such as diarrhoeal illness, pneumonia, measles and malaria, and thus are preventable. The 2005 WHO world health report focussed on maternal and child health and estimated that the cost of universal coverage for essential interventions (malaria control, vaccinations, infant feeding programmes and antibiotics) to be approximately US$53 billion.

In the context of such a background, a dedicated paediatric otolaryngologist would be considered something of a luxury. Many poorer countries have no ENT surgeons at all, let alone one with a sub-specialist interest.

However, diseases of the ears, nose and throat are important in the health of populations in developing countries, and several qualitative differences exist when compared to the developed world. First, healthcare may be administered by a healthcare practitioner other than a medical doctor or ENT surgeon. The scarcity of medically trained personnel, particularly in Africa, has led to the development of nurse practitioners and clinical officers who are trained in the primary care management of some common ENT conditions such as chronic suppurative otitis media (CSOM). Second, disease processes, particularly infective, that are relatively innocuous in the developed world may present in a neglected, more fulminant form, in patients with poor nutrition and poor immune status. When considering diseases of neglect, the cost of treatment, the cost and availability of transport to gain access to treatment and lack of education (another association with poverty), may all conspire against parents seeking early treatment for their children. A further difference is that in the developing world, the practitioner encounters clinical entities endemic to that part of the world that have been eradicated or are rarely seen in developed countries.

Finally, the greatest health threat faced by the developing world, and sub-Saharan Africa in particular, is the human immunodeficiency virus/acquired immunodeficiency syndrome (HIV/AIDS), tuberculosis, malaria (HTM) cluster. The burden of these diseases is disproportionately borne by developing countries, which between them account for over 6 million deaths annually. Of the estimated 42 million people infected with HIV/AIDS, two-thirds are African. Of the 3000 children who die daily from malaria, 90% are in sub-Saharan Africa. The HTM cluster significantly impacts on the presentation of diseases of the ear, nose and throat. All these socioeconomic and geographical factors must be considered as the background to discussion of specific diseases in developing countries.

Specific consideration will now be given to individual clinical scenarios of particular interest to paediatric ENT surgeons.

Ear Disease

Ear disease is common in any paediatric population. In developed countries the common problems presenting to ENT services are otitis media and middle ear effusions. Chronic ear disease is not common and complications of ear disease are rare. In developing countries, the absence of or limited access to ENT services means that otitis media will be managed – or neglected – by whatever primary care services are available, middle ear effusions largely remain unrecognised and available ENT services will be predominantly concerned with management of chronic ear disease and its complications.

Chronic Suppurative Otitis Media

Chronic otitis media (COM) can be defined as the presence of a persistent perforation in the eardrum (see also Chapter 43). When dry it is known as inactive COM, but when infected is known as active COM, terminology that is gradually replacing the traditional one of chronic suppurative otitis media (CSOM). In its simplest definition, this is the presence of chronic infection within the middle ear cleft and mastoid air cell system, with discharge through a perforated tympanic membrane. The WHO defines chronicity as otorrhoea persisting beyond 2 weeks. Although CSOM represents a potential indicator of the overall health status of a regional population, relatively few population surveys have been conducted. Countries where the rate of CSOM exceeds 4% include Australia (Aboriginal population), Guam, Greenland, India, Solomon Islands and Tanzania. Countries with high rates (2–4%) include Angola, Canada (Eskimo population), China, Korea, Malaysia, Mozambique, Nigeria, The Philippines, Thailand and Vietnam. Countries with low rates (1–2%) include Brazil and Kenya.

CSOM is a significant contributor to the morbidity of those affected. In addition, 28,000 deaths per annum occur secondary to complications related to CSOM – mastoiditis and its intracranial complications (meningitis, brain abscess). The major potential sequela of CSOM is an associated hearing deficit. Hearing impairment following CSOM is believed to effect 164 million people worldwide, with the majority living in the developing world.

The management of CSOM in countries with minimal health finance resources and limited ENT-trained personnel represents a major challenge. This has prompted a WHO publication devoted to the subject. The goals of treatment sound simple enough: to eradicate infection and close the tympanic membrane perforation. The former can potentially be achieved by avoidance of precipitants of infection: upper respiratory tract infection and water contamination, with appropriate oral or topical antimicrobials to treat infection when it occurs.

In developing countries things are not so simple. Topical quinolones may not be the most efficacious antimicrobials, but currently have the least ototoxic potential. However, as with everything, cost is often the limiting factor in the prescribing practices of developing countries and it may be necessary to treat patients with cheaper medications of similar efficacy but a poorer side-effect profile: the prolonged use of topical aminoglycoside drops in CSOM is an example of this. Alternatively, simple solutions of antiseptics or acidifying agents such as acetic acid drops may be the only medications available, providing a cheap and effective treatment for some patients. Dry mopping or wicking of the ear is an essential adjunctive procedure that may be performed by non-medical personnel and parents to facilitate optimal ototopical drug delivery, but as a stand-alone procedure, it is no better than no treatment. Such measures can be undertaken through primary care services and, if effective, will render the ear quiescent for a period. In some cases, however, discharge either persists or soon recurs. The application may have been ineffective, the organisms may have been resistant – and in this respect the possibility of tuberculous disease in chronically discharging ears must always be considered in endemic countries – or there may be underlying cholesteatoma. Specialist referral is then required, something that may or may not be available, either for assistance with diagnosis or when surgery is required in the definitive management of these cases and those that present with complications.

Again, it is impossible to treat the disease itself in isolation without addressing the overall living standards of the population. With specific reference to CSOM, the beneficial effects of public health measures have been elegantly demonstrated in the Australian Aborigine population, a high-risk CSOM group. The provision of chlorinated swimming pools to replace contaminated waterholes in "outback" aboriginal communities has improved dramatically several child health parameters including ear health.

Tympanomastoid Surgery

Otorhinolaryngology is a speciality requiring a significant period of training to attain the required level of competence and relatively expensive equipment in order to deliver optimum patient assessment and surgical treatment. Combine these with factors such as lack of training in a country, overburdened services and poor remuneration, and it is not surprising that many developing countries have no ENT specialists at all, either through lack of training or because of emigration of trainees during or after their training has been completed. In those countries that do have them, the ratio of ENT surgeons to population is often of the order of 1:1000,000. This is a stark contrast to European and North American countries, where the ratio of ENT surgeons to population is typically between 1:30,000 and 1:50,000.

In developing countries, ENT surgeons are usually based in the major urban centres and often predominantly serve the private sector. It is a common misconception that every single citizen of an impoverished state is poor. Many developing countries have an affluent sub-population who can afford top-level healthcare and can afford to travel to seek sub-specialist treatment. However, these countries have large rural-based populations, and for them a major difficulty in accessing ENT services, if these are even available in the public sector, is the need to travel vast distances in order to be treated. The travel costs alone may be prohibitive. This can be overcome by using outreach clinics, but a certain level of infrastructure is needed for these to be effective. One of the best examples of such an outreach service is the Rural Ear

Foundation programme in Thailand, which offers same-day clinic assessment and surgery to communities with no access to routine ENT services, typically managing several hundred patients per day.

Surgery is necessary to prevent the potentially devastating complications of active CSOM with or without cholesteatoma. It may also be necessary as an emergency since a significant number of patients will only seek help in the presence of advanced, neglected disease. Depending on the pathology and circumstances, tympanoplasty alone or in combination with cortical mastoidectomy may be sufficient for straightforward CSOM. Cases that require tympanomastoid surgery for cholesteatomatous disease in developing countries are generally managed by open-cavity surgery. Often patients may only be able to afford the time and money for one definitive procedure and a high rate of post-operative out-patient non-attendance can be expected. Therefore, canal wall-up procedures, with the risk of recidivistic disease and need for second-look operations, are inappropriate even though the hearing outcomes after multi-staged canal wall-up procedures may be better than after open-cavity procedures. Where complications are present, such as intracranial abscesses, these must be dealt with in conjunction with definitive mastoid surgery.

Hearing

Hearing impairment is commoner in developing countries (see also Chapters 36 and 37).

1. From the few population-based surveys available, it seems that congenital deafness has a higher incidence, with factors such as consanguinity, maternal infections in pregnancy and lack of adequate antenatal and natal care influencing this.
2. Acquired sensorineural deafness is commoner, particularly in the "meningitis belt" and endemic malaria areas, both from the disease and its treatment. It is also commoner as the result of the infectious diseases of childhood (particularly mumps and measles) in communities where immunisation programmes cover only the "basic schedule" and where cover is incomplete.
3. Ototoxicity is a significant cause of acquired sensorineural hearing loss in the developing world. The cost and availability of medications in this region often determines the prescribing practices of clinicians. In addition, the cost burden of monitoring techniques, such as serum level assay and audiometric equipment, may be prohibitive and limited to specialist centres. The severity of the patient's clinical condition and endemic disease sensitivities often leave the clinician with no alternative but to prescribe drugs with less favourable side-effect profiles, which may include ototoxicity.

One example of this is the increasing use of streptomycin for multi-drug-resistant tuberculosis. Furthermore, patient co-morbidities and the sequelae of the acute disease process under treatment may render some patients vulnerable to ototoxic complications. The unregulated sale of ototoxic medicines and lack of awareness of the risk and mechanisms of ototoxicity have also been suggested by several authors as contributing to the problem in the developing world. It is important to note that all the above causes are potentially preventable.
4. Acquired conductive hearing impairment is also commoner, either because facilities for detection and management of middle-ear effusions in children are not available or from the effects of CSOM.

Universal newborn screening is rapidly becoming the standard of care in the developed world. Such screening programmes in developing countries, if they exist, are usually only found in the more sophisticated communities who are less at risk. For any screening programme to be effective, the disease that is screened for must have an appropriate intervention. If one is to undertake screening for hearing disability in developing communities, access to surgery and hearing aid provision must be available. This is unfortunately not the case and so the development of screening programmes will only eventually follow the appropriate development of services.

The provision of hearing aids represents a significant challenge to developing countries. The WHO has developed suitable audiometric criteria and suggested priorities, but the major problems are those of supply and cost. It has been estimated by the WHO that there are currently about 300 million people worldwide who have significant hearing impairment and who would potentially benefit from a hearing aid; yet current worldwide production is only about 5 million units per year, of which less than 1 million units are sold outside the major "developed" countries. In developing countries, they are simply unaffordable to the majority of affected individuals, even when subsidised, the average cost of a basic aid being US$200–US$500. Financial constraints within public health systems usually preclude provision by the State: Non-Governmental Organisations (NGOs) often fill the void in this regard. The WHO has initiated efforts amongst concerned organisations in different countries, with the aim of mass producing affordable (ideally about US$20), high-quality (minimum performance standards have been defined) hearing aids of simple design, using standard batteries to facilitate easy maintenance. A further consideration is that provision of hearing aid services requires skilled personnel. It is obvious that the solution to aiding the world's most impoverished hearing impaired requires an integrated approach involving both private industry and government. Once more the close relationship of health and economic status is readily apparent.

Adenotonsillar Surgery

Adenotonsillectomy may be available only in certain centres within developing countries, often performed by a Medical Officer, General Practitioner or even a Medical Assistant (see also Chapter 14). Recurrent tonsillitis is probably no more common in developing countries, but the threshold for intervention in cases of recurrent infection or chronic infection is higher than that of developed countries, and is generally reserved for children with severe levels of morbidity or recurrent peritonsillar abscess formation.

The prevalence of paediatric upper airway obstruction with or without obstructive sleep apnoea, the other main indication for adenotonsillectomy, remains undetermined but is a common problem in developing countries. The diagnosis is based largely on history supported by suggestive clinical findings, since access to "gold standard" investigations such as overnight polysomnography is limited or non-existent. Poverty, with attendant poor sanitation and overcrowding, results in greater exposure of infants and children to inhaled pathogens, with a far higher incidence of adenoid and tonsil hyperplasia. Lymphoid tissue hypertrophy is also commonly seen in HIV/AIDS. Lack of awareness of the problem by parents and caregivers, and even by primary care providers, often results in late presentation of neglected disease. In paediatric centres, children presenting with cardiac failure as a consequence of chronic upper airway obstruction is a not uncommon event.

As far as the technical operative procedure of tonsillectomy is concerned, it is probably best performed using "cold steel", and those performing the procedure should be trained in the technique of controlling haemorrhage by placement of ligatures. There seems to be less morbidity with this method compared to diathermy techniques and a lower haemorrhage rate, an important consideration where patients may not easily be able to return to the hospital post-operatively. For this reason, "Day Surgery" is also inappropriate and admission for post-operative observation is generally the normal practice.

HIV/AIDS and Tuberculosis

Any discussion regarding healthcare, adult or paediatric, in developing countries often revolves around the HIV/AIDS pandemic (see also Chapter 10). Approximately 40 million people worldwide are infected, and every day another 11,000 people are infected. In 2005, an estimated 2.3 million children were living with the disease, whilst 570,000 children under the age of 15 years died from HIV/AIDS-related illness. Developing countries bear the greatest disease burden. In these countries and communities, the proportion of HIV-infected infants continues to steadily increase to the extent that in many affected communities more than 50% of infants in the local hospitals at any one time will be infected with HIV. However, some countries are beginning to show signs of stabilizing or even reversing this trend, for instance Uganda. Concerted behaviour-awareness campaigns aimed at modifying sexual practices and improved access to antiretroviral treatment are the mainstays of efforts to combat the pandemic. Unfortunately, in some regions such as Southern Africa, the pandemic continues to escalate and universal access to treatment remains elusive despite considerable progress in this regard. In 2005 only 10% of the Africans and 15% of the Asians who required antiretroviral treatment actually received it. A full discussion of the HIV/AIDS pandemic and the economics behind universal access to antiretroviral therapy is beyond the remit of this chapter, but the cost in human terms makes it a universal problem.

The common acute paediatric ENT infections occur in HIV-infected children, probably with much the same frequency as in non-infected children, but such infections can be more aggressive in the later stages of the disease when children are debilitated by chronic disease and a depressed immune system (AIDS), and they often require more aggressive treatment in terms of dose and duration of antibiotic therapy. Of the chronic problems, middle-ear effusions appear to be commoner, and chronic rhinosinusitis and CSOM are the cause of significant morbidity in infected children. These are both diseases of poverty. Since HIV infection is commoner among the poor, and poverty itself is manifest by the risk factors such as poor nutritional status, contaminated water and inadequate, overcrowded housing, it is difficult to assess the "pure" contribution of HIV infection to their prevalence in infected children. There is no doubt, however, that when these children receive antiretroviral medication, the overall prevalence of such diseases is reduced significantly and the frequency of recurrent episodes in the individual is markedly reduced. Less common are the more usually thought of manifestations of the disease – oral thrush, cervical adenopathy, adenotonsillar hypertrophy, tuberculosis in the head and neck and parotidomegaly. Croup, when it does occur in infected children, is often associated with candidiasis and other unusual organisms, tends to be prolonged and often requires airway intervention – many progressing to tracheotomy when extubation repeatedly fails. There are long lists of the other less common manifestations of HIV infection in children.

Global tuberculosis is on the increase. Approximately 9 million new cases are diagnosed annually and 5500 people die every day from the disease. The resurgence of this old foe has occurred in tandem with the HIV/AIDS pandemic. Indeed, the association between HIV/AIDS, tuberculosis and malaria is so strong that the WHO has coined the term HTM complex to embrace this association. As with all these diseases, the majority of tuberculosis is found in developing regions. ENT practice in these areas has to take this into consideration in patient assessment, since the incidence of extra-pulmonary sites of infection seems to be higher in this pandemic compared to previous ones. Almost as a routine, biopsy has to be considered for any granulating lesion in or around the oral cavity, nose or ears as well as in cases of persistent laryngitis. Although palpable cervical glands are almost universal in children in developing countries, tuberculosis has to be excluded in all cases of persistent significant cervical adenopathy. As mentioned previously, the emergence of multi-drug-resistant tuberculosis has led to increased usage of streptomycin, an aminoglycoside with a significant ototoxic side-effect profile. It is likely that an increase in cochleovestibular disability will be seen as a result of this necessary treatment.

Tracheotomy

Please also refer to Chapters 23 and 28. In developing countries, the capacity to provide adequate housing and community facilities falls far short of the need. Urban centres tend to be surrounded by either semi-formal, sub-economic or informal, shanty settlements that lack adequate facilities. In conflict areas, vast refugee camps, devoid of even the most basic elements such as running water and sanitation, can emerge in short periods of time. Close proximity, overcrowding and poor sanitation and hygiene contribute to respiratory tract disease, which in ENT is seen most commonly as rhinosinusitis, adenotonsillitis and otitis media, but also occasionally as laryngotracheobronchitis (croup), often in mini-epidemics. When conservative measures fail in croup, airway intervention is required; the outcome for the child is then dependent on the quality of care available in the local facilities. Intubation generally has a more favourable outcome than tracheotomy, and in many areas tracheotomy is a death sentence for an infant. Conversely, depending on the clinical situation, failure to perform tracheotomy may also result in death. If tracheotomy is required, the outcome is dependent on the quality of aftercare. Infants and children with a tracheotomy have to remain hospitalised because of lack of facilities to support home-care programmes, even though it is well recognised that a mother is better able to provide the care needed than a busy nurse in an overcrowded ward. In centres where there are good paediatric services, it is possible to develop good tracheotomy programmes. An example is the Red Cross Children's Hospital in South Africa, where about 70–80 paediatric tracheotomies are performed annually and at any one time there are a similar number of paediatric tracheotomised patients in the community, often at great distances from the hospital. A change to a formal stoma technique when performing the procedure and development of a "home care" programme in which parents are taught how to change the tube daily has made tracheotomy-related death in this cohort a rare event.

ENT Aspects of Accidents and Trauma

In developed countries, organisations concerned with child safety have largely ensured, both through pressure and legislation, that manufacturers of potentially harmful substances and objects package and label these in such a manner as to deter access to them by small children. This is seldom the case in developing countries. Potentially corrosive substances are freely available in the local shops where they tend not to be packaged in child-proof containers and may even be decanted into unlabelled containers. As a consequence, corrosive ingestion injury in children is still common. Parent education programmes concerning potential harm from ingestion or inhalation of small objects are at best patchy, and this is another frequent occurrence in these countries.

Childhood trauma, particularly head injury, is another common problem in developing countries. Pedestrian and motor vehicle accidents are frequent as a consequence of the lack of protected play areas in overcrowded settlements, where children normally play in the street. There is poor policing of speed limits and drink and drug driving; old, unsafe vehicles are on the roads. Severe head injuries often involve fracture of the temporal bone, with the attendant risk of facial nerve palsy, cerebrospinal fluid leaks, meningitis and hearing loss. Emergency intubation may be required in severely injured cases and may be undertaken in the field with an inappropriately sized tube – something easily overlooked and not subsequently corrected. Laryngeal injury from intubation is a not uncommon feature of survivors, with all its consequences for ENT services.

Paediatric Head and Neck Tumours

Paediatric head and neck tumours, as elsewhere, are uncommon (see also Chapter 21). One exception is Burkitt's lymphoma, the commonest paediatric malignancy in Central Africa. Given the association of human papilloma virus infection and laryngeal papillomatosis, one would expect a higher rate to be found in countries where HIV/AIDS, also a sexually transmitted disease, is prevalent. There are areas where laryngeal papillomatosis seems to occur more frequently than average, but even in such areas the difference is not as pronounced as one might imagine. In countries affected by the HIV pandemic, tumours such as Kaposi sarcoma will be seen. Infection-related "tumours", such as rhinoscleroma also tend to have a geographical distribution. In general, presentation of head and neck tumours is often late, and diagnostic modalities and treatment options (if available) are expensive. Prognosis is poor in developing countries for children with malignant tumours.

Summary for the Clinician

- The developing world presents a unique and challenging clinical environment. Paediatric patients present with diseases of poverty and neglect, sometimes at an advanced stage. Diagnosing and treating ENT diseases in these countries, particularly where diagnostic and surgical equipment is limited, often requires a different approach to that employed in developed countries. ENT surgeons from developed nations can play a useful part by getting involved in the training of local surgeons and assisting with provision of services under the auspices of NGOs. There are few places where one's clinical and surgical skills are more tested and more needed than the developing world.
- This chapter does not contain a formal list of references; however, a list of useful Public Health reports, websites and other articles is provided.

Bibliography

General

1. Millennium Development Goals 2000. World Health Organisation. Available at: http://www.who.int/mdg/en/. Accessed Jan 1, 2006

2. Report of the National Commission on Macroeconomics and Health. Geneva: World Health Organisation 2004. Available at: http://www.who.int/entity/macrohealth/action/Report%20of%20the%20National%20Commission.pdf. Accessed on Jan 9 2006

Chronic Ear Disease

1. Acuin J (2204) Chronic Suppurative Otitis Media: Burden of Illness and Management Options. Child and Adolescent Health and Development Prevention of Blindness and Deafness. World Health Organisation, Geneva

2. Lehmann D, Tennant MT, Silva DT, et al (2003) Benefits of swimming pools in two remote Aboriginal communities in Western Australia: Intervention study. BMJ 327:415–419

3. Prescott C, Malan JM (1991) Mastoid surgery at the Red Cross War Memorial Children's Hospital 1986–1988. J Laryngol Otol 105:409–412

4. Thorp M, Kruger J, Oliver S, et al (1998) The antibacterial activity of acetic acid and Burow's solution as topical otological preparations. J Laryngol Otol 112:925–928

Hearing Impairment and Deafness

1. Chiodo A, Alberti P (1994) Experimental, clinical and preventive aspects of ototoxicity. Eur Arch Otorhinolaryngol 251:375–392

2. Chukuezi A (1991) Profound and total deafness in Owerri, Nigeria. East Afr Med J 68:905–912

3. Guidelines for hearing aids and services for developing countries (2001) Geneva: World Health Organisation,. Available at: http://www.who.int/entity/pbd/deafness/en/hearing_aids_guidelines.pdf. Accessed Jan 3, 2006

4. Minja B (1998) Aetiology of deafness among children at the Buguruni School for the Deaf in Dar es Salaam, Tanzania. Int J Pediatr Otorhinolaryngol 42:225–231

5. Shine N, Coates H (2005) Systemic ototoxicity: a review. East Afr Med J 82:536–539

HIV/AIDS

1. World Health Organisation (2005) AIDS Epidemic Update: December 2005. World Health Organisation, Geneva

Chapter 14

Tonsils and Adenoids

14

Anne Pitkäranta and Pekka Karma

Core Messages

- The tonsils and adenoids form a substantial part of Waldeyer's ring, the collection of lymphoid tissue that encircles the pharynx, and are the first to sample and react to antigens in the air and food entering the body.
- The main function of the tonsils and adenoids in childhood is in generating B cells, as part of the immune response.
- Acute tonsillitis in children is most commonly viral and self-limiting. More severe viral causes include infectious mononucleosis and cytomegalovirus infection.
- Acute bacterial tonsillitis is most commonly the result of beta-haemolytic streptococcus and is best treated with oral penicillin V, unless the child is allergic to penicillin.
- Peritonsillar abscess is an important suppurative complication of acute bacterial tonsillitis. Non-suppurative complications such as scarlet fever, rheumatic fever and acute glomerulonephritis are now uncommon in developed countries, although still a problem in the developing world.
- Indications for (adeno)tonsillectomy include frequent episodes of acute tonsillitis and obstructive sleep apnoea.
- The commonest and most dangerous post-operative complication after tonsillectomy is haemorrhage, which must be recognised and treated without delay.
- Malignant disease involving the tonsils is extremely rare in children.

Contents

Waldeyer's Ring

The tonsils and adenoids are part of the lymphoid tissues that circle the pharynx known as Waldeyer's ring. This consists of the lymphoid tissue on the base of the tongue (lingual tonsil), two (palatine) tonsils, the adenoids (nasopharyngeal tonsil), and the lymphoid tissue on the posterior pharyngeal wall. (Fig. 14.1) Waldeyer's ring grows throughout childhood until the age of 11 years and after that decreases spontaneously (Arens et al. 2002).

Waldeyer's ring tissue serves as a defence against infection and plays an important role in the development of the immune system, comprising the first organs in the lymphatic system that analyse and react to airborne and alimentary antigenic stimulation. The tonsils and adenoids contain four lymphoid compartments (the crypt-epithelium, the follicular germinal centre with the mantle zone and the interfollicular area), which all participate

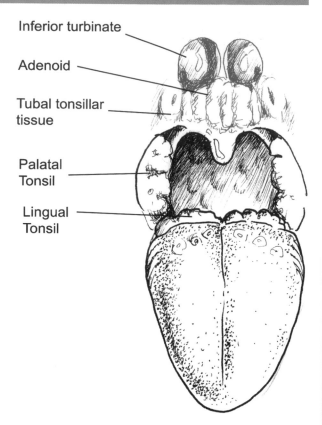

Inferior turbinate

Adenoid

Tubal tonsillar tissue

Palatal Tonsil

Lingual Tonsil

Fig. 14.1 Waldeyer's ring

Table 14.1 Clinically important microbiological causes of pharyngotonsillitis

1. Viruses and Chlamydia
Adenoviruses
Epstein-Barr virus
Enteroviruses (Coxsackie-A, rhinoviruses)
Influenza, parainfluenza viruses
Respiratory syncytial viruses
Cytomegaloviruses
Chlamydia trachomatis
2. Bacteria
Aerobic
Groups A, B, C and G streptococci
Corynebacterium diphtheriae
Arcanobacterium hemolyticum
Anaerobic
Bacteroides species
Fusobacterium species
3. Mycoplasmas
Mycoplasma pneumoniae
4. Fungi
Candida species
5. Parasites
Toxoplasma gondii

in the immune response. The generation of B cells in the germinal centres is the most essential function (Brandtzaeg 2003).

The principal disturbances of the tonsils and adenoids are infection and hyperplasia. Neoplasms of the tonsils and adenoids in children are rare.

Tonsillitis

Acute Tonsillitis

The most common manifestation of acute tonsillitis is sore throat. Tender cervical lymph nodes and fever may often coexist. On physical examination, the tonsils are swollen and erythematous. Exudates may be seen either on the entire tonsillar surface or emanating from tonsillar crypts.

Most cases seen in primary care practice are viral. The main bacterial causative agent is group A beta-haemolytic streptococcus (GABHS, *Streptococcus pyogenes*), but a variety of other organisms can also cause tonsillitis (Table 14.1). The signs and symptoms of viral and bacterial tonsillitis overlap and a precise diagnosis on clinical grounds is difficult.

Viral Tonsillitis

Tonsils are known targets for adenovirus replication, and adenovirus is the most common individual cause of sore throat in infants and small children. Adenovirus tonsillitis, particularly when associated with high fever, may mimic bacterial tonsillitis. It has also been shown that adenovirus tonsillitis may cause leukocytosis and elevated C-reactive protein (Dominquez et al. 2005), which can create differential diagnostic problems.

Coxsackie A viruses can cause epidemic outbreaks of herpangina, where small papules and vesicles develop on the tonsillar surface and the oropharynx.

Viral tonsillitis is usually self-limiting. There is, so far, no rapid sensitive test for adeno- or Coxsackie-virus

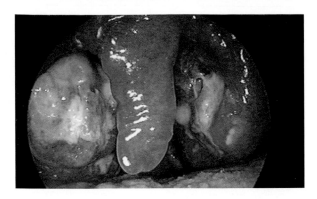

Fig. 14.2 In mononucleosis the tonsils are hyperaemic and pus accumulates in the tonsillar crypts. The debris in the crypts coalesces to form a purulent membrane. The clinical picture resembles of that in streptococcal tonsillitis

infections. No specific treatment for viral tonsillitis exists, and use of antibiotics for viral tonsillitis should be avoided as much as possible.

Epstein-Barr virus (EBV)-associated infectious mononucleosis (glandular fever) is an acute self-limiting disorder that typically occurs in adolescents or young adults as a result of contact with infected saliva, although in many cases primary infection occurs during childhood and may produce clinical symptoms (Macsween and Crawford 2003). Cytomegalovirus infection may also cause a mononucleosis-like syndrome.

Infectious mononucleosis is characterised by sore throat, fever, malaise, lymphadenopathy, hepatosplenomegaly and atypical lymphocytes in peripheral blood. The tonsils may resemble those in GABSH tonsillitis (Fig. 14.2). Confirmation of diagnosis can be based on the clinical picture and positive serology or Paul-Bunnell test. No practical antiviral medication exists and the treatment is symptomatic. Systemic corticosteroids can be used for patients with airway obstruction (Thompson et al. 2005). Maculopapular rash will develop in patients infected with EBV if they receive amoxycillin. No strong evidence-based information predicts the safe return to normal activity, but when the patient is afebrile, well-hydrated and asymptomatic with no palpable liver or spleen, a gradual return to normal activities is permitted.

Bacterial Tonsillitis

Streptococcal tonsillitis (with GABHS) cannot be diagnosed based on the clinical picture alone. A laboratory test is needed to confirm whether GABHS is present in the pharynx. The test may be either a rapid antigen detection test or culture of a throat swab specimen. There is no consensus on whether the sensitivity of the rapid an-

tigen detection test for GABHS is sufficient for diagnosis or whether a confirmatory throat culture is needed. In a recent study it was shown that in children who have tonsillar exudates and no cough, the rapid antigen test may be sensitive enough to meet current paediatric practice guidelines for stand-alone testing (Edmonson and Farwell 2005). However, for children and adolescents with severe symptoms, a negative rapid antigen test should be confirmed with a negative throat culture, unless the physician has ascertained in his/her own practice that a rapid test used is comparable to a throat culture (Bisno et al. 2002).

Children with proven acute GABHS tonsillitis should be treated with antibiotics to eradicate the bacteria from the pharynx, improve clinical symptoms and signs, reduce the transmission of bacteria and prevent suppurative complications and acute rheumatic fever. The first choice is oral penicillin-V (Bisno et al. 2002). Penicillin is effective, safe, has a narrow spectrum and is cheap. Erythromycin (or cephalosporin) is a suitable alternative for children allergic to penicillin. Penicillin (or erythromycin) must be administered for 10 days to achieve eradication of GABHS. Azithromycin for 3 or 5 days may be an alternative in children noncompliant with a 10-day penicillin regimen, although there are no definitive data to allow final evaluation of the efficacy of the newer antibiotics with shorter courses.

Repeated bacteriologic testing of an asymptomatic child after antibiotic treatment is not needed. Asymptomatic contacts of a child with acute GABHS do not need to be tested routinely for GABHS.

Treatment of asymptomatic carriers is needed:
1. if there is a family history of rheumatic fever,
2. if the carrier has a history of acute glomerulonephritis,
3. if the carrier's family is having a "ping-pong" spread of the disease.
4. if the carrier attends a school experiencing a GABHS epidemic (Darrow and Siemens 2002).

The role of anaerobic bacteria in children's tonsillitis is not known, but there is increasing evidence that anaerobes may have been underestimated as the cause of tonsillitis (Brook 2005). An example of anaerobic infection of tonsils is Vincent's angina, which can be diagnosed by taking a scraping from the ulcerative tonsil (or gingiva). Vincent's angina is treated with penicillin and metronidazole. Another example of anaerobic bacteria causing chronic or recurrent tonsillitis is *Fusobacterium necrophorum*, which is best eradicated with clindamycin or metronidazole.

Diphtheria is a very rare condition in the developed world today because of active immunisation. However, it should be considered as a possible diagnosis in tonsillitis among populations of children who have been inadequately immunised or not immunised at all. Membranes may extend outside the tonsils to the larynx, soft palate and oro- or nasopharynx. The borders of the membrane are sharply defined and the membrane is adherent to the underlying tissue. For diagnosis, the membrane should be cultured. Before sending for the culture, the laboratory should be notified about the suspicion of diphtheria. Both antitoxin and antibiotics are mandatory. Penicillin and erythromycin are the drugs of choice. In developing countries, diphtheria remains a common indication for emergency tracheotomy.

Chronic Tonsillitis

Chronic tonsillitis is poorly defined in children but may be described as sore throat of at least 3 months' duration accompanied by tonsillar inflammation. A small percentage of children will have a recurrence of GABHS. Recurrent tonsillitis may have a polymicrobial aetiology; mixed aerobic and anaerobic bacterial infection or penicillin-resistant GABHS may exist. In these children, additional antibiotics, such as clindamycin, are the drugs of choice. If the antibiotics are not effective, tonsillectomy may be indicated.

Complications of Tonsillitis

The complications of tonsillitis may be classified into local, suppurative (peritonsillar, parapharyngeal, and retropharyngeal cellulites and/or abscesses) and systemic, non-suppurative (scarlet fever, acute rheumatic fever, and post-streptococcal glomerulonephritis) complications. The latter types are now rare in Western societies (Del Mar et al. 2004).

Peritonsillar Abscess (Quinsy)

A peritonsillar abscess (PTA) is a collection of pus located between the fibrous capsule of the tonsil and the superior pharyngeal constrictor muscle. The most commonly held theory is that PTA occurs secondary to the penetration of bacteria from the tonsillar crypts through the tonsillar capsule into the peritonsillar space. An alternative theory is that an abscess formation in Weber's salivary glands in the supratonsillar fossa causes PTA (Passy 1994).

The most common symptoms are swallowing difficulties, drooling, trismus and fever. Asymmetric peritonsillar swelling can occur, with deviation of the uvula (Fig. 14.3). Diagnosis is based on physical examination. PTA is an indication for some sort of surgical procedure, since there are no data showing that antibiotics alone are effective in its management. The choices are needle aspiration, incision and drainage under local or general anaesthesia, or

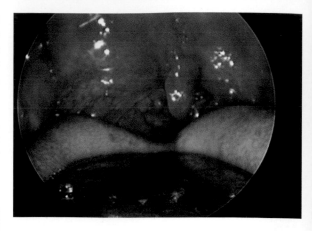

Fig. 14.3 Right peritonsillar abscess; the peritonsillar space, the soft palate and the uvula are swollen. The uvula is displaced to the contralateral side

abscess drainage with simultaneous tonsillectomy (quinsy tonsillectomy). Although all techniques can be used with consistently good results (Johnson and Stewart 2005), in small children, who require general anaesthesia for any procedure, the quinsy tonsillectomy makes most sense. Culture results in peritonsillar abscess may vary, and depend on the microbiological culture technique. Anaerobes are likely to be involved.

Antibiotics are necessary, penicillin (or penicillin with metronidazole) or clindamycin being the best choices. The use of steroids may be beneficial although good evidence is lacking (Johnson and Stewart 2005).

Adenotonsillar Hyperplasia

In children, enlarged adenoids and tonsils play a major role in obstructive sleep apnoea. A history of obstruction (snoring, apnoea), sleep disruption (restless sleep, arousals, daytime symptoms) and suggestive physical findings are indications for adenotonsillectomy in most affected children (Ray and Bower 2005). Obstructive sleep apnoea is discussed in more detail in Chapter 15.

Adenotonsillar hyperplasia may cause dysphagia and swallowing difficulties in some children. Also, the enlarged adenoids and tonsils may decrease nasal airflow causing hyponasal speech.

Mouth Breathing

Nasal obstruction because of adenotonsillar hyperplasia or nasal allergy may cause abnormal dentofacial growth. Downward growth of the mandible and repositioning of the tongue may compensate for the absence of na-

14

sal airflow. This may increase the vertical facial dimension and gonial angle. Absence of contact between the tongue and palate may cause a high, narrow palatal vault and a secondary posterior dental crossbite (Darrow and Siemens 2002). "Adenoidal facies" has been defined as a long, thin face with malar hypoplasia, high-arched palate, narrow maxillary arch, and malocclusion. However, a direct causal relationship between nasal airway obstruction and abnormal craniofacial anatomy has not yet been shown.

Tonsillectomy

Indications

(Adeno)tonsillectomy is a common major surgical procedure performed on children. Convincing scientific evidence for the benefit of tonsillectomy has been demonstrated in children with:

1. seven or more documented episodes of tonsillitis in the preceding year,
2. five or more in each of the two preceding years,
3. three or more in each of the three preceding years (Paradise et al. 1984) and
4. sleep apnoea due to (adeno)tonsillar hypertrophy (Ray and Bower 2005).

These indications account for only 35% of children's tonsillectomies in The Netherlands (Van den Akker et al. 2003). Other indications were swallowing difficulties, tonsillar crypt debris, enlarged cervical lymph nodes, restless sleep, poor appetite, school absence, frequent use of antibiotics, combinations of these (Van den Akker et al. 2003). There is largely anecdotal evidence concerning these indications, also on the use of tonsillectomy in the treatment of guttate psoriasis or periodic fever.

Mallampati scoring (Mallampati et al. 1985) can be used to describe the oropharynx and tonsils, including their size (Table 14.2).

Table 14.2 Description of the oropharynx and tonsils (Mallampati et al. 1985)

Tonsil O:	Tonsils fit within tonsillar fossa
Tonsil 1+:	Tonsils <25% of space between pillars
Tonsil 2+:	Tonsils <50% of space between pillars
Tonsil 3+:	Tonsils <75% of space between pillars
Tonsil 4+:	Tonsils >75% of space between pillars

Clinical signs: Heavy snoring, quality of sleep, dysphagia, reduced growth, cardiopulmonary disorders, speech; hot potato voice

Because of the limited evidence of the usefulness of surgery in children with mild symptoms and without frequent throat infections or sleep apnoea, the decision to perform tonsillectomy must always be made on an individual basis by the surgeon together with the patient and the family, who must be fully informed of the risks involved.

In many cases, tonsillectomy and adenoidectomy are combined. This should only occur when there are indications for both operations.

Techniques

Tonsillectomies are usually performed under general anaesthesia in children. There are several tonsillectomy techniques currently in use, but the superiority of one over another has not been clearly demonstrated (Pinder and Hinton 2005) (Table 14.3).

Removal of the tonsils has traditionally been performed by so-called "cold steel dissection" tonsillectomy (Fig 14.4a, b). After dissection, haemostasis is achieved with ligatures or diathermy (Fig. 14.4c). Diathermy uses an electric current to coagulate blood vessels, or to cut tissue. There are two main diathermy types: bipolar and monopolar. In bipolar diathermy, electric current passes through the tissue between the tips of a pair of forceps. In monopolar diathermy, current passes away from the instrument and is dispersed safely to an electrode with a large surface area placed on the patient's thigh. In bipolar dissection tonsillectomy, currently the preferred technique in many departments, the tonsil is removed and haemostasis secured simultaneously. In this technique the tips of the diathermy forceps should be as fine as possible, to avoid burning the surrounding tissue.

Table 14.3 Different techniques

Tonsillectomy
– Cold knife (suture – diathermy)
– Bipolar diathermy (scissors)
– Laser – CO_2, KTP, Diodi
– Ultrasonic scalpel
– Ligasure
– Radiofrequency technique
(as surgery – as diathermy; Coblation tonsillectomy)
Tonsillotomy
- Laser
- Radiofrequency (tonsillar reduction - radiofrequency)

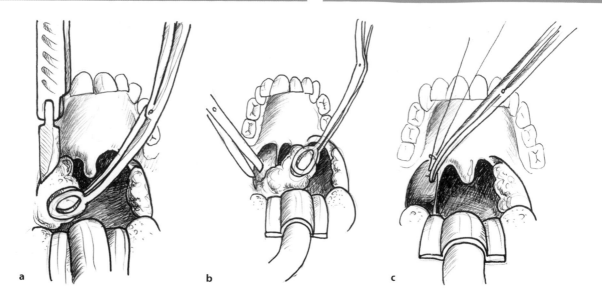

Fig. 14.4a–c Cold-knife tonsillectomy (drawings by Hannu Tapiovaara). **a** The superior pole of the tonsil is pulled medially. The mucosa overlying the superior pole is incised at the junction between the tonsil and the mucosal fold. Scissors or a clamp can be used to identify the avascular dissection plane between the tonsillar capsule and the tonsillar fossa. **b** Dissection between the tonsillar capsule and fossa proceeds from superior to inferior. **c** After tonsil removal, haemostasis is established with ligation (or cauterisation)

14

Other tools are:

1. The harmonic scalpel, which uses ultrasonic energy to vibrate its blade at 55,000 cycles per second, transferring energy to the tissue, and providing simultaneous cutting and coagulation.
2. Monopolar radiofrequency, whereby energy is transferred to the tonsil tissue through probes inserted in the tonsil.
3. Bipolar radiofrequency ablation (Coblation; Belloso et al. 2003) produces an ionised saline layer that disrupts molecular bonds without using heat. As the energy is transferred to the tissue, ionic dissociation occurs.
4. The Ligasure technique (Lachanas et al. 2005), which uses a special instrument that is both a haemostatic device and a dissection tool with integrated active feedback control of energy denaturing the tissue.
5. Carbon dioxide lasers can be used to remove tonsil tissue by vaporisation. Tonsillotomy (intracapsular partial tonsillectomy) can be done with either a carbon dioxide laser (Hultcrantz et al. 2005) or radiofrequency (Bäck et al. 2001).

In some units, children are discharged from hospital within 4–6 hours after surgery, once the main risk of reactionary bleeding has passed. The exceptions are children under 2 years of age, children with obstructive sleep apnoea whose breathing needs to be monitored post-operatively, or children with severe associated medical prob-

lems. However, large variations exist in the tonsillectomy day-case rate across countries. In Europe, the day-case tonsillectomy rate is increasing, but in some countries, children still spend several nights in a hospital.

Post-operative pain is significant after tonsillectomy, and may be severe enough to delay the discharge from hospital, the resumption of normal diet and normal activities. Paracetamol (acetaminophen), with codeine in older children without sleep apnoea is recommended. Increased risk of bleeding, although rare, must be considered if medications containing ibuprofen are used. Post-operative pain may be decreased by anaesthesiologists starting pain killers perioperatively. Perioperative dexamethasone may decrease post-operative nausea and vomiting.

Complications

Tonsillectomy is not without complications, and the risks must always be taken into account while considering the operation. The most important potential complication is bleeding. It is important to exclude a family history of abnormal bleeding and bruising before embarking on surgery. Post-operative bleeding can vary from a minor to a life-threatening haemorrhage. Reactionary haemorrhage, within 6–8 hours after the operation, is estimated to occur in 0–3.5% of tonsillectomies. Occurrence of secondary haemorrhage varies markedly in the literature, from 0 to 33%. Differences in post-operative bleeding rates may be real, or may simply reflect differences in reporting. Bleeding may be so severe that its control in the operating room is needed. Bleeding vessels can be cauterised or ligated. Strenuous activity and hard food should be avoided until the tonsillar fossae have healed.

More rare complications such as infection, dental injury, nasopharyngeal stenosis, patulous Eustachian tube, hypernasality, lingual nerve palsy and cautery burns have also been reported (Randall and Hoffner 1998). Clinical variant Creutzfelt-Jacob disease could, in theory, be associated with transfer of prions to the patient on surgical instruments, although today no definitive data of positive cases exist (Frosh et al. 2004).

Evaluation of the Adenoids

The adenoid pad in the child's nasopharynx is a normal structure with specific immunologic function. The size of adenoid tissue may vary from child to child. Adenoid tissue can react with immune-associated events and agents, as has been shown in children with adenotonsillar enlargement after successful treatment of childhood malignancies (Karadeniz et al. 2005). Respiratory infections affect the size of the adenoid; children with successful medical treatment for rhinosinusitis show reduction of adenoid size (Georgalas et al. 2005).

Fibre-optic nasendoscopy has been shown to be a reliable technique for evaluation of the child's adenoid size (Cassano et al. 2003). In a cooperative child, examination of the nasopharynx with a post-nasal mirror can be performed. A lateral radiograph for evaluating the size of the adenoid in children is no longer thought appropriate because of radiation dose and inherent inaccuracy. Acoustic rhinometry is not reliable for such a posterior structure (Fisher et al. 1994). Clinical symptoms, nasal obstruction, snoring, sleep-related disorders, mouth breathing, hyponasal speech and failure to thrive are important when evaluating the size of adenoids. Parental estimation of snoring on a visual analogue scale correlates with adenoid size at operation (E. Fisher, personal communication).

Adenoidectomy

Indications

Adenoidectomy remains one of the most commonly performed surgical operations in the paediatric age group. Considering this and the amount of research, it is amazing that no all-encompassing indications exist.

While the positive effect of adenoidectomy has been shown in improving the physical condition and quality of life of children with obstructive adenoid tissue (obstructive sleep apnoea, nasal airway obstruction), children with recurrent and chronic rhinosinusitis, and those with otitis media with effusion persisting after tympanostomy tubes (Maw and Bawden 1994; American Academy of Pediatrics 2004; see also Chapter 42), the value of adenoidectomy in recurrent acute otitis media and preventing abnormal craniofacial growth is constantly debated in the literature (Table 14.4). There is growing evidence that adenoidectomy should not be recommended as the first choice of treatment for recurrent acute otitis media in children (Koivunen et al. 2004). For children referred to an otorhinolaryngologist because of orthodontic indications, adeno(tonsillectomy) can be considered if the adeno(tonsillar) tissue is markedly hyperplastic or hypertrophic. Dysphagia associated with failure to thrive and unintelligible hyponasal speech are rare indications for adenoidectomy.

It is uncertain whether such an entity as chronic adenoiditis exists, and the relationships between chronic rhinitis and recurrent rhinosinusitis and the adenoids are poorly understood. However, before considering endoscopic sinus surgery, most clinicians prefer to perform adenoidectomy in children with persistent or recurrent rhinosinusitis (Darrow and Siemens 2002).

There is large unexplained international variation between adeno(tonsillectomy) rates. In addition to the correct indications, the effectiveness of the procedure may also depend on stringency in making the correct diagnoses for rhinosinusitis and otitis media in children.

Table 14.4 Indications to consider adenoidectomy

Snoring
Obstructive sleep apnoea
Otitis media with effusion (>3 months) in children with other medical problems
Otitis media with effusion relapses after tympanostomy
Nasal obstruction
Associated speech problems
Rhinitis/recurrent (>3/6 months)/chronic (>3 months) rhinosinusitis?
Recurrent acute otitis media?
Abnormal craniofacial growth?
Mouth breathing?

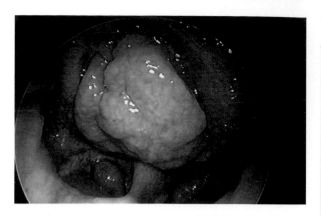

Fig. 14.5 A mirror view of the adenoid in the nasopharynx of a 6-year-old boy during surgery. The inferior turbinates can be seen through the choanae, below the adenoids in this picture

Table 14.5 Complications of adenoidectomy

| Post-operative bleeding |
| Regrowth of adenoid tissue |
| Hypernasality |
| Atlantoaxial subluxation |
| Dental injury |
| Nasopharyngeal stenosis |
| Eustachian tube injury |
| Cautery burns |

Techniques

Traditionally, the adenoid pad (Fig. 14.5) has been removed by curettage. Power-assisted (endoscopic shaver) and electrocautery or suction-diathermy techniques have been shown to be as effective and less bloody (Elluru et al. 2002), but may be slower. However, the necessary equipment needed for new techniques is expensive, and more experience is required to attain proficiency.

The mouth gag is inserted to retract the tongue forward and open the mouth. Whatever the method, the palate is inspected and palpated for evidence of submucous cleft. The catheter is inserted in the nose, retrieved through the mouth, and pulled anteriorly to retract the soft palate forward and to allow access to the nasopharynx. The nasopharynx is inspected with a mirror. The removal of the adenoid tissue can then be performed by using a curette, a suction coagulator or a shaver instrument. For children who are at risk for velopharyngeal insufficiency, a partial adenoidectomy can be performed, leaving the inferior part of the adenoid intact for sufficient velopharyngeal closure.

The child can start normal activity and diet as soon as he or she desires. The post-operative pain medication can be the same as after tonsillectomy, usually paracetamol (acetaminophen) is sufficient.

Complications

Complications after adenoidectomy exist (Table 14.5; Randall and Hoffner 1998). Post-operative bleeding may occur, although not as often as after tonsillectomy. The practical way of controlling the haemorrhage, if cauterisation is not helpful, is post-nasal packing. It can be applied for a few hours or even overnight. The regrowth of the adenoid tissue or symptomatic tubal tonsil hypertro-

phy after adenoidectomy may require revision surgery, although not very often (Buchinsky et al. 2000; Emerick and Cunningham 2006). In atlantoaxial subluxation or dislocation, especially in children with Down syndrome who have an increased risk (Pueschel 1998), a neurosurgical or an orthopaedic consultation may be needed, as well as the dentist in cases of dental injury. Other complications are nasopharyngeal stenosis, transient or persistent velopharyngeal insufficiency, and Eustachian tube injury if the torus tubarius has been cauterised or damaged by a curette. Although electrocautery during adenoidectomy can result in substantial local temperature change, complications appear to be independent of adenoidectomy techniques (Henry et al. 2005).

Neoplasms of the Tonsils and the Adenoids

In children it is relatively common that tonsils are somewhat different in size. However malignancies are very rare (see also Chapter 21). In a study with 2012 children who underwent tonsillectomy on the basis of asymmetry between tonsils, a malignant lymphoma was found in only one tonsil, but was suspected prior to surgery (Dohar and Bonilla 1996).

Summary for the Clinician

- The tonsils and adenoids are part of the lymphoid tissues, known as Waldeyer's ring, that circle the pharynx. These tissues serve as a defence against infection and play an important role in the development of the immune system. The principal disturbances of the tonsils and adenoids are infection and hyperplasia. Most episodes of tonsillitis are self-limiting viral infections, which may include infectious mononucleosis. The main bacterial causative agent in tonsillitis is group A beta-haemolytic streptococcus (GABHS). Children with proven acute GABHS tonsillitis should be treated with antibiotics, the first choice being oral penicillin-V. Chronic tonsillitis is poorly defined in children. (Adeno)tonsillectomy is a common major surgical procedure performed on children. Evidence for the benefit of tonsillectomy has been shown in children with seven or more documented episodes of tonsillitis in the preceding year, five or more in each of the two preceding years, or three or more in each of the three preceding years, and in children with sleep apnoea due to (adeno)tonsillar hypertrophy. The positive effect of adenoidectomy has been shown in improving the physical condition and quality of life of children with obstructive adenoid tissue and of children with respiratory infectious problems.

References

1. American Academy of Family Physicians, et al (2004) Otitis media with effusion. Pediatrics 113:1412–1429
2. Arens R, McDonough JM, Corbin AM, et al (2002) Linear dimensions of the upper airway structure during development. Am J Respir Crit Care Med 165:117–122
3. Belloso A, Chidambaram A, Morar P, et al (2003) Coblation tonsillectomy versus dissection tonsillectomy: postoperative hemorrhage. Laryngoscope 113:2010–2013
4. Bisno AL, Gerber MA, Gwaltney JM (2002) Practice guidelines for the diagnosis and management of group A streptococcal pharyngitis. Infectious Diseases Society of America. Clin Infect Dis 35:113–125
5. Brandtzaeg P (2003) Immunology of tonsils and adenoids: everything the ENT surgeon needs to know. Int J Pediatr Otorhinolaryngol 67:S69–S76
6. Brook I (2005) The role of anaerobic bacteria in tonsillitis. Int J Pediatr Otorhinolaryngol 69:9–19
7. Buchinsky FJ, Lowry MA, Isaacson G (2000) Do adenoids regrow after excision? Otolaryngol Head Neck Surg 123:576–581
8. Bäck L, Paloheimo M, Ylikoski J (2001) Traditional tonsillectomy compared with bipolar radiofrequency thermal ablation tonsillectomy in adults: a pilot study. Arch Otolaryngol Head Neck Surg 127:1106–1112
9. Cassano P, Gelardi M, Cassano M, et al (2003) Adenoid tissue rhinopharyngeal obstruction grading based on fiberendoscopic findings: a novel approach to therapeutic management. Int J Pediatr Otorhinolaryngol 67:1303–1309
10. Darrow DH, Siemens C (2002) Indications for tonsillectomy and adenoidectomy. Laryngoscope 112:6–10
11. Del Mar CB, Glasziou PP, Spinks AB (2004) Antibiotics for sore throat. Cochrane Database Syst Rev 2:CD000023
12. Dohar JE, Bonilla JA (1996) Processing of adenoid and tonsil specimens in children: a national survey of standard practices and five-year review of the experience at the Children's Hospital of Pittsburgh. Otolaryngol Head Neck Surg 115:94–97
13. Dominquez O, Rojo P, de las Hera S, et al (2005) Clinical presentation and characteristics of pharyngeal adenovirus infections. Pediatr Infect Dis J 24:733–734
14. Edmonson MB, Farwell KR (2005) Relationship between the clinical likelihood of group A Streptococcal pharyngitis and the sensitivity of a rapid antigen-detection test in a pediatric practice. Pediatrics 115:280–285
15. Elluru RG, Johnson L, Myer CM (2002) Electrocautery adenoidectomy compared with curette and power-assisted methods. Laryngoscope 112:23–25
16. Emerick KS, Cunningham MJ (2006) Tubal tonsil hypertrophy. A cause of recurrent symptoms after adenoidectomy. Arch Otolaryngol Head neck Surg 132:153–156
17. Fisher E, Lund VJ, Scadding GK (1994) Acoustic rhinometry in rhinological practice: discussion paper. J R Soc Med 87:411–413
18. Frosh A, Smith LC, Jackson CJ, et al (2004) Analysis of 2000 consecutive UK tonsillectomy specimens for disease-related prion protein. Lancet 364:1260–1262
19. Georgalas C, Thomas K, Owens C, et al (2005) Medical treatment for rhinosinusitis associated with adenoidal hypertrophy in children: an evaluation of clinical response and changes on magnetic resonance imaging. Ann Otol Rhinol Laryngol 114:638–644
20. Henry LR, Gal TJ, Mair EA (2005) Does increased electrocautery during adenoidectomy lead to neck pain? Otolaryngol Head Neck Surg 133:556–561
21. Hultcrantz E, Linder A, Markström A (2005) Long-term effects of intracapsular partial tonsillectomy (tonsillotomy) compared with full tonsillectomy. Int J Pediatr Otorhinolaryngol 69:463–469
22. Johnson RF, Stewart MG (2005) The contemporary approach to diagnosis and management of peritonsillar abscess. Curr Opin Otolaryngol Head Neck Surg 13:157–160
23. Karadeniz OA, Citak EC, Conly NA, et al (2005) Thymic and adenotonsillar enlargement after successful treatment of malignancies. Pediatr Hematol Oncol 22:423–435
24. Koivunen P, Uhari M. Luotonen J, et al (2004) Adenoidectomy versus chemoprophylaxis and placebo for recurrent acute otitis media in children aged under 2 years: randomized controlled trials. BMJ 328:487–451
25. Lachanas VA, Prokopakis EP, Bourolias CA, et al (2005) Ligasure versus cold knife tonsillectomy. Laryngoscope 115:1591–1594
26. Macsween KF, Crawford DH (2003) Epstein-Barr virus – recent advances. Lancet Infect Dis 3:131–140

27. Mallampati SR, Gatt SP, Guigino LD (1985) A clinical sign to predict difficult tracheal intubation: a prospective study. Can Anaesth Soc J 32:429–434

28. Maw AR, Bawden R (1994) Does adenoidectomy have an adjuvant effect on ventilation tube insertion and thus reduce the need for re-treatment? Clin Otolaryngol 19:340–343

29. Paradise JL, Bluestone CD, Bachman RZ, et al (1984) Efficacy of tonsillectomy for recurrent throat infection in severely affected children. N Engl J Med 310:674–683

30. Passy V (1994) Pathogenesis of peritonsillar abscess. Laryngoscopy 104:185–190

31. Pinder D, Hilton M (2005) Dissection versus diathermy for tonsillectomy. Cochrane Database Syst Rev 4:CD002211

32. Pueschel SM (1998) Should children with Down syndrome be screened for atlantoaxial instability? Arch Pediatr Adolesc Med 152:119–122

33. Randall DA, Hoffner ME (1998) Complications of tonsillectomy and adenoidectomy. Otolaryngol Head Neck Surg 118:61–68

34. Ray RM, Bower CM (2005) Pediatric obstructive sleep apnea; the year in review. Curr Opin Otolaryngol Head Neck Surg 13:360–365

35. Thomson SK, Doerr TD, Hengerer AS (2005) Infectious mononucleosis and corticosteroids: management practices and outcomes. Arch Otolaryngol Head Neck Surg 131:900–904

36. Van den Akker EH, Schilder AGM, Kemps YJM, (2003) Current indications for (adeno)tonsillectomy in children: a survey in The Netherlands. Int J Pediatr Otorhinolaryngol 67:603–607

Chapter 15

The Causes and Effects of Obstructive Sleep Apnoea in Children

15

Ray W. Clarke

"It is not surprising that children suffering from adenoidal obstruction should be mentally dull and apathetic, and incapable of sustained attention even when at play. This condition is traditionally termed "aprosexia". Fortunately, it is susceptible of marked improvement following operation" (Wilson 1955).

Core Messages

- ■ Causes and Effects
- – Obstructive sleep apnoea (OSA) is common in children.
- – OSA is characterised by reduction (hypopnoea) or cessation (apnoea) of oronasal airflow despite continuing thoracic and abdominal respiratory effort.
- – Untreated OSA can cause failure to thrive, recurrent aspiration, chest infections and cor pulmonale.
- – Children with untreated OSA may go on to develop OSA in adult life.
- – Occasional snoring in children is physiological, but there is mounting evidence that prolonged snoring may be a marker for prolonged airway obstruction. In particular, there may be adverse neuropsychological effects and otolaryngologists need to be alert to the possibility of undiagnosed OSA in these children.
- ■ Diagnosis
- – The diagnosis of OSA is largely clinical.
- – A short home video of the child sleeping can provide useful evidence to aid the diagnosis of OSA.
- – Good-quality sleep studies are not widely available for children. Standardisation varies.
- – Establishing a firm evidence base for treatment and protocols for intervention in children has been difficult due to uncertainty over diagnostic criteria.

- ■ Quality of Life Issues
- – OSA has a significant adverse effect on quality of life for both parents and children.
- – Quality of life measures improve considerably following adenotonsillectomy.
- – Comorbidity is common. OSA is especially prevalent in children with complex disorders, in syndromic children and in children with developmental delay. These children are challenging to treat.
- ■ Treatment
- – Adenotonsillectomy is the mainstay of treatment of OSA in children.
- – Anaesthesia and peri-operative care pose particular difficulties in children with OSA.
- – Dental malocclusion may be a cause of OSA and should be treated.
- – Adequate treatment of rhinitis with intranasal steroids can greatly help children with OSA.
- ■ The Child With Comorbidity
- – Continuous positive airway pressure has a role especially in children with significant comorbidity.
- – Palatal, maxillomandibular and tongue base surgery as developed in adults have all proved disappointing in the management of childhood OSA.
- – Tracheostomy is effective, but is associated with significant morbidity.

Contents

15

Pathophysiology of Childhood Obstructive Sleep Apnoea

Introduction

The defining feature of obstructive sleep apnoea (OSA) is that reduction (hypopnoea) or cessation (apnoea) of oronasal airflow occurs despite continuing thoracic and abdominal respiratory effort (Guilleminault et al. 2005). OSA is at one end of a spectrum of disorders ranging from mild and innocuous snoring to multiple sequential episodes of prolonged nocturnal apnoea. Both adults and children are affected.

The aetiology, presentation, management and expectations from treatment are very different in the two groups, with the result that OSA in children is a discrete clinical entity.

Prevalence

Good epidemiological data are sparse. Prevalence figures vary due to the diagnostic difficulties discussed below. What studies there are suggest that the prevalence of OSA in children is between 1 and 5%. It is more common in prematurity. The typical child is aged 2–5 years and, apart from adenotonsillar hypertrophy (Fig. 15.1), is otherwise healthy. There are racial differences, with higher incidences among black and Hispanic children. Boys are more often affected than girls (Ali et al. 1991; Brunetti et al. 2001; Enright et al. 2003; Gislason and Benediktsdottir 1995; Kotagal 2005; Rosen et al. 2003).

Aetiology

A range of causes of nasal and pharyngeal airway obstruction in children (Tables 15.1 and 15.2) may contribute to OSA. OSA is common in children with developmental

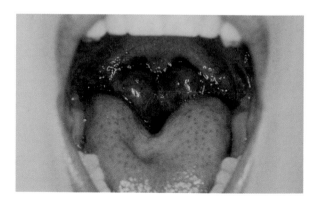

Fig. 15.1 Tonsillar hypertrophy

Table 15.1 Local causes of obstructive sleep apnoea (OSA) in children

Oropharyngeal	Nasal/nasopharyngeal
Enlarged tonsils	Rhinitis
Retrognathia	Adenoids
Macroglossia	Septal deviation
Glossoptosis	Rare nasopharyngeal masses

Table 15.2 Systemic diseases and syndromes causing OSA (see also Chapter 8)

Diseases	Syndromes
Cerebral palsy	Down syndrome
Reticuloses	Prader-Willi syndrome
Sickle cell disease	Apert syndrome
Glycogen storage diseases	Treacher-Collins syndrome
Achondroplasia	Crouzon syndrome

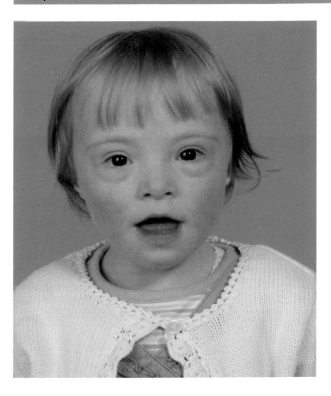

Fig. 15.2 Down syndrome

delay, neurological impairment, and in craniofacial dysmorphism where midfacial hypoplasia and generalised hypotonia contribute. In Down syndrome (Fig. 15.2), macroglossia may also be a factor (Table 15.2).

Mechanisms

OSA is essentially a manifestation of pharyngeal airway obstruction. The patency of the pharyngeal airway is maintained in part by muscle tone, hence the tendency for this type of obstruction to worsen during sleep as muscles relax and the pharyngeal structures become flaccid. Continuing respiratory efforts give rise to cyclical vibrations of the pharyngeal walls (snoring) interspersed with episodes of partial (hypopnoea) and complete (apnoea) closure of the pharyngeal airway. The resultant hypoxaemia leads to a rise in sympathetic output, causing peripheral vasoconstriction, with tachycardia and a rise in blood pressure. Hypoxaemia causes reflex wakening (arousal) and the cycle is repeated.

The physiology of sleep is well documented in adults. Normal sleep brings about an increase in upper airway resistance and a decrease in tidal volume. This decreased tidal volume is especially marked in rapid eye movement (REM) sleep. The physiology of sleep in children – particularly the very young – is less well understood (Kota-gal 2005). Children undergo significant maturation and change in sleep patterns, especially in the first 2 years of life.

Diagnosis of OSA

The Spectrum of Airway Obstruction

Snoring is a manifestation of airway obstruction. It may occur alone – primary snoring (PS) – or in association with hypopnoeas, infrequent apnoeas or as part of overt OSA. Sleep-related airway obstruction in children that is not severe enough to be categorised as OSA is common, but there is confusion about terminology and definitions (Guilleminault et al. 2005). The term upper airways resistance syndrome (UARS) is widely used in adult medicine to describe a form of sleep-disordered breathing characterised by apnoeas and hypopnoeas of a frequency and duration not sufficient to meet the diagnostic criteria for full-blown OSA. Nevertheless, UARS in adults is a discrete clinical entity with significant adverse effects. The accepted diagnostic criteria for UARS in adults are not applicable in children, but some authors use the term "sleep-associated" gas exchange abnormalities" (SAGEA) to describe hypoxaemia and hypercarbia in the absence of overt apnoeas (Gozal 1998). The term "obstructive hypoventilation" is also used (Anonymous 1996; Anonymous 2002). It is again characterised by partial airway obstruction, but the frequency and severity of apnoeas is insufficient to warrant a diagnosis of OSA. Children who may be categorised as having PS, obstructive hypoventilation or SAGEA may not present for treatment. These disorders can lead to significant clinical symptoms as a result of nighttime arousals and pulmonary hypoventilation (Gozal et al. 2001; Gozal and O'Brien 2004).

Lack of precision in the literature with regard to these definitions has bedevilled attempts to establish a firm evidence base for the diagnosis and treatment of childhood OSA. The exact characterisation of where a particular child is on the spectrum requires sleep studies; moreover, measurements of respiratory physiological parameters may vary from night to night.

In clinical practice, the term OSA is used imprecisely. The differentiation is more important in research studies when accurate categorisation is important for comparison of results between centres.

Diagnostic Criteria

Otolaryngologists make the diagnosis of OSA largely on the basis of clinical findings. In the USA, more precise diagnostic criteria may be needed as healthcare providers often insist on formal confirmation of the diagnosis by laboratory-based studies. As discussed above, attempts to define OSA in children with the same precision as is used in adult sleep research have proved difficult because of age-related changes and the normal variability of sleep patterns in children. Guilleminault et al. (2005) provide a detailed account of currently accepted guidelines and discuss the difficulties brought about by lack of standardisation between sleep laboratories. In adult medicine, the accepted definition of OSA is precise, based on the finding of a designated number of apnoeic episodes during a sleep cycle (Anonymous 1997). The lack of widely available and reproducible children's sleep laboratory measurements even in research settings makes definition more uncertain. Consensus on normative sleep data in children is poor. Brief apnoeas may be physiological in infancy – particularly in prematurity. Cessation of oronasal airflow for 6 s is seconds may be innocuous in adolescence, but pathological in a pre-school child. While an apnoea is easily defined as a complete interruption of oronasal airflow, a brief cessation is normal at the end of a breath cycle; categorisation of exactly what constitutes apnoea and what a hypopnoea is remains unclear, is not always defined and varies with age; Guilleminault defines an apnoea as absent oronasal airflow for two attempted breaths and a hypopnoea as a reduction in oronasal flow by 50% or more for a minimum of two breaths. (Guilleminault et al. 2005).

Presentation

Clinical Features

Snoring is a constant feature of OSA. Affected children are restless sleepers. Parents often report that the child adopts an unusual sleeping posture, is unsettled throughout the night, disturbs the bedclothes and seems never to get into a deep restful sleep. Apnoeas, which can be very disconcerting for parents, are common, but by no means always recognised by parents. More often the parents will witness mini-arousals, which they describe as "gasping for breath" or "waking himself up". Agitation, night sweats and nocturnal drooling are sometimes seen. OSA children tend to mouth-breathe during both wakefulness and sleep.

In severe cases there is evidence of airway obstruction when the child is awake. This may manifest as stertorous breathing, tachypnoea, sternal recession and feeding difficulties in the very young. OSA should be differentiated from airway obstruction caused by laryngomalacia in infants. The sound in OSA is lower pitched (i.e. stertor rather than stridor; see Chapter 21).

Differential Diagnosis

If there is a typical history with witnessed apnoeas, "gasps", arousals and obvious struggling for breath, the diagnosis is clear and treatment can be planned. Infants, syndromic children and children with neurodevelopmental delay can be particularly challenging. Apnoeic spells can be "central" due to pathological variations in respiratory drive. Problems with settling into sleep are not uncommon, particularly in infants and in children with neurodevelopmental delay. Nocturnal anoxia may be due to cardiac pathology or epilepsy. The parasomnias (e.g. night terrors and sleep-walking) may cause confusion (Goodwin et al. 2004). Occasionally a child with epileptic fitting may be misdiagnosed as suffering from episodes of obstructive hypoxaemia.

Many parents now have a camcorder or a digital camera with facilities for a brief "movie" clip. These can provide useful images of the child during sleep. It is important to look for the characteristic continuing respiratory efforts despite cessation of breathing.

Effects of OSA

The adverse effects of OSA are due a combination of factors: hypoxaemia and hypercapnea, prolonged respiratory muscle effort and the cognitive and neuropsychological deficits brought about by poor-quality sleep.

Untreated OSA may lead to failure to thrive and recurrent upper respiratory infections. In children with neurodevelopmental delay, the hypoxic episodes can be compounded by aspiration with repeated chest infections (Guilleminault et al. 1976, 2004; O'Brien et al. 2004). In severe cases, prolonged hypoxaemia and hypercarbia may give rise to pulmonary oedema, rapidly progressive pulmonary hypertension and right-sided heart failure (cor pulmonale). There is evidence to link childhood OSA with hypertension that persists into adult life (Marcus et al. 1998). Pectus excavatum secondary to chronic sternal recession is nowadays rarely seen (Fig. 15.3). The plethoric facies of polycythaemia secondary to prolonged hypoxaemia is also rarely seen. In "The Posthumous Papers of the Pickwick Club" Charles Dickens provides a classic description of a boy with OSA – Joe – as a "fat and red-faced boy in a state of somnolency" (Dickens 1837).

Chronic OSA may give rise to hypoplasia of the midface. The "adenoidal facies" (Fig. 15.4) characteristic of pharyngeal airway obstruction may persist into adulthood. There is increasing evidence to link untreated childhood OSA with snoring and sleep-related breathing disorders in adults (Gozal and O'Brien 2004).

The cognitive and neuropsychological consequences of OSA are now well known. OSA children have demonstrable deficits in attention span and general intellectual ability when compared with age-matched controls. Gozal has demonstrated poorer school performance in children who snore but do not have overt sleep apnoea when compared with age-matched controls (Gozal 1998). School performance improves following adenotonsillectomy in appropriately selected cases. Neurocognitive deficits in primary snoring are now widely reported and the traditional advice that snoring in children is entirely benign and does not warrant treatment may need to be revised (O'Brien et al. 2004).

The daytime somnolence so characteristic of adult OSA may manifest in children as hyperactivity, irritability, behaviour disorders and fatigue. This, as well as a disturbed sleep pattern, contributes to the often profound adverse effect of OSA on quality of life for both the child and family. This effect is particularly marked in the families of children with special needs, where sleep patterns are often disturbed independent of airway obstruction (Quine 2001). Adequate treatment of OSA can bring about marked improvement in quality of life (De Serres et al. 2002; Goldstein et al. 2002; Gozal and O'Brien 2004; Mitchell et al. 2004; Tarasiuk et al. 2004).

Management

Investigations

There is considerable controversy as to the role of investigations in the diagnosis and management of OSA. Most otolaryngologists will make a clinical diagnosis and will plan treatment accordingly based on a good history and examination. Supplementary evidence can be obtained by a camcorder, a period of observation by an experienced children's nurse or by the use of an overnight transcutaneous oxygen saturation monitor (Owen et al. 1995). Some units arrange for home overnight oxygen saturation monitoring either at home or on a children's ward using a transcutaneous monitor (pulse oximeter).

Sleep Studies (Polysomnography)

Several studies show that the accuracy of both clinical examination and pulse oximetry is limited and many authors recommend polysomnography or sleep studies (Anonymous 1996; Anonymous 1999a, b; Anonymous 2002; Goldstein et al. 2004; Nixon and Brouillette 2002; Nixon et al. 2004).

Sleep studies involve the simultaneous measurement of multiple physiological variables during sleep. These include oxygen saturation, the volume and frequency of oronasal airflow, spirometric volumes and flow rates, and respiratory muscle excursions. Measurements of end-tidal carbon dioxide are particularly useful evidence of alveolar hypoventilation. Cardiovascular measures such

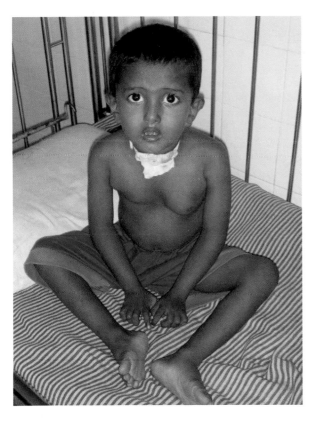

Fig. 15.3 Boy with pectus exavatum due to prolonged OSA

as pulse electrocardiography (ECG) and blood pressure and cortical activity measured by electroencephalography are typically recorded as well. Analysis of the resultant traces enable the investigator to compute the frequency of apnoeas and hypopnoeas and to correlate their presence with other events in the sleep cycle (e.g. snoring, arousals and REM sleep). Good-quality sleep studies are difficult to obtain in children. The sleep period subjected to analysis is often unphysiological as the child may be admitted to an unfamiliar environment, and interpretation of findings is variable. Sleep studies may help establish the diagnosis in difficult cases. In children with a central or neurological cause for apnoeas, the sleep studies will demonstrate the lack of association between apnoeas and continuing respiratory effort. They can define where on the spectrum of sleep-related airway obstruction a child is (i.e. does she have innocuous PS, snoring with some evidence of hypoxaemia or full-blown OSA?). Outcome analysis for research studies is also greatly enhanced by sleep studies. They may help predict which children require more intensive peri-operative monitoring and aftercare.

Unfortunately, despite valiant efforts to standardise diagnostic criteria and ensure that comparable measurements are used in different centres, there is still variation in the interpretation of sleep studies (polysomnography). It is unclear what type of respiratory event should be scored and tabulated. Some workers regard a single episode of apnoea per hour as diagnostic of OSA, some require up to five such events. A hypopnoea is defined as a 50% reduction in oronasal flow for two breaths. Some laboratories use a reduction in oxygen saturation of 3% as signifying an obstructive event, and some – including federal guidelines in the USA (Medicare) – require a change of 4% (Kotagal 2005).

In children with complex comorbidity or where heroic interventions such as tongue-base reduction surgery or maxillofacial distraction are contemplated, sleep studies may help refine selection of children likely to have a good outcome, although evidence on this is uncertain.

The difficulties associated with formal polysomnography have generated interest in a variety of lesser and more easily obtained "mini-sleep" studies. Some are available for home use and rely on video analysis combined with oxygen saturation monitoring (Brouillette et al. 2000; Nixon et al. 2002).

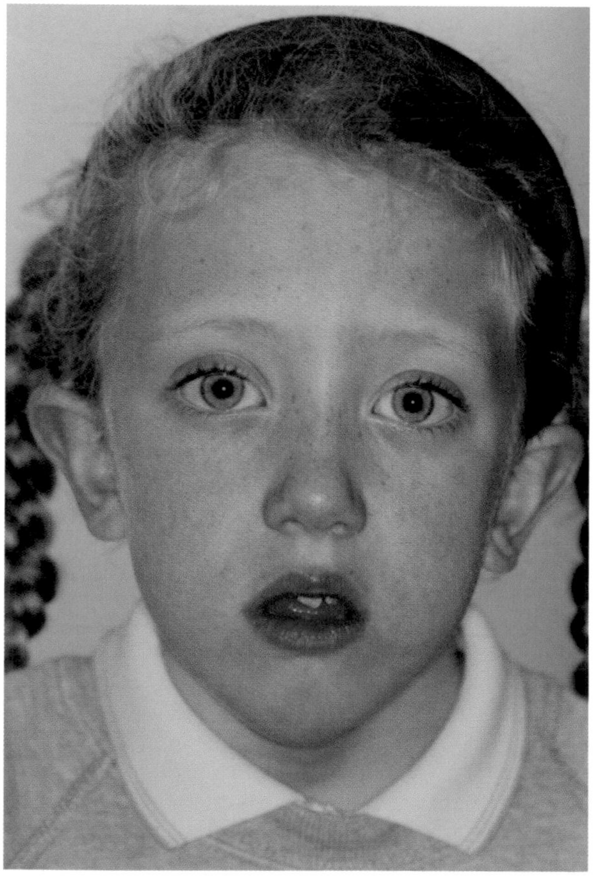

Fig. 15.4 Adenoidal facies

Pre-Operative Investigations

Some anaesthesiologists find it helpful to have a pre-operative ECG and in some cases a chest x-ray to help predict which children will require more intensive peri-operative management (Koomson et al. 2004; Rosen et al. 1994). In severe cases, a chest x-ray may show atelectasia, pulmonary hypertension, right ventricular hypertrophy and cardiomegaly. A plain x-ray of the post-nasal space can help to delineate the adenoidal pad, but this can nowadays be better demonstrated by flexible endoscopy. Computed tomography scanning and dynamic magnetic resonance imaging may demonstrate the site of airway obstruction, but these are rarely needed in clinical practice.

Endoscopy (Sleep Nasendoscopy)

Some authors recommend pernasal endoscopy of the upper airway during sleep or during the sleep induced by sedation/anaesthesia (sleep nasendoscopy) to help delineate the level of obstruction. In order to mimic the physiology of normal sleep, this is undertaken under sedation with the help of a skilled anaesthetist. A flexible endoscope is introduced transnasally and the airway inspected during several cycles of breathing. Obstruction may be at the level of the velopharynx, the tonsils, the tongue base or the supraglottis (Caulfield 2007). Such knowledge may help treatment planning and guide expectations from treatment. Not all OSA is due to adenotonsillar obstruction. A full evaluation of the child's airway may require rigid tracheobronchoscopy, depending on the clinical presentation, for example if there is coexisting stridor.

Paediatric Evaluation

If there is diagnostic doubt, and particularly if the child has suspected neurological or cardiovascular disease or a craniofacial syndrome, the help of a paediatrician can be invaluable in planning treatment. Children with cerebral palsy, Down syndrome and children with craniofacial syndromes (e.g. Crouzon's syndrome) will usually be under the care of a multidisciplinary team, and liaison with this team is essential in planning treatment.

Treatment

General Principles

Childhood OSA is in the main a rewarding and simple condition to treat. Most children will improve dramatically following tonsillectomy, adenoidectomy, or more often both. Other surgical interventions are used and are sometimes appropriate, but are often disappointing, unpredictable, technically challenging and associated with significant morbidity (Anonymous 2002; Cohen et al. 2002; Coleman 1999; Woodson and Fujita 1992).

Pharmacological Treatment

Rhinitis in children is common, but often unrecognised and undertreated (see Chapter 34). Even if there is adenotonsillar hypertrophy, there may be coexistent rhinitis; it is often prudent to give the child a therapeutic trial of intra-nasal steroids (Brouillette et al. 2001). Both systemic steroids and prolonged antibiotic therapy have been advocated for children with tonsillar enlargement, but the safety of adenotonsillectomy is now such that surgery will usually be preferable.

Dental Devices

Adult OSA patients often improve with the use of a customised dental device to hoist the tongue base forward (Dort et al. 2006). This approach is often not well tolerated by children, but worth pursuing in a child with dental malocclusion or mild retrognathia. A paediatric dental surgeon or orthodontist with a special interest in this type of work is best equipped to assess the child's needs and prescribe appropriately.

Continuous Positive Airway Pressure

Continuous positive airway pressure (CPAP) is widely used in the management of nocturnal airway obstruction in adults. The principle relies on a continuous stream of air usually delivered through a face-mask to act as a pneumatic splint and maintain patency of the otherwise flaccid pharyngeal airway. There may be compliance problems in children, but the device can be used at home and is particularly useful in children with complex medical needs or in those with severe OSA who have had a poor response to surgery (Fig. 15.5).

Many children's hospitals and clinics now manage home CPAP programmes (Guilleminault et al. 2005). The help of a respiratory physician or anaesthetist is invaluable. CPAP is not without side effects and can cause nasal drying, vestibulitis headaches and epistaxis.

Postural Therapy

Children with retrognathia or micrognathia are prone to obstruct the airway due to backward prolapse of the tongue base (glossoptosis). Despite the general advice to nurse young children on their backs to reduce the risk of sudden infant death, these children are best laid prone. In children with Pierre-Robin sequence (Fig. 15.6), careful positioning may obviate the need for invasive intervention such as a nasopharyngeal airway or tracheotomy (Bath and Bull 1997).

Nasopharyngeal Airway

A modified endotracheal tube introduced transnasally with the distal end positioned just above the free margin of the soft palate may maintain a patent nasopharyngeal airway in children with glossoptosis. If parents are adequately trained to clean and change such an airway, the Pierre-Robin child (Fig. 15.6) can often be discharged home and monitored for weeks or even months until the retrognathia improves and (s)he can manage without airway support.

Adenotonsillectomy

Adenotonsillectomy is by far the most widely performed procedure for OSA in children. Symptomatic improvement is rapid. Polysomnography before and after adenotonsillectomy confirms improved apnoea and oxygen saturation scores. In judiciously chosen cases, the procedure will bring about marked improvement in quality of life measures for parent and child .

OSA children by definition have airway obstruction. This can make for challenges in peri-operative management. Otherwise healthy children rarely present endotracheal intubation difficulties, but they may be difficult to extubate, slow to recover from anaesthesia and show a marked sedating respond to opioid analgesia. Severe cases may have segmental atelectasis or incipient right-heart failure. They may have an impaired ventilatory response to carbon dioxide and are at increased risk of respiratory complications.

An experienced anaesthetist skilled in the management of children is an essential member of the team treating these children. Local protocols vary and it may be prudent to arrange for a period of aftercare in a high-dependency unit, or in severe cases – particularly syndromic children, cerebral palsy children and the very young (under 3 years) – to plan for a short post-operative stay in the paediatric intensive care unit.

There is some evidence to support the use of pre-operative atropine. Peri-operative glucocorticoids (dexamethasone 1 mg/kg) may help reduce post-operative morbidity. Children with severe OSA tend to do best when they have surgery in the morning rather than later in the day. (Koomson et al. 2004).

Nasal Surgery

Nasal septal surgery may be considered for severe septal deflections. While each case should be judged on its merits, it is wise to wait if at all possible until the adolescent growth spurt is complete. Polyposis (see Chapter 35) and gross turbinate hypertrophy may obstruct the nasal airway and require intervention.

Maxillomandibular Surgery

Maxillary and mandibular osteotomies are used in the management of adult OSA. Osteotomies to facilitate maxillary protrusion or to elongate the mandible and help hoist the tongue base forward are considered

in severe cases in consultation with a paediatric maxillofacial surgeon who has an interest in this work. Results are unpredictable. To date, this modality of treatment is not part of the routine management of OSA in children except on a carefully considered individual basis (Coleman et al. 1999).

Maxillofacial and paediatric craniofacial surgeons are getting better and better results with the technique of "distraction osteogenesis". This involves the placement of an interposed prosthesis into the growing facial skeleton, which is then sequentially expanded over a period of months. Often used for aesthetic reasons, this technique can facilitate the reversal of tracheotomy in children with airway obstruction due to craniofacial syndromes.

Palatal Surgery

Uvulopalatopharyngoplasty was pioneered by Fujita (Fujita et al. 1981) for the treatment of adult OSA. It is still widely used primarily for symptomatic treatment of snoring in adults. The principle is to enlarge the oropharyngeal inlet and leave less flaccid tissue to collapse during inspiration, thus reducing apnoeas and hypopnoeas. Various less invasive procedures are also used,

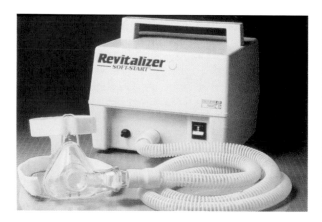

Fig. 15.5 Continuous positive airway pressure

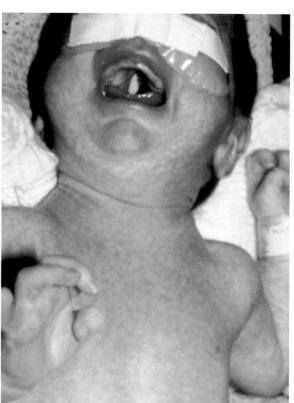

Fig. 15.6 Nasopharyngeal airway in a child with Pierre-Robin sequence

mainly to stiffen or reduce the bulk of the soft palate. The procedures are painful and risk post-operative nasal regurgitation as they interfere with palatal muscular function.

In children, initial enthusiasm for palatal surgery has been tempered as results in the main are disappointing. Adenotonsillectomy is usually the preferred first intervention and palatal surgery is particularly poor in cases where adenotonsillectomy has failed.

In infants with retrognathia it may be useful to plicate the anterior and posterior tonsil pillars together – including a tonsillectomy if there is a substantial volume of tonsillar tissue – with a single absorbable suture on each side to enlarge the oropharyngeal airway. Otherwise, palatal surgery has little to offer in childhood OSA.

Tongue-Base Surgery

Techniques to hoist the tongue base forward and increase the calibre of the oropharyngeal and hypopharyngeal airway are used in adult OSA, with some success in selected cases (Woodson and Fujita 1992). Attempts to replicate this success in children have proved difficult. In centres experienced in the management of complex paediatric OSA and in limited individual cases techniques such as hyoid suspension, partial glossectomy and genioglossus advancement may be offered, but again they are not part of the routine armoury of interventions in children, and evidence of their usefulness is limited.

Tracheotomy

Tracheotomy is a tried and trusted technique to bypass upper airway obstruction. It is very rarely considered for uncomplicated OSA, but in children with severe multisystem disease it may be a last resort. Tracheotomy is sometimes requested in children with severe neurological dysfunction. It should be considered an extreme measure and the implications and potential complications (see Chapter 28) need to be discussed in detail with the parents or carers, the child's medical attendants and – if old enough – with the child (Fig. 15.7).

Challenges in OSA Management

OSA and Obesity

Obesity is traditionally associated with adult OSA. In contrast, children with severe OSA are often thin with failure to thrive. Nonetheless, obesity is more common now in children, and more and more obese children are presenting with OSA (Frühbeck 2005; Mayor 2005). A high proportion of obese adolescents have abnormal

polysomnograms, and otolaryngologists should be alert to the possibility of unrecognised OSA in these children.

OSA in Special Needs Children

Syndromic children, children with neurological impairment and children with developmental delay are particularly prone to OSA. These children have a much higher incidence of problems settling into sleep and of sleep disorders in general. They may be especially challenging for the otolaryngologist both from a diagnostic and therapeutic perspective. Often, airway obstruction is multisegmental and recalcitrant to treatment.

OSA occurs in about half of Down's children (Clarke 2005). Pharyngeal hypotonia, a small pharynx and macroglossia may all play a part. Down's children may also have cardiac anomalies and are particularly at risk of pulmonary hypertension. Otolaryngologists should be vigilant and consider active and early intervention. Tonsillectomy can be particularly rewarding, adenoidectomy is often technically challenging and rarely as helpful.

Cerebral palsy may be complicated by severe pharyngeal hypotonia. OSA is especially difficult to manage in these children and will require a multidisciplinary approach.

Craniofacial syndromes are associated with (Table 15.2) OSA. In severe cases, tracheotomy may be needed. These

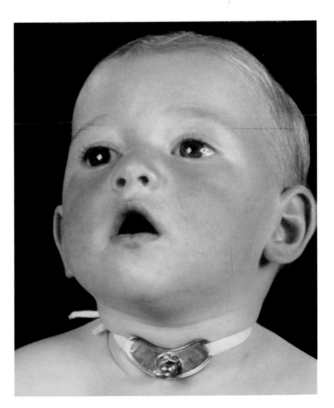

Fig. 15.7 Tracheotomy

children are best managed in a regional centre where the expertise to deal with the multiple problems associated with craniofacial anomalies is available.

Summary for the Clinician

- OSA in children is common and of great clinical importance. Although good-quality sleep studies are not widely available for children and the diagnosis remains mainly clinical, the link between the clinical picture and significant levels of desaturation is now widely accepted. OSA is acknowledged to have adverse effects on the child's health and quality of life.

- Adenotonsillectomy is the definitive treatment in most cases, and it improves the quality of life for both children and parents, but needs to be performed in a safe environment, with an experienced medical and nursing team. OSA is both more prevalent and more complex in children with other disorders, where there may be a role for CPAP and even tracheostomy.

15

References

1. Ali N, Pierson D, Stradling J (1991) The prevalence of snoring, sleep disturbance and sleep related breathing disorders and their relation to daytime sleepiness in 4–5 year old children. Am Rev Respir Dis 143:A381

2. Anonymous (1996) Standards and indications for cardiopulmonary sleep studies in children. Am J Respir Crit Care Med 153:886–878

3. Anonymous (1997) The International Classification of Sleep Disorders, Revised: Diagnostic and Coding Manual. American Sleep Disorders Association, Rochester, Mn, pp 195–197

4. Anonymous (1999) Cardiorespiratory sleep studies in children: establishment of normative data and polysomnographic predictors of morbidity. Am J Respir Crit Care Med 160:1381–1387

5. Anonymous (1999) Sleep-related breathing disorders in adults: recommendations for syndrome definitions and measurement techniques in clinical research. The Report of an American Academy of Sleep Medicine Task Force. Sleep 22:667–689

6. Anonymous (2002) Clinical practice guidelines: diagnosis and management of childhood obstructive sleep apnea syndrome. Pediatrics 109:704–712

7. Bath AP, Bull PD (1997) Management of upper airway obstruction in Pierre Robin sequence. J Laryngol Otol 111:1115–1117

8. Brouilette RT, Morielli A, Leimnais A, Waters KA, Luciano R, Ducharme FM (2000) Nocturnal pulse oximetry as an abbreviated testing modality for pediatric obstructive sleep apnea. Pediatrics 105:405–412

9. Brouilette RT, Manoukian JJ, Ducharme FM, Oudjhane K, Earle LG, Ladan S, et al (2001) Efficacy of fluticasone nasal spray for pediatric obstructive sleep apnea. J Pediatrics 138:838–834

10. Brunetti L, Rana S, Lospalluti ML, et al (2001) Prevalence of obstructive sleep apnea in a cohort of 1207 children from the south of Italy. Chest 120:1930–1935

11. Clarke RW (2005) Ear, nose and throat problems in children with Down syndrome. Br J Hosp Med (Lond) 66:504–506

12. Caulfield H (2007) Obstructive sleep apnoea in children. In: Scott Brown's Otolaryngology, 7th edition. Hodder Arnold, London, in press

13. Cohen SR, Holmes RE, Machado L, Magit A (2002) Surgical strategies in the treatment of complex obstructive sleep apnoea in children. Paediatr Respir Rev 3:25–35

14. Coleman J (1999) Oral and maxillofacial surgery for the management of obstructive sleep apnea syndrome. Otolaryngol Clin North Am 32:235–241

15. De Serres LM, Derkay C, Sie K, et al (2002) Impact of adenotonsillectomy on quality of life in children with obstructive sleep disorders. Arch Otolaryngol Head Neck Surg 130:190–194

16. Dickens C (1837) The Posthumous Papers of the Pickwick Club. Chapman Hall, London

17. Dort LC, Hadjuk E, Remmers JE (2006) Mandibular advancement and obstructive sleep apnoea: a method for determining effective mandibular protrusion. Eur Respir J 27:1003–1009

18. Enright PL, Goodwin JL, Sherrill DL, Quan JR, Quan SF (2003) Blood pressure elevation associated with sleep-related breathing disorder in a community sample of white and Hispanic children: the Tucson Children's Assessment of Sleep Apnea study. Arch Pediatr Adolesc Med 157:901–904

19. Frühbeck G (2005) Facing changes in the epidemiological trends of childhood obstructive sleep apnoea: potential impact of the obesity epidemic (Rapid Response). BMJ 330:978–979

20. Fujita S. Conway W, Zorick F, Roth T (1981) Surgical correction of anatomic abnormalities in obstructive sleep apnea syndrome: uvulopalatopharyngoplasty. Otolaryngol Head Neck Surg 89:923–934

21. Gislason T, Benediktsdottir B (1995) Snoring, apnoeic episodes and nocturnal hypoxemia among children 6 months to 6 years old: an epidemiologic study of lower limits of prevalence. Chest 107:936–966

22. Goldstein NA, Fatima M, Campbell TF, Rosenfeld RM (2002) Child behaviour and quality of life before and after tonsillectomy and adenoidectomy. Arch Otolaryngol Head Neck Surg 128:770–775

23. Goldstein NA, Pugazhendhi V, Rao SM, Weedon J, Campbell TF, Goldman AC, et al (2004) Clinical assessment of pediatric obstructive sleep apnea. Pediatrics 114:33–43

24. Goodwin JL, Kaemingk KL, Fregosi RF, et al (2004) Parasomnias and sleep disordered breathing in Caucasian and Hispanic children: the Tucson Children's Assessment of Sleep Apnea Study. BMC Med 2:14

25. Gozal D (1998) Sleep-disordered breathing and school performance in children. Pediatrics 102:616–620

26. Gozal D, Pope DW Jr (2001) Snoring during early childhood and academic performance at ages thirteen to fourteen years. Pediatrics 107:1394–1399

27. Gozal D, O'Brien LM (2004) Snoring and obstructive sleep apnoea in children: why should we treat? Paediatr Respir Rev 5:S371–S376

28. Guilleminault C, Eldridge F, Simmons FB, et al (1976) Sleep apnea in eight children. Pediatrics 58:23–30

29. Guilleminault C, Li KK, Khramtsov A, Pelayo R, Martinez S (2004) Sleep disordered breathing: surgical outcome in prepubertal children. Laryngoscope 114:132–137

30. Guilleminault C, Lee JH, Chan A (2005) Pediatric obstructive sleep apnea syndrome. Arch Pediatr Asolesc Med 159:775–785

31. Koomson A, Morin I, Brouillette R, et al (2004) Children with severe OSAS who have adenotonsillectomy in the morning are less likely to have postoperative desaturation than those operated in the afternoon. Can J Anesth 51:62–67

32. Kotagal S (2005) Childhood obstructive sleep apnoea. BMJ 330:978–979

33. Marcus CL, Greene MG, Carroll JL (1998) Blood pressure in children with obstructive sleep apnea. Am J Respir Crit Care Med 157:1098–1103

34. Mayor S (2005) Obesity in children in England continues to rise. BMJ 330:1044

35. Mitchell RB, Kelly J, Call E, Yao N (2004) Quality of life after adenotonsillectomy for obstructive sleep apnea in children. Arch Otolaryngol Head Neck Surg 130:190–194

36. Nixon GM, Brouillette RT (2002) Diagnostic techniques for obstructive sleep apnoea: is polysomnography necessary? Paediatr Respir Rev 3:18–24

37. Nixon GM, Kermack AS, Davis GM, et al (2004) Planning adenotonsillectomy in children with obstructive sleep apnea: the role of overnight oximetry. Pediatrics 113:19–25

38. O'Brien LM, Mervis CB, Holborrok CR, Bruner JL, Klaus CJ, Rutherford J, et al (2004) Neurobehavioural implications of habitual snoring in children. Pediatrics 114:44–49

39. Owen GO, Canter RJ, Robinson A (1995) Overnight pulse oximetry in snoring and non-snoring children. Clin Otolaryngol 20:403–406

40. Quine L (2001) Sleep problems in primary school children: comparison between mainstream and special school children. Child Care Health Dev 27:201–221

41. Rosen GM, Muckle RP, Mahowald MW, et al (1994) Postoperative respiratory compromise in children with obstructive sleep apnea syndrome: can it be anticipated? Pediatrics 93:784–788

42. Rosen CL, Larkin EK, Kirchner L, Emancipator JL, Bivins SF, Surovex SA, et al (2003) Prevalence and risk factors for sleep disordered breathing in 8 to 11 year old children: association with race and prematurity. J Pediatrics 142:383–389

43. Tarasiuk A, Simon T, Tal A, Reuveni H (2004) Adenotonsillectomy in children with obstructive sleep apnea syndrome reduces health care utilization. Pediatrics 113:351–356

44. Woodson BT, Fujita S (1992) Clinical experience with lingualplasty as part of the treatment of severe obstructive sleep apnea. Otolaryngol Head Neck Surg 107:40–48

45. Wilson TG (1955) Diseases of the Ear, Nose and Throat in Children. Heinemann, London

Chapter 16

Cleft Lip and Palate

John Boorman

Core Messages

- This chapter considers the embryology, presentation and management of children with cleft lip and palate.
- The management is multidisciplinary and involves plastic and reconstructive surgeons, maxillofacial and dental surgeons, and otolaryngologists.
- Equally important is the expertise of speech and language therapists and teachers in managing the complex problems that these children present.

Contents

Embryology

Clefts of the lip and palate occur as a result of the failure of fusion of the maxillary and frontonasal processes during embryonic development. At around 5 weeks of gestation, the palate anterior to the incisive foramen fuses progressively through the anterior hard palate, alveolus and lip. The failure of this fusion process produces a cleft lip, which can be either unilateral or bilateral. At about 7 weeks of gestation, a fusion process moves caudally from the incisive foramen through the hard palate and the soft palate to the tip of the uvula. Failure of this fusion process produces a cleft palate. The part of the palate anterior to the incisive foramen that fuses first is often referred to as the primary palate for that reason, but occurs as part of a cleft lip, not a cleft palate. A midline cleft of the upper lip is a very unusual anomaly and is often associated with other midline developmental problems such as absence of the corpus callosum and holoprosencephaly (failure of the hemispheres to divide).

Aetiology

The aetiology is multifactorial, having both genetic and environmental components. Monozygotic twins can be discordant for clefts. Hundreds of syndromes have been described that include clefting of the lip and/or palate as a component. These include single gene and chromosomal defects. The majority of clefts, however, occur without any obvious genetic component or family history. Environmental influences that have been associated with cleft lip and palate include steroids, tobacco, alcohol, folic acid deficiency and the use of anti-epileptic drugs during pregnancy.

Prevalence

In the UK, as with much of the Western world, the prevalence of cleft lip and palate is approximately 1.6 per 1,000 live births, or 1 in 600. Of these, roughly 40% will have a cleft palate without a cleft lip and the remaining 60% will be more or less equally divided between cleft lip and cleft lip and palate. With regard to cleft lip and to cleft lip with cleft palate, clefting is more common on the left side than the right, which in turn is more frequent than the bilateral deformity. Figures are approximately 60% left, 30% right and 10% bilateral. The reason for this imbalance between the left and the right sides in cleft lip is not clear. Cleft lip with or without a cleft palate [CL{P}] is a distinct condition from a cleft palate occurring without a cleft lip [CP]. [CL{P}] is approximately twice as common in boys as in girls whilst [CP] is roughly 1.5 times more common in girls than in boys. In addition, where there is a familial tendency for cleft palate, there is normally no higher prevalence of [CL{P}] and vice versa. [CL{P}] shows a higher racial variation, with a low incidence in

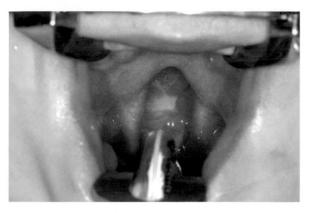

Fig. 16.1 Cleft palate without cleft lip

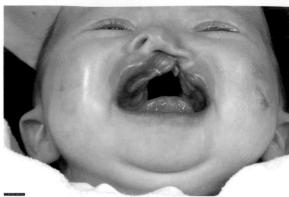

Fig. 16.2 Cleft lip and palate. As in this case, clefts on the left are commoner than those on the right, which are commoner than bilateral clefts

the black population, but a relatively high incidence in the Asian population. Prevalence of cleft palate is less affected by race, but more likely to be associated with syndromes. Cleft lip varies in severity from a microform abnormality, where the only sign may be a vertical groove running along the line of the philtral column on one side or a slight asymmetry of the nostril, up to the complete cleft involving the floor of the nose, alveolus and primary palate. The cleft usually passes between the lateral incisor and the canine and it is not infrequent that there is a missing, deformed, or extra tooth in the line of the cleft. Similarly, cleft palates vary in severity from a bifid uvula, which may be regarded as a microform cleft palate, through to a complete cleft involving the uvula, soft palate and hard palate up to the incisive foramen. Because of the timing and direction of palate fusion, it is not possible to get a cleft in the hard palate without one in the soft. Figure 16.1 shows cleft palate, without cleft lip; Fig. 16.2 shows cleft lip and palate.

Presentation

Now that in most UK maternity centres examination of the face has become a mandatory part of the 20-week foetal anomaly scan, most, if not all significant cleft lips should be diagnosed at this time. Indeed, it is possible to identify cleft lips on foetal ultrasound as early as 15 weeks, and as the technology improves, this may well become easier. It is very rare for a cleft palate to be diagnosed on an ultrasound scan without the presence of a cleft lip. The present technology cannot visualise the secondary palate reliably, only the alveolus (which is part of the primary palate) and therefore of a cleft lip.

On the diagnosis of a cleft, the regional cleft centre should be notified and counselling can be arranged speedily. This allows for the family to be prepared for the birth of a baby with a cleft and avoids the inevitable shock at the time of birth that would otherwise occur. In some cases, particularly bilateral complete clefts, there may be associated anomalies detected on the ultrasound scan, and consideration will be given to karyotyping to look for chromosomal abnormalities and syndromes that may not be compatible with normal life.

Clefts not detected antenatally should be apparent on neonatal examination soon after birth. Oral examination will allow the presence or absence of a cleft palate to be determined with certainty and an adequate digital examination will detect almost all clefts of the palate. Some lesser clefts of the palate, however, will present with "nasal" speech or glue ear in childhood.

Robin Sequence

Robin sequence consists of a small mandible, glossoptosis, a cleft palate and respiratory difficulties. It is thought that the small mandible maintains the tongue in a high position in the mouth and that this prevents the palatal shelves from fusing normally. The cleft is typically described as being wide and U-shaped in comparison to other cleft palates, but this is by no means always the case. Robin sequence has more than one cause and may be associated with several syndromes. The mandible may have the potential for catch-up growth after birth, or it may be genetically programmed to remain small.

The effect of the tongue malposition is to impair the airway and increase the work of breathing. Babies with this condition are not typically blue, nor are their oxygen saturations significantly affected. What will be apparent, however, are signs of upper-airway obstruction, such as sub-costal and intercostal recession. If this condition is not managed properly, then the babies will have great difficulty feeding and will fail to thrive.

The historical treatment for Robin sequence was to nurse the baby prone in a Burston frame. This works in mild cases, but the signs of respiratory distress are not clearly seen in the prone baby, nor is it very easy for the baby to interact with its surroundings in such a position. The modern management of Robin sequence uses a nasopharyngeal airway that extends to the level of the base of the tongue and holds it forward. This provides for a satisfactory airway and will, in almost all cases, allow for normal oral feeding and weight gain. It is best if this treatment is instituted early (within the first week or two of life) as the child will progress more quickly and spend less time overall in hospital. The family can be taught to change the airway at home or, if not, the child can be brought back to the ward if a tube falls out in order that a new one be inserted. The airway may need to be left in for many weeks, but after that the child is usually able to maintain its airway satisfactorily. Should the child fail to make satisfactory progress in terms of feeding and weight gain after satisfactory placement of the nasopharyngeal airway, it strongly suggests that there is an additional problem, for instance tracheomalacia or a neurological abnormality, which would require separate management. Other methods of managing the airway, such as suturing the tongue to the lower lip or mandible, tracheotomy, or mandibular distraction, should rarely, if ever, be indicated in Robin sequence babies.

Feeding

The presence of a cleft palate reduces the efficiency of sucking and the baby will have difficulty in breast feeding or using a normal bottle. The easiest way to manage this problem is with a soft, squeezy bottle so that the parent can reduce the work of suction required by the baby but it can still go through the actions of feeding, which aids the development of the muscles in the area that will later be important for communication. Expressed breast milk is ideal, otherwise formula can be used. It should be noted that babies with a cleft palate have been found to have an unusually high incidence of intolerance to cow's milk. The reason for this is not clear, although it may be the presence of the cow's milk in the nose and nasopharynx that increases problems compared with a non-cleft baby.

Surgery for Cleft Lip and Palate

Clefts of the lip and palate are usually operated on in infancy. The typical age for repairing a cleft lip is at 3 months and is based on the old "rule of tens", which states that the baby should weigh at least 10 lbs (4.5 kg), be at least 10 weeks of age and have a haemoglobin level of at least 10 g/dl. Palate repair in the UK is typically carried out between 6 and 12 months of age. The advantage of doing it earlier is to provide an intact palate by the time that the child is babbling and saying its first words. There is evidence that children who have a normal babble are more likely to develop normal speech without hypernasality. The drawback of early surgery is that it appears to impair the growth of the maxilla and may therefore result in the need for orthognathic surgery in early adult life.

In the repair of the cleft lip, the lip has to be lengthened by some type of Z plasty or flap. The most important aspect is to correct the underlying muscle abnormality, particularly in the orbicularis oris muscle, which is discontinuous across the cleft and therefore inserts abnormally on the lateral side into the base into the alar base and on the medial side at the columella base. In addition, other muscles around the lip such as the levators and the nasalis muscle are also out of position and need to be corrected. The nasal asymmetry that is seen with a significant unilateral cleft can also be corrected at the time of lip repair, and studies for up to 20 years follow up have shown that this does not significantly impair growth. Many surgeons will free the septum on both sides and let it swing into a more vertical, straight position. In general, the alveolar cleft is not closed at this time. There is frequently a malposition of the segments and a significant gap between them and closure would be impracticable. Therefore, the aim normally is to close the nasal floor but not the alveolus itself, which is left until the mixed-dentition phase at around the age of 8–10 years.

In cleft palate surgery, the muscles are again the most important structures, as they cannot form a normal sling across the palate, and insert instead into the cleft edge, the hard palate and the aponeurosis formed by the tensor palati tendon. There are five muscles in the soft palate, although one of them, the tensor palati, exists as an aponeurotic sheet formed after the tendon has curled around the hook of the hamulus to enter the palate. This muscle is important in swallowing and in Eustachian tube function. It has little relevance to velopharyngeal closure for speech. The levator palati is the most important muscle for speech. It is the only elevator of the soft palate. The musculus uvulae is a longitudinal muscle. The palatopharyngeus has a significant vector to extend the palate. The importance of muscle correction has been increasingly recognised over the years and the trend is for a very radical repositioning of the levator muscle in particular. Its nerve supply, which comes from the pharyngeal plexus, enters the muscle lateral to the soft palate and is therefore not damaged by this surgery, although the lesser palatine nerve may well be injured.

The closure of the hard palate is usually done at the same time as the soft palate, but can be done at a different stage, almost always later. The advantage of a delayed hard palate closure is that the palate has had more time to grow prior to the operation and the resultant scarring, which is inevitable, may be the cause of the poor maxillary growth. In addition, if the soft palate has been repaired, the hard palate shelves tend to move closer together and a less radical procedure may be needed to close them. Closure may be done at any age from 2 to 16 years. If the hard palate is closed at the time of the soft palate repair, then flaps will normally have to be elevated from the hard palate. In the past, the traditional method in the UK was the Veau Wardill Kilner "push back" procedure, which attempted to lengthen the soft palate using the VY principle. This, however, leaves significant defects in the soft palate, both interiorly and laterally, and has been blamed for the severe upper dental arch distortions and very poor maxillary growth, which were frequently seen. The trend now is to do less radical surgery on the hard palate, and the Von Langenbeck method, whereby mucoperiosteal flaps are raised and moved medially with no effort at lengthening, is much more in favour and appears to cause less in the way of growth disturbance.

One recent method that appeared to show promising results is the Furlow double-reversing Z plasty for the soft palate. This consists of creating two Z plasties – one on the oral and one on the nasal mucosa. The posteriorly based flap in each case is made to include the muscle, and thus both muscle bundles are transposed posteriorly and indeed can be overlapped. This, however, does not provide such a radical muscle correction as the intravelar veloplasty. Prophylactic antibiotics are frequently used at the time of cleft palate surgery in order to prevent streptococcal infection.

The early complications of cleft palate surgery include bleeding, which may necessitate a return to theatre in 1–2% of cases, and some airway obstruction, which is usually transient. The longer-term complications are really twofold, namely fistula formation and velopharyngeal incompetence. Fistulae are the result of wound breakdown, infection, undue tension or poor blood supply in the flaps. They are not always symptomatic, but food can escape through them into the nose and cause irritation and nasal regurgitation, particularly of yoghurt and chocolate.

Velopharyngeal Insufficiency

Velopharyngeal insufficiency (VPI) is the term used to describe the failure of the sphincter formed by the soft palate and the pharyngeal walls. The sphincter should close for swallowing, vomiting and all the consonants in the English language apart from /m/n/ and /ng/. During speech, if the sphincter does not close appropriately then air escapes into the nose, producing nasal escape and/or turbulence. In addition, the resonance of the speech becomes hypernasal. As a consequence of the failure of this sphincter, the child may attempt to halt the airstream by closing the anterior nares in a nasal grimace, or develop compensatory articulation such as a pharyngeal fricative or a glottal stop. VPI is seen in approximately 20–25% of children following a cleft palate repair. It cannot be cured by speech therapy and will normally require further surgery or, if that is not possible, some form of speech bulb or palatal lift appliance. In a pre-lingual child, the presence of regurgitation of food down the nose in the absence of a fistula is a symptom of VPI. In general, the closure of the velopharyngeal sphincter for speech is a more delicate and faster movement than that for swallowing, and regurgitation of food through the mechanism is an indication of relatively severe dysfunction.

Sub-mucous Cleft Palate and Bifid Uvula

Sub-mucous cleft palate is usually a variant of cleft palate that is described as having a classic triad of features: a bifid uvula, a palpable notch at the posterior end of the hard palate where the posterior nasal spine should be and a visible lucent strip that appears somewhat bluish in the mid-line of the soft palate, representing a muscle diastasis (Fig. 16.3). The prevalence of sub-mucous cleft palate may be around 1 in 1,000 of the population, but they are not all symptomatic. It has been estimated that about 50% of them will speak normally with no evidence of VPI. Many children with sub-mucous cleft palate will not be diagnosed at birth, but present later on with either the speech pattern of VPI, or glue ear because of the associated dysfunction of the Eustachian tube.

The situation is complicated by the fact that not all of these children present with classic features. The condition of occult sub-mucous cleft palate, in which none of the features of sub-mucous cleft palate are seen, but where, on nasendoscopy, one can detect an abnormality in the sphincter, has been described.

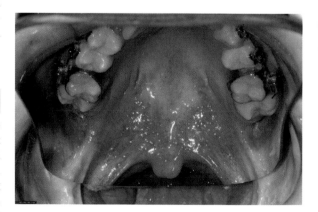

Fig. 16.3 Sub-mucous cleft, with bifid uvula. The cleft in the hard palate is not visible and is identified by palpation with a finger. It is a sound rule always to palpate the hard palate before adenoidectomy

16

Bifid uvula in itself is a relatively common variant, being seen in 1–2% of the normal population without any apparent effect on speech. Notching of the hard palate, however appears to be a much rarer finding in the normal population. In a study we carried out of over 1700 school children in Sussex, we identified no notching of the posterior hard palate. This suggests that the notching of the posterior hard palate is a fairly strong sign of an underlying abnormality and should alert the examiner. In a child presenting with glue ear, or for whom an adenoidectomy may be being considered, an inspection of the palate is mandatory. If the child has any features suggestive of a sub-mucous cleft palate or even a bifid uvula, it is probably wise to seek referral for a more detailed assessment of velopharyngeal function by the local cleft palate service. An adenoidectomy carried out on a patient with borderline velopharyngeal function will almost certainly precipitate them into significant velopharyngeal incompetence and the need for further surgery.

Assessment of VPI

In assessing a patient with velopharyngeal incompetence, we wish to know whether there are any relevant factors in the medical history such as known syndromes, family history or other anomalies – particularly cardiac, which might point to a syndromic diagnosis. We want to know also about the middle ear, in particular Eustachian tube function, which may be associated with a cleft palate, either overt or sub-mucous, and the history of any feeding difficulties in infancy, which would be an early indicator of VPI. We would also want to know whether the child's adenoids or tonsils had been removed. Clinical examination of the palate is important, to look for the palate to look for the presence of a sub-mucous cleft and the position of the levator muscles. When the child says "Aah" and the palate lifts, dimples form on the oral mucosa, approximately two-thirds of the way back from the back of the hard palate to the base of the uvula. This is effectively the locus of action of the levator muscles. In the case of a previously repaired cleft where the muscles have not been adequately corrected, we may see that the lift of the soft palate is inadequate and that the dimples are situated anteriorly or are widely separated. A similar pattern of muscle activity is seen in an unrepaired sub-mucous cleft palate. Examination of the face may reveal a typical appearance of a child with velocardiofacial syndrome, who will tend to have a worse prognosis from the treatment of VPI. They may also give a history of learning difficulties.

Although examination of the palate may give some idea of its length, it is not normally possible to visualise the nasopharynx or the contact, or lack of it, between the palate and the posterior pharyngeal wall. Lateral videofluoroscopy provides the best objective way of assessing palate function for velopharyngeal closure. Children from the age of 4 years, or sometimes younger, will usually cope with this perfectly well and are asked to repeat standard sentences whilst a video recording is made. This allows us to determine the position of the levator muscles and the degree to which they are acting. Other videofluoroscopic views can be used, but they are harder to interpret and require a barium coating of the nasopharynx, which reduces their usefulness in young children. Nasendoscopy using narrow, flexible endoscopes, can normally be carried out from the age of 5 years onwards. It is customary to instil local anaesthetic into the nose, together with a vasoconstrictor to make the endoscope easier to pass. Again, the child is asked to repeat syllables and sentences whilst the recording is made. Endoscopy allows a view of the complete velopharyngeal sphincter including lateral wall movement, and this may be very useful, particularly in deciding which type of pharyngoplasty to carry out. However, it is not possible to tell on nasendoscopy whether any palate lift that is observed is active or has been produced passively by the tongue.

Treatment of VPI

Whilst the traditional treatment for VPI has been a pharyngoplasty, there are several associated potential complications such as a difficulty in breathing through the nose, snoring, catarrh and obstructive sleep apnoea. The preference now is, where possible, to try and improve the palate function by means of a muscle correction. In the unrepaired sub-mucous cleft palate patient this means a primary repair, whereas in the previously repaired cleft palate, this is a re-repair of the soft palate concentrating on correction of the abnormally anterior muscle insertions. This can be combined with a lengthening of the soft palate by means of Z plasties. In cases where pre-operative investigations have demonstrated poor levator muscle position and function, this should be the first procedure and will be successful in 90% of patients. Where this fails, or in patients who have normal or very good soft palate function, a pharyngoplasty is the operation of choice provided that the patient does not already exhibit features of obstructive sleep apnoea. Pharyngoplasties fall into two main groups: midline pharyngeal flaps and sphincter pharyngoplasty. There is no evidence that one type is better than the other. An alternative procedure is to build up the posterior pharyngeal wall, which may be done either with flaps taken from the lateral pharyngeal wall or by implanting some tissue into a sub-muscular pocket via an oral approach.

Velocardiofacial Syndrome

This syndrome, also known as 22Q11 deletion syndrome, Catch 22 syndrome or Sphrintzen syndrome, is associated, in over 90% of cases, with a deletion at the Q11 region of chromosome 22, which can be detected on fluorescent in situ hybridisation. This syndrome has a wide variety of features – the main ones of which are VPI, a typical facial appearance, severe cardiac abnormalities and significant learning difficulties. It is an autosomal dominant condition. Some of these children have overt clefts, but submucous clefts are more likely, and indeed the majority of them have no cleft at all. Their VPI is made worse by the cranial base angle, which is rather more obtuse than normal, and the relative hypoplasia of their adenoids as part of their immunological deficiencies. Both of these factors combine to increase their chances of VPI and make it harder to treat. It is an important condition to be aware of and, as it is autosomal dominant, it can be inherited by any future offspring. Curiously, most of the cases that are seen are de novo mutations and not inherited.

Stickler syndrome is another autosomal dominant condition. It is seen in association with Robin sequence and is associated with a significant risk of retinal detachment in young adult life; an early referral to an ophthalmologist is thus mandatory.

Summary for the Clinician

- Cleft lip and palate can be sporadic or familial and may be syndromic. It cannot always be diagnosed antenatally. Particular attention needs to be paid to management of the airway, feeding and speech development. The surgery should be performed by experts working as a multi-disciplinary team.

References

1. Berkowitz S (1996) Cleft Lip and Palate – Perspectives in Management. Singular, San Diego
2. Clinical Standards Advisory Group (1998) Cleft Lip and/or Palate. HMSO, London
3. Kummer AW (2001) Cleft Palate and Craniofacial Anomalies – Effects on Speech and Resonance. Singular, San Diego
4. Millard DR (1980) Cleft Craft – The Evolution of its Surgery. Little Brown, Boston
5. Shaw B, Semb G, Nelson P, et al (2001) The Eurocleft project 1996–2000. IOS Press, Amsterdam

Chapter 17

Salivary Gland Disease in Childhood

17

Peter D. Bull

Core Messages

- Salivary gland disease in children is uncommon, but mirrors the conditions found in adults with the addition of a number of congenital disorders.
- Proper management requires an understanding of the embryology and pathology of the lesions and a recognition that malignant disease can occur in this young age group.

Contents

Introduction

The salivary glands include:
1. The parotid glands.
2. The submandibular salivary glands.
3. The sublingual glands.
4. The minor salivary glands distributed throughout the oral and pharyngeal mucosa.

The same disorders affect the salivary glands in children and adults, but the relative incidences differ.

History, Investigations

History

In taking the history, ask:
1. How long has it been going on?
2. How quickly does it flare up?
3. How frequently does it happen?
4. Is it painful?
5. Is it worse on eating?
6. Has there been any weakness of the face?

Inflammatory and infective conditions tend to flare up quickly. They may be recurrent and are usually painful. The skin may be reddened. A slowly enlarging mass is more probably benign; rapid enlargement of a lump, especially with facial weakness, is highly suggestive of malignancy.

Examination

Examination must include inspection in a good light. The presence of swelling of the salivary glands should be noted and bimanual examination of all the glands should be made. The pharynx and oral cavity must be inspected for parapharyngeal swelling and the state of the salivary ducts – is there trauma, is there a good salivary flow? It helps to milk the parotid duct forwards to assess flow properly, and giving the patient fruity lozenges to suck will stimulate saliva production. Minute assessment of facial nerve function is essential.

Investigation

For many conditions, no further investigation is required. The need for particular blood tests will be discussed with each condition. Imaging may be of benefit. Ultrasonography, particularly with high-definition scanning, is non-invasive and readily available and will differentiate solid from cystic lesions and give information about blood flow in a mass.

Computed tomography (CT) scanning exposes the child to ionising radiation but gives good detail, particularly of deeper structures that may be difficult to see on ultrasonography. Magnetic resonance scanning is slower than CT and may require general anaesthesia or sedation to avoid movement artefact, but it avoids ionising rays. Sialography, by introducing radio-opaque contrast medium into the duct, gives information about the glandular duct system and will show stones, strictures and sialectasis, but may not be tolerated by young children.

Congenital Disorders

The absence of salivary glands is extremely rare and may be complete or partial. Complete absence leads to xerostomia and dental decay. (Hodgson et al. 2001)

Congenital Cysts and Fistulae

These are dealt with in detail elsewhere (Chapter 19). Cystic hygroma and dermoids may involve in particular the parotid and submandibular glands. First-arch duplication anomalies result in either a cyst or a fistula with an external opening. The track is lined with skin and is almost always deep to the facial nerve. Surgery of these conditions necessitates a transparotid exploration of the facial nerve and dissection of the track.

Ranulas in the floor of the mouth are sometimes congenital, but more often present later and arise from extravasation of saliva from the sublingual glands. Treatment is by excision of the sublingual gland. Simple drainage almost always results in recurrence.

Inflammatory Disorders of the Salivary Glands

Viral Infections

Mumps sialadenitis remains the commonest acute inflammatory condition affecting the salivary glands as well as other organs. A mild pyrexial illness is accompanied by painful enlargement of one or more of the salivary glands, most often the parotid, in 40% of cases.

MMR vaccine is now used in 92% of developed countries, but a decline in vaccination uptake has resulted in recent epidemics among teenagers in Britain. If the diagnosis is uncertain, S and V antigen levels can be measured in blood samples. (Galazka et al. 1999)

Bacterial Disease

Acute suppurative sialadenitis can occur at any age, including the neonatal period (Fig. 17.1). The diagnosis is usually obvious and the presence of pus will determine the need for surgical drainage; the superficial position of the facial nerve must be remembered in children. The organisms most commonly responsible are *Staphylococcus aureus* and *Streptococcus pyogenes*, and the pus should be cultured for antibiotic sensitivity.

Atypical Mycobacterial Disease of Salivary the Glands

Infection with non-tuberculous mycobacteria occurs in young children (Fig. 17.2). It is rare beyond the age of 6 years. Initially the infection affects the peri- or intrasalivary lymph nodes, but caseation will result in spread to salivary parenchyma. (Jervis et al. 2001; Dhooge et al 1993)

Features

An enlarged node or discrete swelling over the parotid or submandibular area appears, often acutely. The child is not unwell and usually there is little or no pain. The overlying skin becomes inflamed with a dusty violaceous

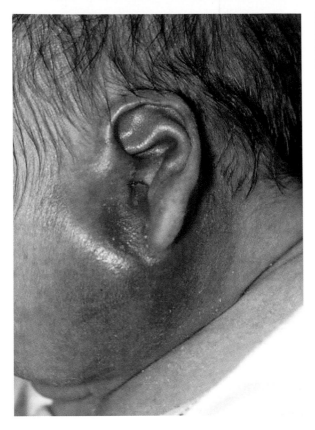

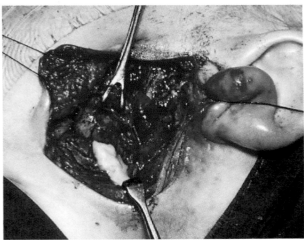

Fig. 17.2 Caseation in a case of atypical mycobacterial infection of the left parotid gland

Fig. 17.1 Acute bacterial suppurative parotitis in a neonate

discoloration and may ultimately break down to leave a chronically discharging sinus. Without treatment, this chronic abscess may take many months to heal.

Investigations

If pus is available, culture should be requested, although the non-tuberculous mycobacteria are difficult to grow. If there is doubt about the diagnosis, a Mantoux test should be done. A chest x-ray is advisable. Fine-needle aspiration (under general anaesthesia if necessary) may reveal the diagnosis by obtaining pus for culture or cells for cytology.

Treatment

If left without treatment, the condition will eventually heal. The organisms are not sensitive to conventional antibiotic regimes, but are usually responsive to combination therapy with azithromycin and ciprofloxacin, continued for many weeks. If there is actual or impending necrosis, surgery to remove the inflammatory mass with preservation of the facial nerve is curative.

Recurrent Parotitis of Childhood

Often taken to be mumps in the first attack, this is the commonest condition affecting the salivary glands in children. The usual presentation is at 5–6 years of age. One (sometimes both) parotid gland will be swollen and painful. The saliva expressed from the duct will be turbid and may grow *Str. pneumonia* or *Haemophilus influenzae*.

Treatment is by rehydration, sialogues such as citrus fruit sweets and gentle massage of the gland towards the duct opening. Antibiotics are probably only necessary if the child is systemically unwell and determined by the results of the microbiology culture. The frequency of attacks reduces with age and by puberty nearly all cases have resolved. There is rarely, if ever, need for open surgery. The immune status of the child with recurrent parotitis should be assessed. (Cohen et al. 1992)

Sjogren's Syndrome

This is a systemic autoimmune disorder that usually involves the salivary glands (Fig. 17.3). It is rare in children, and three-quarters of the cases in this age group will be girls. Parotid enlargement is usual (62% of cases in childhood vs 13% in adults) and rheumatoid factor is positive in 70%. Treatment is aimed at oral and dental care and should be by a multidisciplinary team, including rheumatologist, dentist and immunologist. (Anaya et al 1995; Bartunkova et al. 1999)

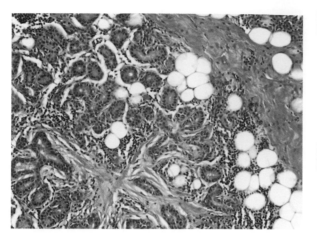

Fig. 17.3 Sjogren's disease showing lymphocytic infiltration

Human Immunodeficiency Virus/Acquired Immune Deficiency Syndrome

Involvement of the parotid glands and the presence of intra-glandular lymphoepithelial cysts are features of human immunodeficiency virus (HIV) infection in childhood. Such cysts should alert the clinician to the diagnosis of HIV infection. Surgery to the cysts is not required unless neoplasia is suspected. (Schiott 1992)

Sarcoidosis

Sarcoidosis can present in the teenage years, and affects the parotid glands in 10% of cases. The presentation may be acute, with fever, uveitis and parotid swelling.

Obstructive Disorders

Salivary Gland Calculi

Salivary gland stones are uncommon in childhood and most occur in the submandibular gland because the mucoid nature of the saliva predisposes to stasis and increased viscosity. (Bull 2001)

Presentation

The gland becomes acutely swollen and painful, usually during eating. It will subside in an hour or so but recurs when the child next eats. Inspection of the salivary duct may reveal an impacted stone. If this stone is more proximal in the duct, it may be felt on bimanual palpitation, or in the body of the gland.

Treatment

If the stone is visible and accessible, it can be removed from the duct by the oral route. A new development is the removal of the stone by ductal endoscopy, using a very fine, semi-rigid endoscope and extraction forceps (Karl Storz, Germany).

Ranula

From the Latin for small frog, ranula is a cystic swelling in the floor of the mouth. It is caused by obstruction of the sublingual gland and sometimes extravasation of the saliva. It may follow surgery for relocation of the submandibular ducts for dribbling. If extension occurs through the mylohyoid muscle in the floor of the mouth, a cystic swelling in the neck is formed, referred to as a plunging ranula. (Dhaif et al. 1998)

Treatment

Aspiration or drainage is followed by a high recurrence rate, but excision of the sublingual gland is usually curative.

Salivary Gland Tumours in Childhood

Fewer than 5% of all salivary gland tumours occur under the age of 16 years, so they are rare. Unfortunately, because of this rarity, they may not be recognised for what they are and are often managed badly. Tumours of salivary origin present as an enlarging mass in a salivary gland and may be benign or malignant. In children, 80% of salivary tumours are in the parotid. Rapid growth suggests malignancy and facial weakness makes it almost certain. (Bull 1999; Orvidas et al. 2000)

Benign

In the parotid, haemangiomas (Fig. 17.4) are not usually present at birth, but appear at a few weeks of age. Many will also have a cutaneous component. They are endothelial, not truly of salivary origin and initially grow rapidly. Involution usually starts by 12–18 months and is usually complete by 5 years. Such haemangiomas must not be confused with vascular malformations, which are present at birth and do not involute.

Pleomorphic salivary adenomas (Fig. 17.5) account for 30% of paediatric salivary gland tumours, mostly in the parotid, and less commonly in the submandibular gland. However, all types of benign salivary tumours may occur in children. Treatment is by the same careful resection

age group are likely to be malignant, although usually low grade.

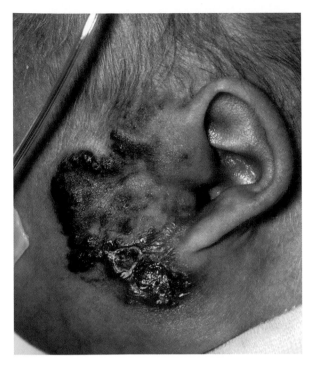

Fig. 17.4 Capillary haemangioma of the parotid region

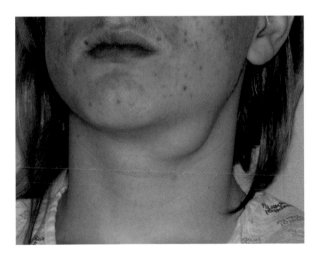

Fig. 17.5 Benign pleomorphic salivary adenoma in left submandibular gland

with facial nerve preservation. Post-operative radiotherapy must not be used to salvage an inadequate operation.

Malignant

While the overall incidence of salivary tumours is low, 60% of solid non-vascular tumours occurring in a young

Presentation

Most malignant tumours of salivary gland origin present simply as an enlarging mass, although growth may be more rapid than with pleomorphic salivary adenomas. Facial weakness and increasing pain are highly indicative of malignancy.

Pathology

The commonest malignant tumour type in children is mucoepidermoid carcinoma, accounting for about 50% of malignant cases in this age group. This is followed by acinic cell tumours (20%). Again, all cell types will occur in childhood.

Treatment

Wide excision is required. Prior agreement to facial nerve sacrifice must be obtained and performed if there is invasion of the nerve. Nerve grafting may be more successful in children and should be attempted if the nerve has to be resected. With good initial surgery, the recurrence rate is minimised. The cases should be managed in conjunction with a paediatric oncologist.

Complications of Parotid Surgery

Facial Nerve Damage

The risk of this can be minimised by the use of facial nerve monitoring by electrodes in the facial muscles recording action potentials. Magnification by use of the microscope or loupes is invaluable in allowing good visualisation of the nerve. It goes without saying that extensive experience and training in parotid surgery is essential if a surgeon is to operate on children.

Frey's Syndrome

The incidence may be less in children than in adults. It can be minimised by an interposed sternomastoid muscle clap at the time of operation. The risk is that any recurrence of the tumour may be more difficult to detect. If severe, it may be treated by injection of botulinum toxin.

Summary for the Clinician

● In children, congenital disorders of the salivary glands include first-arch duplication anomalies and lymphangioma. There is a susceptibility to infection, including atypical (non-tuberculous) mycobacterial disease. Solid tumours can occur, and in a young age group (i.e. under 16 years) have a 60% risk of malignancy.

References

1. Hodgson TA, Shah R, Porter SR (2001) The investigation of major salivary gland agenesis: a case report. Pediatric Dentistry 23(2):131–134

2. Cohen HA, Gross S, Nussinovitch M, Frydman M, Varsano I (1992) Recurrent parotitis. Archives of Disease in Childhood 67(8):1036–1037, Comment in: Arch Dis Child. (1993) 68(1):151

3. Galazka AM, Robertson SE, Kraigher A (1999) Mumps and mumps vaccine: a global review. Bulletin of the World Health Organization 77(1):3–14

4. Jervis PN, Lee JA, Bull PD (2001) Management of Non-tuberculous Mycobacterial peri-sialadenitis in Children. Clinical Otolaryngology and Allied Sciences 26,243–248

5. Dhooge I, Dhooge C, De Baets F, Van Caauwenberge P (1993) Diagnostic and therapeutic management of atypical mycobacterial infections in children. European Archives of Oto-Rhino-Laryngology 250(7):387–91

6. Anaya JM, Ogawa N, Talal N (1995) Sjogren's syndrome in childhood. Journal of Rheumatology 22(6):1152–8

7. Bartunkova J, Sediva A, Vencovsky J, Tesar V (1999) Primary Sjogren's syndrome in children and adolescents: proposal for diagnostic criteria. Clinical & Experimental Rheumatology 17(3):381–386

8. Schiott M (1992) HIV associated salivary gland disease: a review. Oral Surgery, Oral Medicine, Oral Pathology 73:164–167

9. Dhaif G, Ahmed Y, Ramaraj R (1998) Ranula and the sublingual salivary glands. Review of 32 cases. Bahrain Medical Bulletin 20(1):3–4

10. Bull PD (2001) Salivary stones Hospital Medicine 62(7):396–399

11. Bull PD (1999) Salivary gland neoplasia in childhood International Journal of Pediatric Otolaryngology 49 Suppl. 1:235–238

12. Orvidas LJ, Kasperbauer JL, Lewis JE, Olsen KD, Lesnick TG (2000) Pediatric Parotid Masses. Archives of Otolaryngology, Head and Neck Surgery Volume 126(2):177–184

17

Drooling – Salivary Incontinence (Sialorrhoea)

Peter D. Bull

18

- While all babies dribble until their oral and swallowing reflexes mature, it is not normal in the older child, who has usually gained control by the age of 4 years or so.
- Persistent and uncontrollable dribbling or drooling is socially unacceptable even in children, and is a source of embarrassment to the parents.
- Drooling may lead to ostracism and social isolation, and as children get older and develop insight, they too will become distressed by it.

Contents

Introduction

While all babies dribble until their oral and swallowing reflexes mature, it is not normal in the older child, who has usually gained control by the age of 4 years or so. Persistent and uncontrollable dribbling or drooling is socially unacceptable even in children, and is a source of embarrassment to the parents. It may lead to ostracism and social isolation, and as children get older and develop insight, they too will become distressed by it.

The word "drool" is a dialect and US contraction of the older word "drivel", from which derives "dribble". To the English ear, "drool" carries connotations of lack of intellect and may be better avoided.

The cause of the excessive dribbling is a poor swallowing reflex associated with poor oromotor and lingual control. The volume of saliva produced is no greater than in any other child. It is seen mainly in children with cerebral palsy, but also in children with progressive neurodegenerative disease and bulbar palsy. Dribbling leads to damage to clothes, and in doing school work, saliva will spoil the child's books and drawings because of the need to bend over the work. It will also produce excoriation of the skin of the chin, especially in cold winter weather.

Innervation

The salivary glands receive their autonomic innervation via the VIIth and IXth cranial nerves (Figs. 18.1 and 18.2).

Assessment

It is helpful to arrange a multidisciplinary assessment whenever possible, and the team should include a speech and language therapist, physiotherapist, orthodontist, orthotist and otolaryngologist. It is important to assess:

1. the level of awareness by the child
2. head posture and control
3. dental health
4. dental occlusion and lip seal
5. safety of the swallowing mechanism
6. nasal obstruction

All of these may worsen the dribbling if not favourable.

It is also important to assess the amount of dribbling and frequency of changing bibs or clothes as a baseline and an indication of the severity of the condition.

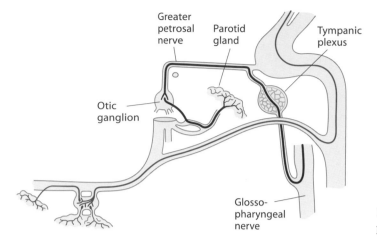

Fig. 18.1 Autonomic secretomotor supply to the parotid gland

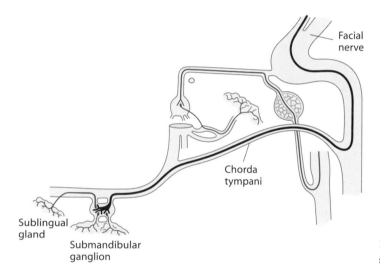

Fig. 18.2 Autonomic secretomotor supply to the submandibular gland

18

Non-Surgical Management

Posture Control

By maintaining an upright head posture, gravity will play a lesser role. With the head flexed and mouth open, all of us will dribble. The advice of the physiotherapist and orthotist is invaluable in improving posture.

Improvement of lip seal by orthodontic treatment as required will reduce the salivary incontinence (Domaracki and Sisson 1990). Correction of nasal obstruction, by allowing closure of the mouth, will benefit the degree of lip seal.

Drug Treatment

Anti-cholinergic drugs, by blocking the secretomotor impulses to the salivary glands, will reduce salivation and permit the child to deal with the reduced amount of saliva produced. The use of such drugs is limited by side effects such as confusion, excessive dryness and blurred vision (Jongerius et al. 2003).

Scopolamine can be applied as transdermal patches, administering 1 mg every 72 h, or the patches can be cut up to provide a smaller dose.

Glycopyrrolate can be given orally in a dose of 0.04 mg/kg three times daily, but has a higher incidence of anticholinergic side effects than scopolamine (Mier et al. 2000).

Botulinum toxin can be injected into the submandibular glands to produce cholinergic blockade of the parasympathetic secretomotor fibres. In children, this will need to be done under general anaesthetic, possibly with ultrasound control if the glands are not palpable. The procedure will need to be repeated every few months, but the results can be good.

Surgical Management

Submandibular duct relocation remains the mainstay of the surgical control of dribbling as described by Crysdale (1992). The submandibular glands provide up to 85% of resting saliva and relocating the ducts into the region of the tonsil will direct the saliva to the back of the pharynx, where it will trigger a swallowing reflex. Obviously if the swallow is not secure from aspiration, this procedure is contraindicated. With good patient selection, up to 80% of patients achieved long-term control of dribbling (Mankarious et al. 1999; Panarese et al. 2001).

An island of mucosa in the anterior floor of mouth is developed and the submandibular ducts are dissected out as far back as the lingual nerves (Fig. 18.3). The mucosal bridge joining the ducts is divided and each duct is fed through a submucosal tunnel to the base of the tonsil, where it is sutured into place. The risk of ranula formation is reduced if the sublingual glands are excised at the same time.

If the child is so handicapped as to have an unsafe swallow, excision of the submandibular salivary glands is the procedure of choice, in order to prevent salivary aspiration. Although very effective, the drawback to this procedure is the risk of excessive dryness, leading to dental caries, and the presence of external scarring.

An older approach is the operation originally described by Wilkie (1970), who excised both submandibular glands and ligated both parotid ducts intra-orally. This led to xerostomia and parotid swelling and was no more effective than submandibular duct relocation.

Division of autonomic nerves to the salivary glands had a period of popularity, but is not effective in the long term. Chorda tympani section results in loss of taste, which is unacceptable in a child who may already have feeding problems. Tympanic neurectomy to denervate the parotid glands is technically difficult to achieve fully and, as the submandibular glands produce most of the resting saliva, is aimed at the wrong target.

There is an excellent review of the problem of salivary incontinence by Hockstein and his colleagues (2004).

Summary for the Clinician

- Management of salivary incontinence in children calls for patience and understanding and an incremental approach to medication, physical therapy and surgery. It is never possible to overcome the effects of gravity, but improvement will be very welcome to the child and his family.

References

1. Crysdale WS (1992) Drooling. Experience with team assessment and management. Clin Pediatr 31:77–80
2. Domaracki LS, Sisson LA (1990) Decreasing drooling with oral motor stimulation in children with multiple disabilities. Am J Occup Ther 44:680–684
3. Hockstein NG, Samadi DS, Gendron K, et al (2004) Sialorrhea: a management challenge. Am Fam Physician 69:2628–2634
4. Jongerius PH, van Tiel P, van Limbeek J, et al (2003) A systematic review for evidence of efficacy of anticholinergic drugs to treat drooling Arch Dis Child 88:911–914
5. Mankarious LA, Bottrill IA, Huchzermyer PM, et al (1999) Long-term follow-up of submandibular duct rerouting for the treatment of sialorrhea in the pediatric population. Otolaryngol Head Neck Surg 120:303–307
6. Mier RJ, Bachrach SJ, Lakin RC, et al (2000) Treatment of sialorrhea with glycopyrrolate: a double-blind, dose-ranging study. Arch Pediatr Adolesc Med 154:1214–1218
7. Panarese A, Ghosh S, Hodgson D, McEwan J, Bull PD (2001) Outcomes of submandibular duct re-implantation for sialorrhoea. Clin Otolaryngol 26:143–146
8. Wilkie TF (1970) The surgical treatment of drooling. A follow-up report of five years experience. Plast Reconstr Surg 45:549–554

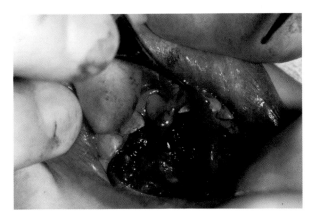

Fig. 18.3 Both submandibular ducts have been dissected prior to posterior relocation

Chapter 19

Congenital Cysts, Sinuses and Fistulae

19

Fiona B. MacGregor

Core Messages

- Pre-auricular sinuses. Excise the tract in continuity with adjacent cartilage to avoid recurrence.
- First branchial arch anomalies: recurrent parotid and/or periauricular abscess formation in a child may be due to an underlying first branchial arch anomaly.
- Third and fourth arch anomalies: consider performing a barium swallow in a child with a history of recurrent thyroiditis.
- Thyroglossal duct cysts. If there is a midline cyst in the neck and an ultrasound scan confirms a normal thyroid gland, then a Sistrunk's procedure should be performed to avoid recurrence (5% will subsequently turn out to be dermoid cysts).
- Nasal dermoid cysts: look carefully for a punctum on the nose in a child presenting with swelling and/or infection in the nasal area.

Contents

Introduction

An understanding of human developmental anatomy is important in appreciating the congenital abnormalities that can occur within the head and neck region in children. Although some cysts, sinuses and fistulae are immediately apparent at presentation, others are not, and children may be examined on several occasions before a diagnosis is made. Appropriate medical and surgical treatment at an early stage will help to avoid recurrence. This chapter will outline the underlying developmental anatomy, and discuss the presentation, investigation and treatment of the lesions most commonly encountered by paediatric otolaryngologists and head and neck surgeons.

Developmental Anatomy

The most typical feature of the head and neck in an early embryo is the series of branchial arches that begin to develop during the 4th week of gestation and gives the embryo its characteristic external appearance. Four well-defined pairs of arches appear, while the fifth and sixth are believed to be rudimentary. The arches are separated from each other on the external surface of the embryo by ectodermal clefts, and internally within the pharynx by endodermal pouches. Each arch contains a cartilaginous rod (which forms the skeleton of the arch), a muscular component, a nerve and an artery (Mandell 2000).

During the 5th week of gestation, the ventral aspect of the second arch grows caudally to overlap the third and fourth arches resulting in the formation of the cervical sinus. This sinus then usually disappears by the 7th week, giving the neck a smooth contour. The first pouch and cleft become closely related and ultimately form much of the middle ear, mastoid and eustachian tube. The second pouch remains in part as the tonsillar fossa. The third pouch contributes to the thyroid gland and inferior parathyroid, and the fourth to the superior parathyroid gland (Fig. 19.1).

The external ear begins to develop at week 6 of gestation in the form of three otic folds or hillocks on the first arch and three on the second arch. These ultimately fuse to form the developing auricle.

The thyroid gland appears as an epithelial proliferation in the floor of the pharynx at a point later indicated by the foramen caecum. The thyroid gland then descends down in front of the pharyngeal gut as a bi-lobed diverticulum. During this migration, the gland remains connected to the tongue by a narrow canal called the thyroglossal duct. By the end of the 7th week, the thyroid has reached its final destination anterior to the trachea; the duct involutes and disappears with time. The thyroid gland

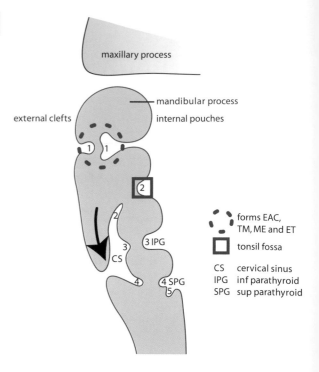

Fig. 19.1 The branchial apparatus at 6 weeks gestation showing the external clefts and internal pouches. *EAC* External auditory canal, *TM* tympanic membrane, *ME* middle ear, *ET* Eustachian tube, *CS* cervical sinus, *IPG* inferior parathyroid gland, *SPG* superior parathyroid gland

begins to function at approximately the end of the 3rd month.

Classification of Congenital Branchial Abnormalities in the Neck

A cyst is an epithelium-lined structure without an external opening. A sinus is a blind tract with an opening either externally through the skin (representing persistence of a branchial cleft) or internally into the foregut (representing persistence of a branchial pouch). A fistula is a tract that communicates between the skin externally and the foregut internally and therefore represents persistence of a connection between a branchial cleft and its corresponding pouch.

Pre-Auricular Sinuses

These are thought to result from abnormal development of the otic hillocks of the first and second branchial arches rather than from a defect of the first branchial cleft.

19

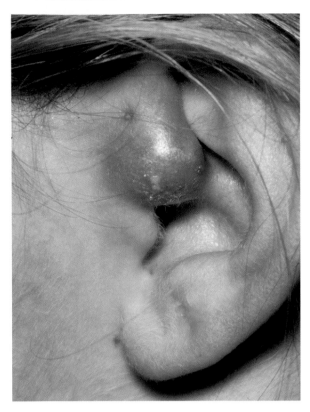

Fig. 19.2 Infected preauricular sinus

Presentation

A punctum is found within a triangular area of skin anterior to the ear close to the anterior border of the ascending limb of the helix. An epithelium-lined sinus extends deeply from this towards the tragal cartilage (Fig. 19.2).

The sinus may become infected and the patient can present with pain, discharge and even abscess formation. These abnormalities may be associated with skin appendages, which usually occur along the line extending from the external auditory canal to the lateral oral commissure.

Investigations

The diagnosis is clinical and investigations are not routinely required.

Management

This abnormality is frequently asymptomatic and treatment is not required, but if there has been recurrent infection, excision may be necessary. These sinuses may be associated with subcutaneous branching and a tortuous course, and the treatment of choice is wide local excision down to and including the perichondrium and adjacent tragal cartilage (Lam et al. 2001). The deep limit is the temporalis fascia. To avoid damage to the facial nerve, remain posterior to the superficial temporal artery.

Complications

The recurrence rate is higher when cartilage is not excised or where there is a history of previous incision and drainage. (Gur et al. 1998).

Key point: Excise the tract in continuity with adjacent cartilage to avoid recurrence.

First Branchial Arch Anomalies

There are several (complicated) classifications of these anomalies, the most frequently quoted being that of Work (1972). It is important, however, to appreciate that none of the classifications described predicts accurately the anatomical relationship of any abnormality to the facial nerve. This is a crucial point in the management of these patients.

Presentation

First branchial arch anomalies usually present as a periauricular swelling or sinus, a mass in the external auditory canal or discharge from the ear in the presence of a normal tympanic membrane. Patients may also present with a mass or sinus opening in the region of the lower pole

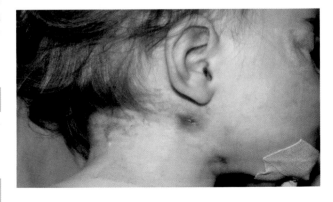

Fig. 19.3 Recurrent infection in the peri-auricular/parotid region secondary to first arch anomaly

of the parotid gland, which can be mistaken for recurrent parotitis or a parotid tumour (Fig. 19.3). The average time to diagnosis after initial presentation is 4 years and regrettably usually follows several surgical interventions (Ford et al. 1992).

Investigations

Imaging is probably of limited benefit, although a computed tomography (CT) or magnetic resonance imaging (MRI) scan may give some information about the deep extent of a mass lesion and its proximity to the facial nerve and middle ear. Ultrasound should distinguish a cystic from a solid swelling.

Treatment

Acute infection should be treated, and surgery considered once infection has resolved. Because of the potential close anatomical relationship of any tract or cyst to the facial nerve, a parotidectomy incision should be performed with formal dissection of the facial nerve and its branches to avoid inadvertent damage. Complete excision of the abnormality should then be performed. The tract has been found to run lateral to, medial to or even directly through the main trunk of the facial nerve. Very occasionally, a tract may be found running into the middle ear and even along the eustachian tube towards the nasopharynx (Mandell 2000).

Complications

Surgery may be challenging and complex because of the close relationship to the facial nerve and the frequency of pre-operative infection and previous surgical interventions. The involvement of an experienced surgeon is required and the use of a facial nerve monitor is recommended.

Key point: Recurrent parotid and/or periauricular abscess formation in a child may be due to an underlying first branchial arch anomaly.

Second Branchial Arch Anomalies

Second branchial cleft fistulae and sinuses extend from an external skin opening in the mid or lower neck along the anterior border of the sternocleidomastoid muscle, and run superiorly along the carotid sheath, passing over the hypoglossal nerve and beneath the posterior belly of the digastric muscle between the internal and external carotid arteries. A sinus will end in a blind sac along this course, while a fistula will continue upwards and open into the tonsil fossa (Karmody 2002).

Presentation

These commonly present in early childhood, and 78% are recognised by the age of 5 years. Patients may have no symptoms or may present with recurrent pain and discharge from the external skin opening.

Investigations

The diagnosis of a second arch sinus or fistula is clinical in the presence of a skin punctum, but a sinogram provides a good demonstration of the course of any tract.

Treatment

Sinuses and fistulae are treated by complete excision of the tract. An elliptical skin incision should be made around the external opening and the tract followed up to the tonsil fossa if necessary. Insertion of a lacrimal probe or instillation of methylene blue can define the course of the lesion. In young children, one horizontal skin incision is usually adequate, but in older children and adults, a stepladder technique may be required.

Third and Fourth Arch Anomalies

These are uncommon and present in a similar fashion to each other.

Presentation

Most third and fourth branchial pouch anomalies present in childhood or early adulthood with recurrent cervical abscesses or thyroiditis (Fig. 19.4). Females are more

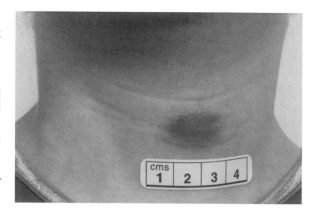

Fig. 19.4 Ten-year-old girl with recurrent thyroiditis secondary to fourth branchial pouch sinus

frequently affected and 97% are left-sided (the reason for this is not well understood). Occasionally the abnormality presents in the neonate with a large neck cyst or abscess resulting in airway obstruction. An opening in the pyriform sinus may be visualised by flexible laryngoscopy (Rea et al. 2004).

Investigations

A barium swallow should confirm a tract extending downwards from the pyriform sinus. This should be performed once any infection has settled to avoid missing a tract occluded by oedema. A CT scan is sometimes performed to further determine the extent of the abnormality.

Management

Pre-existing infections should be treated with antibiotics and with incision and drainage if required. Complete surgical excision (including hemithyroidectomy if appropriate) remains the treatment of choice. The tract should be removed in its entirety, the fistulous opening in the pyriform sinus should be closed and the ipsilateral lobe of thyroid should be excised. The insertion of a fine vascular catheter into the sinus can be helpful in subsequently locating the tract within the neck. There have been recent reports of successful treatment with the application of diathermy to the fistulous opening in the pyriform sinus, thus avoiding the necessity for open surgery (Pereira et al. 2004).

Complications

There is the risk of potential damage to adjacent neurovascular structures and knowledge of the expected anatomy is important – in particular the recurrent laryngeal and the hypoglossal nerves. If the tract is not excised in its entirety, then it may recur.

Key point: Consider performing a barium swallow in a child with a history of recurrent thyroiditis.

Branchio-Oto-Renal Syndrome

This is a rare autosomal dominant syndrome (with variable penetrance) where children can exhibit branchial cleft cysts, sinuses and fistulae in association with structural defects of the middle or inner ear. These children can also have renal malformations, therefore a renal assessment should be performed on any child presenting with branchial arch anomalies and deafness.

Thyroglossal Duct Cyst

Thyroglossal duct cysts account for around 70% of congenital abnormalities in the head and neck region. Persistent ducts and cysts occur because of a failure of the thyroglossal duct to involute between the 8th and 10th week of gestation, and a cyst can therefore occur anywhere along the duct's natural course from the foramen caecum to the thyroid gland. The duct assumes an intimate anatomical association with the hyoid bone, and in approximately 30% of cases, a tract has been found posterior to this structure. This has important implications in the treatment of this disorder (see below).

Presentation

They most commonly present in the first two decades of life. Cysts usually appear as a midline cervical mass and lie in close proximity to the hyoid bone. Patients can present with a smooth, cystic swelling in the midline of the neck, which moves on swallowing and tongue protrusion. Thyroglossal duct cysts can become infected, resulting in a red, painful midline swelling, which can discharge (Maddalozzo et al. 2001; Fig. 19.5).

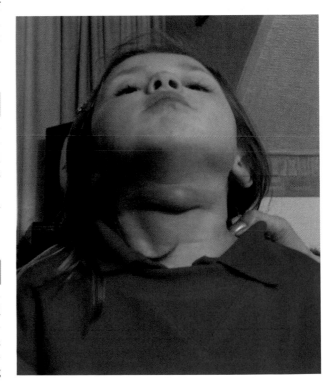

Fig. 19.5 Infected thyroglossal duct cyst

Investigations

An ultrasound examination should be performed to establish the presence of a cystic structure in the neck and to confirm that there is a separate and normal-looking thyroid gland (Brewis et al. 2000). This will prevent the rare possibility of inadvertent removal of an ectopic thyroid gland resulting in post-operative hypothyroidism.

Treatment

A Sistrunk's procedure is the treatment of choice (Sistrunk 1920). This is performed through a horizontal skin crease incision at the approximate level of the hyoid bone, taking a skin ellipse around any discharging sinus. The cyst and its associated tract are then dissected out in continuity with the middle portion of the hyoid bone and a wedge of muscle superior to the hyoid bone extending up to the foramen caecum.

Complications

Hypoglossal nerve injury is unlikely, but conceivable. This can be prevented by transecting the hyoid at the level of the lesser cornu and maintaining all subsequent dissection medial to the anterior belly of digastric. Insertion of a drain will also prevent accumulation of a haematoma. Recurrence rates are low when a Sistrunk's procedure is performed (0–3%), but can be as high as 50% if an inadequate surgical procedure is performed initially.

Key point: If there is a midline cyst in the neck and an ultrasound examination confirms a normal thyroid gland, then a Sistrunk's procedure should be performed to avoid recurrence (5% will subsequently turn out to be dermoid cysts).

Lingual Thyroid

If the primitive thyroid gland fails to descend during development, it can enlarge and function within the tongue base.

Presentation

The thyroid mass usually increases in size as the child develops and may manifest as a mass lesion in the tongue base causing dysphagia, dysphonia and airway compromise (Fig. 19.6).

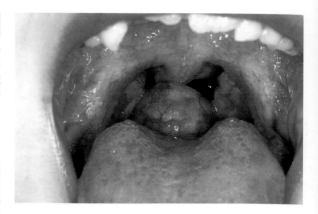

Fig. 19.6 Lingual thyroid

Investigations

A radioisotope scan is required to confirm the diagnosis and to determine the amount of functioning thyroid tissue present. Thyroid function tests should also be performed.

Management

In a euthyroid and asymptomatic child, no treatment is required. If the child has functional symptoms then thyroid replacement therapy should be commenced to see if regression of the mass occurs. If this results in an acceptable improvement in symptoms, then medical therapy can continue. An inadequate response requires surgical excision of the mass followed by thyroid replacement. Surgery carries no risk to the parathyroid glands, which are derived from the third and fourth arches (Muntz and Gray 2002).

Complications

There is an increased risk of thyroid carcinoma in lingual thyroid tissue, so careful follow-up is recommended.

Dermoid Cyst

A dermoid cyst is the result of inclusion of epithelial cells along the lines of embryonic closure. The cyst contains ectodermal and mesodermal elements, resulting in the presence of hair follicles and sebaceous glands. The cyst can therefore fill with sebaceous material, which can become infected.

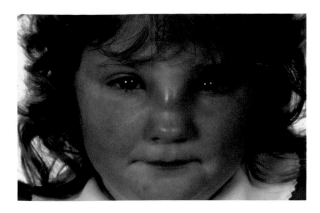

Fig. 19.7 Infected nasal dermoid with inferiorly placed midline punctum (reproduced, with the permission of the BMJ publishing group, from MacGregor and Geddes 1993, Fig. 2)

Presentation

Forty percent of dermoid cysts are clinically apparent at birth, and most of the remainder present by the age of 5 years. There is a slight male predominance. Dermoid cysts are the second most common midline neck mass after a thyroglossal duct cyst. Unlike a thyroglossal duct cyst, a dermoid cyst does not move on swallowing or tongue protrusion, as it is not attached to the underlying structures.

Investigations

This is usually a clinical diagnosis, but if there is any doubt an ultrasound scan may be useful.

Treatment

Local excision.

Nasal Dermoid Cysts

This is a specific group of dermoid cysts that can be difficult to diagnose and a challenge to treat.

Presentation

Children typically present with a small punctum over the bridge of the nose, often with hair extruding from the opening. However, there may be a cyst or swelling anywhere between the forehead and nasal tip, and a tract can extend through the crista galli. The cyst and/or tract may become infected and is rarely associated with complications such as periorbital cellulitis or meningitis (Fig. 19.7).

Investigations

A CT scan and MRI can both provide helpful information as to the extent of the nasal dermoid cyst. In particular, a bifid crista galli on CT suggests intracranial extension and an intracranial mass or cyst may be apparent on MRI.

Management

Infection should be treated appropriately and then complete surgical excision performed. A small, localized cyst may be removed through an incision over the nasal dorsum. An external rhinoplasty incision is the method of choice for access to more extensive lesions, whilst providing an acceptable cosmetic result. Rarely, when there is significant intracranial involvement, a more extensive craniofacial approach is required (Bloom et al. 2002).

Key point: Look carefully for a punctum on the nose in a child presenting with swelling and/or infection in the nasal area.

Summary for the Clinician

- 1. An understanding of the underlying embryological anatomy of these disorders will aid in diagnosis and management.
- 2. Consider the diagnosis of an underlying congenital cyst, sinus or fistula in recurrent infection or abscess formation in the head and neck region in children
- 3. It is important to make the correct diagnosis, then perform the appropriate procedure at initial surgery to avoid recurrence

References

1. Bloom DC, Carvalho DS, Dory C, et al (2002) Imaging and surgical approach of nasal dermoids. Int J Pediatr Otorhinolaryngol 62:111–122
2. Brewis C, Mahadevan M, Bailey CM, et al (2000) Investigation and treatment of thyroglossal cysts in children. J Roy Soc Med 93:18–21
3. Ford GR, Balakrishnan A, Evans JNG, et al (1992) Branchial cleft and pouch anomalies. J Laryngol Otol 118:19–24

4. Gur E, Yeung A, Al-Azzawi M et al (1998) The excised pre-auricular sinus in 14 years of experience: is there a problem? Plast Reconstr Surg 102:1405–1408

5. Karmody CS (2002) Developmental anomalies of the neck. In: Bluestone CD, Stool SE (eds) Pediatric Otolaryngology, 4th edn. Saunders, Philadelphia, pp 1648–1663

6. Lam HCK, Soo G, Wormald PJ, et al (2001) Excision of the preauricular sinus: a comparison of two surgical techniques Laryngoscope 111:317–319

7. MacGregor FB, Geddes NK (1993) Nasal dermoids: the significance of a midline punctum. Arch Dis Child 68:418–419

8. Maddalozzo J, Venkatesan TK, Gupta P (2001) Complications associated with the Sistrunk procedure. Laryngoscope 111:119–123

9. Mandell DL (2000) Head and neck anomalies related to the branchial apparatus. Otolaryngol Clin North Am 33:1309–1332

10. Muntz HR, Gray SD, Stool Sylvan E, et al. (2002) Congenital malformations of the mouth and pharynx. In: Bluestone CD, Stool SE (eds) Pediatric Otolaryngology, 4th edn. Saunders, Philadelphia, pp 917

11. Pereira KD, Losh GG, Oliver D, et al (2004) Management of anomalies of the third and fourth branchial pouches. Int J Pediatr Otorhinolaryngol 68:43–50

12. Rea PA, Hartley BE, Bailey CM (2004) Third and fourth branchial pouch anomalies. J Laryngol Otol 118:19–24

13. Sistrunk WE (1920) The surgical treatment of cysts of the thyroglossal tract. Ann Surg 71:121–124

14. Work WP (1972) Newer concepts of first branchial cleft defects. Laryngoscope 82:1581–1593

19

Chapter 20

Airway Endoscopy and Assessment in Children

20

Sonia Ayari-Khalfallah and Patrick Froehlich

Core Messages

- Airway endoscopy may use fibre-optic or rigid instruments.
- Flexible endoscopy can provide a view of the nasal fossae, choanae, pharynx and larynx, even in the neonate, without the need for general anaesthesia. It also allows a dynamic view of laryngeal and upper airway function. It may also be used during general anaesthesia.
- Rigid endoscopy is performed under general anaesthesia, when careful anaesthetic technique is required.
- Direct microlaryngoscopy, using a suspension laryngoscope, allows inspection of the larynx and pharynx, with excellent illumination and magnification; it allows surgical and therapeutic intervention.
- Under general anaesthesia, bronchoscopy and oesophagoscopy are also possible to complete the examination.
- Imaging may useful to complement the endoscopy findings.

Contents

Introduction

Recent advances in airway endoscopy have made it an essential tool in the management of several pathologies of the pharyngolarynx, oesophagus and trachea. It can be performed using a flexible fibroscope or a rigid endoscope, and may require back-up examinations – notably by x-ray.

Flexible pernasal laryngoscopy (FL) is feasible even neonatally, using a small-calibre (diameter 1.8–2.1 mm) fibroscope (Fig. 20.1). It can be performed during outpatient consultation, with prior local anaesthesia of the nasal fossae, with or without associated vasoconstriction, depending on the child's age. For non-cooperative children, analgesic gas (50% nitrogen monoxide, 50% oxygen) can be administered in outpatient consultation with few side effects (Boulland et al. 2005). Flexible laryngoscopy can also be performed under general anaesthesia in the operating theatre; this facilitates examination, since the patient does not move, and may be the only resort

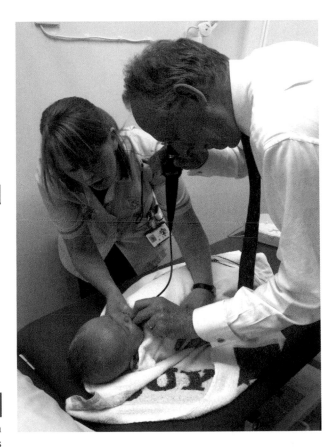

Fig. 20.1 Flexible fibroscopic endoscopy in a conscious infant. The endoscope is passed through the nose, after application of a topical anaesthetic, to view the upper airways as far as the vocal cords

with a totally non-cooperative child or in case of certain physical disabilities; it can also reveal certain sleep pathologies.

FL can be connected to a video camera to provide an enlarged image on screen, with recording for subsequent comparative examination.

FL is liable to be reflexogenic, inducing laryngospasm, especially in ex-premature infants or infants affected by cardiac pathology. To avoid this, the fibroscope should be kept out of contact with the epiglottis; no attempt should be made to pass it through the glottis.

Paediatric FL raises a cost issue, the fibroscope here being much more expensive than adult models. Being finer, it is also more fragile and less resistant to the various decontamination procedures that involve total immersion in disinfectant solutions, with soaking-disinfection-rinsing cycles of as long as 1 h (Midulla et al. 2003). Progress could be made here by using a disposable sterile sheath, thus improving fibroscope turnover and cost-effectiveness, and increasing the life of the instrument by reducing the number of decontamination cycles.

FL enables assessment of the nasal fossae (mucosa, concha, secretions, tumours and malformations), choana permeability and nasopharynx (adenoid vegetation hypertrophy and tumours). It further enables dynamic and morphological analysis of the pharyngolarynx, exploring vocal fold and soft palate mobility and the quality of the contact between the soft palate and the posterior pharyngeal wall in case of velar insufficiency. It can disclose pharyngomalacia, in the form of pharyngeal wall collapse during inspiration, or laryngomalacia, in the form of collapse of the supraglottic larynx during inspiration. In some cases, it is possible to relate the respiratory noise, noted during examination, to an observed obstacle.

Rigid Endoscopy

Please also refer to Chapter 48 – Appendix: Developmental Data- for Bronchoscope Sizes. Rigid endoscopy is performed under general anaesthesia in the operating theatre. During general anaesthesia, various techniques of ventilation are possible: spontaneous ventilation, mechanically controlled ventilation after intubation, intermittent apnoea ventilation and transglottic or transtracheal jet ventilation (Jaquet et al. 2006). In spontaneous as compared to mechanically controlled ventilation, endoscopy is not hindered by any intubation probe, however small in calibre; it does, however, require a balance, which can be difficult to strike in young infants, between spontaneity of ventilation and a state of anaesthesia deep enough to prevent laryngospasm or bronchospasm when the endoscope is introduced. Another disadvantage lies in the inhalation of anaesthetic gas by the medical and paramedical team (Gentili et al. 2004). Even so, it is our

technique of choice. Intermittent apnoea provides the surgeon with a satisfactory view, but one that is often of short duration. Jet ventilation, via a small-calibre transglottic or transtracheal cannula (which is not always easy to install) provides satisfactory ventilation, with a high ventilation frequency of 150–300 breaths/min and an in-breath pressure of 1–3 bar (Jaquet et al. 2006); however, it also entails a risk of barotrauma with possible pneumothorax or pneumomediastinum, especially if an obstruction such as laryngeal spasm occurs, blocking the escape of gases under pressure in the trachea. It is also possible for the intratracheal cannula to be accidentally placed in the oesophagus, for example during repositioning of the laryngoscope, with equally serious effects. The other ventilation techniques are also subject to this kind of complication, and early detection and prevention of airway obstruction is to be recommended.

The anaesthetic techniques used are gas (sevofluorane) and/or intravenous (propofol, rapifen, mivacurium or remifentanil). To avoid gas inhalation by the surgeon, some teams use an exclusively intravenous approach; others combine both. Sevofluorane, being a bronchodilator, is useful in case of bronchopulmonary spasticity. Muscular paralysis and mechanically controlled ventilation are also useful for obtaining complete oesophageal relaxation during oesophageal endoscopy (see also chapter 3).

Endoscopy begins with direct laryngoscopy. Local anaesthesia (5% xylocaine at 1 spray per 3 kg body-weight) is applied to the pharyngolaryngeal mucosa, often with an associated analgesic intravenous bolus to reduce the risk of spasm when the rigid endoscope is being introduced. There are various models of laryngoscopes (Fig. 20.2), varying in their proximal opening and in their length, closed circumferentially or with a lateral slot to accommodate a bronchoscope or oesophagoscope. The optic cable may be clipped directly onto the laryngoscope, or else run through a lateral channel in a light-conducting stem. The direct laryngoscope may include a lateral insufflation channel for anaesthetic gas or oxygen during spontaneous ventilation and a lateral aspiration channel for laser surgery fumes. Various kinds of thoracic support can be fitted to the laryngoscope, for laryngeal suspension (Fig. 20.3). The suspension laryngoscope can be used with a 400-mm-lens operating microscope. Direct microlaryngoscopy has the advantage of leaving both of the surgeon's hands free and of enabling greater precision thanks to the enlarged microscopy image. A rigid telescope, using the Hopkins lens system (Fig. 20.4), can also be passed through the laryngoscope, with telescopes of various diameters (2.7 or 4 mm) and angled lenses (0°, 30° or 70°). Small-diameter (2.7 mm) telescopes are fragile and require delicate handling. Like a microscope, they can be connected to a video camera system. Here again there have been advances in technology, with integrated image digitisation modules in the camera itself. Some cameras come with three charge-coupled devices for separate processing of the three primary colours, providing high-fidelity colour restitution and a very satisfactory image quality. The camera can be connected up to an image and video storage system. The camera heads can usually be dipped in suitable disinfectant solutions; otherwise, systems using sterile sheaths are available (Fig. 20.5).

Direct laryngoscopy thus enables the pharynx (tonsils, soft palate, tongue base, hypopharynx and mouth of the oesophagus) and larynx to be analysed. Ventilation conditions permitting, the telescope may go beyond the glottis to visualise the subglottis and trachea. In some pathologies, laryngoscopy may be enough; otherwise, complementary rigid bronchoscopy is required, the size of the bronchoscope depending on the body weight and age of the child. The outside diameter of the bronchoscope varies with the manufacturer. Passing a rigid telescope that is connected to a camera, through the bronchoscope

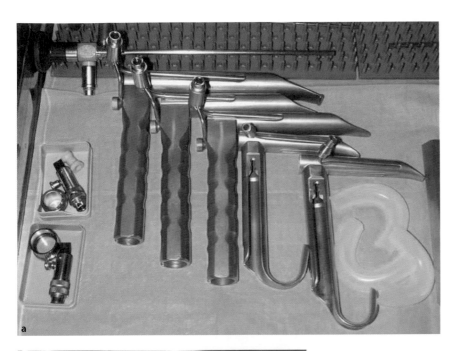

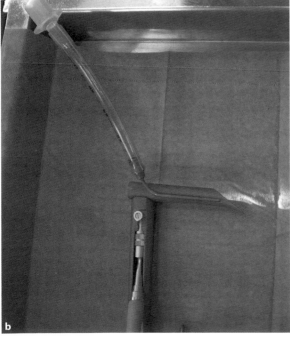

Fig. 20.2a,b Various kinds of laryngoscope

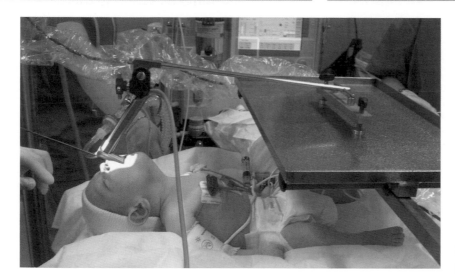

Fig. 20.3 Suspension microlaryngoscopy in an anaesthetised infant

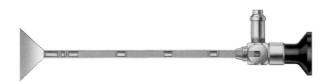

Fig. 20.4 A Storz rigid telescope, using the Hopkins rod system

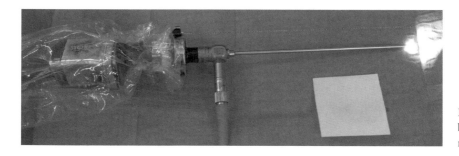

Fig. 20.5 A video camera, covered by a sterile sheath, attached to a rigid telescope

20

again enhances the analysis of the tracheobronchial tree, down to the lobar or even segmentary branches. Finally, the oesophagus can be analysed using a rigid oesophagoscope, the size of which again depends on the child's age. Here again, extra precision can be obtained by the use of telescopes and video cameras.

During endoscopy, the entire upper airway can be analysed both visually and by palpation (checking for cricoarytenoid joint mobility, compressibility of a tumour and assessing the subglottic diameter) using an intubation tube. Samples may be taken for bacteriology, virology, mycology or histopathology throughout the airway.

In therapeutic airway endoscopy, various tools can be used. There is a range of micro-instruments: forceps, scissors, palpators and knives, adapted to airway endoscopy.

Carbon dioxide, potassium tintanyl phosphate or erbium-yttrium aluminium garnet lasers may be employed. There are microdebriders, for use in various congenital or acquired pathologies (Naiman et al. 2003; Zalzal and Collins 2005); dilating balloons for use in oesophageal or tracheal stenosis (Monnier et al. 2005); basket probes to remove tracheobronchial or oesophageal foreign bodies; tracheal or bronchial stents for certain kinds of severe malacia (Geller et al. 2004). Topical medications may be applied, such as mitomycin-C, to prevent intraluminal scarring (Perepelitsyn and Shapshay 2004). Intralesional injections may be used, for example of corticosteroids, for the treatment of subglottic angioma (Meeuwis et al. 1990), or cidofovir for laryngeal papillomatosis (Mandell et al. 2004; Naiman et al. 2003).

Supplementary Examinations

Imaging may be a useful complement to endoscopy. If endoscopy reveals tracheomalacia or bronchomalacia, imaging is necessary to rule out extrinsic compression by vascular malformations, especially abnormalities of the aortic arches, or by tumours. Simple intrinsic tracheomalacia may also be identified, especially in cases of oesophageal atresia (Briganti et al. 2005). In cases of right aortic arch, a chest radiograph can show the typical contralateral deviation of the trachea to the right; the presence of two arches may be suspected when there is compression of the trachea at the level of the arches, particularly on the lateral view (Hernanz-Sculman 2005). The anterior view of the barium oesophagogram shows anomalies on the oesophageal margin (such as opposing notches on the left and right margins as the result of a double aortic arch); the lateral view may show a broad impression on the posterior margin of the oesophagus, from a double aortic arch or aberrant subclavian artery, or an anterior notch at the level of the carina in cases of aberrant retrotracheal left pulmonary artery (Oddone et al. 2005). The bi-dimensional echocardiogram with Doppler can accurately diagnose some vascular anomalies, and it is important to rule out any important associated cardiac pathology . Contrast spiral computerised tomography (CT) scan of the chest using three-dimensional reconstruction will define the exact vascular anatomy and can visualise tumours such as bronchogenic cysts and malignant tumours (Oddone et al. 2005). Imaging can be performed in real time, with extremely short acquisition times, allowing "virtual endoscopy" (Briganti et al. 2005; Ferretti and Coulomb 2000). Virtual endoscopy reproduces real endoscopic images and can be useful if the child is at high risk from general anaesthesia, but this technique cannot provide information on the state of the mucosa. It offers possible applications for preparing, guiding and controlling interventional endoscopy procedures.

A chest magnetic resonance image (MRI) can be substituted for a CT scan for the diagnosis of vascular abnormalities and tumours (Faust et al. 2002; Oddone et al. 2005). The advantages of the spiral CT over an MRI are its speed and frequent lack of the need for sedation. The advantages of MRI include its lack of the need for iodinated intravenous contrast and the absence of radiation exposure.

Twenty-four-hour pH-metry tests for gastroesophageal reflux, and may be indicated when there are endoscopic signs of reflux, such as supraglottic laryngeal oedema, or in pathologies frequently involving reflux, such as severe laryngomalacia, laryngeal dyskinesias or neurological pharyngomalacia, when it may aggravate the clinical symptomatology (Garabedian 1996).

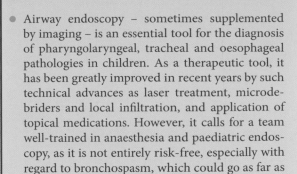

Summary for the Clinician

- Airway endoscopy – sometimes supplemented by imaging – is an essential tool for the diagnosis of pharyngolaryngeal, tracheal and oesophageal pathologies in children. As a therapeutic tool, it has been greatly improved in recent years by such technical advances as laser treatment, microdebriders and local infiltration, and application of topical medications. However, it calls for a team well-trained in anaesthesia and paediatric endoscopy, as it is not entirely risk-free, especially with regard to bronchospasm, which could go as far as to cause cardiorespiratory arrest.

References

1. Boulland P, Favier JC, Villevieille T, et al (2005) Mélange équimolaire oxygène-protoxyde d'azote (MEOPA) Rappels théoriques et modalités pratiques d'utilisation. Ann Fr Anesth Reanim 24:1305–1312

2. Briganti V, Oriolo L, Buffa V, et al (2005) Tracheomalacia in oesophageal atresia: morphological considerations by endoscopic and CT study. Eur J Cardiothorac Surg 28:11–15

3. Faust RA, Rimell FL, Remley KB (2002) Cine magnetic resonance imaging for evaluation of focal tracheomalacia: innominate artery compression syndrome. Int J Pediatr Otolaryngol 65:27–33

4. Ferretti G, Coulomb M (2000) Imagerie 3D et virtuelle de l'arbre respiratoire proximal. Rev Pneumol Clin 56:132–139

5. Garabedian EN (1996) Sémiologie et approche diagnostique de la pathologie pharyngolaryngeé et trachéale In: Garabédian EA, Bobin S, Monteil P, Triglia JM (eds) ORL de l'Enfant. Flammarion Médecine – Sciences, Paris, pp 163–167

6. Geller KA, Wells WJ, Koempel JA, et al (2004) Use of the Palmaz stent in the treatment of severe tracheomalacia. Ann Otol Rhinol Laryngol 113:641–647

7. Gentili A, Accorsi A, Pigna A, et al (2004) Exposure of personnel to sevoflurane during paediatric anaesthesia: influence of professional role and anaesthetic procedure. Eur J Anaesthesiol 21:638–645

8. Hernanz-Schulman M (2005) Vascular rings: a practical approach to imaging diagnosis. Pediatr Radiol 35:961–979

9. Jaquet Y, Monnier P, Van Melle G, et al (2006) Complications of different ventilation strategies in endoscopic laryngeal surgery: a 10-year review. Anesthesiology 104:52–59

10. Mandell DL, Arjmand EM, Kay DJ, et al (2004) Intralesional cidofovir for pediatric recurrent respiratory papillomatosis. Arch Otolaryngol Head Neck Surg 130:1319–1323

11. Meeuwis J, Bos CE, Hoeve LJ, et al (1990) Subglottic hemangiomas in infants: treatment with intralesional corticosteroid injection and intubation. Int J Pediatr Otorhinolaryngol 19:145–150

12. Midulla F, de Blic J, Barbato A, et al (2003) Flexible endoscopy of paediatric airways. Eur Respir J 22:698–708

13. Monnier P, George M, Monod ML, et al (2005) The role of the CO_2 laser in the management of laryngotracheal stenosis: a survey of 100 cases. Eur J Anaesthesiol 262:602–608

14. Naiman AN, Ceruse P, Coulombeau B, et al (2003) Intralesional cidofovir and surgical excision for laryngeal papillomatosis. Laryngoscope 113:2174–2181

15. Oddone M, Granata C, Vercellino N, et al (2005) Multimodality evaluation of the abnormalities of the aortic arches in children: techniques and imaging spectrum with emphasis on MRI. Pediatr Radiol 35:947–960

16. Perepelitsyn I, Shapshay SM (2004) Endoscopic treatment of laryngeal and tracheal stenosis – has mitomycin C improved the outcome? Otolaryngol Head Neck Surg 131:16–20

17. Zalzal GH, Collins WO (2005) Microdebrider-assisted supraglottoplasty. Int J Pediatr Otorhinolaryngol 69:305–309

20

Chapter 21

Emergency Management of the Paediatric Airway

21

Michael Kuo and Michael Rothera

Contents

Anatomical and Physiological Considerations

In managing upper-airway problems in neonates, infants and children, it is important to understand the differences between the anatomy and physiology of their respiratory system and that of adults. It is obvious that the neonate's airway is considerably smaller than that of an adult. The average diameter of the subglottis in a full-term baby is around 3.5 mm, that of an adolescent around 7 mm and in an adult around 10–14 mm. The impact of a reduction in the diameter of the airway upon its cross-sectional area (Fig. 21.1) is increased by the direct relationship of this area to the square of the radius (cross-sectional area = πr^2). The clinical implication of this is further magnified by the inverse relation of resistance of flow to the radius^4 in a tubular structure, as defined by Poiseuille's law, originally describing laminar flow of a fluid in a cylindrical tube (resistance $\alpha l \times \partial / \pi r^4$, where l is the length of the tube, r is the radius and ∂ is the density of the gas). Figure 21.2 illustrates the dramatic differences in the impact of 1 mm of mucosal oedema in an adult, a child of 6–8 years of age and a neonate. An adult will barely notice the change, a

child will have significant difficulty, and for a neonate, it may have a fatal outcome.

Safe per-operative management of the airway-compromised child also requires understanding of paediatric respiratory physiology. Neonates have a higher rate of oxygen consumption than adults (6 l/kg/min vs. 3 l/kg/min). This is attributable to a higher metabolic rate and increased energy requirement for temperature homeostasis, due to a relatively high surface area to weight ratio. Lung capacity in the child is also smaller, and therefore the child is less able to tolerate long periods of apnoea. However, in favour of the child, the increased compliance of the lung and thorax tends to facilitate assisted tubeless anaesthesia with spontaneous respiration.

Clinical and Radiological Assessment of the Acutely Compromised Upper Airway

Obtaining the history is often difficult in cases of acute airway obstruction because parents are understandably distressed. Few symptom complexes are entirely pathog-

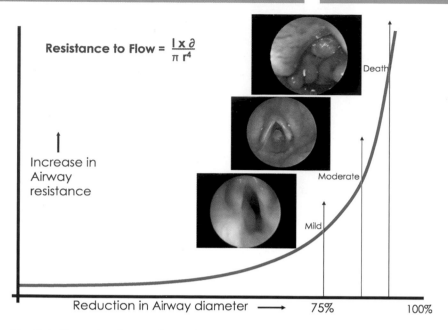

$$\text{Resistance to Flow} = \frac{l \times \partial}{\pi\, r^4}$$

Increase in
Airway
resistance

Reduction in Airway diameter ⟶   75%   100%

Death

Moderate

Mild

Fig. 21.1 Illustration showing the rapid rise in airway resistance with reducing airway diameter, as dictated by Poiseuille's law

Approx age	From	To	Resistance $\propto 1/r^4$	Area $= \pi r^2$	Myer-Cotton Grade
0 - 9/12	2mm	1mm	↑ 16x	↓ 75%	III
6 - 8 yrs	3mm	2mm	↑ 5x	↓ 55%	II
12 - 14 yrs	4mm	3mm	↑ 3x	↓ 44%	I

Fig. 21.2 The effect upon airway resistance of 1 mm of oedema on airways of different sizes at different ages (adapted from Hartnick and Cotton 2003, see Fig. 6)

21

nomonic of specific diagnoses, but general enquiries can give excellent clues to the likely pathology. The neonatal history, particularly including birth trauma and neonatal endotracheal intubation, is important to establish whether the child has an underlying airway compromise, such as vocal fold paralysis or subglottic stenosis. A history of obstructive sleep apnoea indicates a baseline adenotonsillar hypertrophy. Rapid onset of airway obstruction often suggests an infective process. Infection of any point of the upper airway can cause airway obstruction. Obstructive adenotonsillar hypertrophy can arise from acute infection, particularly in infectious mononucleosis. Laryngotracheobronchitis (croup) is characterised by inspiratory stridor and a barking cough as well as features of acute infection such as pyrexia and tachypnoea.

The practical aim of the history and examination is to locate accurately the likely site of the obstruction, to gauge its severity and to predict its likely short-term progression. The quality and timing of the noise of breathing often give much information on the likely location of the obstruction (Table 21.1). Noisy breathing that is worse when a baby is asleep than when awake is likely to be due to pharyngeal obstruction, which also has a characteristic sound known as stertor. Conversely, noisy breathing that is worse with exertion is more likely to be laryngotracheobronchial in nature. The timing of stridor further refines the area of suspicion. Inspiratory stridor suggests an extrathoracic or supraglottic obstruction, while expiratory stridor suggests an intrathoracic obstruction. Biphasic stridor tends to indicate obstruction at the glottic or subglottic laryngeal level, such as in vocal fold paralysis, subglottic stenosis and subglottic haemangioma, although it is also a feature of laryngotracheobronchitis (Holinger 1992).

The volume of the noise associated with breathing is not a robust indicator of the severity of airway obstruction. This caveat is particularly important to observe where the obstruction is physically soft in nature, for example with subglottic haemangioma, soft subglottic cysts and laryngeal papillomatosis. Fixed obstructions, such as bilateral vocal fold paralysis, often give a louder and harsher sound despite the obstruction being less severe and less immediately life-threatening. Decreasing volume may also reflect tiring of the child and indicate impending respiratory collapse. More revealing clinical signs of the severity of upper airway obstruction in babies and children are pre-tracheal tug, intercostal and sternal recession, shallow respiration and tachypnoea. In small babies, the use of accessory muscles of respiration results in a characteristic "head-bobbing", and increased air hunger causes nasal flaring. Overt cyanosis is a late event in paediatric upper airway obstruction and should be relied upon as a marker of distress only to predict imminent respiratory collapse.

Dysphagia and odynophagia often manifest themselves as drooling in children. Drooling in association with noisy breathing indicates an acute pharyngeal obstruction such as acute tonsillitis or a supraglottic lesion such as epiglottitis or foreign body impaction at that level. The widespread uptake of the Hib vaccine has dramatically reduced the incidence of acute epiglottitis; however, it should always remain in the differential diagnosis of acute airway obstruction, as vaccine failure resulting in acute epiglottitis is well documented (Tanner et al. 2002).

The role of radiology in the assessment of acute paediatric airway obstruction is limited. Traditional teaching has it that a lateral neck radiograph should never be taken in a patient with suspected epiglottitis to avoid the risk of losing the airway in an environment suboptimal for airway resuscitation. The acquisition of high-quality plain film imaging with portable equipment is difficult. However, as auscultation of the lungs is complicated in cases of upper airway obstruction by the transmission of upper airway sounds, it has a role in excluding additional lower-airway pathology. The potential of radiological investigation to provide information that might influence treatment must be weighed against the risk of treatment delay and temporary removal of the child to an environment not optimal for monitoring and resuscitation. However, there are special circumstances where radiology may play

Table 21.1 Clinical signs and symptoms typical of airway obstruction at different levels of the upper respiratory tract

Location of obstruction	Typical clinical sign/symptom
Pharynx	"Hot potato" voice Drooling Odynophagia Stertor Worse while asleep
Supraglottis	"Hot potato" voice Drooling Odynophagia Inspiratory stridor
Glottis	Hoarse voice/rasping cry Normal swallowing Barking cough Inspiratory or biphasic stridor
Tracheobronchial tree	Normal voice Normal swallowing Barking cough Expiratory stridor/wheeze

a major role in influencing treatment. These are when there is a high index of suspicion of certain pathologies. In suspected retropharyngeal abscess formation, for example, a soft-tissue lateral cervical radiograph can confirm the diagnosis and indicate the inferior extent of the pathology. In interpreting these x-rays, one needs to be aware that the rule in adults of the retropharyngeal space not normally exceeding the width of the body of the vertebra can not always be applied: in the screaming child, particularly with some neck flexion, this appearance may be normal. In the case of a suspected airway foreign body, radio-opaque foreign bodies are easy to identify and localise using plain radiography in two planes. However, with suspected radio-lucent foreign bodies, particularly in a bronchus, inspiratory and expiratory radiographs may demonstrate air-trapping or even mediastinal shift in the expiratory films, due to ball-valving obstruction of expiration (Brown et al. 1963).

Resuscitation and Pre-Operating-Room Management

It cannot be emphasised enough that the child with a compromised airway needs to be handled not only expediently, but in a calm environment. Not only are the parents understandably anxious at the distress of their child, but above all the child needs to be kept calm and not irritated, so as not to exacerbate the airway obstruction. For example, numbers of relatives and hospital personnel in the resuscitation room should be kept to a safe minimum. As far as possible, the child should be observed and examined while resting in a parent's arms. Fibre-optic laryngoscopy, which would be considered almost mandatory, both in the assessment of an adult with acute upper airway obstruction and in the elective assessment of the paediatric airway, can be contraindicated in the acutely compromised paediatric airway: instrumentation of this nature must be carried out with great care, if at all. Procedures such as intravenous cannulation of the child should be carried out only when absolutely necessary and in an environment where, should respiratory arrest be precipitated, appropriate resuscitation facilities and expertise are at hand. Early involvement of the anaesthetic team is essential to provide a rapid response if transfer to the paediatric intensive care unit or the operating theatre is demanded.

Central to the resuscitation of the child with acute upper airway obstruction, is the reduction in resistance of air flow. This can be achieved by reducing mucosal oedema and reducing the density of the inspired gas. Nebulised adrenaline (5 ml of 1:1000 adrenaline repeated hourly if indicated) can dramatically reduce the local mucosal oedema in the short term, allowing safe transfer of the child. Similarly, dexamethasone (300 μg/kg) reduces mu-

cosal oedema, but its slower onset of action means that its principal role is the prevention of late mucosal swelling after airway intervention.

Poiseuille's law also indicates that resistance to flow can be reduced by reduction of the viscosity of the fluid or the density of the gas flowing through the tubular structure. Reduction in the density of the inspired gas can be achieved by replacing nitrogen with the less dense helium. Heliox, a mixture of 21% oxygen and 79% helium, can significantly reduce the work of breathing in a child who is tiring because of prolonged breathing through an obstructed airway.

Endoscopy Under General Anaesthesia

The endoscopic examination of a child with an acute airway obstruction requires intimate coordination and teamwork between the anaesthetist, the laryngologist and the operating room nurse, who must be entirely familiar with the ventilating bronchoscope in all its sizes and methods of assembly. A regularly checked Storz ventilating bronchoscope set (Fig. 21.3) is an essential piece of equipment and must be available in all hospitals that serve children. Induction of anaesthesia should be carried out in the operating theatre and should not be attempted until all of the bronchoscopy equipment has been assembled and checked. This is necessary because in certain situations, such as retrognathia, tongue-base lesions or supraglottic oedema, intubation with the naked eye may be impossible and fibre-optic intubation is extremely difficult due to the small size of endotracheal tube required. If urgent intubation is needed in these circumstances, a 0° Hopkins rod telescope can be inserted through an endotracheal tube and intubation carried out, using a far lateral approach, through the glossotonsillar sulcus, under direct vision (Fig. 21.4). Similar temporary access to the trachea can be achieved by inserting the ventilating bronchoscope in the same way.

If at all possible, however, the paediatric airway should be examined without having been instrumented or intubated. General anaesthesia is induced either by intravenous propofol or, more commonly, by inhalation of sevoflurane in oxygen. Intravenous atropine (15 μg/kg) is often given prior to induction to reduce secretions and to depress vagal reflexes, which produce bradycardia with laryngeal stimulation, especially if halothane is used as the volatile agent (Hartnick and Cotton 2003). The larynx is anaesthetised topically with 2% lignocaine, and anaesthesia maintained by sevoflurane in oxygen through a nasopharyngeal airway, of a size and length appropriate for the child's age. See also Chapter 3, Anaesthesia for Paediatric ENT.

Once anaesthetised, laryngoscopy is performed with a Parsons laryngoscope, which is designed with a slit on one

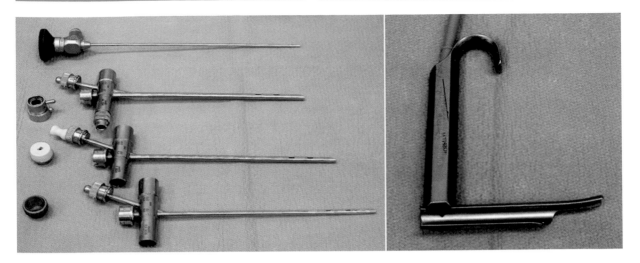

Fig. 21.3 Storz ventilating bronchoscopes and the Parsons laryngscope are essential pieces of equipment for safe management of the paediatric airway

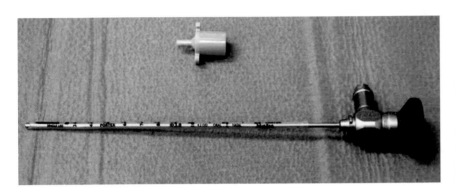

Fig. 21.4 Use of a Hopkins rod telescope within an endotracheal tube for difficult intubations. This is particularly useful when approaching the larynx from the glossotonsillar sulcus, for example in babies with micrognathia

side of the laryngoscope to allow introduction of the ventilating bronchoscope. Supraglottic oedema can obscure the laryngeal inlet and mucosal swelling can worsen an already precarious airway. With the larynx under direct vision, application of 1:10,000 adrenaline on neurosurgical patties will usually overcome this soft obstruction. A comprehensive laryngotracheobronchoscopy can then be carried out. Where appropriate, the size of the airway should be measured and documented (Fig. 21.5). This is achieved by inserting an endotracheal tube, the initial size of which will correspond to the size of the ventilating bronchoscope. Successively larger tubes are placed until no air leak is perceptible with a positive pressure of 30 cmH$_2$0. The largest tube that permits a leak is then taken to be the size of the airway. Finally, assessment of vocal cord movement is essential to complete the examination. The authors' preference is for the placement of a fibre-optic nasolaryngoscope while the anaesthesia is reversed. This allows clear observation of vocal cord movement without risk of laryngospasm or injury due to the presence of rigid endoscopic equipment in the mouth on awakening.

Surgical Management of the Acutely Obstructed Paediatric Airway

Surgical management of the acutely obstructed airway depends on the diagnosis made on endoscopy and/or radiology. Emergency tracheostomy is rarely required due to better endoscopic techniques. Where the diagnosis was not clear pre-operatively, the imperative is to make a diagnosis and secure the airway by endotracheal intubation if necessary. Further definitive treatment should be delayed pending a full discussion of the options with the parents. Exceptions to this general principle are where definitive endoscopic treatment will obviate the need for endotracheal intubation, for example by excision of obstructing laryngeal papillomata, balloon dilatation of evolving subglottic stenosis or marsupialisation of subglottic cysts (Axon et al. 1995). Safe removal of tracheobronchial foreign bodies requires optical forceps together with the Storz ventilating bronchoscope and should be carried out without delay. Acute tonsillectomy for airway obstruction secondary to infectious mononucleosis

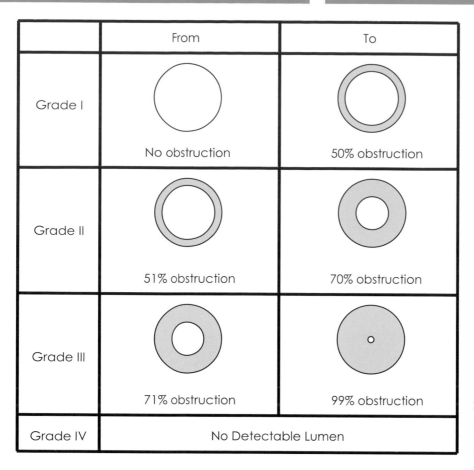

	From	To
Grade I	No obstruction	50% obstruction
Grade II	51% obstruction	70% obstruction
Grade III	71% obstruction	99% obstruction
Grade IV	No Detectable Lumen	

Fig. 21.5 Subglottic stenosis is usually graded according to the scheme proposed by Myer and Cotton (Myer et al. 1994)

remains contentious, but can be carried out safely (Stevenson et al. 1992).

Summary for the Clinician ↓

- A child with severe upper airway obstruction presents both doctors and parents with perhaps the most hair-raising clinical scenario imaginable. An understanding of the principles of airway anatomy and physiology underpin the successful assessment and management of such a child. Most worrying for the surgeon is the prospect of an emergency tracheostomy in a baby with an unsecured airway, but timely use of inhaled and systemic drugs, effective team working with the anaesthetic team and familiarity with the essential Storz ventilating bronchoscope renders this a very small risk, and should allow the airway to be properly assessed and, if necessary, secured, to allow transfer to a specialist unit.

References

1. Axon PR, Hartley C, Rothera MP (1995) Endoscopic balloon dilatation of subglottic stenosis. J Laryngol Otol 109:876–879
2. Brown BS, Ma H, Dunbar JS, et al (1963) Foreign bodies in tracheobronchial tree in childhood. J Can Assoc Radiol 14:158–171
3. Hartnick C, Cotton R (2003) Stridor and airway obstruction. In: Bluestone CD, Stool SE, Alper CM, et al (eds) Pediatric Otolaryngology. Saunders, Philadelphia, pp 1437–1447
4. Holinger LD (1992) Evaluation of stridor and wheezing. In: Holinger LD, Lusk RP, Green CG (eds) Pediatric Laryngology and Bronchoesophagology. Lippincott-Raven, Philadelphia, pp 41–48
5. Myer CM 3rd, O'Connor DM, Cotton RT (1994) Proposed grading system for subglottic stenosis based on endotracheal tube sizes. Ann Otol Rhinol Laryngol 103:319–323
6. Stevenson DS, Webster G, Stewart IA (1992) Acute tonsillectomy in the management of infectious mononucleosis. J Laryngol Otol 106:989–991
7. Tanner K, Fitzsimmons G, Carrol ED, et al (2002) Haemophilus influenzae type b epiglottitis as a cause of acute upper airways obstruction in children. BMJ 325:1099–1100

21

Congenital Disorders of the Larynx, Trachea and Bronchi

22

Martin Bailey

Core Messages

- The diagnosis of mild laryngomalacia can be confirmed in the outpatient clinic by flexible fibre-optic laryngoscopy.
- Microlaryngoscopy and bronchoscopy, under general anaesthesia, is necessary if the stridor in laryngomalacia is severe, if there is failure to thrive or if there are any atypical features.
- In laryngomalacia, the stridor is usually improved immediately following aryepiglottoplasty.
- In the EXIT procedure (EXtrauterine Intrapartum Treatment), tracheostomy is undertaken with the foetus still on placental circulation.
- Although outpatient flexible, fibre-optic laryngoscopy may indicate the diagnosis of vocal cord palsy, a formal microlaryngoscopy and bronchoscopy under general anaesthesia is essential to exclude other coexisting airway pathology.
- Investigation of the child with aspiration and stridor requires a careful microlaryngoscopy and bronchoscopy; no other diagnostic method can replace it.

Contents

Introduction

The exact incidence of congenital abnormalities of the airway is uncertain, but a figure has been quoted for congenital laryngeal anomalies of between 1:10,000 and 1:50,000 births (Van den Broek and Brinkman 1979). Furthermore, some of these children will have more than one anomaly in the airway (Shugar and Healey 1980).

Larynx

The larynx is divided into three regions: supraglottis, glottis and subglottis. The supraglottic larynx comprises the epiglottis, aryepiglottic folds, false cords and ventricles.

The glottis consists of the vocal cords (also referred to as vocal folds). The subglottis extends from the undersurface of the vocal cords to the inferior border of the cricoid cartilage.

Supraglottis

Laryngomalacia

Laryngomalacia is characterised by partial or complete collapse of the supraglottic structures on inspiration. It is the commonest cause of congenital stridor, but its pathophysiology remains somewhat obscure. However, there are characteristic anatomical abnormalities that are undoubtedly primarily responsible for the supraglottic collapse that occurs on inspiration: the epiglottis is rather long and curled (omega-shaped) and the aryepiglottic folds are tall and bulky, while at the same time being short anteroposteriorly and rather tightly tethered to the epiglottis. The result is a tall, narrow supraglottis with a deep interarytenoid cleft (Fig. 22.1). The epiglottis is soft and may curl and collapse, and the redundant mucosa and submucosa of the aryepiglottic folds may prolapse anteromedially into the airway. It has been suggested that there may also be an element of neuromuscular immaturity and consequent uncoordinated arytenoid movements.

The characteristic high-pitched, fluttering inspiratory stridor is usually present at or shortly after birth. It is highly variable, typically being most noticeable when the infant is active or upset, and may disappear when the child is asleep. The severity of the stridor tends to increase as the child becomes more active during the first 9 months of life, and then gradually diminishes, until by the age of 2 years, it has generally disappeared. Very rarely, stridor may persist into late childhood.

The diagnosis can be confirmed in the outpatient clinic by flexible fibre-optic laryngoscopy. The supraglottic col-

lapse on inspiration which is typical of laryngomalacia is easily seen, but may obscure the vocal cords and the examination certainly provides no view below the glottis: a second, coexisting airway pathology therefore cannot be excluded. For this reason, a microlaryngoscopy and bronchoscopy under general anaesthesia is necessary if the stridor is severe, if there is failure to thrive or if there are any atypical features. It is of course also necessary if an adequate view cannot be obtained with the fibrescope.

In approximately 90% of reported cases, the condition is mild, no intervention is needed and the parents can be reassured accordingly (Lane et al. 1984). In severe laryngomalacia, however, there is serious respiratory obstruction with substantial sternal and intercostal recession, feeding difficulties that may be compounded by reflux enhanced by the high negative intrathoracic pressures generated, and consequent failure to thrive. Matters are made worse if there are other factors increasing the level of cardiorespiratory embarrassment, such as congenital cyanotic heart disease. Cor pulmonale may ensue and, in cases of severe sternal recession, a permanent pectus excavatum may develop.

Restoration of an adequate airway can be achieved by performing an endoscopic aryepiglottoplasty (sometimes termed a supraglottoplasty; Jani et al. 1991). In this procedure, the larynx is visualised with the aid of an operating microscope; anaesthesia is maintained via a nasotracheal tube, which also serves to protect the interarytenoid mucosa. Using cup forceps and microscissors (or alternatively the carbon dioxide laser), each aryepiglottic fold is first divided to release it from the edge of the epiglottis, and the redundant mucosa and submucosal tissue are then excised from over the arytenoids, together if necessary with part or all of the cuneiform cartilages. The stridor is usually improved immediately following the surgery, and if significant stridor and feeding difficulties persist, an underlying hypotonic neurological disorder is likely (Toynton et al. 2001).

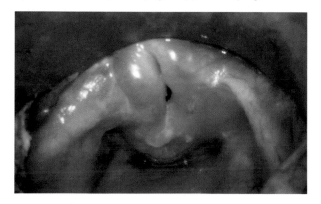

Fig. 22.1 Laryngomalacia (Reprinted with permission from Bull TR, Color Atlas of ENT Diagnosis, Thieme 2003, p. 214)

Saccular Cysts and Laryngocoeles

Congenital saccular cyst is an unusual lesion that may present with respiratory obstruction in infants and young children. Like a laryngocoele, it represents an abnormal dilatation or herniation of the saccule of the ventricle of the larynx; however, it differs from a laryngocoele in that there is no opening into the larynx and it is filled with mucus instead of air. It is considered to form as the result of a developmental failure to maintain patency of the orifice between the saccule and the ventricle, and may be of anterior or lateral type. The anterior saccular cyst extends medially and posteriorly from the saccule and so protrudes into the laryngeal airway between the true and false vocal cords. The lateral saccular cyst is commonest

22

in infants, and expands posterosuperiorly into the false cord and aryepiglottic fold (Cotton and Prescott 1999).

A laryngocoele is classified as internal if it is contained entirely within the laryngeal framework, external if it pierces the thyrohyoid membrane, and combined if there are both internal and external components. It is an uncommon lesion that usually occurs in middle age, but may rarely be seen in infancy, when it can produce respiratory distress that typically becomes worse on crying due to increased distension of the laryngocoele with air. However, a laryngocoele may obstruct and fill with mucus or become infected (laryngopyocoele), thus becoming indistinguishable from a saccular cyst.

Diagnosis is confirmed by endoscopy, except in an external laryngocoele, where no abnormality may be seen except on imaging. Saccular cysts are best treated at the initial endoscopy by wide endoscopic marsupialisation. If the cyst recurs, then the procedure of choice is a lateral cervical approach extending through the thyrohyoid membrane at the superior margin of the ala of the thyroid cartilage, with sub-perichondrial resection of a portion of the upper part of the ala. The cyst can be completely excised through this "window" using short-term intubation to secure the airway post-operatively

Lymphangioma

Lymphangiomas are cystic malformations (sometimes termed cystic hygromas) that result from abnormal development of the lymphatic vessels. In the head and neck they may be macrocystic (usually infrahyoid), microcystic (usually suprahyoid) or a combination of the two. Occasionally a microcystic lymphangioma may extend into the tongue base, valleculae and supraglottis, and airway obstruction may result. If the lymphangioma is very extensive, a tracheotomy may be required, but where supraglottic involvement is less severe it may be possible to debulk the lesion by endoscopic vaporisation using the carbon dioxide laser (April et al. 1992; see also Chapter 12).

Bifid Epiglottis

Bifid epiglottis is a rare laryngeal anomaly in which the epiglottis fails to fuse in the midline and so has a cleft extending down to its tubercle. It may be seen as a feature of Pallister-Hall syndrome, the cardinal elements of which are hypothalamic hamartoblastoma, hypopituitarism, imperforate anus and post-axial polydactyly. It usually presents with feeding difficulties due to aspiration and with stridor due to collapse and enfolding of the two halves of the epiglottis. Endoscopy establishes the diagnosis, and treatment options include amputation of the epiglottis and tracheotomy.

Glottis

Laryngeal Webs

This will be discussed in detail in Chapter 24.

Laryngeal Atresia

Laryngeal atresia is incompatible with life unless there is an associated tracheo-oesophageal fistula (TOF) that permits ventilation via a tube in the oesophagus, or unless an emergency tracheotomy is performed in the delivery room. However, cases are now being recognised antenatally on ultrasound imaging and managed with a so-called EXIT procedure (EXtrauterine Intrapartum Treatment), whereby tracheotomy is undertaken following elective Caesarian section with the neonate still on placental circulation.

Cri-du-Chat Syndrome

This syndrome is primarily characterised by a cat-like mewing cry in infancy, microcephaly, downward-slanting palpebral fissures, mental retardation and hypotonia. It is due to partial deletion of the short arm of chromosome 5. At endoscopy, observation during phonation reveals that the posterior part of the glottis remains open, giving it a diamond-shaped appearance. There is no respiratory embarrassment, and the cry becomes less abnormal as the child grows older.

Vocal Cord Paralysis

Vocal cord paralysis is the second most common congenital anomaly of the larynx after laryngomalacia. It is worth noting that up to 45% of patients may have other, coexisting airway pathology, and so although outpatient flexible fibre-optic laryngoscopy may indicate the diagnosis, a formal microlaryngoscopy and bronchoscopy under general anaesthesia is nevertheless essential. Laryngeal ultrasound can be an accurate and reproducible method of assessing vocal cord movement, and may be useful in monitoring a child with known vocal cord palsy and in the diagnosis of the very sick child who may be unfit for endoscopy under general anaesthesia. About half the cases are unilateral and half bilateral.

Unilateral vocal cord paralysis is usually not congenital, most cases being acquired as a result of surgical injury to the left recurrent laryngeal nerve, often following correction of a congenital cardiac anomaly. The vocal cord lies in an intermediate position, and patients present with mild stridor, dysphonia and sometimes aspiration. Surgical intervention is not usually necessary. The voice can be expected to improve as time passes, when either recovery occurs or the other vocal cord compensates.

In contrast, bilateral vocal cord palsy is usually the result of a congenital abductor paralysis; the vocal cords lie in the paramedian position with consequent inspiratory stridor, and a tracheotomy is necessary in approximately half the cases, most of whom have other associated airway pathology. A classical cause of congenital bilateral vocal cord palsy is hydrocephalus with the Arnold-Chiari malformation. Once the diagnosis is made, prompt correction of the raised intracranial pressure with a shunt often improves vocal cord movement and a tracheotomy may thus be avoided. However, most cases of congenital bilateral vocal cord paralysis are idiopathic, and the approach to management is greatly influenced by the fact that up to 58% will eventually recover, with 10% taking more than 5 years to do so and one reported case of recovery at the age of 11 years (Daya et al. 2000). This suggests strongly that the problem is often one of delayed maturation in the vagal nuclei and argues convincingly in favour of a conservative management philosophy.

The infant with an inadequate airway and failure to thrive will require a tracheotomy. If vocal cord movement does not develop and the airway does not become adequate as a result of laryngeal growth, then an endoscopic laser cordotomy or arytenoidectomy should be considered at the age of 11+ years following a full discussion with the patient and parents regarding the trade-off between airway and voice. If it is considered imperative to achieve decannulation earlier, perhaps because of poor social circumstances, then an endoscopic laser cordotomy can be undertaken as early as 2 years of age. If that fails, then an external arytenoidectomy via a laryngofissure may be done at the age of 4–5 years, with the prospect of an 84% decannulation rate (Bower et al. 1994); however, there is a small risk of aspiration as well as loss of voice quality, and the procedure is irreversible.

Subglottis

Congenital Subglottic Stenosis

Congenital subglottic stenosis is due to defective canalisation of the cricoid cartilage and/or conus elasticus, resulting in a small, elliptical, thickened cricoid and/or excessive submucosal soft tissue (Holinger 1999). Typically, there is gross thickening of the anterior lamina of the abnormal cricoid (Fig. 22.2); alternatively, there may be anterior fusion of the vocal cords with subglottic extension, as seen in 22q11 (Shprintzen) syndrome. Severe stenosis will present with airway obstruction soon after birth. Milder degrees of stenosis present as inspiratory or biphasic stridor as the child becomes older and more active, or as recurrent "croup" due to superimposed oedema from upper respiratory tract infections.

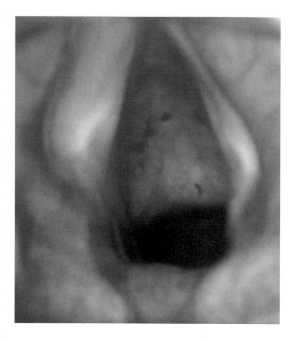

Fig. 22.2 Congenital subglottic stenosis, showing anterior cricoid thickening

Diagnosis requires a microlaryngoscopy and bronchoscopy. If the airway is not severely compromised, then surgery may not be required, especially as a congenital stenosis can be expected to enlarge with growth. Congenital cartilaginous stenosis represents a strict contraindication to dilatation or laser resection; any type of endoscopic treatment is liable to worsen the initial condition, and attempted dilatation is inevitably ineffective as the thickened ring of cricoid cartilage cannot be expanded.

If the airway is severely compromised, then a tracheotomy is needed. This can sometimes be avoided in specialist centres where there are facilities for single-stage airway reconstruction in which an endotracheal tube is used as a stent, usually for a period of 5–7 days.

The surgical options have evolved from the classical castellated laryngotracheoplasty designed by Evans (Evans and Todd 1974) in the early 1970s to achieve laryngeal framework expansion. This was superseded during the early 1980s by the laryngotracheal reconstruction (LTR) devised primarily by Cotton (1978). LTR involves augmentation of the laryngotracheal complex by anterior and/or posterior midline incision of the cricoid, with insertion of costal cartilage grafts to expand the airway. This technique has now been supplemented by the partial cricotracheal resection (PCTR), which was introduced into the paediatric age group by Monnier et al. (1993) in the early 1990s. This involves resection of the stenotic segment with end-to-end anastomosis of the tracheal stump to the thyroid cartilage.

Results from the most experienced centres (Cotton et al. 1989; Ochi et al. 1992; Ndiaye et al. 1999) show an overall decannulation rate in excess of 80% following LTR. The latest results from the two centres with the largest experience in PCTR show a decannulation rate of 98% for primary surgery and 94% for salvage surgery after failed previous airway reconstruction (Monnier et al. 2001; Rutter et al. 2001).

For more detail on the management of post-intubation laryngeal stenosis, the reader is referred to Chapter 25.

Subglottic Haemangioma

This will be discussed in detail in Chapter 24.

Laryngeal and Laryngotracheo-Oesophageal Cleft

Posterior laryngeal clefts result from failure of the posterior cricoid lamina to fuse, and in the more extensive laryngotracheo-oesophageal clefts there is also incomplete development of the tracheo-oesophageal septum. The classification devised by Benjamin and Inglis (1989) has been widely adopted because it relates well to symptoms and treatment. A type I cleft may extend down to the level of the vocal cords; a type II cleft extends below the vocal cords into the cricoid (Fig. 22.3); a type III cleft extends down into the cervical trachea; the fortunately rare type IV cleft extends into the thoracic trachea and may even reach the carina. Approximately 25% of patients with a laryngeal cleft will also have a TOF, but conversely, the incidence of laryngeal cleft in patients with a TOF is low. Abnormalities of the tracheal ring structure in cleft pa-

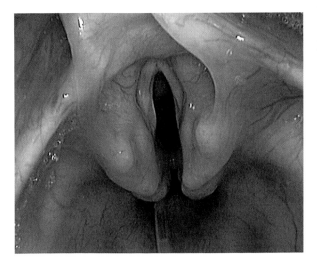

Fig. 22.3 Laryngeal cleft (type II)

tients may result in associated tracheomalacia, which can add to the difficulties of management.

The majority of laryngeal cleft patients have other associated congenital abnormalities, of which TOF is the commonest, but which may include gastro-oesophageal reflux, tracheobronchomalacia, congenital heart disease, dextrocardia and situs inversus. Laryngeal clefts are characteristic of two syndromes: Opitz-Frias syndrome (G syndrome), which comprises hypertelorism, cleft lip and palate, laryngeal cleft and hypospadias, and Pallister-Hall syndrome, which consists of congenital hypothalamic hamartoblastoma, hypopituitarism, imperforate anus and post-axial polydactyly, and may include a laryngeal cleft.

As might be expected, symptoms become more severe the longer the cleft. Type I clefts present with cyanotic attacks on feeding and recurrent chest infections. Stridor (similar to that of laryngomalacia) may be a feature secondary to prolapse of the cleft edges into the airway. Type II and III clefts produce dramatic aspiration with recurrent pneumonia, sometimes with stridor and an abnormal cry. Type IV clefts cause severe aspiration, cyanosis and incipient cardiorespiratory failure.

Investigation of the child with aspiration and stridor requires a careful microlaryngoscopy and bronchoscopy, and no other diagnostic method can replace it. Suspension microlaryngoscopy allows the use of two probes to part the arytenoids, and without this manoeuvre the diagnosis may be missed, as redundant mucosa tends to prolapse into the defect and obscure it.

The approach to treatment depends entirely upon the length of the cleft. A short type I cleft with no aspiration requires no treatment. Minimal aspiration may be managed by thickening the feeds. Significant aspiration requires endoscopic repair of the cleft in two layers, using a nasogastric feeding tube until the suture line has healed. A very short type II cleft may also be repaired endoscopically, albeit with difficulty, and using a nasogastric tube. However, a long type II or a type III cleft needs to be approached anteriorly through an extended laryngofissure, with a low tracheotomy to cover the procedure; a nasogastric tube will tend to erode through the suture line, and so a gastrostomy is required (usually combined with a Nissen fundoplication to control reflux reliably). These children take many months to learn to swallow following successful cleft repair and so long-term gastrostomy feeding is necessary. Surgical repair of the cleft is undertaken in three layers in an effort to optimise healing: the two mucosal layers are reinforced by an interposition graft of tibial periosteum or temporalis fascia. The type IV cleft presents an altogether more difficult surgical challenge. Because of the length of the cleft, a tracheotomy is unhelpful in stabilising the airway, and the repair must therefore be undertaken using a single-stage technique with endotracheal extubation taking place 7–10 days post-operatively. Type IV clefts require an anterior cervicothoracic approach via a median sternotomy, with repair on extracorporeal membrane oxygenation. Post-operatively, tracheomalacia may prevent extubation and so a tracheotomy may be needed once the cleft has healed soundly.

Mortality remains significant, being around 14% overall (Evans et al. 1995), rising to 66% for type IV laryngo-tracheo-oesophageal clefts and up to 100% for full-length clefts ending at the carina (Shehab and Bailey 2001). A large part of the mortality is from causes unrelated to the cleft, and notable morbidity is produced by other associated congenital abnormalities and often by delay in reaching the correct diagnosis. Management should be in a major paediatric centre where a full multi-disciplinary team is available with full neonatal and paediatric intensive care facilities.

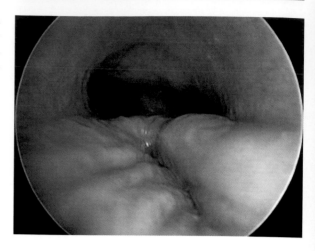

Fig. 22.4 Tracheo-oesophageal fistula seen at bronchoscopy

Trachea and Bronchi

Agenesis

Tracheal agenesis may be complete (full-length) or partial, but in either case there is no continuity between the larynx and the bronchi. Occasionally, short-term survival may be possible if there is a broncho-oesophageal fistula, which can permit some airflow into the lungs, but surgical efforts to use the oesophagus as a tracheal replacement have not been successful and long-term survival has not proved possible. The majority of cases are complicated by other severe congenital abnormalities.

Agenesis of one main bronchus and its associated lung is not as rare as tracheal agenesis and is survivable, although such children often have other coexisting congenital anomalies and are at risk from chest infections because of their much-reduced respiratory reserve. Bilateral bronchial and pulmonary agenesis is extremely rare and is, of course, incompatible with life. Occasionally, localised atresia occurs in a peripheral bronchus, resulting in a distal mucocoele that may need to be resected if it is causing severe compression of the surrounding lung.

Stenosis

This is also discussed in Chapter 26. Bronchial webs may be ruptured with a bronchoscope or by balloon dilatation. Stenosis of a main bronchus is often associated with an adjoining vascular anomaly, and segmental resection with end-to-end anastomosis may be necessary.

Tracheomalacia and Bronchomalacia

These will be discussed in detail in Chapter 27.

Tracheo-Oesophageal Fistula

TOF is a fairly common congenital malformation of the neonatal air and food passages that usually occurs in association with oesophageal atresia. Eighty-seven percent of cases have oesophageal atresia with a TOF communicating between the distal oesophagus and the mid- to lower trachea or a main bronchus. The remainder have oesophageal atresia without a TOF (6%), atresia with a proximal TOF (2%), atresia with a proximal and distal TOF (1%) or a TOF without atresia ("H-type fistula"; 4%). Approximately 50% of infants with a TOF have additional congenital malformations, and 10–20% have tracheomalacia (Spitz 1997).

Children who present to the paediatric otolaryngologist are invariably those with an H-type fistula. Because there is no oesophageal atresia, they are the least symptomatic of the group, with no swallowing difficulty, but small amounts of fluid pass through the fistula into the trachea and produce symptoms and signs of recurrent minor aspiration. The diagnosis is usually established by a barium swallow, but even thin contrast may not pass through a tiny fistula. In such cases, bronchoscopy is required to identify the tracheal opening, which is typically characterised by a V-shaped mucosal fold around it in the posterior wall of the trachea (Fig. 22.4). Usually the fistula is too small to allow passage of a fine spaghetti suction catheter, but methylene blue introduced into the oesophagus will be seen to seep into the trachea at this point. Treatment is by ligation and division of the fistula. This is discussed further in Chapter 30.

Vascular Compression

It is estimated that 3% of the population have an anomaly of the great vessels, but only a few of these have symptomatic airway compression (Smith et al. 1984). Such vascular anomalies are classified into vascular rings, which completely encircle the trachea and oesophagus, and vascular slings, which exert non-circumferential pressure.

Vascular Ring

The commonest vascular ring is a double aortic arch. In this abnormality, the ascending aorta divides into two arches, one of which passes to the right of the trachea and the other to the left, reuniting posterior to the oesophagus to form the descending aorta on the left. The left arch is usually smaller than the right, and the configuration of the main branches is variable, but the result is compression of both the trachea and oesophagus, producing stridor, dyspnoea, dysphagia and a brassy cough.

A less common and less constricting ring is produced when there is a right-sided aortic arch and descending aorta associated with an aberrant left subclavian artery. In this situation the ring is completed by the ligamentum arteriosum, which passes to the left of the trachea, connecting the descending aorta to the pulmonary trunk.

Patients with vascular rings tend to present earlier in life than those with vascular slings and with more severe airway symptoms. A barium swallow is diagnostic, showing a characteristic double impression upon the column of contrast, and an echocardiogram will confirm the anomaly. Surgical treatment is almost always necessary, by dividing the lesser component of the ring, but there is invariably a localised area of tracheomalacia produced by the compression, which may persist for months or even years.

Vascular Sling

The commonest vascular sling is an aberrant innominate artery. The artery arises further to the left and more posteriorly than usual, and crosses the anterior surface of the trachea obliquely just above the carina from the left inferiorly, to the right superiorly.

Cases of vascular sling usually present during the 1st year of life with less severe airway obstruction than that caused by vascular rings. Typically, there is expiratory stridor, cough, recurrent chest infections and sometimes reflex apnoea. The bronchoscopic appearances are diagnostic, with a characteristic sloping, pulsatile compression of the trachea 1–2 cm above the carina, which is most marked on its anterolateral aspect. Upward pressure with the tip of the bronchoscope compresses the artery against the sternum and obliterates the right radial pulse. In severe cases, surgical relief of the obstruction is necessary: this can be achieved either by arteriopexy, in which the vessel is suspended anteriorly from the sternum, or by reimplanting it further to the right on the aortic arch.

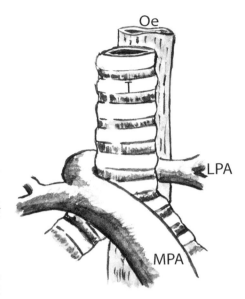

Fig. 22.5 Diagram of a pulmonary artery sling. *LPA* Left pulmonary artery, *MPA* main pulmonary artery, *Oe* oesophagus, *T* trachea

A "pulmonary artery sling" is produced by an anomalous left pulmonary artery, which arises on the right and passes between the trachea and oesophagus, compressing both (Fig. 22.5). This may be associated with lower-end tracheal stenosis, which sometimes also involves the carina and right main bronchus. Surgical reanastomosis may be needed to relieve the compression.

Enlargement of the pulmonary artery in association with a cardiac defect can also produce compression of the distal trachea and its bifurcation. An aberrant right or, more rarely, left subclavian artery passing posterior to the oesophagus will compress the oesophagus alone, and so produces dysphagia but no stridor.

Anomalous Bifurcations

The right upper lobe bronchus may take origin from the right lateral wall of the trachea above the carina, and is then often termed a "pig bronchus", or "bronchi suis". It is usually an asymptomatic, incidental finding, but may sometimes be associated with tracheal stenosis. Minor alterations to the distal bronchial branching pattern are not unusual and likewise do not usually cause problems.

Congenital Cysts and Tumours

Tracheogenic and bronchogenic cysts are thought to originate from evaginations of the primitive tracheal bud, and are sometimes termed reduplication anomalies. They may occur anywhere along the tracheobronchial tree. They are lined with respiratory epithelium, filled with mucus, and their walls may contain any elements of the normal tracheobronchial wall. Bronchogenic cysts may communicate with the airway.

Some patients are symptom-free, but large cysts or those that become infected cause non-pulsatile compression of the airway and present with symptoms, signs and endoscopic appearances otherwise similar to those produced by vascular compression (see above). Computed tomography (CT) or magnetic resonance imaging (MRI) will demonstrate the lesion clearly, and treatment is by thoracotomy and surgical excision.

Thymomas or teratomas may produce airway compression in the neck or mediastinum. CT or MRI is needed to define the size and situation of the mass prior to surgical excision. This is discussed in more detail in Chapter 12.

Summary for the Clinician

- Endoscopy to diagnose many of these conditions is dependent upon skilled paediatric anaesthesia. Management of congenital disorders of the larynx, trachea and bronchi requires the multidisciplinary resources of a major children's centre.

References

1. April MM, Rebeiz E, Friedman EM, et al (1992) Laser surgery for lymphatic malformations of the upper aerodigestive tract. An evolving experience. Arch Otolaryngol Head Neck Surg 118:205–208

2. Benjamin B, Inglis A (1989) Minor congenital laryngeal clefts: diagnosis and classification. Ann Otol Rhinol Laryngol 98:417–420

3. Bower CM, Choi SS, Cotton RT (1994) Arytenoidectomy in children. Ann Otol Rhinol Laryngol 103:271–278

4. Cotton RT (1978) Management of subglottic stenosis in infancy and childhood. Review of a consecutive series of cases managed by surgical reconstruction. Ann Otol Rhinol Laryngol 87:649–657

5. Cotton RT, Gray SD, Miller RP (1989) Update of the Cincinnati experience in pediatric laryngotracheal reconstruction. Laryngoscope 99:1111–1116

6. Cotton RT, Prescott CAJ (1999) Congenital anomalies of the larynx. In: Cotton RT, Myer CM (eds) Practical Pediatric Otolaryngology. Lippincott-Raven, Philadelphia, pp 497–513

7. Daya H, Hosni A, Bejar-Solar I, et al (2000) Pediatric vocal fold paralysis – a long-term retrospective study. Arch Otolaryngol Head Neck Surg 126:21–25

8. Evans JNG, Todd GB (1974) Laryngotracheoplasty. J Laryngol Otol 87:589–597

9. Evans KL, Courtney-Harris R, Bailey CM, et al (1995) Management of posterior laryngeal and laryngotracheoesophageal clefts. Arch Otolaryngol Head Neck Surg 121:1380–1385

10. Holinger LD (1999) Histopathology of congenital subglottic stenosis. Ann Otol Rhinol Laryngol 108:101–111

11. Jani P, Koltai P, Ochi JW, Bailey CM (1991) Surgical treatment of laryngomalacia. J Laryngol Otol 105:1040–1045

12. Lane RW, Weider DJ, Steinem C, et al (1984) Laryngomalacia: a review and case report of surgical treatment with resolution of pectus excavatum. Arch Otolaryngol 110:546–551

13. Monnier P, Lang F, Savary M (2001) Traitement des sténoses sous-glottiques de l'enfant par résection crico-trachéale: expérience lausannoise dans 58 cas. Ann Otolaryngol Chir Cervicofac 118:299–305

14. Monnier P, Savary M, Chapuis G (1993) Partial cricoid resection with primary tracheal anastomosis for subglottic stenosis in infants and children. Laryngoscope 103:1273–1283

15. Ndiaye I, Van den Abbeele T, Francois M, et al (1999) Traitement chirurgical des sténoses laryngées de l'enfant. Ann Otolaryngol Chir Cervicofac 116:143–148

16. Ochi JW, Evans JNG, Bailey CM (1992) Pediatric airway reconstruction at Great Ormond Street: a ten-year review, I: laryngotracheoplasty and laryngotracheal reconstruction. Ann Otolo Rhinol Laryngol 101:465–468

17. Rutter MJ, Hartley BEJ, Cotton RT (2001) Cricotracheal resection in children. Arch Otolaryngol Head Neck Surg 127:289–292

18. Shehab ZP, Bailey CM (2001) Type IV laryngotracheoesophageal clefts – recent 5 year experience at Great Ormond Street Hospital for Children. Int J Pediatr Otorhinolaryngol 60:1–9

19. Shugar MA, Healy GB (1980) Coexistent lesions of the pediatric airway. Int J Pediatr Otorhinolaryngol 2:323–327

20. Smith RJ, Smith MC, Glossop LP, et al (1984) Congenital vascular anomalies causing tracheoesophageal compression. Arch Otolaryngol Head Neck Surg 110:82–87

21. Spitz L (1997) Diseases of the oesophagus. In: Kerr AG (ed) Scott-Brown's Otolaryngology. Butterworth-Heinemann, Oxford, pp 1–21

22. Toynton SC, Saunders MW, Bailey CM (2001) Aryepiglottoplasty for laryngomalacia: 100 consecutive cases. J Laryngol Otol 115:35–38

23. Van den Broek P, Brinkman WFB (1979) Congenital laryngeal defects. Int J Pediatr Otorhinolaryngol 1:71–78

22

Chapter 23

Acquired Disorders of the Larynx in Children

23

Neville P. Shine and Christopher Prescott

Core Messages

- If a child develops symptoms that suggest acquired laryngeal disease, it is imperative to make a rapid definitive diagnosis and to begin management with the minimum of delay.
- Infections include laryngitis (both viral and bacterial) and more "specific" infection such as herpes, tuberculosis, candidiasis and diphtheria, as well as laryngotracheobronchitis and the less common supraglottitis/epiglottitis.
- Gastro-oesophageal reflux is an increasingly recognised problem in children. It may produce laryngeal inflammation and oedema as well as the respiratory complications of aspiration.
- Laryngeal trauma can be either external or internal. The latter includes both corrosive ingestion or steam/flame inhalation as well as intubation trauma and its consequences.
- Vocal abuse can be regarded as laryngeal trauma.
- Foreign body ingestion/inhalation should always be considered, particularly in the younger child.
- Recurrent laryngeal nerve palsy is often a difficult diagnosis to make in a child.
- As far as tumours are concerned, recurrent respiratory papillomatosis is the most common, but other benign and malignant tumours do occur in the paediatric larynx.
- The debate concerning tracheotomy vs. tracheostomy continues, but whichever technique is adopted, the outcome for the child is determined by the quality of care for both the stoma and the tube.

Contents

Infections

Laryngitis

Laryngitis is an inflammatory process affecting the larynx. Acute infective laryngitis is the most frequent form of laryngitis seen in clinical practice in the primary care setting. In children it is usually associated with an upper respiratory tract infection. The vast majority of cases are of viral aetiology, the usual causative agents being rhinovirus, adenovirus, parainfluenza virus or respiratory syncytial virus. Rarely nowadays, since the introduction of widespread vaccination, laryngitis may also occur during the course of measles and *Bordetella pertussis* infection. Most cases are relatively benign and self-limiting, resolving spontaneously with only supportive treatment necessary. Occasionally, a child is referred with persistent hoarseness after a typical sounding episode of laryngitis, and then flexible laryngoscopy is required to exclude any other pathology. In the absence of such pathology, the usual finding is of some persistent oedema of the laryngeal mucosa, particularly of the vocal cords. This will generally settle over time.

Laryngotracheobronchitis (Croup)

This is a common childhood illness that most frequently occurs between the ages of 6 months and 5 years, with a peak at 2 years (Fig. 23.1). Presentation at less than 6 months or older than 5 years is uncommon and warrants a high index of suspicion of underlying laryngeal or tracheal abnormalities or pathology, for example subglottic haemangioma and congenital or acquired subglottic stenosis.

The most common pathogen is parainfluenza virus with types I–III accounting for 75% of cases. Respiratory syncytial and influenza viruses are commonly implicated in the remaining cases. The resulting inflammatory, soft-tissue oedema and induration affects predominantly the subglottis, although, as the name suggests, the larynx, trachea and bronchi can all be affected. The subglottis is the narrowest part of the paediatric airway and progressive oedema at this site results in stridor and airway obstruction. The disease follows a course of 5–7 days, beginning with an upper respiratory tract infection phase, which is followed by the development of the classical "croupy" cough (characteristically "barking" in nature) and the on-

set of stridor. Often these symptoms are worse at night and it is not unusual for these children to present to the emergency department in the early hours of the morning. The clinical diagnosis is relatively straightforward, but if an anterior–posterior soft-tissue x-ray of the neck is obtained, the classical "steeple sign" of subglottic narrowing will be seen (Fig. 23.2).

In the acute presentation of the disease, the adequacy of the airway is the crucial concern. Most cases can be managed by the administration of oral dexamethasone, followed by a period of observation with humidified air, a calm nursing environment and supportive hydration. Often these cases can be managed in the emergency department and following the above treatment can be safely discharged home. Occasionally, other measures are necessary in cases of progressive airway obstruction or non-resolving obstruction with a tiring child. Nebulised racemic adrenaline in oxygen is frequently used in such cases and, although the efficacy of such treatment has not been proven, it is the authors' experience that such treatment may spare some children invasive airway intervention.

Airway obstruction is best assessed clinically by the characteristics of the stridor as illustrated in (Fig. 23.3). The one danger of this method is that in Grade 4 there may be so much limitation of airflow that a stridulous sound cannot be produced. The usefulness of this grading system (which should only be applied to croup) is that it translates into appropriate management:

1. Grades 1–2: Nebulised adrenaline inhalations together with systemic steroids.
2. Persistent grade 3: If nebulised adrenaline inhalations do not cause regression to grade 2 and if the child is

23

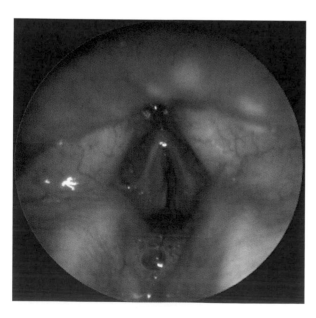

Fig. 23.1 Acute laryngotracheobronchitis (croup)

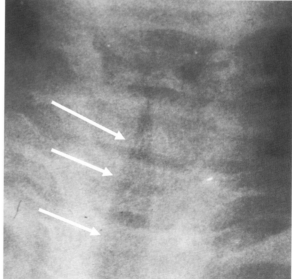

Fig. 23.2 Anterior–posterior neck x-ray in croup demonstrating the "steeple sign" (*white arrows*)

becoming exhausted from the effort to breathe, then airway intervention, intubation or tracheotomy, is required.

3. Grade 4: An emergency situation requiring airway intervention.

Airway intervention is usually by intubation. The size of endotracheal tube selected should be one whole size smaller than anticipated for the age and size of the child (half a size smaller for infants up to 6 months). Ideally, the intubation should be done under controlled circumstances – general anaesthetic is preferable – and the opportunity taken to view and assess the larynx. Typically, the laryngeal mucosa is not particularly inflamed and the most notable feature is the manner in which the vocal cords blend into the immediate subglottic soft-tissue induration. The endotracheal tube should be felt to "slide in easily". If it does not, it is best to avoid trying to force the tube through the narrowed segment, so an even smaller tube should be tried. The appropriate size of tube cannot be judged from the presence of a "leak" past the tube, since the oedema closes up all the spaces around it. Tracheotomy is indicated if the only tube that will "slide in easily" is too small for the child's ventilatory requirements or is likely to block up with secretions.

Once airway intervention has become necessary, intubation is usually required for several days. Extubation may be possible even before a leak can be demonstrated around the tube. If intubation is prolonged beyond 3–4 days, then laryngoscopy should be repeated. The main reason for this is to check that there is no intubation trauma (see below). If the mucosa remains intact but the airway is still inadequate, then intubation with the same-size tube can be repeated. If, however, the mucosa is ulcerated in the tube contact areas and the airway is inadequate, then a tracheotomy should be considered. This is mandatory if the ulceration is circumferential, particularly within the cricoid ring.

Bacterial Laryngitis/Tracheitis

Bacterial laryngitis and tracheitis is uncommon (Fig. 23.4). In general, these children present with a shorter history of stridor and a deteriorating airway than with viral laryngotracheobronchitis, are more pyrexial and are more systemically unwell. The commonest offending pathogen is *Staphylococcus aureus*.

The priority of treatment is the securing of a compromised or potentially imperilled airway, and airway intervention is usually required. This should be undertaken preferably under general anaesthetic in the operating theatre. Laryngotracheobronchoscopy can then be performed to confirm the clinical diagnosis and obtain specimens for bacterial culture and antibiotic sensitivity. The laryngeal mucosa will be seen to be far more inflamed than in viral laryngotracheobronchitis and the tracheal secretions to be more purulent and tenacious. Tracheotomy may need to be considered in preference to intubation in order to facilitate aspiration of these tenacious, obstructing secretions. Appropriate intravenous antibiotic should be administered. Humidification and frequent aspiration of the tenacious secretions is essential to maintain the patency of the tube. The infection should

LARYNGO-TRACHEO-BRONCHITIS

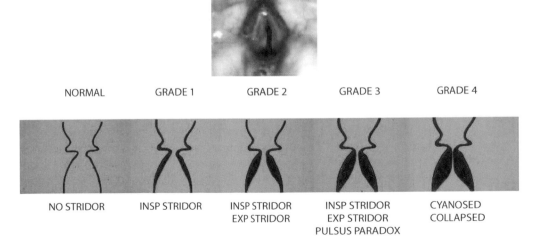

Fig. 23.3 Croup grading system. *INSP* Inspiratory, *EXP* expiratory

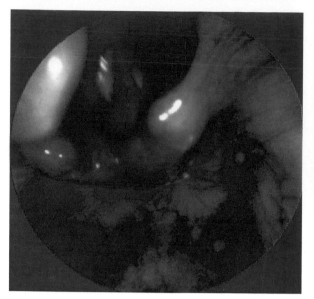

Fig. 23.4 Bacterial laryngitis

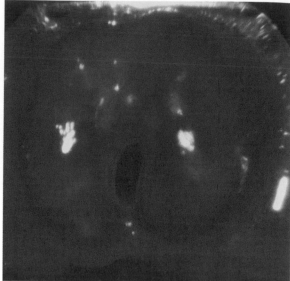

Fig. 23.5 Supraglottitis (epiglottitis)

gradually resolve over 4–5 days, after which, extubation can be attempted.

Supraglottitis (Epiglottitis)

Classically this condition resulted from acute *Haemophilus influenzae* infection of the supraglottic soft tissues around the laryngeal inlet (Fig. 23.5), but the incidence of typical cases is rapidly declining as the use of *Haemophilus* vaccination becomes more widespread. It can still occur in unvaccinated children or vaccine failures, and an increasing number of cases resulting from infection by other bacteria and viruses are being seen.

Supraglottitis is a condition that tends to affect older children than croup – the peak incidence is in the 2- to 4-year-old age group – and the presentation is more dramatic. Usually this is a "toxic" child with rapid onset of sore throat, dysphagia, stridor and airway obstruction. The child often adopts a "sniffing the morning air position" in an attempt to maintain an airway. The danger is the rapid progression of inflammatory swelling to the point of potentially fatal, near-total or total airway obstruction. Usually by the time these children arrive in the Emergency Unit, the situation is critical and, if considered, the diagnosis is obvious. If there is doubt and a lateral neck x-ray is taken (with an appropriate clinician in attendance at all times, prepared for emergency intubation), the shadow of the swollen epiglottis will be seen, the classical "thumbprint sign". It is imperative that definitive management of a precarious airway should not be delayed by the acquisition of x-rays.

Nebulised racemic adrenaline inhalations in oxygen should be commenced, but airway intervention is usually required. Prior to this, no manoeuvres provoking an acute obstruction of the precipitous airway, such as taking blood or examination of the upper aerodigestive tract, should be undertaken. The services of a skilled anaesthetist should be employed for laryngoscopy and intubation under general anaesthetic. Classically, the diagnosis is made from the "cherry red", grossly swollen appearance of the epiglottis seen with *H. influenzae*, infection but this is not always the case when other bacteria/viruses are implicated. An endotracheal tube can usually be passed, since the inflammatory swelling affects predominantly the supraglottic tissues of the laryngeal inlet. Appropriate intravenous antibiotics should be administered and the condition usually settles sufficiently to permit extubation after 2–3 days. Laryngoscopy prior to this confirms resolution of the supraglottic oedema permitting safe extubation.

Unusual Laryngeal Infections

Herpetic Laryngitis

Although uncommon, several case reports have documented infection of the larynx by herpes simplex virus (Figs. 23.6 and 23.7). It occurs in both immunocompetent and immunocompromised children. The presence of ulcerative gingivostomatitis with symptoms similar to acute epiglottitis or croup suggests the possibility of herpetic disease. At laryngoscopy, sloughing ulcers will be

23

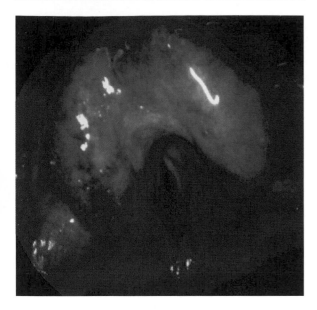

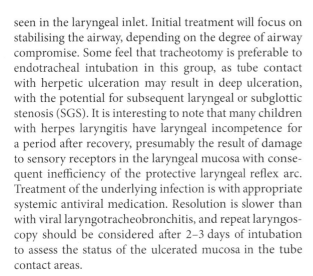

Fig. 23.6 Herpes supraglottitis

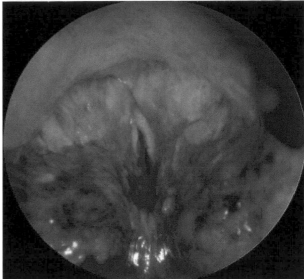

Fig. 23.7 Herpes laryngitis

seen in the laryngeal inlet. Initial treatment will focus on stabilising the airway, depending on the degree of airway compromise. Some feel that tracheotomy is preferable to endotracheal intubation in this group, as tube contact with herpetic ulceration may result in deep ulceration, with the potential for subsequent laryngeal or subglottic stenosis (SGS). It is interesting to note that many children with herpes laryngitis have laryngeal incompetence for a period after recovery, presumably the result of damage to sensory receptors in the laryngeal mucosa with consequent inefficiency of the protective laryngeal reflex arc. Treatment of the underlying infection is with appropriate systemic antiviral medication. Resolution is slower than with viral laryngotracheobronchitis, and repeat laryngoscopy should be considered after 2–3 days of intubation to assess the status of the ulcerated mucosa in the tube contact areas.

Candidiasis

As the worldwide human immunodeficiency virus (HIV) pandemic continues and an increasing number of infected infants and children are being seen, there is an increasing incidence of unusual laryngeal infections in affected children, of which the commonest is that caused by *Candida albicans*. Laryngeal candidiasis can be deduced in an HIV-positive infant or child with stridor who has been noted to have oral thrush. A combination of topical and systemic antifungal agents should be used, but resolution is slow. Laryngoscopy may be required for diagnosis when there is persistent stridor or deterioration in the

airway. This is undertaken preferably under anaesthetic with appropriate precautions, and biopsy specimens can then be taken. An initial period of intubation can be considered when airway intervention is required, but many of these children will require tracheotomy because of slow resolution.

Tuberculosis

Tuberculous (TB) laryngitis, caused by infection with *Mycobacterium tuberculosis*, is also occasionally seen in particularly endemic areas such as the Indian subcontinent and sub-Saharan Africa, usually, but not always, coexistent with active pulmonary TB. Whilst rare in children, this disease is once more on the rise, inextricably linked to the HIV pandemic. Symptoms are variable but may include hoarseness, stridor and airway obstruction (Fig. 23.8). Diagnosis may be suggested by typical chest radiology appearances of tuberculosis with concurrent granulomatous or inflammatory disease of the larynx; however, laryngeal TB may occur without any obvious evidence of pulmonary disease. Diagnostic confirmation may be achieved by identifying the presence of acid-fast bacilli in sputum, gastric washings or from biopsy of laryngeal tissue. Sputum culture may require several weeks and rapid polymerase chain reaction testing may give false negative results. Therefore, if the clinician has a high index of suspicion, multiple or repeat specimens may be required to ascertain the diagnosis.

As treatment is primarily medical, of prolonged duration and with slow resolution, those cases with significant

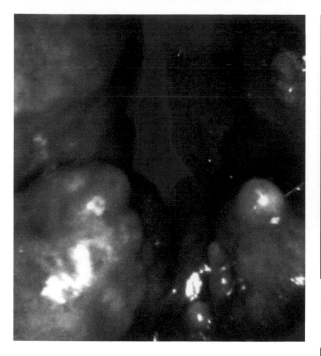

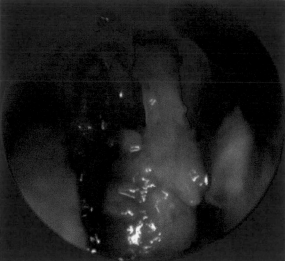

Fig. 23.9 Diphtheria affecting the larynx

Fig. 23.8 Tuberculous laryngitis

airway obstruction must be considered for tracheotomy. Medical treatment is as for the pulmonary form of the disease, guided by local infectious disease guidelines.

The presence of an atypical laryngeal infection such as TB or candidiasis mandates further investigation regarding immune status, including testing for HIV.

The slow resolution of these unusual laryngeal infections can be anticipated, and it may be several months, even on appropriate treatment, before there is sufficient resolution to permit decannulation.

Gastro-Oesophageal Reflux Disease – Laryngeal Manifestations

This topic is also discussed in Chapter 30. Gastric content reflux has the potential to cause inflammatory change in the mucosa throughout the upper aero-digestive tract and, when aspirated, in the lower respiratory system, and is being increasingly implicated, with good evidence, in many ENT disorders. In the paediatric larynx, reflux manifests primarily with inflammatory oedema, particularly located posteriorly (Fig. 23.10), and secondarily in prolonged healing after surgical procedures.

When suspected, investigations include barium swallow, radiolabelled milk scan, identification of fat-laden

Diphtheria

Diphtheria still occurs, usually in areas where immunisation is incomplete or where "vaccine chain" control measures have failed, so that the vaccine has denatured and become ineffective. It should be suspected at laryngoscopy when inflammation is associated with a sloughing membrane, and appropriate specimens should be taken for microbiological examination (Fig. 23.9). Tracheotomy is the preferred method of airway intervention when this is required. The causative organism – *Corynebacterium diphtheria* – is penicillin sensitive and this should be administered for 14 days. The outcome depends not only on maintaining the airway, but also on the cardiac and neurological toxins produced by the bacteria. Antitoxin should be administered, but unfortunately, these days, is difficult to obtain.

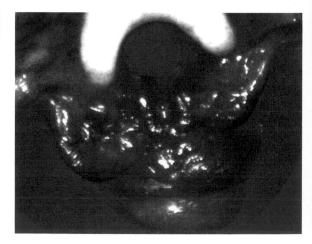

Fig. 23.10 Posterior inflammatory oedema

macrophages in sputum or tracheal aspirate specimens and oesophageal pH monitoring, currently the "gold standard". However, demonstration of significant reflux has to be correlated with the clinical picture before considering treatment, since in a significant proportion of children, particularly infants, reflux is a common occurrence without causing apparent disease/disorder.

Paediatric laryngeal disorders in which reflux can be implicated as a causative/aggravating factor include laryngomalacia, laryngitis, laryngotracheobronchitis and, more recently, respiratory tract papillomatosis.

In laryngomalacia, the majority of those infants whose condition is not severe enough to require intervention, gradually improve over time. However, some experience periods of deterioration with onset of significant obstruction. Although this is usually associated with a respiratory tract infection, the possibility of reflux-induced oedema of the prolapsing posterior soft tissues must be considered and often, when this is identified, such cases respond to antireflux medication and avoid the need for intervention. Infants with the more severe degrees of laryngomalacia who require intervention often have apparent swallowing disorders and, if investigated, many will be found to have reflux. Whether this is due to an associated motility problem or due to the increased negative intrathoracic pressures generated during obstructed inspiration is unclear. Most improve after surgical intervention (supraglottic trimming/supraglottoplasty), but treatment for reflux may need to be considered.

Laryngitis and laryngotracheobronchitis in children are usually associated with a respiratory tract infection. When they become a recurrent problem, the possibility of reflux as the cause or as an exacerbating factor needs to be considered and investigated and, if identified, should be treated. Current recommendation is for a 3-month course of treatment with a proton-pump inhibitor, followed by a period of "watchful waiting" to determine whether or not there is regression to symptomatic effects that may then require a further period of treatment or surgical antireflux intervention.

The possibility of a link between reflux and recurrent respiratory papillomatosis is discussed in Chapter 29. It is certainly something that should be considered in older children with the disease, and treated if identified.

Prior to undertaking any open surgery to the larynx in children, investigation to exclude reflux should be considered. Since most such children have a tracheotomy, a simple, useful method is to test the tracheal aspirate with litmus, identification of any acidity confirming reflux with aspiration. Identified reflux should be controlled prior to surgery and treatment maintained until well after healing, as experience has been that delayed healing due to inflammatory induration and granulation tissue formation is usually associated with reflux and aspiration.

Laryngeal Trauma

External Trauma

The paediatric larynx is well protected from blunt traumatic injury by its high position in the neck, the protection afforded by the mandible and sternum, and its relative elasticity. Where blunt trauma does occur, fractures are uncommon but shearing of the endolaryngeal mucosa from the pliant laryngeal cartilage can cause significant oedema or haematoma formation, with potentially life-threatening respiratory embarrassment (Fig. 23.11). Other injuries that may occur include recurrent laryngeal nerve (RLN) injuries (unilateral or bilateral), arytenoid cartilage dislocations or laryngotracheal separation.

Typical mechanisms of injury seen are "clothesline" injuries sustained during sporting activities, following a motor accident or from accidental or intentional hanging. When the described mode of injury is incongruous with the clinical findings or bruising consistent with strangulation is noted, the possibility of nonaccidental injury should also be entertained.

Massive disruption of the airway following significant trauma to the neck may result in death prior to the arrival of emergency services or transfer to the hospital setting. In less severe cases, the patient may arrive in the emergency department with variable symptoms. Dysphonia/aphonia, stridor, respiratory distress and drooling in a patient known to have sustained blunt trauma to the neck should be managed with a high index of suspicion for an impending airway problem. The presence of neck bruising, haematoma, neck tenderness, and crepitus all suggest a potential laryngeal injury.

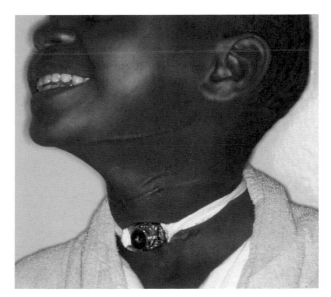

Fig. 23.11 External laryngeal trauma

The mode of injury must be ascertained as the possibility of associated traumatic pathology affecting the cervical spine, chest and pelvis must be considered and initial management should be in keeping with the Advanced Trauma Life Support (ATLS) guidelines.

Where necessary, the airway should be secured by means of endotracheal intubation or tracheotomy. If the cervical spine has not been cleared of pathology due to the severity of the patient's condition, then a cervical spine injury should be presumed and in-line traction used during intubation. Once the endangered airway has been secured, ventilation must be optimised and management of associated injuries such as pneumothoraces must be undertaken. Haemodynamic resuscitation should be instituted as necessary. Associated injuries to the great vessels in the neck must be considered and investigated as appropriate.

Once the overall condition has been stabilised, direct laryngoscopy and pharyngo-oesophagoscopy must be carefully performed with the patient under general anaesthetic. This evaluation regarding the nature and extent of injury will help decide the need and approach for definitive surgical intervention. Further valuable information regarding the cartilage underlying the endolaryngeal mucosa can be gained by computed tomography (CT) scans of the larynx. Table 23.1 shows the classification of laryngeal injuries formulated by Schaeffer (1992).

Definitive treatment of the disrupted larynx should be undertaken with a view to restoring the anatomical and functional integrity of the organ, reducing fractures and dislocations, debriding devitalised tissue and exposed cartilage, and restoring the mucosal integrity.

Mild injuries, grades 1 and 2, may require no more than observation and medical treatment consisting of upright nursing (to reduce soft-tissue oedema), steroids and antibiotic cover to prevent supervening infection. More severe injuries will require tracheotomy, if not already performed at acute presentation, and open surgical exploration by means of laryngofissure. Stenting may be required with anterior commissure involvement, multiple displaced fractures or multiple severe lacerations. These

serve to maintain the shape of the repaired larynx, stabilise the repair and reduced tissues and fractures, and help prevent stenosis. Surgery should be complemented by appropriate adjuvant medical therapy including steroids to minimise oedema, antibiotics to prevent chondritis, and proton-pump inhibitors to prevent acid reflux in the vicinity of the laryngeal tissues.

Internal Trauma

Inhalation Burns

All children with significant burns of the head and neck should be suspected of having sustained inhalation burns should their voice change or stridor develop, at which time laryngoscopy should be performed – by flexible laryngoscopy, unless an anaesthetic is planned to manage the burn injuries (Fig. 23.12). As in all potential airway injuries, regardless of aetiology, assessment by flexible endoscopy should proceed with caution lest it exacerbate any respiratory embarrassment. Appropriate facilities for securing an emergency airway should be readily available.

Minor laryngeal burns with mucosal oedema can be managed with nebulised racemic adrenaline. More severe burns with airway compromise require laryngoscopy under anaesthetic to assess the larynx to determine whether intubation is an appropriate method of airway intervention or whether a tracheotomy would be preferable. In flame burns, bronchoscopy should be performed in addition to laryngoscopy, the presence of carbon particles in the trachea indicating the likelihood of lower airway involvement and anticipated pulmonary complications. Intubation is appropriate when the ulcerating burns do not involve the tube contact areas of the larynx; other-

Table 23.1 Classification of laryngeal injury

Grade	Injury
Grade 1	Mild laryngeal oedema, no fracture
Grade 2	Laryngeal oedema with associated mucosal disruption, no exposed cartilage, fracture thyroid cartilage (not displaced)
Grade 3	Massive laryngeal oedema, displaced fracture thyroid cartilage, fixed cord
Grade 4	As for grade 3 with 2 or more fracture lines

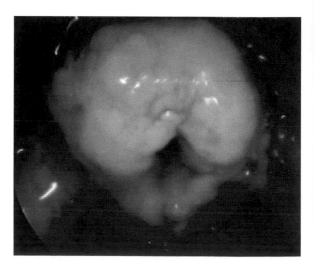

Fig. 23.12 Steam inhalation burns of the larynx

wise tracheotomy is the preferred option. The difficulty arises when there are both extensive internal laryngeal burns and significant burns anteriorly in the neck, posing potential problems for any tracheotomy. The risks of intubation injury exacerbating the burn injury have to be considered and an appropriate plan of management worked out with the burn management team.

Corrosive Ingestion

Chemical burns arise from ingestion of corrosive chemicals, in either granular or liquid form. Typically, the corrosive ingested is alkaline (60–80% of cases), for example caustic soda or "lye water" (a solution of potassium hydroxide made from wood ash and rain water, used in developing countries in food preparation and for making soap). Other noxious substances may be acid, for example pool or battery acid, or industrial-strength bleach. The corrosive will act upon all tissues with which it comes into contact and, following ingestion, areas of injury can include the oral cavity, pharynx, oesophagus and larynx. When corrosive agents are ingested, hold-up at the cricopharyngeal sphincter may result in spill over into the laryngeal inlet. The laryngeal protective reflexes usually limit consequent burns to the supraglottic structures, but subsequent inflammation may result in airway compromise (Fig. 23.13).

Any suggestion of corrosive ingestion in a child must be treated seriously, the history from the caregiver being crucial. Important elements include the type of corrosive (if known), the amount ingested and any subsequent vomiting, as this causes a repeat exposure to the noxious agent. If possible, try to obtain the bottle containing the offending corrosive as this allows for accurate identifica-

tion of the type and concentration of agent involved. Unfortunately, in some cases, the corrosive has been placed in a soft drinks bottle, which has led to the accidental ingestion. In these cases, pH testing can assist in identification of an acid or alkali corrosive. In addition, the local Poisons Centre should be contacted for further advice.

The priority concern on initial presentation to the trauma unit is for the patient's airway since this can be compromised by swelling of the tongue, pharyngeal soft tissues and the larynx. Such swelling may progress over several hours following the initial ingestion so an initial reassuring examination must not lull the clinician into a false sense of security. Stertor, "hot potato" voice, drooling, stridor and dysphonia are ominous signs.

In cases of significant laryngeal injury where airway intervention is required, early tracheotomy is preferable as resolution may take several weeks and endotracheal intubation may prolong the inflammation associated with the burn injury. Although no firm evidence exists supporting the use of adjunctive medical treatment, many consider the use of steroids, antibiotics and proton-pump inhibitors to be of benefit in these cases. Laryngoscopic evaluation at 2- to 3-week intervals is required to assess resolution. Superficial burns usually heal with return to normal anatomy with a normal voice; however, disruption of sensory receptors in the laryngeal mucosa may compromise the laryngeal protective reflex arc, resulting in a period of laryngeal incompetence. Deep burns usually result in necrosis, with loss of varying amounts of supraglottic tissues, and disruption of the anatomy is compounded by fibrosis and contracture with later healing, and the outcome for the voice and the airway can only be assessed with the passage of time. Corrosive injury to the pharynx and oesophagus is more common than laryngeal damage, but outside the scope of this chapter.

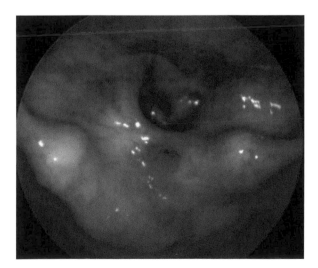

Fig. 23.13 Laryngeal stenosis following healing after corrosive ingestion

Intubation Injury

This topic is also discussed in Chapter 25. Endotracheal intubation, even in skilled hands, can potentially traumatise the endolaryngeal mucosa either directly by injury or indirectly from subsequent pressure necrosis (Fig. 23.14). In the majority of cases this does not result in any deleterious clinical sequelae, but in some children, a sequence of events is initiated at intubation, progresses through mucosal ulceration and underlying chondritis and culminates in healing by fibrosis with contracture. The cricoid ring, the narrowest portion of the paediatric airway, is the most significant site for injury, since subsequent subglottic stenosis (SGS) may occur here. Several factors predispose certain intubated paediatric patients to this iatrogenic insult, not least the presence of an endotracheal tube that is of an inappropriate size. It is the size of the endotracheal tube relative to the patient's airway that determines its appropriateness.

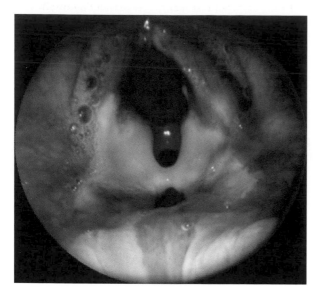

Fig. 23.14 Intubation trauma – fibrin deposits and adhesion bands

Unsurprisingly, such injuries are seen most frequently in neonates (see Chapter 25 post-intubation laryngotracheal stenosis). A suitably sized tube is one that exerts no pressure on the laryngeal mucosa at the tube contact sites. An inappropriately sized tube is one that compresses the mucosa against the laryngeal skeleton at the tube contact sites, interrupts its blood perfusion and results in varying depths of necrosis and ulceration at these sites. Prolonged intubation and excessive tube movement may also contribute to such a situation. The onset of this process can be rapid, especially in low-perfusion-pressure situations such as shock or cardiac surgery, and in such cases, necrotic ulceration can occur after even a few hours of intubation (Gould and Howard 1985; Gould 1988). The main focus of the clinician managing the intubated paediatric patient should be the avoidance of such injuries.

Anaesthetists tend to rely on the presence of a "leak" past the tube to judge when an endotracheal tube is of an appropriate size (see "Croup" above for an example of an exception to this). However, not all of them remember, when a period of post-operative intubation is required, to downsize the tube at the end of a surgical procedure during which they have required a tighter fit for the purpose of ventilation. An intubated child needs to have the "leak" assessed on a daily basis because one of the earliest indications of tube injury problems is swelling, with consequent loss of that leak. Downsizing of the tube is then indicated to prevent progression of injury. This daily assessment is especially important when the details of the intubation are unknown (e.g. emergency intubation in trauma or collapse situations), because it is frequently in such patients that subsequent problems arise. It is also important in "poor perfusion" situations such as, for example, cardiac surgery, severe infections and shock.

Once the process of intubation injury starts, the longer the inappropriate tube remains in place, the worse the depth of necrosis that will occur and the worse the extent of granulation tissue that will form in the consequent ulceration, which in turn translates into more fibrosis and more subsequent contracture. Depending on local circumstances, guidelines for timing of laryngoscopy after intubation need to be developed. A reasonable guideline would be within 24 h if a "leak" has never been present (exception – croup) or within 24 h after loss of the "leak" if it is not restored when the tube is downsized.

Identification of necrosis and ulceration means that serious consideration has to be given to tracheotomy, especially when the necrosis or ulceration is circumferential in the cricoid ring. Parenteral antibiotics should be administered to combat any superinfection within the cartilage, and proton-pump inhibitors considered to obviate the risk of acid reflux exacerbating the inflammatory process. The role of systemic steroids in reducing granulations and minimising incipient organisation of fibrotic tissue is not proven, but it is advocated by several authors. More recently, application of mitomycin C (a cytotoxic agent said to have action against fibroblasts and therefore the potential to inhibit the fibrotic process) to the ulcerated or granulating subglottic tissue has shown promise in preventing subsequent stenosis.

Once injury has occurred, resolution is generally protracted and the final outcome for the airway and the voice will depend on the depth of necrosis, the extent of granulation tissue formation, the degree of fibrosis resulting from this and the extent to which it contracts. Laryngoscopy at 2- to 3-week intervals is required to assess progress. If it becomes apparent that an SGS is developing, particularly if it appears to be complete, dilatation and further application of mitomycin C should be considered in an attempt to limit the final stricture, as the outcome of any subsequent surgery relates to the degree of stenosis.

Established SGS has been graded by Cotton as:
1. Grade 1: less than or equal to 50% of the subglottic lumen.
2. Grade II: between 51% and 70% of the subglottic lumen.
3. Grade III: between 71% and 99% of the subglottic lumen.
4. Grade IV: no detectable lumen.
For a diagram of the Cotton grades see Chapter 25.

The goal of treatment of SGS is to establish a safe airway with good voice. The approach taken to the management depends not only on factors such as the age of the patient, the aetiology, the age and maturation of the stenosis and its grade, but also, importantly on the patient's general condition.

23

Early in the course of neonatal SGS, an anterior cricoid split procedure may avoid the need for tracheotomy and upper airway reconstruction. In this procedure, the cricoid is incised with a vertical incision extending superiorly into the inferior half of the thyroid cartilage and inferiorly through the upper tracheal ring, to release the stenosed cricoid ring. The infant is kept intubated for at least 1 week before attempting extubation to allow healing of the splinted airway, and steroids are given prior to extubation to minimise oedema and optimise the potential for success. Infants who develop respiratory distress post-extubation require endoscopic evaluation under general anaesthesia. Exuberant granulation tissue may require debulking, and dilatation may be beneficial. If these measures do not resolve the problem, a further period of intubation should be tried before resorting to tracheotomy.

Thereafter, adopting a "wait and see" approach as the child grows may result in sufficient growth of the lumen of the stenotic segment to permit decannulation, thus avoiding the need for an open procedure. Some would advocate lasering of stenosing granulation tissue to diminish the severity of the ultimate stricture in cases that are identified early, when scar tissue is not fully organised. Over-aggressive use of the laser must be avoided as it may provoke deep scarring and a worsening of the stenosis.

When these measures fail, open surgery may be required. The principle of these techniques is to incise the strictured cricoid, releasing the stricture anteriorly, adding posterior and even lateral incisions in more severe cases to achieve further release. Autologous interposition cartilage grafts are placed to complete the augmentation procedure, which is then stented either by an endotracheal tube (single-stage procedure) or some other form of stent. These procedures require not only a skilled surgical team with the support of specialist paediatric anaesthetists, but also good intensive care nursing post-operatively to achieve the best results. As with all surgery on the paediatric airway, appropriate antibiotic, proton-pump inhibitor and steroid therapy should be instituted as required.

Vocal Abuse

This topic is also discussed in Chapter 6. Many children are "screamers", and hence liable to the consequences of vocal abuse. This usually takes the form of fluctuating oedema of the vocal cords associated with fluctuating voice change or "thickening" of the vocal cords with more persistent voice change, but the occasional child progresses to form frank "screamer's" nodules with established hoarseness. The status of the vocal cords is best assessed at awake, flexible laryngoscopy, but in centres with appropriate equipment, videostroboscopy can be attempted. Examination of the larynx is important to exclude other pathology.

The mainstay of management is speech therapy, but in children, once the pattern of vocal abuse has been established it can be very hard to break, and therapy should persist for at least 12–18 months. As a general rule, vocal cord surgery is not indicated. However, in a child with established vocal cord nodules who has been able to correct the vocal abuse, this may need consideration.

Foreign Bodies

The inadvertent passage of objects or food into the childhood airway is a potentially lethal event when complete airway obstruction occurs (Fig. 23.15). Fortunately, this is uncommon. Younger children, particularly boys, are more commonly affected. Most units have a large collection of the enormous variety of objects of all shapes and sizes that have been inhaled by children. In the acute phase, the type of foreign body (FB) is less important than the size, the site of impaction and the completeness of the obstruction.

Large obstructing FBs may lodge in the laryngeal inlet, thus causing acute, potentially fatal airway compromise. In such cases, the outcome will be dictated by the use of appropriate on-scene first aid by whoever is present (e.g. parents or babysitters). A combination of back blows and chest compression is the recommended first-aid management if positioning and tongue/jaw lift do not relieve the obstruction. For survivors arriving in an Emergency Room with a deteriorating airway, topical local anaesthetic spray with restraint of the child may enable sufficient visualisation with an anaesthetic laryngoscope to permit removal of the FB with whatever forceps are available. In such a situation, it would be a good precaution to

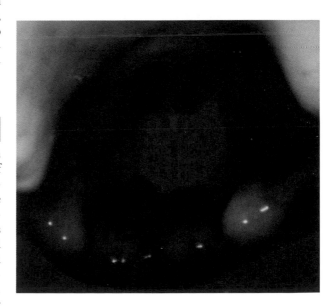

Fig. 23.15 Foreign body impacted in the larynx

have infiltrated the neck with local anaesthetic and have an emergency tracheotomy pack opened and ready for use in case of failure and a totally obstructed airway.

In the slightly less acute situation, laryngoscopy under general anaesthetic is the preferred option for assessment and removal of the FB. If not found in the larynx, then tracheoscopy/bronchoscopy and, if warranted, oesophagoscopy should be done.

Sharp or thin, flat objects can lodge in the larynx to cause hoarseness and stridor rather than fatal airway obstruction. Most FBs (≈90%), however, migrate distally into the trachea (characterised by an audible slap on inspiration accompanied with a palpatory thud and asthmatoid wheeze) or one of the main-stem bronchi, where symptoms may be minimal after an initial choking phase.

The history is of great importance. An episode of choking and coughing during eating may be reported by the older child or witnessed by the caregiver. Following this, symptoms may progress, remain stable or may regress into a period of quiescence before the development of late complications. Presentation days or weeks after the aspiration can occur, typically, in the case of retained laryngeal FBs, with voice change and/or stridor. More distal retained FBs may present with persistent cough, wheezing or pneumonitis and attendant respiratory distress. In up to 50% of late presentations, no history of observed or reported aspiration can be obtained. It is therefore prudent to maintain suspicion of FB aspiration in all cases of chronic laryngeal and respiratory symptoms. Any suggestion of FB inhalation requires laryngoscopy and bronchoscopy for both diagnosis and treatment, when the presence of a FB can be confirmed. In the larynx, the longer the FB has been in place, the greater the degree of ulceration and inflammatory swelling, and in some cases even removal of the FB does not provide an adequate enough airway so that short-term tracheotomy may be required.

Neurological Conditions

Recurrent Laryngeal Nerve Palsy

Acquired RLN palsy may be broadly classified as occurring secondary to trauma (birth, surgical, external), infectious conditions or to be idiopathic when no other causes can be identified. The RLN supplies all the intrinsic muscles of the larynx except the cricothyroid, which is supplied by the external branch of the superior laryngeal nerve. It also supplies sensation caudal to the vocal fold. The course of the left RLN is longer than the right and its course extends into the thorax, thus exposing it to a greater chance of injury. Unilateral RLN palsy is therefore more common on the left side, and overall unilateral palsy is slightly more common than bilateral palsy.

RLN palsy is the second commonest cause of neonatal stridor and can be unilateral or bilateral. Birth trauma is said to account for this when associated with a traumatic birth requiring forceps-assisted delivery, but it is difficult to separate this as the cause from congenital RLN palsy. Causes for the latter are often speculative, for example the lie of the foetus has resulted in abnormal tractional forces on the nerve. Some cases are associated with intracranial abnormality or the Arnold-Chiari malformation, and in this regard, expeditious treatment of identified hydrocephalus usually results in reversal of the RLN deficit. In general terms, 50% of cases will recover spontaneously within 6 months after birth and a further 25% by 9 months. Of the remainder, some will recover during the following months, a few will recover even several years later, whilst a minority will have a permanent palsy.

Surgical trauma in children can result in injury to either or both RLNs, but the left side is at greatest risk. The procedures most frequently associated with such injuries are congenital cardiac anomaly and tracheoesophageal fistula surgery. Less frequently, excision of congenital neck masses such as cervical teratomas, thyroid tumours and cystic hygromas can inadvertently injure the RLN on either side. External trauma, either blunt or penetrating, although rare in children, can occasionally damage the RLN.

The advent of widespread vaccination programmes has dramatically reduced the incidence of infection-related RLN palsy. Whooping cough, poliomyelitis, tetanus, rabies, infectious mononucleosis and syphilis have all been implicated.

Idiopathic cases are diagnosed by exclusion following a full clinical work-up to exclude alternate diagnoses.

The presentation of RLN palsy is dependent on the age of the child and whether the palsy is unilateral or bilateral. In general, a unilateral vocal cord palsy results in a weak voice/cry, possibly associated with stridor, with or without symptoms consistent with aspiration. The presence of an associated superior laryngeal nerve deficit increases the possibility of the latter. Bilateral RLN palsy results in the vocal cords lying in either a median or paramedian position. Therefore, the voice or cry will be only minimally affected, with good protection of the lower tracheobronchial tree but with a precarious airway. Diagnosis is best achieved while the patient is awake using a flexible fibre-optic endoscope to view the larynx, although assessment under general anaesthesia to rule out any other associated laryngeal, tracheal or oesophageal pathologies may need to be considered. If awake, flexible, fibre-optic evaluation of the larynx is not possible, diagnosis can be made during light general anaesthesia, but may be difficult as the degree of general and topical anaesthesia required to permit adequate laryngeal visualisation may immobilise the cords.

By and large, unilateral RLN palsy does not require any treatment in children. The contralateral side usually compensates adequately for phonation and airway protection. In rare cases, injection of the affected cord may be required for a stronger voice or to prevent distal soiling. Thyroplasty techniques have been used in the paediatric population, but concerns remain about such procedures in the immature larynx.

Bilateral palsies nearly always require tracheotomy. Although the airway may be stable at presentation, if the cords are significantly medialised, only a minor degree of inflammation, such as that seen during respiratory tract infection, may precipitate a life-threatening airway obstruction. In general, they have a worse prognosis for full recovery than unilateral lesions. A significant proportion of bilateral cases, possibly 50–70%, although the exact figure is not well defined, will resolve spontaneously. Spontaneous resolution can occur even several years after the initial event. Surgery to improve the airway enough to allow decannulation should be deferred to allow time for a natural resolution. The timing of surgical intervention is controversial, but the longer it can be delayed, the better. One must balance the possibility of spontaneous resolution and the tolerability of tracheotomy to the patient and parents for a prolonged period, against the desire to expedite decannulation, the effects of surgery on voice outcome and protection of the lower tracheobronchial tree. Laser cordotomy, laser arytenoidectomy and Woodman's procedure are all recognised techniques, but appropriate timing and patient selection are vital for a successful outcome.

For discussions of benign and malignant tumours, management of emergency airway problems in children, and tracheotomy/tracheostomy and respiratory papillomatosis see Chapters 12, 21, 28 and 29, respectively.

Summary for the Clinician

- Symptoms suggesting laryngeal disease in a child need to be taken seriously and a clear diagnosis made at an early stage. Infective conditions can include relatively rare, but serious disease. Gastro-oesophageal reflux is becoming more commonly recognised as a problem. The larynx may be damaged by both external and internal trauma: the latter can be produced both by ingestion of caustic substances and by laryngeal intubation. If direct tracheal intubation is required, the techniques of both tracheostomy (with construction of a formal stoma) and tracheotomy are practised: each technique has its advantages and disadvantages.

Suggestions for Further Reading

Infection

1. Hatherill M, Reynolds L, Waggie Z, Argent A (2001) Severe upper airway obstruction caused by ulcerative laryngitis. Arch Dis Child 85:326–329
2. Leung AK, Kellner JD, Johnson DW (2004) Viral croup: a current perspective. J Pediatr Health Care 18:297–301
3. McEwan J, Giridharan W, Clarke RW, Shears P (2003) Paediatric acute epiglottitis: not a disappearing entity. Int J Pediatr Otorhinolaryngol 67:317–321
4. Shah RK, Roberson DW, Jones DT (2004) Epiglottitis in the Hemophilus influenzae type B vaccine era: changing trends. Laryngoscope 114:557–560

Reflux

1. Bach KK, McGuirt WF Jr, Postma GN (2002) Pediatric laryngopharyngeal reflux. Ear Nose Throat J 81:27–31
2. Carr MM, Nagy ML, Pizzuto MP, Poje CP, Brodsky LS (2001) Correlation of findings at direct laryngoscopy and bronchoscopy with gastroesophageal reflux disease in children: a prospective study. Arch Otolaryngol Head Neck Surg 127:369–374
3. Gilger MA (2003) Pediatric otolaryngologic manifestations of gastroesophageal reflux disease. Curr Gastroenterol Rep 5:247–252

Trauma

1. Merritt RM, Bent JP, Porubsky ES (1998) Acute laryngeal trauma in the pediatric patient. Ann Otol Rhinol Laryngol 107:104–106
2. Myer CM 3rd (2004) Trauma of the larynx and craniofacial structures: airway implications. Paediatr Anaesth 14:103–106
3. Schaefer SD (1992) The acute management of external laryngeal trauma. A 27-year experience. Arch Otolaryngol Head Neck Surg 118:598–604

Intubation Injury

1. Gould SJ, Howard S (1985) The histopathology of the larynx in the neonate following endotracheal intubation. J Pathol 146:301–311
2. Gould SJ (1988) The pathology of neonatal endotracheal intubation and its relationship to subglottic stenosis. J Laryngol Otol 17:S3–S6

Foreign Bodies

1. Bloom DC, Christenson TE, Manning SC, Eksteen EC, Perkins JA, Inglis AF, Stool SE (2005) Plastic laryngeal foreign bodies in children: a diagnostic challenge. Int J Pediatr Otorhinolaryngol 69:657–662

Papillomatosis

1. Chadha N, James A, Chadha N (2005) Adjuvant antiviral therapy for recurrent respiratory papillomatosis. Cochrane Database Syst Rev 4:CD005053
2. Derkay C (2005) Cidofovir for recurrent respiratory papillomatosis (RRP): a re-assessment of risks. Int J Pediatr Otorhinolaryngol 69:1465–1467
3. Silverman DA, Pitman MJ (2004) Current diagnostic and management trends for recurrent respiratory papillomatosis. Curr Opin Otolaryngol Head Neck Surg 12:532–537

Tracheostomy

1. Prescott CA (1992) Peristomal complications of paediatric tracheostomy. Int J Pediatr Otorhinolaryngol 23:141–149

Laryngeal Webs and Subglottic Hemangiomas

24

Michael J. Rutter

Core Messages

- Nondynamic, congenital laryngeal anomalies such as laryngeal webs and subglottic hemangiomas present with an endoscopic degree of obstruction disproportionate to their clinical presentation.
- Congenital anterior glottic webs are usually thick, and not easily managed endoscopically
- Congenital anterior glottic webs are amenable to open reconstruction of the anterior commissure, while acquired webs are better managed with placement of a laryngeal keel.
- Subglottic hemangiomas are frequently associated with a degree of subglottic stenosis.
- Open excision of a subglottic hemangioma is an alternative to tracheotomy or endoscopic debulking.

Contents

Introduction

Within the anatomic confines of the larynx, a variety of pathologies may compromise air flow, causing airway obstruction. This chapter describes two such anomalies – laryngeal webs and subglottic hemangiomas. This chapter includes a description of these disorders followed by a synopsis of diagnostic guidelines and current management strategies.

Laryngeal webs are either congenital or acquired. Congenital webs are comparatively rare and result from an embryologic failure of laryngeal canalization. Patients typically present with an abnormal cry at birth and some may have symptoms of airway obstruction. In contrast, acquired webs are generally posttraumatic in origin. They may be iatrogenic in nature or result from direct trauma or inhalational injuries. Laryngeal webs have been described in the supraglottic, glottic, and subglottic regions, and may occur anteriorly or posteriorly. As anterior glottic webs comprise more than 95% of cases, the present discussion will be confined to these anomalies.

Congenital Anterior Glottic Webs

Congenital anterior glottic webs comprise two distinct subtypes: the rare gossamer-thin web that is confined to the glottis alone (Cotton and Tewfik 1985) and the much more frequently occurring thick anterior web with subglottic extension (Drolet et al. 1999). The thick anterior web has a characteristic thin luminal edge, but a much thicker base that extends into the subglottis. In lateral xerographs of the airway, the web appears as a "subglottic sail" (Fig. 24.1). The thick anterior web may be considered as a type of partial laryngeal atresia rather than as a true web. In severe cases, it may present with complete airway obstruction at birth due to complete laryngeal

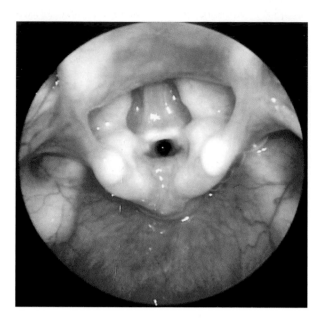

Fig. 24.1 Endoscopic view of an extensive anterior laryngeal web with subglottic extension

atresia. A complete laryngeal atresia generally results in congenital high airway obstructive syndrome (see Chapter 9) unless there is a concomitant tracheoesophageal fistula, allowing decompression of the tracheobronchial tree. Although complete laryngeal atresia is the most severe form of glottic webbing, the condition comprises a spectrum, with the least severe form presenting with minor blunting of the anterior commissure. There is no generally accepted classification; however, anterior glottic webs are considered as minor, moderate, severe, or complete. These webs do not improve spontaneously, and the web grows in proportion to the rest of the larynx.

Anterior glottic webs are rare, comprising 5% of congenital laryngeal anomalies. Since most congenital anterior glottic webs occur with associated subglottic stenosis, this anomaly may be considered a subset of congenital subglottic stenosis. Although there is currently no known gene that causes congenital glottic webbing, a significant association between this anomaly and chromosome 22q11.2 deletion syndrome (velocardiofacial syndrome) has been noted (McElhinney et al. 2002; Miyamoto et al. 2004). Given that more than 50% of patients with an anterior glottic web have chromosome 22q11.2 deletion syndrome, it is prudent to refer all patients with congenital anterior glottic webbing for genetic evaluation.

Diagnostic Guidelines

Infants presenting with congenital anterior glottic webs have an abnormal cry or even aphonia. If a patient with

an anterior glottic web presents with significant airway compromise in the first few hours or days of life, it is likely that the web is severe. In such cases, urgent airway intervention is required. Nevertheless, because infants are remarkably tolerant of congenital airway compromise, even patients with moderate to severe glottic webbing may initially show only subtle airway symptoms. As with most causes of congenital airway stenosis, symptoms exacerbate over the first few months of life. In infants with moderate to severe webbing, biphasic stridor and retraction of the chest wall, particularly when upset or feeding, become increasingly evident. Failure to thrive, apnea, and cyanosis are characteristic of more severe airway compromise.

Awake, flexible laryngoscopy should be performed initially. This may be diagnostic or may at least exclude laryngomalacia or vocal cord palsy from the differential diagnosis. A definitive evaluation requires rigid or flexible bronchoscopy. Both the severity of the web and its subglottic extension are evaluated. Whereas flexible bronchoscopy provides an excellent view of the anterior commissure, rigid bronchoscopy is more advantageous in evaluating the associated degree of subglottic stenosis, and angled (70°) telescopes provide better images of the web. In children with severe webs, care must be taken not to compromise further an already compromised airway, and spontaneous ventilation with the infant maintaining their own airway is preferable to intubation or emergency tracheotomy.

Radiological evaluation is a secondary consideration. While any infant stable enough to have a high-kilovolt airway film should have this film prior to bronchoscopic evaluation, it is performed primarily to exclude congenital tracheal stenosis. A lateral airway xerograph (Fig. 24.2) provides a superb image of the web, but the required radiation involved is unjustifiable and it is no longer widely available. Similarly, although high-resolu-

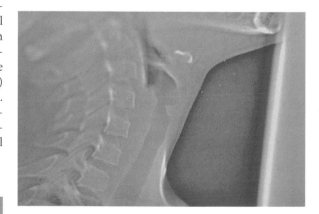

Fig. 24.2 Lateral xerograph of the airway illustrating the "subglottic sail"

24

tion computed tomography (CT) of the airway with sagittal reconstruction provides excellent images, it requires significant radiation and adds little to the information provided by bronchoscopy. Magnetic resonance imaging (MRI) is time consuming, and in an infant with a compromised airway, the necessary sedation is too great a risk to include in standard evaluation.

Management Strategies

Management of the infant with the rare true gossamer-thin anterior glottic web is quite different from management of the far more frequent thick web with subglottic extension. The infant with a thin glottic web may never be diagnosed, as it is suspected that in a child with neonatal airway compromise due to such a web, intubation for airway stabilization may brush aside the web and completely resolve the problem. In an infant presenting with a thin anterior web on bronchoscopy, simple division of the web with a sickle knife under suspension laryngoscopy using a small Lindholm laryngoscope is both quick and curative.

In infants presenting with a thick glottic web, an initial decision must be made as to whether repair should be performed early in the neonatal period or later in childhood. In children with a mild or moderate web and in whom no clinical airway compromise is present, late repair is preferable, as this is technically easier to perform in a larger larynx. Late repair is usually done by age 4 years, so as to improve the quality of a child's voice prior to school age. In children with a more severe degree of glottic compromise, repair may be performed early, or alternatively, a tracheotomy placed and late repair planned.

Options for repair of a congenital anterior glottic web include open keel placement and open reconstruction of the anterior commissure. Endoscopic procedures such as laser division of the web or endoscopic keel placement are not advocated. Laser division is likely to result in web reformation and does not adequately manage the inherent subglottic stenosis that is usually present. Similarly, endoscopic keel placement does not deal with subglottic stenosis. Moreover, it is technically demanding in an infant, although it may be an appropriate option in an older child.

Open repair may be performed as a single- or two-stage procedure. If a tracheotomy is already present, the latter is preferable. Otherwise, a single-stage procedure (i.e., without tracheotomy) should be a consideration if intensive care facilities permit. Single-stage reconstruction is an option whether a keel is placed or the anterior commissure is reconstructed.

Open keel placement requires adequate exposure of the larynx and complete laryngofissure. This is best accomplished with an assistant providing endoscopic glottic visualization during the laryngofissure to ensure that the split is performed exactly in the midline. Partially incising or grooving the thyroid cartilage between the superior and inferior thyroid notches facilitates meticulous midline placement of the laryngofissure. The laryngofissure is carried down through the cricoid cartilage, as the "sail" of the web extends to the lower border of the cricoid cartilage anteriorly. If a segment of age-appropriate endotracheal tube is placed in the glottic lumen, through the cricoid split, at this point, the surgeon can evaluate whether the cricoid will close easily over the endotracheal tube. More commonly, the cricoid will not easily close over the endotracheal tube, and an anterior cartilage graft is required to repair the associated subglottic stenosis. Thyroid ala is a useful cartilage graft in these infants, and a small graft may be obtained from a superior lateral thyroid alar margin (not involving the laryngofissure). Alternatively, a costal cartilage graft may be used. Leaving an open cricoid split is also an option, but with a keel in place this will not heal as readily. Once the graft is placed with its superior aspect level with the upper border of the cricoid cartilage, an appropriate size laryngeal keel (e.g., the Montgomery Keel) is selected, trimmed, and placed, extending from the upper border of the anterior cricoid graft (if such a graft is present) to the superior thyroid notch. The upper limit of the keel should not be so high as to disrupt the insertion of the epiglottic petiole.

The posterior (intraglottic) limb of the keel should extend far enough to cover the raw split edges of the web, but should not abut the mucosa of the posterior glottis. The keel is sutured into place, and the complex suture technique recommended by Montgomery (Montgomery and Montgomery 1990) is used to secure the keel. The airway is closed over an endotracheal tube in a single-stage procedure or over a suprastomal stent or no stent in a two-stage procedure. The more severe the subglottic stenosis, the more likely will be the need for a suprastomal stent and a two-stage procedure.

The keel is removed within 10 days to 4 weeks, with longer stenting periods used for more severe webs and two-stage procedures. Stent removal requires an open procedure. The resultant open laryngofissure requires closure with laterally placed mattress sutures, as the cartilage edges of the laryngofissure are friable and easily damaged if sutures pull out. For this reason, antibiotic coverage and antireflux measures are advised during the period that the keel is in place and for an additional few days following keel removal.

An alternative to the use of a keel is open reconstruction of the anterior commissure (Fig. 24.3). Since this approach is possible in children in whom at least 25% of the lumen is patent, it is an option even for those with a moderately severe web. This technique is reliant on the mobility of the remnant vocal fold mucosa over the vocal ligament. It is therefore usually not suitable for salvage repair of a web when scar tissue is present, such as occurs

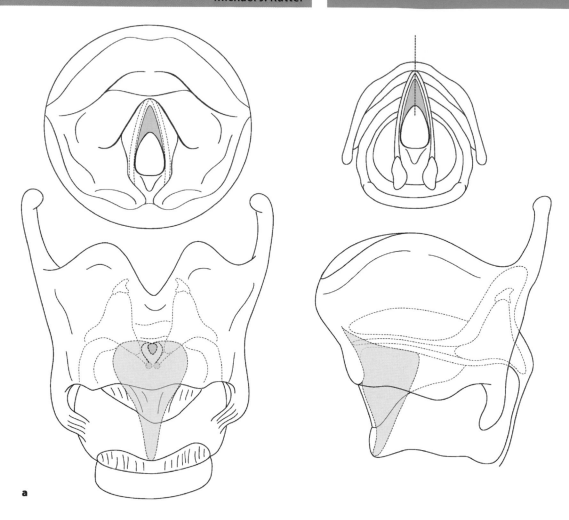

Fig. 24.3 a Endoscopic (*top left and right*) and three-dimensional profiles (*bottom left and right*) of an anterior glottic web (*shaded*). **b** *see next page*

following unsuccessful laser web division. The laryngofissure is performed in a fashion similar to the technique used when placing a keel. The cut edge of the mucosa overlying the cord is remarkably mobile if there has been no previous trauma or surgery to induce scar tissue; it may thus be sutured anteriorly to the cut edge of the thyroid cartilage to recreate an anterior commissure. A 6.0 PDS suture is placed through the thyroid cartilage near the edge of the laryngofissure at the level of the vocal ligament. This ligament lies at the junction of the lower third and upper two-thirds of the laryngofissure in an infant. The suture is then placed through the mucosal edge and into the airway lumen. In a mattress fashion, it is brought back through the mucosa and thyroid cartilage 0.5 mm parallel to the initial pass of the suture and then secured. A second pexing suture is placed below the initial suture to further mucosalize the raw incised edge of the web.

The same procedure is then performed on the opposite vocal ligament. The larynx is loosely approximated over an age-appropriate endotracheal tube. If the cricoid easily approximates, the larynx is closed. More commonly, however, the cricoid does not easily approximate. In such cases, placement of an anterior cartilage graft is appropriate. A keel is not required, and the child is intubated for 2–5 days.

Acquired Anterior Glottic Webs

Acquired anterior glottic webs are even less common than congenital webs and are posttraumatic in origin. These webs have two main etiologies: (1) anterior neck trauma, which is often associated with a fractured larynx, and (2) iatrogenic damage, which is often associated

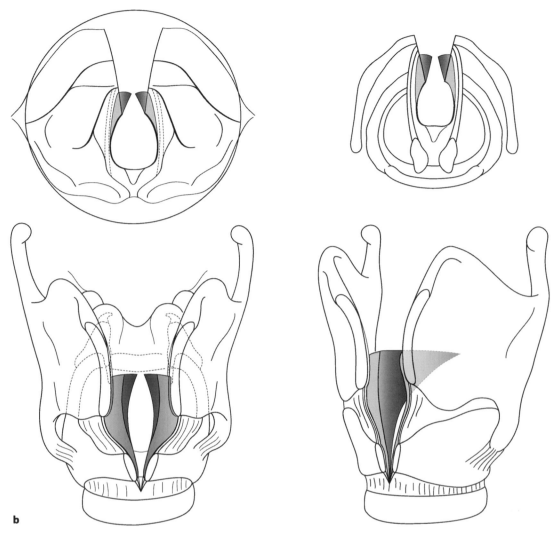

b

Fig. 24.3 *(Continued)* **b** Views of the anterior glottic web following laryngofissure. **c** *see next page*

with injudicious use of a laser at the anterior commissure while managing laryngeal papillomatosis. It is rare for prolonged intubation to induce anterior glottic stenosis unless there is also associated subglottic stenosis.

Management Strategies

The management of acquired anterior glottic stenosis differs significantly from that of the congenital anterior glottic web. The latter has normal mucosa within the remaining glottic inlet, and during reconstruction there may be sufficient mobility of the mucosal layer to reconstruct the anterior commissure without requiring use of a laryngeal keel. In contrast, acquired anterior glottic stenosis is, by definition, associated with fibrosis and scarring. The mucosa is fibrotic and therefore rarely amenable to

reconstruction of the anterior commissure. Reconstruction with placement of a laryngeal keel is thus mandatory, while the raw surfaces on either side of the laryngofissure remucosalize, as described earlier.

In an older child, an alternative to open placement of a laryngeal keel is endoscopic keel placement; however, the latter is technically more challenging. Several techniques have been described, but surgeons at our institution have found that using an endoscopically guided technique combined with an open approach to the neck is precise and reliable (Fig. 24.4). This technique involves initially suspending the larynx with a laryngoscope, and endoscopically dividing the web with a sickle knife. With the patient still suspended, the neck is then prepped and draped, and a small incision is made over the thyroid cartilage. A 4.0 prolene suture on a small straight needle is then passed through the midline of the lower thyroid car-

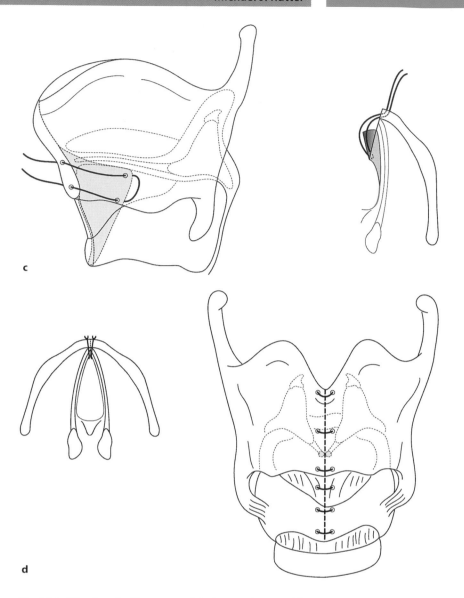

Fig. 24.3 *(Continued)* **c** Placement of the laryngeal mucosal "pexing" suture. **d** Reconstructed anterior commissure following closure of the laryngofissure

tilage, below vocal cord level, and visualized in the airway. An assistant grasps the needle (laparoscopic needle-holding forceps are useful) and withdraws the needle from the mouth. The surgeon then places a hollow, large-bore needle through the midline of the upper thyroid cartilage, above cord level, until it is visualized in the airway. Next, the assistant trims a thin silastic sheet so that it will cover the raw surfaces of the web and passes the straight needle though the inferior and superior borders of the silastic sheet in the midline. The small needle is then passed into the lumen of the large-bore hollow needle and withdrawn back into the neck incision. The suture is secured over a segment of a plastic intravenous cannula, and multiple throws are placed on the suture. The neck wound is then

closed and the child is intubated for 24 h. The keel is removed 7–14 days later, with the neck incision being reopened to remove the suture securing the keel.

Hemangiomas of Infancy

Natural History

Hemangiomas of infancy are benign vascular tumors that are characterized by endothelial hyperplasia and increased numbers of mast cells. These tumors occur more commonly in Caucasian newborns and have a higher incidence in females and premature infants (Fishman and Mulliken

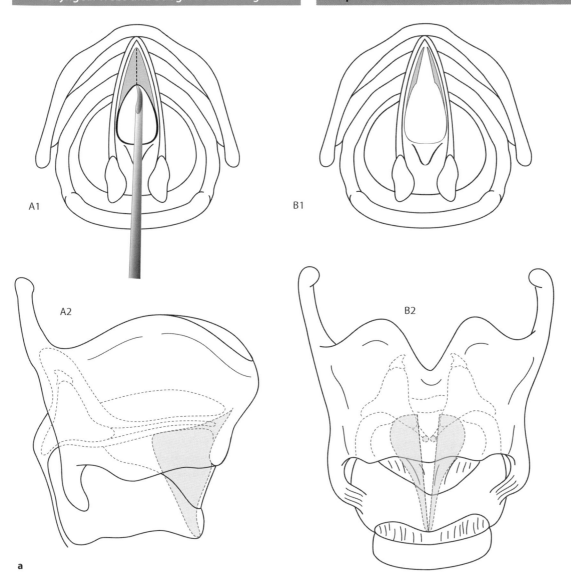

A1

B1

A2

B2

a

Fig. 24.4 **a** Anterior glottic web before (**A1** and **A2**) and after (**B1** and **B2**) endoscopic division. **b** *see next page*

1998; Drolet et al 1999). Hemangiomas of infancy follow a predetermined course of proliferation and spontaneous involution, although they exhibit a wide variation in the rate, duration, and degree of growth and tumor regression. The proliferative phase begins during the first few weeks of life and generally continues for 4–10 months. After a period of quiescence during which the growth rate of lesions stabilizes, the involuting stage begins.

Subglottic Hemangiomas

Hemangiomas most commonly present cutaneously, but can also occur in any body site. Of hemangiomas occur-

ring within the tracheobronchial tree, almost all are in the subglottis. The natural history of these hemangiomas mirrors that of cutaneous lesions; however, subglottic hemangiomas expand and involute more rapidly, with involution beginning before 12 months of age and spontaneous regression typically occurring within 18–24 months. Although 50% of children with subglottic hemangiomas have associated cutaneous lesions, subglottic hemangiomas are rare. They are seen more frequently in patients with cervicofacial hemangiomas that cover a beard distribution including the chin, jawline, and pre-auricular areas (Orlow et al. 1997). These patients should be closely monitored for airway involvement. Subglottic hemangiomas are the most common neoplasm of the

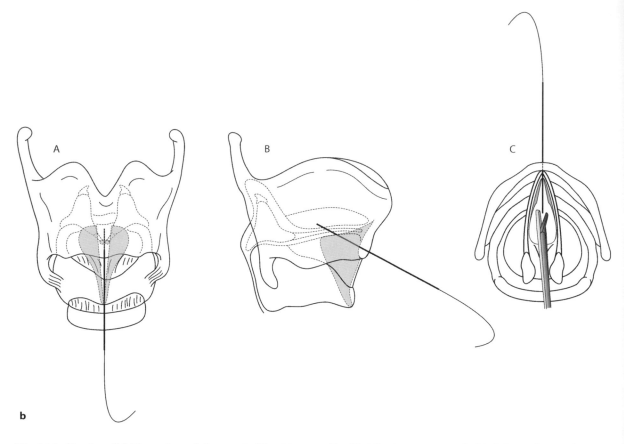

Fig. 24.4 *(Continued)* **b** Three views of placement of the skinny needle with 4.0 nylon suture attached inferior to the anterior commissure, and with the needle being grasped with an endoscopic needle holder in **c**. **c** *see next page*

airway in infants, and when untreated have a 40–70% mortality rate.

Diagnostic Guidelines

Most infants with a subglottic hemangioma present between 2 and 4 months of age, and more females than males are affected. The earlier the presentation, the more likely is the need for intervention. As the hemangioma increases in size, progressive deterioration of the airway occurs. Symptoms include biphasic stridor with retractions, especially when upset or when feeding, and a barking cough similar to that seen with croup. Airway compromise while feeding may cause failure to thrive. When airway obstruction is severe, apnea, cyanosis and "dying spells" may occur.

Optimally, initial evaluation is carried out with awake transnasal flexible laryngoscopy. Although this may allow for visualization of the compromised subglottis, more importantly, it should exclude other causes of neonatal stridor, particularly laryngomalacia and vocal cord paralysis.

A child with progressive stridor and a normal glottic and supraglottic examination requires a formal laryngoscopy and bronchoscopy performed under general anesthesia in the operating room. Preoperative plain (high-kilovolt) airway films are advisable to evaluate the subglottic airway, and classically, a subglottic hemangioma will cause an asymmetric narrowing of the subglottis. Laryngoscopy and bronchoscopy are best performed with the infant breathing spontaneously. As mentioned earlier in this chapter, it is remarkable how tolerant infants are to congenital or slowly progressive subglottic airway compromise. In light of this tolerance, there may be an 80–90% compromise of the subglottic lumen by the time the child presents for rigid bronchoscopy.

Unlike subglottic stenosis, a subglottic hemangioma is spongy and easily compressible, allowing straightforward intubation with a small endotracheal tube to maintain the airway if required. This characteristic also allows adequate evaluation of the distal airway with a small Hopkins rod telescope, such as a 2.8-mm telescope. The characteristic findings are of an asymmetrical subglottic sessile mass severely compromising the airway, with the

24

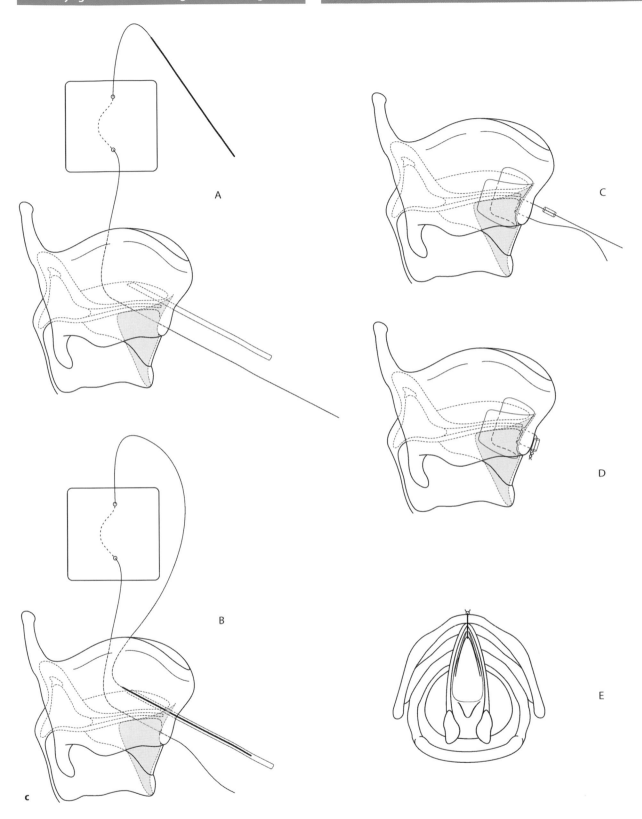

Fig. 24.4 *(Continued)* **c** Placement and securing of an endoscopically placed laryngeal keel

base of the tumor lying posterolaterally, more commonly left sided than right sided. The mass may occasionally extend up to true cord level, but rarely involves the anterior subglottis or anterior commissure; more than one hemangioma may be present. Although there may be abnormal vascularity of the mucosa overlying the hemangioma, more commonly the hemangioma is submucosal, but may still have a characteristic reddish or bluish hue. Because of this it may be confused with a submucosal subglottic cyst. If the child has been intubated prior to evaluation, the diagnosis may be challenging, and a period of extubation prior to repeat bronchoscopy may be required to confirm the diagnosis. Biopsy is not generally indicated.

Once the diagnosis is made, additional airway imaging may be of value in selected cases. It is unusual for a subglottic hemangioma to extend beyond the subglottic region. Contrast-enhanced MRI or CT evaluation of the neck and chest may, however, establish the extent of the hemangioma and reveal whether there is mediastinal involvement that could complicate management. This is generally characteristic of a child with extensive hemangiomatous disease.

Management Strategies

Airway compromise frequently occurs before involution, thus necessitating intervention. A wide range of interventions and treatment modalities has been reported (Rahbar et al. 2004). These approaches are often combined, depending on individual needs, the severity of airway compromise and surgeon's preferences. The relative merits and drawbacks of each of these therapies have been widely reported and remain controversial. Also, several techniques used in the past have now been abandoned; these techniques include external beam radiation, gold seed irradiation, cryotherapy, and chemotherapy with interferon alfa-2A.

Observation

Observation is appropriate for an older child in whom there is a small and minimally symptomatic subglottic hemangioma. This situation is most frequently seen in a child with cutaneous disease and mild symptoms of stridor that warrants an evaluation of the subglottis. If there is less than a 50% compromise of the airway in a minimally symptomatic child, observation with close follow-up is appropriate, and re-evaluation is warranted should symptoms progress or persist beyond 18 months.

Pharmacotherapy

The only medications currently recommended are high-dose systemic steroids, and two suggested dose regimens are provided (Table 24.1). Nevertheless, the side-effects of prolonged use are significant and include failure to thrive, osteopenia, and adrenal suppression. If a response is not rapid and if the child cannot be weaned down to an acceptable maintenance dose within several weeks, other interventions should be explored. In the child who presents within the first 6 weeks of life, the hemangioma is likely to grow rapidly and steroids are unlikely to be beneficial.

Endoscopic Surgical Management

Endoscopic techniques include intralesional steroid injection and prolonged intubation, microdebrider submucosal dissection, and both carbon dioxide and potassium

24

Table 24.1 Two suggested dosage regimens for steroid treatment of subglottic hemangioma

Steroid	Dose	Duration	Response
Cincinnati Protocol			
Dexamethasone	1.0–2.0 mg/kg/72 h	10 days initial therapy, then wean	If no response within 10 days, stop. If symptoms not greatly improved within 3 weeks, stop. If unable to wean to half initial dose within 6 weeks, then rapidly wean and stop
Boston Protocol[a]			
Prednisone	2–3 mg/kg/day	1 week initial therapy, then wean	If no response within 7 days, stop. If symptoms not greatly improved within 3 weeks, stop

[a]Derived from Rahbar et al. (2004)

titanyl phosphate laser ablation. All of these techniques rely on subtotal removal of the hemangioma, while attempting to inflict minimal damage to the mucosa or cricoid cartilage. All are quite effective, but are associated with a low, though significant, incidence of acquired subglottic stenosis, especially when multiple treatments are required (Cotton and Tewfik 1985). It is my belief that a majority of subglottic hemangiomas are associated with a mild congenital subglottic stenosis (see open excision) and that endoscopic intervention and the requisite postoperative intubation carries a small innate risk of inducing an "acquired on congenital" subglottic stenosis.

Tracheotomy

Tracheotomy placement offers a stable, safe airway during the growth and involution phases of a hemangioma; it can usually be removed at between 18–30 months of age without requiring any other surgical intervention and with preservation of normal vocal function. There is, however, a recognized mortality rate associated with tracheotomy placement for subglottic compromise in neonates. Furthermore, given the option of tracheotomy placement or an alternative intervention, a parent will rarely opt for tracheotomy placement.

Some children in whom a tracheotomy has been placed still require surgery to achieve decannulation. In these children, the hemangioma may not have fully involuted or may have involuted leaving residual fibrofatty tissue, which precludes decannulation without surgical excision. Tracheotomy may also be undesirable in a child with extensive cutaneous hemangioma overlying the anterior neck.

Open Surgical Excision

In our institution, we are increasingly offering open excision as an alternative to tracheotomy in infants who present at a young age with a large and rapidly growing subglottic hemangioma (Vijayasekaran et al. 2006). In such cases, our experience indicates that endoscopic management is not sufficient. We have also found open excision of value in achieving decannulation in children when involution has not occurred by 2 years of age. While still offering endoscopic management of smaller lesions, our positive experience with open excision has made this our preferred management stratagem for the symptomatic subglottic hemangioma.

Open excision is performed through a standard transverse neck incision, with exposure of the hemangioma through a vertical laryngofissure extending to the first or second tracheal ring. A temporary tracheotomy placed through the 4th and 5th tracheal rings permits control of the airway during the procedure. The laryngofissure is best performed with an assistant providing endoscopic guidance to allow as accurate a midline split of the anterior commissure as possible. Once the thyroid alae and cricoid cartilages are retracted laterally, the subglottic hemangioma is displayed, and the neighboring mucosa infiltrated with epinephrine. A mucosal flap may then be elevated to expose the hemangioma. The hemangioma may then be peeled off the posterior cricoid plate, and removed. This is usually a surprisingly bloodless procedure. The mucosal flap is the repositioned and secured with a 6.0 absorbable suture; the child is then intubated, and the temporary tracheotomy closed. If the cricoid cartilage will not easily close over a 3.5-mm endotracheal tube (in an infant), then associated subglottic stenosis coexists, and an anterior cartilage graft is required. This may be readily harvested from the upper aspect of the thyroid ala, taking care not to involve the laryngofissure incision. The laryngofissure is then closed, taking care to carefully reapproximate the anterior commissure. The thyroid alar graft (if required) is then secured between the cut edges of the cricoid cartilage, the neck closed, and the child transferred to the intensive care unit. Extubation occurs between 2 and 4 days postoperatively.

The most likely complication is anterior glottic webbing or cord asymmetry as a consequence of the laryngofissure or its closure. This may be avoided by meticulous laryngofissure and subsequent closure, or by avoiding complete laryngofissure altogether. While early in our series, we invariably required complete laryngofissure, as we have become more familiar with the technique, we have evolved to the point where most hemangiomas may be removed through an incision extending up to, but not through, the anterior commissure.

Summary for the Clinician

- Within the anatomic confines of the larynx, a variety of pathologies may compromise air flow, causing airway obstruction. This chapter has described two such anomalies – laryngeal webs and subglottic hemangiomas. This chapter included a description of these disorders followed by a synopsis of diagnostic guidelines and current management strategies.

References

1. Cotton RT, Tewfik TL (1985) Laryngeal stenosis following carbon dioxide laser in subglottic hemangioma. Report of three cases. Ann Otol Rhinol Laryngol 94:494–497

2. Drolet B, et al (1999) Hemangiomas in children. N Engl J Med 341:173–181

3. Fishman SJ, Mulliken JB (1998) Vascular anomalies: a primer for pediatricians. Pediatr Clin North Am 45:1455–1477

4. McElhinney DB, et al (2002) Chromosomal and cardiovascular anomalies associated with congenital laryngeal web. Int J Pediatr Otorhinolaryngol 66:23–27

5. Miyamoto RC, et al (2004) Association of anterior glottic webs with velocardiofacial syndrome (chromosome 22q11.2 deletion). Otolaryngol Head Neck Surg 130:415–417

6. Montgomery WW, Montgomery SK (1990) Manual for use of Montgomery laryngeal, tracheal, and esophageal prostheses: update 1990. Ann Otol Rhinol Laryngol Suppl 150:2–28

7. Orlow SJ, et al (1997) Increased risk of symptomatic hemangiomas of the airway in association with cutaneous hemangiomas in a "beard" distribution. J Pediatr 131:643–646

8. Rahbar R, et al (2004) The biology and management of subglottic hemangioma: past, present, future. Laryngoscope 114:1880–1891

9. Vijayasekaran S, et al (2006) Open excision of subglottic hemangiomas to avoid tracheostomy. Arch Otolaryngol Head Neck Surg 132:159–163

24

Chapter 25

Post-Intubation Laryngotracheal Stenosis

David Albert

25

Core Messages

- Ventilation of premature neonates continues to result in damage to the larynx, particularly at the level of the cricoid cartilage.
- The use of surfactant has reduced the number of neonates requiring ventilation.
- Careful management of the correctly sized endotracheal tube will reduce the incidence of laryngotracheal stenosis (LTS).
- After failed extubation, possible contributing factors such as gastro-oesophageal reflux and chest infection should be controlled. The possibility of coexisting problems such as tracheomalacia and vascular rings should also be considered.
- Endoscopy under general anaesthesia is the "gold standard" investigation. It should involve a team approach, with an experienced surgeon and paediatric anaesthetist.
- There is a place for endoscopic removal of granulations and cysts; use of the laser should be discouraged. There may be a place for balloon dilatation of early stenosis.
- The Cotton grading system is widely used to assess the degree of LTS.
- At the stage of failed extubation, when the reintroduced endotracheal tube is still of an appropriate size for the infant, a period of up to 2 weeks of "laryngeal rest", with an undisturbed endotracheal tube and control of reflux and infection, may allow successful extubation once a "leak" has been noted around the tube.
- A cricoid split procedure, endoscopic or through a neck incision, may allow successful extubation 1 week later.
- When extubation is not successful after these measures, or when an infant has already received a tracheotomy, allowing firm stenosis to develop, augmentation grafting using costal cartilage is the standard surgical treatment.
- In some cases of severe stenosis, resection of the stenosed segment may be possible.

Contents

Introduction

Definition

The older term "subglottic stenosis" has largely been replaced by laryngotracheal stenosis (LTS) to highlight the glottic component of the stenosis, which is particularly important when considering resection.

Pathology and Aetiology

Ventilation of the premature neonate for respiratory distress syndrome usually requires intubation. Although ideally, a small endotracheal tube (ETT) should reduce the incidence of LTS, these tend to kink and block and may be inadequate to ventilate the stiff lungs. The pressure of the tube on the subglottic cricoid cartilage causes ischaemia and ulceration. The situation may be worsened by movement, frequent intubations, reflux and general debility. If the subglottis is congenitally small, as in Down syndrome, the situation is worse. Infection also seems to play a part. Some ulcers can heal without stenosis (Gould and Howard 1985), but if there is underlying chondritis, stenosis occurs, usually from fibrous scar rather than excessively thickened cartilage. Synovitis of the cricoarytenoid joint can lead to cricoarytenoid fixation. Initially, the fibrous scar is immature and soft, but in time it becomes firm and organised. If the infant has a tracheotomy and the ETT, with its stenting effect, is withdrawn, damage to the perichondrial envelope of the cricoid cartilage may destabilise the complex mechanical forces within the matrix of the cartilage and cause it to collapse into its own lumen (Verwoerd et al. 1991).

Incidence

Although the incidence of LTS is relatively low, at about 2–5%, there is quite a variation between reported series. There is a male preponderance. Preventative measures have tended to reduce incidence for a given gestational age, but as younger and smaller neonates are surviving, including those who are medically challenged, the overall incidence does not seem to be changing much.

Prevention

The use of surfactant has reduced the number of moderately premature neonates requiring ventilation, but not the most premature. There is greater awareness of the risk of damage. If a shouldered tube is used, this must be checked to make certain that the shoulder does not pass through the cords. However, with any tube through the larynx, there will always be some risk of damage. Tubes impregnated with steroids or mitomycin have been suggested, but are not in routine use. If endotracheal biofilms are discovered, it may be that EDTA could help break these up and reduce the effect of infection.

Assessment of LTS

History

The initial intubation may have been traumatic or suggestive of an underlying narrowing. The general condition of the neonate is important in planning extubation, noting in particular the neonate's dependence on ventilation, oxygen requirements, cardiac status and any surgery that could have complicated the situation with a cord palsy. The need for high positive airway pressures might suggest an underlying tracheomalacia.

Examination

If the child is extubated but stridulous, check for micrognathia, macroglossia or other syndromic features that could be contributing to upper airway obstruction. Biphasic stridor may suggest tracheomalacia. In the tracheostomised child, the ability to vocalise suggests that the larynx is at least patent, but inability to maintain effective respiration with the tube occluded could either be because of the tube size or a suprastomal occlusion from anterior wall collapse or granuloma, as well as an inadequate laryngeal airway.

Pre-Endoscopy Investigations

These may include lateral neck x-rays to show the larynx and subglottis, plain or filtered x-rays of the chest to show the lower airway, and occasionally a barium swallow looking for a vascular ring or tracheomalacia. In general, however, radiology does not give a reliable assessment of subglottic stenosis.

Endoscopy

This is the gold standard and requires a careful, safe, team approach with an experienced paediatric anaesthetist and adequate photo-documentation. Age-appropriate endoscopes and bronchoscopes are essential. Endoscopic surgery has improved dramatically from the days of operating with the aid of a microscope. The view on a quality monitor using a Hopkins rod wide-angle telescope and three-chip video camera is superb. The technique is similar to endoscopic sinus surgery, with the left hand holding the telescope, leaving the right hand free for instrumentation.

Table 25.1 Cotton Grades (see Fig. 25.1)

Grade	Amount of lumen obstructed
I	Less than or equal to 50% of the subglottic lumen
II	Between 51% and 70% of the subglottic lumen
III	Between 71% and 99% of the subglottic lumen (see Fig. 25.2)
IV	No detectable lumen

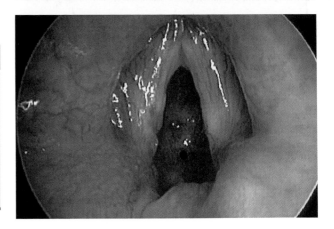

Fig. 25.2 An example of Cotton grade III stenosis, with "pinhole" lumen, at an interval after tracheotomy and removal of the stenting effect of the endotracheal tube

Classification	From	To
Grade I	No Obstruction	50% Obstruction
Grade II	51% Obstruction	70% Obstruction
Grade III	71% Obstruction	99% Obstruction
Grade IV	No Detectable Lumen	

Fig. 25.1 Diagram of Cotton staging of laryngotracheal stenosis

Grading

The Cotton grading system is used universally and is based on the degree of stenosis compared to an age-related normal value (Table 25.1, Figs. 25.1, 25.2).

Scenarios

Failed Extubation

This is the commonest situation, with a request to the ENT surgeon to see an ex-premature neonate who has failed extubation. Ideally, neonatal units should develop good relationships with a paediatric ENT surgeon so that potential problems and strategies to avoid LTS can be discussed at an early stage. Extubation should be attempted when the neonate is generally well: ideally, with an audible leak around the tube. If extubation fails, try to determine whether this is due to general lower respiratory factors such as bronchopulmonary dyplasia or due to upper airway obstruction. If the latter is suspected, consider conditions both above and below the larynx, such as Pierre Robin and tracheomalacia, which may respond to continuous positive airway pressure. Intubation-related damage such as oedema, granulations, subglottic cysts and stenosis are, however, the usual culprits and need to be assessed by endoscopy. Soft oedema may settle with a period of laryngeal rest, a period of undisturbed "therapeutic" intubation, or occasionally an endoscopic anterior cricoid split, using a sickle knife, to decompress the larynx. Discrete lesions can be removed at endoscopy. Firm stenosis will require open surgery to split the anterior cricoid and insert a small anterior cartilage graft. Persisting extubation failure is often due to a combination of factors such as poor cardiorespiratory function, laryngeal oedema and undisclosed tracheobronchomalacia. These neonates may need to remain intubated for a while to allow problems in the lower respiratory tract to be treated, or may eventually need a tracheotomy. Dependence on a tracheostomy has a higher morbidity and mortality than in older children and may allow quite mild stenosis to progress to near-complete occlusion, once the ETT, with its stenting effect, has been withdrawn.

Existing Tracheostomy

Patients referred with a tracheostomy and established stenosis need an assessment of the stenosis and of their general status. If they are otherwise well, it is often preferable to expand or resect the stenotic area at the same time as closing the tracheostomy, using a single-stage technique. In this technique, a cartilage graft is placed to expand the subglottis and, if necessary, support any stomal collapse. The reconstruction is then supported with a period of endotracheal intubation. If the child has other medical problems including poor respiratory function or a poor upper airway, it is often preferable to reconstruct the larynx leaving the tracheostomy in place with the reconstruction supported with an indwelling stent.

Recurrent Croup/Progressive Stridor

These patients present with croup or stridor and can have significant stenosis but are coping without a tracheostomy. A single-stage reconstruction (as outlined below) is ideal as it avoids the need for a tracheostomy.

Management of Early Soft Stenosis

Laryngeal Rest

A period of laryngeal rest, with a formal period of about 2 weeks undisturbed intubation may allow extubation of infants with early, soft, stenosis as an alternative to cricoid split (Graham 1994; Hoeve et al. 1995). This is based on histological studies of non-surviving intubated neonates (Gould and Howard 1985), which showed that quite severe subglottic ulcers could heal without scarring and stenosis. It certainly makes good sense to avoid the vicious circle of too frequent trials of extubation, each of which is followed by the trauma of re-intubation, often with increasingly narrow tubes. Laryngeal rest may work best in the mildly oedematous larynx with some ulcers, but no firm stenosis.

Removal of Granulations

One important reason to perform a careful endoscopy in failed extubation is to look for the characteristic "seal flipper" granulations that embrace the ETT whilst it is in place, but then prolapse into the lumen at extubation. They are easily removed allowing successful extubation.

Avoidance of the Laser

There is virtually no lesion in developing stenosis that benefits from the use of the laser. Careful sharp dissection using appropriate micro-instrumentation causes far less collateral damage, and any bleeding is easily stopped with adrenalin.

Endoscopic Procedures

Subglottic cysts and granulations should be carefully de-roofed or removed using micro-cupped forceps. If extubation is to be attempted it is best to apply topical adrenalin to the area and administer intravenous dexamethasone (0.25 mg/kg) as a single dose.

Radial Dilatation

Congenital stenosis responded poorly to dilatation in the early days of paediatric laryngeal surgery, prompting Evans and Todd (1974) to develop the laryngotracheoplasty operation. Early, soft and developing stenosis does respond to dilatation, but the pressure needs to be applied radially using cardiothoracic balloons. The pressure needs to be carefully monitored and sometimes endoscopic radial cuts need to be made if there is an element of firmer stenosis.

Endoscopic Decompression/Cricoid Split

If there is considerable oedema and an element of developing stenosis, the above measures may not be sufficient and a cricoid split should be considered (Fig. 25.3). This can be performed endoscopically, but surgical emphysema may result if it is too extensive. The aim is to allow

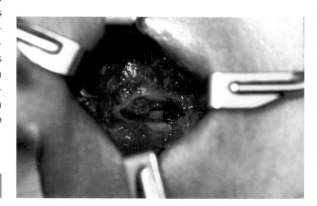

Fig. 25.3 Cricoid split procedure: The cricoid cartilage has been divided vertically in the midline through a horizontal, skin crease incision, and gently pulled apart, revealing the endotracheal tube in the lumen of the larynx. The infant's head is to the right of the photograph

25

the oedema to disperse rather than to allow separation of the cricoid laminae.

Mitomycin

This antineoplastic fibrinolytic is useful if initially successful dilatation is complicated by granulations that may heal with concentric stenosis.

Conventional External Cricoid Split

Conventional anterior cricoid split (anterior cricoidotomy) is followed by 1 week of intubation and has a 70–80% rate of successful extubation.

Management of Firm Established Stenosis

Expectant Waiting/Natural Resolution

Established stenosis does not improve with time and may progress in the presence of a tracheostomy due to the presence of infected secretions.

Augmentation Grafting

This is the commonest treatment method of established stenosis using rib cartilage (Fig. 25.4) and a single- or two-stage procedure. The single-stage procedure (Prescott 1988) supports the reconstruction with an ETT during a period of intubation in the intensive care unit. The traditional two-stage procedure uses an indwelling stent in the

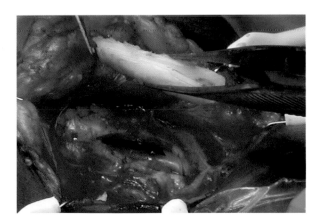

Fig. 25.4 Augmentation graft, using rib cartilage: the harvested and shaped piece of costal cartilage is shown next to the vertical incision in the anterior segment of the cricoid cartilage into which it will be placed and secured by sutures. In the one-stage procedure, no tracheotomy is necessary and the endotracheal tube is removed after a period in intensive care

subglottis and sometimes through the vocal cords, as well as a tracheostomy.

Resection

In severe stenosis with a margin below the vocal cords, a resection of the stenosis is possible with an anastomosis. The anterior half of the cricoid is included in the resection, but the posterior lamina is retained. This is thinned with a drill to receive the distal tracheal segment to which it is sutured. Anteriorly, the anastomosis is enlarged with a notch or a separate cartilage graft to prevent anastomotic stenosis.

Prevention of Post-Operative Restenosis – Salvage Techniques

The results of surgery for severe stenosis can be improved by careful attention to any granulations or restenosis. Mitomycin, radial dilatation and the selective use of endoscopically placed stents or Montgomery T-Tubes all have a place in preventing restenosis.

Summary for the Clinician

- A safe and accurate assessment is vital to plan treatment. Endoscopic treatment (minimally invasive laryngeal surgery) has the potential to reduce the amount of open surgery. A careful audit of results will identify the situations in which this more conservative approach is appropriate.

References

1. Evans JNG, Todd GB (1974) Laryngotracheoplasty. J Laryngol Otol 88:589–597
2. Gould SJ, Howard S (1985) The histopathology of the larynx in the neonate following endotracheal intubation. J Pathol 146:301–311
3. Graham JM (1994) Formal reintubation for incipient neonatal subglottic stenosis. J Laryngol Otol 108:474–478
4. Hoeve LJ, Eskici O, Verwoerd CDA (1995) Therapeutic reintubation for post-intubation laryngotracheal injury in preterm infants. Int J Pediatr Otorhinolaryngol 31:7–13
5. Prescott CAJ (1988) Protocol for management of the interposition cartilage graft laryngotracheoplasty. Ann Otol Rhinol Laryngol 97:239–242
6. Verwoerd CDA, Bean JK, Adriaansen FC, Verwoerd-Verhoef HL (1991) Trauma of the cricoid and interlocked stress. Acta Otolaryngol 111:403–409

Chapter 26

Congenital and Acquired Tracheal Stenosis in Children

26

Emmanuel Le Bret and E. Noel Garabédian

Core Messages

- Congenital tracheal stenosis is more common than acquired tracheal stenosis and its management is more straightforward.
- Congenital stenosis presents with respiratory difficulty since birth or, more commonly, with collapse and apnoea at home. Intubation and ventilation may have been attempted and found to be difficult. Transfer to a specialist unit is needed for long-term management.
- Computed tomography (CT) and magnetic resonance imaging (MRI) provide the quality of imaging necessary for initial assessment and the planning of treatment. Three-dimensional reconstructions of CT and MRI scans allow "virtual bronchoscopy" and visualisation of the relationship between the airway and other structures.
- Flexible and rigid tracheobronchoscopy is the standard method of assessing the state of the airway.
- Surgical management depends on the degree of narrowing of the trachea, the length of the narrow segment, the anatomy of the bronchial tree and the presence of concomitant lesions and malformations.

- Surgical management depends on the length of the stenotic segment:-
- Short segments are managed by resection and end-to-end anastomosis.
- Segments of up to two-thirds of the tracheal length should be managed by slide tracheoplasty.
- Longer segments are usually managed by slide tracheoplasty, although patch tracheoplasty is an alternative.
- Acquired laryngotracheal stenosis is more common than acquired tracheal stenosis on its own.
- The main cause of acquired stenosis is endotracheal intubation. It may also be related to the presence of a tracheotomy tube.
- Careful endoscopic assessment is required before planning treatment.
- Dilatation has a place in the management of the early, acute stenosis.
- Tracheal resection and tracheoplasty using rib cartilage are both successful methods of managing acquired tracheal stenosis.

Contents

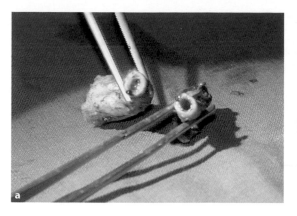
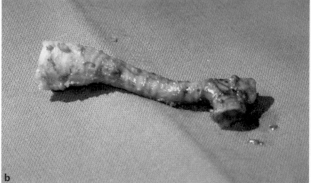

Fig. 26.1a,b Congenital stenosis with complete cartilage ring

Congenital Stenosis

The vast majority of paediatric tracheal stenosis is congenital and relates to the presence of complete tracheal rings, so that the entire circumference of the airway is cartilaginous (Fig. 26.1).

Assessment of the Lesion

Presenting Symptoms and Management

The clinical presentation of congenital tracheal stenosis is highly variable. A substantial minority of the patients have only inspiratory and/or expiratory stridor as their primary symptoms. There may be a history of minor respiratory difficulties since birth, or shortly after birth, or of repeated and stubborn respiratory infections. In some cases, difficulties in intubation or impossibility of extubation will have led to the diagnosis. The majority, however, present to their local hospital *in extremis* after collapse at home. Active resuscitation by parents has frequently been required and most have been intubated with difficulty and prove hard to ventilate. Some patients have proved impossible to ventilate, and have needed extra-corporeal membrane oxygenation (ECMO; Goldman et al. 1996). As soon as the patient's ventilatory state is stable, the child should be transferred to a specialist unit.

Investigation, Imaging

Diagnostic evaluation may include chest radiography, airway tomography, computed tomography (CT) scanning or magnetic resonance imaging (MRI). Contrast bronchography was used in the past, but has been generally replaced by modern three-dimensional imaging techniques. Mandatory evaluations include flexible and rigid bronchoscopy (Fig. 26.2), the latter is probably the gold standard for measuring the minimal diameter of the airway and the length of the stenotic segment.

Newer imaging technology has allowed the performance of virtual bronchoscopy, whereby an intraluminal view of the airway may be reconstructed from CT images (Fig. 26.3; Burke et al. 2000).

Three-dimensional reconstructions of CT scans or MRI scans also allow excellent visualisation of the relationship between the airway and the mediastinal cardiovascular structures (Fig. 26.4).

The complete evaluation of the child with a narrowed airway must also include a search for associated cardiovascular anomalies with echocardiography.

Description of the Lesions

There are at least four elements that affect severity: the narrowness of the trachea, the extent of tracheal involvement, the anatomy of the bronchi and the presence of associated lesions.

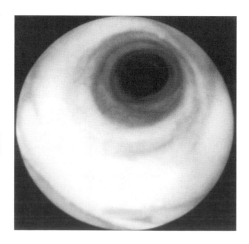

Fig. 26.2 Endoscopic view of "O" rings (Grillo 2004a)

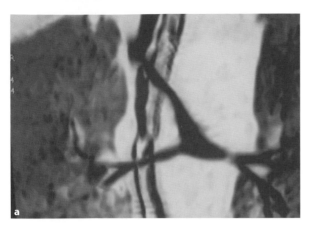
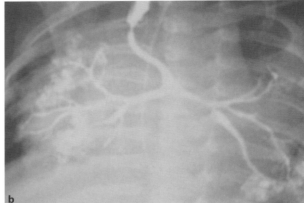

Fig. 26.3a,b Computed tomography (CT) scan (**a**) and bronchography (**b**) of a similar case

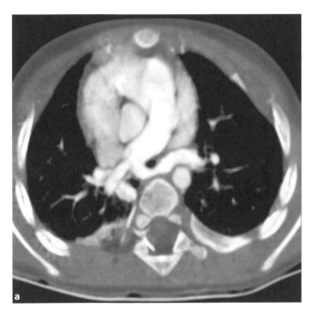
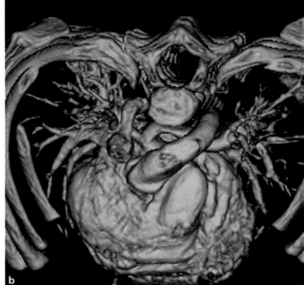

Fig. 26.4a,b CT scan (**a**) and three-dimensional reconstruction (**b**) of pulmonary artery sling associated with tracheal hypoplasia

The Narrowness of the Trachea

The trachea can be so narrow that ventilation is impossible and ECMO support can be required. There is a big difference between a trachea of 1 mm internal diameter and one of 2.5 mm internal diameter (Elliott et al. 2003).

The Extent of Tracheal Involvement

This is the classic description of severity, often stated in terms of percentage of the length of trachea (Cantrel and Guild 1964). Tracheal hypoplasia has been classified into three principal types (Fig. 26.5):

1. Generalised hypoplasia. The larynx is of normal diameter but the entire trachea or much of the trachea is narrowed (1–3 mm diameter in the newborn) to a point just above the carina. The main bronchi are often normal in diameter, but may be more transverse than usual, and there is frequently bronchomalacia. In some cases, the bronchi are also stenotic and composed of "O" rings of cartilage.

2. Funnel-like narrowing. The trachea begins with a normal diameter, but then funnels down over a variable length to a tight stenosis. The location of the funnelling and of the tight stenosis varies widely. It may be located proximally, with a more distal normal segment. In many cases, the stenosis is long, involving

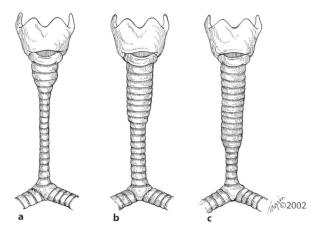

Fig. 26.5 **a** Generalised tracheal hypoplasia, **b** funnel shape of variable length and **c** segmental hypoplasia (Grillo 2004a)

more than half of the trachea and can extend to the main bronchi.

3. Segmental stenosis. Segmental stenosis may occur at any level in the trachea and may be of any length, but it occurs most often in the lower trachea. Bronchial anomalies may be present, such as a misplaced right upper lobe bronchus (bronchus suis), which takes off from the trachea above an area of segmental stenosis (Grillo 2004a).

The Anatomy of the Bronchi

This feature is often ignored, yet may militate against the use of particular types of repair. In very small babies, the bronchi are often involved. Associated bronchial hypoplasia or bronchomalacia has emerged as a significant risk factor.

Tracheal stenosis may also be present above an anomalous right upper lobe bronchus, with tighter stenosis or "bridge bronchus" below the lobar bronchus (Fig. 26.6). These patients are more difficult to correct surgically than when the trachea has a more normal pattern (Grillo 2004a).

Associated Lesions

In over 50% of the patients, congenital tracheal stenosis is accompanied by other malformations, including cardiac anomalies, hyaline membrane disease, pulmonary anomalies, inguinal hernias, imperforate anus, radial aplasia and megaureter.

Segmental stenosis may be associated with an aberrant left pulmonary artery, the so-called "pulmonary artery sling" (Fig. 26.7).

The left pulmonary artery originates from the proximal portion of the right artery and passes behind the trachea to the left lung. In most of these patients, "O" rings of cartilage are found in the stenotic segment. The length of tracheal stenosis most often extends beyond the region of the anomalous pulmonary artery sling (Fiore et al. 2005; Loubakov et al. 2004). Where stenosis is not present, there may instead be a malacic segment at the level of the artery. The artery can also obstruct the right main bronchus.

Surgical Treatment

Gas Exchange During Reconstruction

Once the diagnosis of tracheal stenosis is made, a surgical strategy for tracheal reconstruction is chosen from several options, discussed below. Regardless of the particular approach chosen, airway management during the recon-

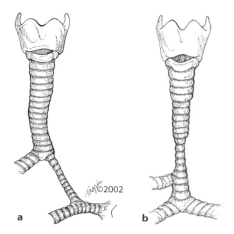

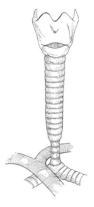

Fig. 26.6 **a** Bridging bronchus and **b** bronchus suis (Grillo 2004a)   Fig. 26.7 Pulmonary artery sling

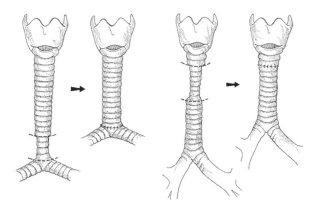

Fig. 26.8 Resection and end-to-end anastomosis (Grillo 2004a)

struction is of paramount importance. In adults requiring tracheobronchial reconstruction, there are well-established techniques for providing cross-field ventilation, thus allowing avoidance of cardiopulmonary bypass. Because the paediatric airway is so much smaller, especially in infants, cardiopulmonary bypass is much more commonly used.

Very-Short-Segment Tracheal Stenosis

Classical primary resection and end-to-end anastomosis is the treatment of choice (Islam et al. 2001). Exposure is achieved by cervicotomy or by sternotomy. The technique includes a large mobilisation of the trachea, resection of the stenotic segment and anastomosis of the tracheal ends with interrupted PDS single-layer sutures (Fig. 26.8; Friedman et al. 1990).

The maximal length that can be resected is still controversial (Longaker et al. 1990). It seems that for some authors, 30% of the tracheal length represents the maximum that can safely be resected (Wright et al. 2002), but for others, the maximal length is the entire trachea (Jacobs et al. 1996).

Recently, balloon dilatation has become an accepted modality and the results are encouraging (Brown et al. 1987; Jaffe 1997). This can be combined with posterior lasering to release complete tracheal rings (Maeda et al. 2000; Othersen et al. 2000). Not enough patients have yet been treated this way to recommend this method, but it is undoubtedly worth exploring. Various stents have been employed (Filler et al. 1998; Jacobs et al. 2000), but we can see few indications for their use in children, where definitive repair is of greater value, permitting rather than constraining growth (Couraud et al. 1990), as is inherent in the use of stents.

Medium-Length Stenoses (up to Two-Thirds of Tracheal Length)

For these lesions, slide tracheoplasty should be the initial treatment of choice (Goldman et al. 1996). The technique was first described by Tsang et al. (1989) and since then has been used by several authors (Dayan et al. 1997; Garabedian et al. 2001; Grillo 1994; Kutlu and Goldstraw 1999).

The trachea and the main bronchi are extensively mobilised, the stenotic segment is transected at its midpoint, the upper and lower segments are incised vertically (anteriorly in the distal segment and posteriorly in the proximal segment), the corners of the segments are trimmed to spatulate them, and the two ends are slid together and sutured (Fig. 26.9). With this technique, the circumfer-

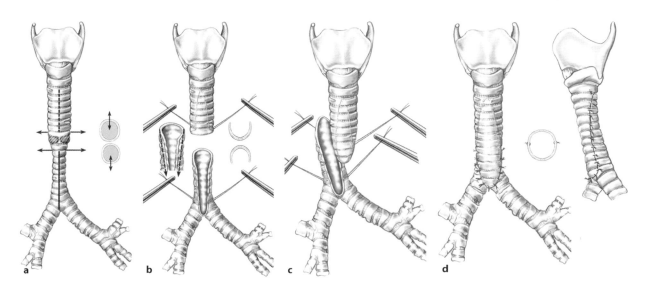

Fig. 26.9a–d Slide tracheoplasty (Garabedian et al. 2001)

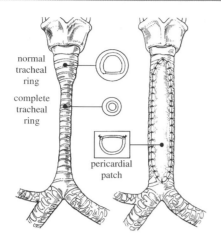

normal
tracheal
ring

complete
tracheal
ring

pericardial
patch

Fig. 26.10 Tracheoplasty with pericardial patch (Backer et al. 2001)

ence of the trachea is doubled and the cross-sectional area quadrupled. Only native tissue is used and tracheal growth has been seen to be satisfactory (Macchiarini et al. 1997).

Slide tracheoplasty can be combined with short-segment resection in cases when tracheal hypoplasia is associated with a critical degree of stenosis (Garabedian et al. 2001). In addition, Slide Tracheoplasty can be performed in the presence of tracheal bronchus (Le Bret 2006) or if the hypoplasia involves the origin of the main bronchi (Le Bret 2006).

Long and Very Long Tracheal Stenoses

It is for this group that the greatest number of options exist, and for this group that the greatest controversy remains. We believe, as the Great Ormond Street team believe (Elliott et al. 2003), that slide tracheoplasty with or without resection should always be the first option.

Slide tracheoplasty can even be applied in case of tracheal hypoplasia associated to cricoïd stenosis (Le Bret 2006). However, other techniques have been developed to treat very long tracheal stenoses.

Patch Tracheoplasty

The basic principles of patch tracheoplasty are simple. Cardiopulmonary bypass is usually necessary. The trachea is opened longitudinally anteriorly from above to below the stenosis. The anterior defect is then enlarged with a patch.

Several materials have been employed over the years, but the most common and successful have been autologous pericardium (Fig. 26.10; Backer et al. 2001; Idriss et al. 1984), rib cartilage (Matute et al. 2001), tracheal autograft (Fig. 26.11; Backer et al. 2001), tracheal allograft (Elliott et al. 1996) and most recently, carotid artery (Dodge-Khatami et al. 2002; Martinod et al. 2005). Heterograft tissue and prosthetic material do not work. None of the materials has been shown to be clearly superior and each has its proponents. For each material, a period of postoperative mechanical ventilation is required to allow healing of the graft and stabilisation of the airway. Some authors recommended the use of suspension sutures on the outside of the pericardial patch (Bando et al. 1996) or the use of tracheal stenting to maintain the patch open and to avoid acquired tracheomalacia.

Post-Operative Complications and Their Management

Granulation Tissue Formation

Granulations occur as a part of the healing process of tracheal epithelium. They may result in significant and even life-threatening obstruction of a relatively narrow airway.

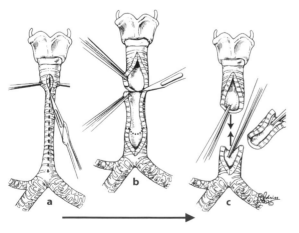

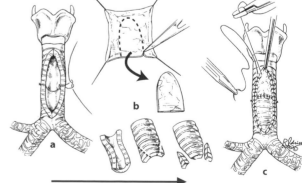

Fig. 26.11 Free tracheal autograft (Backer et al. 2001)

Attention to technical detail during repair is probably helpful in reducing the incidence, and we would suggest that wherever possible, sutures should be placed deep to the tracheal mucosa in an attempt to diminish the stimuli to granulation formation.

The management of granulations is usually described as bronchoscopic avulsion with grasping forceps or lasering. For others (Elliott et al. 2003), post-operative regular balloon dilatation has dramatically reduced the incidence of granulation-related airway obstruction.

Malacia

The management of malacia can be very challenging. Treatment of tracheobronchomalacia is discussed in Chapter 27. Briefly, three strategies can be employed: prolonged ventilatory support with continuous positive airway pressure or bi-level positive airway pressure (Essouri et al. 2005), tracheostomy and stenting.

Infection

While very rare, infection can be catastrophic. During the initial surgery, the unsterile tracheal contents are exposed to the mediastinum, often during a period of immunologic compromise, and cardiopulmonary bypass.

Recurrent Stenosis

If recurrent stenosis does occur, balloon dilatation and/or stenting can be performed.

Acquired Stenosis

Acquired isolated tracheal stenosis in infancy and childhood is much less common than acquired laryngotracheal stenosis (see Chapter 25). However, it has become a common problem, primarily because of improved survival of premature infants with respiratory distress requiring prolonged endotracheal intubation. In addition, insults to the tracheal mucosa from caustic aspiration, instrumentation and infections can cause endotracheal scarring and compromise the size of the tracheal lumen. Unlike congenital tracheal stenosis, repair or reconstruction of acquired stenosis is frequently complicated by recurrent scarring, poor healing because of vascular compromise or infection, and life-threatening anastomotic disruption. Thus, conservative (non-operative) therapy is appropriate for many of these lesions. When conservative therapy fails, however, a more aggressive, but highly individualised, approach is indicated.

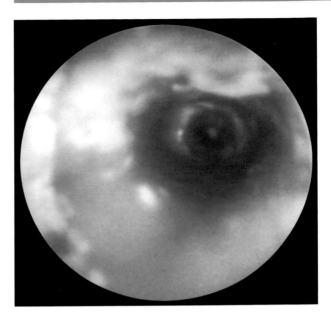

Fig. 26.12 Endoscopic view of acquired tracheal stenosis

Aetiologies and Localisation of Acquired Tracheal Stenosis in Children

One of the largest series of acquired tracheal stenosis in children was reported in 1991 by Weber et al. In a 10-year period, 62 patients (4 weeks to 14 years of age) were treated for acquired tracheal stenosis. The causes of stenosis were endotracheal intubation (71%), caustic aspiration (5%), recurrent infection (8%), bronchoscopic perforation (5%) and gastric aspiration (4%).

In a younger child, the aetiology of post-intubation tracheal stenosis is more likely to be a problem related to, and directly above, the tracheotomy tube. In an older child, the aetiology is likely to derive from short-term intubation with too large an endotracheal tube, or an over-inflated, cuffed endotracheal tube.

In the same series (Weber et al. 1991), the subglottic or upper trachea was involved in 76% of cases, the mid portion in 13% and the distal or carinal area in 11%.

Patient Assessment

Regardless of the aetiology or age, a careful endoscopy must be performed to ascertain whether the stenosis is anterior, posterior or circumferential in nature (Fig. 26.12). Sizing of the airway is imperative to allow for pre-operative planning and post-operative comparison. Flexible nasopharyngoscopy should evaluate vocal fold mobility, and a flexible endoscope passed through the tracheotomy tube will establish if tracheomalacia is present.

Treatment

Endoscopic Procedures

Endoscopic dilatation (balloon or serial dilatators) is appropriate for tracheal stenoses that are in the acute phase. If the stenosis is progressing or the narrow segment has become a chronic scar, more aggressive treatment will be necessary. Carbon dioxide or potassium titanyl phosphate lasers can be utilised to ablate a single quadrant of the tracheal stenosis, followed by dilatation in an attempt to enlarge the airway (Garabedian et al. 1990; Ward 1992). This technique works well for short-segment stenoses limited to one or two rings, and lesions that have an obvious thin lip of scar tissue or are limited to only one quadrant of the trachea. However, only 30% of the circumference should be resected at one time, and care must be taken not to come too close to the perichondrium. Therefore, repeated small incisions may be more successful than aggressive resection, which may lead to worsening of the obstruction. If the lesion has failed to respond to laser therapy, or involves a longer segment, open surgical intervention will be necessary.

Open Surgical Procedure

Open surgical treatment of tracheal stenosis generally involves a tracheal resection. This procedure is very well established in adults, but it is rarely done in children. In a series of 208 patients with tracheal stenosis, Grillo et al. (1995) reported treating only three children, the youngest being 12 years old. Specific cases of a predominantly anterior tracheal stenosis may be best treated by a tracheoplasty and anterior cartilage expansion.

Tracheal Resection

This is usually performed via a horizontal cervical incision overlying the third tracheal ring, and incorporating the tracheotomy stoma if one is present (Alstrup and Sorensen 1984). A shoulder bag is used to extend the neck. The strap muscles are separated in the vertical midline and the trachea is exposed. Lateral dissection of the trachea should take place in a subperichondrial plane to avoid injury to the recurrent laryngeal nerves. If a tracheotomy is present, the stoma can be utilised as the starting point to opening the trachea in a superior direction in the vertical midline. If a tracheotomy is not present, endoscopy can be performed to precisely identify the stenosis and place a needle into the airway immediately superior and inferior to the stenosis. At each of these sites, a horizontal intercartilagenous incision is made, and extended laterally to 3 and 6 o'clock. Then the posterior membranous tracheal wall is incised horizontally, layer by layer, until the tissue "party wall" between the trachea and oesophagus is identified. The lateral and posterior incisions are then connected with care to hug the trachea in the subperichondrial plane. The stenotic segment is then removed (Fig. 26.13). The posterior anastomosis is created with interrupted absorbable sutures; then the shoulder roll is removed. The patient is then intubated orally. The anterior and lateral sutures are then performed also with interrupted absorbable sutures. Care is taken to place the suture material outside the

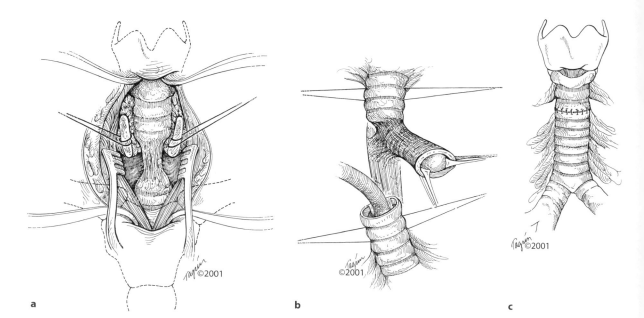

Fig. 26.13a–c Tracheal resection (Grillo 2004b)

26

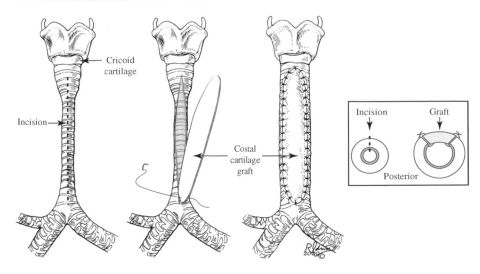

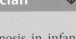

Fig. 26.14 Tracheoplasty with rib cartilage (Tsugawa et al. 2003)

lumen, because troublesome granulomas can form around intraluminal suture material. A drain is placed in the neck, and the wound closed in two layers.

The majority of patients can be extubated in the operating room and monitored closely in the hospital for 1 week. For smaller children, it may be wise to wait 24–48 h before extubation. In children, it is especially important to avoid endotracheal intubation post-operatively. If this should be necessary, non-cuffed, soft tubes must be used, not extending below the anastomosis. Follow-up endoscopy should be performed. Complications can include restenosis, anastomotic breakdown, pneumomediastinum and wound infection.

Tracheoplasty with Rib Cartilage

This technique has been described by Tsugawa et al. (2003) for congenital tracheal stenosis (Fig. 26.14) and applied by others (Majeski et al. 1980; Pashley et al. 1984) for acquired tracheal stenosis in children. Briefly, the area of stenosis is exposed anteriorly, and the trachea is opened longitudinally. Intraluminal scar and granulation are excised, usually with a curette or electrocautery, and a previously obtained piece of rib cartilage, with perichondrium intact, is fashioned. This allows the perichondrium to be placed facing the lumen. After placement of a silicone T tube, the rib cartilage graft is sutured in place with interrupted absorbable suture. Usually the T tube can be removed after 3 or 4 months, with excellent healing.

Summary for the Clinician

• Tracheal narrowing and stenosis in infants and children can be broadly categorised into congenital and acquired disorders. Congenital disorders are first seen early in life with varying degrees of respiratory distress when there is no history of previous airway instrumentation, prolonged intubation, infection or aspiration. Because the tracheal tissue is generally healthy, management is usually straightforward, with any number of satisfactory techniques. Acquired tracheal stenosis, on the other hand, is frequently complicated by injury, infection, mucosal sloughing, rapid granulation and scar formation, and recurrence of narrowing after treatment. Thus, the management of these patients usually involves long-term treatment, requires a variety of techniques and needs individual management based on the level of stenosis, the cause and previous therapy.

References

1. Alstrup P, Sorensen R (1984) Resection of acquired tracheal stenosis in childhood. J Thorac Cardiovasc Surg 87:547–549
2. Backer CL, Mavroudis C, Gerber M, et al (2001) Tracheal surgery in children: an 18-year review of four techniques. Eur J Cardiothorac Surg 19:777–784
3. Bando K, Turrentine MW, Sun K, et al (1996) Anterior pericardial tracheoplasty for tracheal stenosis: Intermediate to long term out comes. Ann Thorac Surg 62:981–989

4. Brown SB, Hedlund GL, Glasier CM, et al (1987) Tracheo-bronchial stenosis in infants: successful balloon dilatation therapy. Radiology 164:475–478

5. Burke AJ, Vining DJ, McGuirt WJ, et al: (2000) Evaluation of airway obstruction using virtual endoscopy. Laryngoscope 110:23–29

6. Cantrel JR, Guild HC (1964) Congenital stenosis of the trachea. Am J Surg 108:297–305

7. Couraud L, Moreau JM, Velly JF (1990) The growth of circumferential scars of the major airways from infancy to adulthood. Eur J Cardiothoracic Surg 4:521–526

8. Dayan SH, Dunham ME, Backer CL, et al (1997) Slide tracheoplasty in the management of congenital tracheal stenosis. Ann Otol Rhinol Laryngol 106:914–919

9. Dodge-Khatami A, Nijdam NC, Broekhuis E, et al (2002) Carotid artery patch plasty as a last resort repair for long segment congenital tracheal stenosis. J Thorac Cardiovasc Surg 123:826–828

10. Elliott M, Roebuck D, Noctor C, et al (2003) The management of congenital tracheal stenosis. Int J Pediatr Otorhinolaryngol 67S1:S183–192

11. Elliott MJ, Haw MP, Jacobs JP, et al (1996) Tracheal reconstruction in children using cadaveric homograft trachea. Eur J Cardiothoracic Surg 10:707–712

12. Essouri S, Nicot F, Clément A, et al (2005) Non invasive positive pressure ventilation in infants with upper airway obstruction: comparison of continuous and bilevel positive pressure. Intensive Care Med 31:574–580

13. Filler RM, Forte V, Chait P (1998) Tracheobronchial stenting for the treatment of airway obstruction. J Pediatr Surg 33:304–311

14. Fiore AC, Brown JW, Weber TR, et al (2005) Surgical treatment of pulmonary artery sling and tracheal stenosis. Ann Thorac Surg 79:38–46

15. Friedman E, Perez-Atayde AR, Silvera M, et al (1990) Growth of tracheal anastomoses in lambs. Comparison of PDS and Vicryl suture material and interrupted and continuous techniques. J Thorac Cardiovasc Surg 100:188–193

16. Garabédian EN, Denoyelle F, Grimfeld A, et al (1990) Indication of the carbon dioxide laser in tracheobronchial pathology of the infant and young child: 14 cases. Laryngoscope 100:1225–1228

17. Garabedian EN, Le Bret E, Corre A, et al (2001) Tracheal resection associated with slide tracheoplasty for long segment congenital tracheal stenosis involving the carina. J Thorac Cardiovasc Surg 121:393–395

18. Goldman AP, Macrae DJ, Edberg KE, et al (1996) Extracorporeal membrane oxygenation (ECMO) as a bridge to definitive tracheal surgery in children. J Pediatr 128:386–388

19. Grillo HC (1994) Slide tracheoplasty for long segment congenital tracheal stenosis. Ann Thorac Surg 58:613–621

20. Grillo HC (2004a) Congenital and acquired tracheal lesions in children. In: Grillo HC (ed) Surgery of the Trachea and Bronchi. Decker, Hamilton, Ontario, Canada, pp 173–206

21. Grillo HC (2004b) Tracheal reconstruction. In: Grillo HC (ed), Surgery of the trachea and bronchi. Decker, Hamilton, Ontario, Canada, pp 665–680

22. Grillo HC, Donahue DM, Mathisen DJ, et al (1995) Postintubation tracheal stenosis. Treatment and results. J Thorac Cardiovasc Surg 109:486–493

23. Idriss FS, Deleon SY, Ilbawy MN, et al (1984) Tracheoplasty with pericardial patch for extensive tracheal stenosis in infants and children. J Thorac Cardiovasc Surg 88:527–536

24. Islam S, Masiakos PT, Doody DP, et al (2001) Tracheal resection and reanastomosis in the neonatal period. J Pediatr Surg 36:1262–1265

25. Jacobs JP, Haw MP, Motbey JA, et al (1996) Successful complete tracheal resection in a three month infant. Ann Thorac Surg 61:1824–1827

26. Jacobs JP, Quintessenza JA, Botero LM, et al (2000) The role of airway stents in the management of pediatric tracheal, carinal and bronchial disease. Eur J Cardiothorac Surg 18:505–512

27. Jaffe RB (1997) Balloon dilatation of congenital and acquired stenosis of the trachea and bronchi. Radiology 203:405–409

28. Kutlu CA, Goldstraw P (1999) Slide tracheoplasty for congenital funnel-shaped tracheal stenosis (a 9-year follow-up of the first case) Eur J Cardiothorac Surg 16:98–99

29. E. Le Bret, E.N. Garabedian, N. Teissier, E. Belli, N. Gharbi, J. Bruniaux, R. Roussin, A. Sigal-Cinqualbre, A. Serraf. Slide Crico-Tracheoplasty in infant. J Thorac Cardiovasc Surg 2006;132:179–80

30. E. Le Bret, E.N. Garabedian, N. Teissier, E. Belli, N. Gharbi, J. Bruniaux, R. Roussin, A. Sigal-Cinqualbre, A. Serraf. Slide Tracheo-Bronchoplasty in infant. J Thorac Cardiovasc Surg 2006;132:181–3

31. E. Le Bret, N Teissier, E Belli, A Sigal-Cinqualbre, V. Couloignier, P Narcy S Demontoux, N Gharbi, R Roussin, T Vanden Abbeele, A Serraf,. Slide tracheoplasty in presence of tracheal bronchus in infant. J Thorac Cardiovasc Surg 2006;132:e15–6

32. Longaker MT, Harrison MR, Adzick S (1990) Testing the limits of neonatal tracheal resection. J Pediatr Surg 25:790–792

33. Loubakov T, Sebening C, Springer W, et al (2004) A case of Pulmonary artery sling associated with long-segment funnel trachea and bronchus suis. Ann Thorac Surg 78:1839–1842

34. Macchiarini P, Dulmet E, de Montpreville V, et al (1997) Tracheal growth after slide tracheoplasty. J Thorac Cardiovasc Surg 113:558–566

35. Maeda K, Yasufuku M, Yamamoto T (2000) A new approach to the treatment of congenital tracheal stenosis: balloon tracheoplasty and expandable metallic stenting. J Pediatr Surg 36:1646–1649

36. Majeski JA, Schreiber JT, Cotton R, et al (1980) Tracheoplasty for tracheal stenosis in the pediatric burned patient. J Trauma 20:81–86

26

37. Martinod E, Seguin A, Holder-Espinasse M, et al (2005) Tracheal regeneration following tracheal replacement with an allogenic aorta. Ann Thorac Surg 79:942–949

38. Matute JA, Romero R, Garcia-Casillas MA, et al (2001) Surgical approach to funnel shape congenital tracheal stenosis. J Pediatr Surg 36:320–323

39. Othersen HB, Hebra A, Tagge EP (2000) A new method of treatment for complete tracheal rings in an infant: endoscopic laser division and balloon dilatation. J Pediatr Surg 35:262–264

40. Pashley N, Jaskumas JM, Waldstein G (1984) Laryngotracheoplasty with costochondral grafts – a clinical correlate of graft survival. Laryngoscope 94:1493–1496

41. Tsang V, Murday A, Gilbe C, Goldstraw P (1989) Slide tracheoplasty for congenital funnel shaped tracheal stenosis. Ann Thorac Surg 48:632–635

42. Tsugawa C, Nishijiwa E, Muraji T, et al (2003) Tracheoplasty for long segment congenital tracheal stenosis: analysis of 29 patients over two decades. J Pediatr Surg 38:1703–1706

43. Ward RF (1992) Treatment of tracheal and endobronchial lesions with the potassium titanyl phosphate laser. Ann Otol Rhinol Laryngol 101:205–208

44. Weber TR, Connors RH, Tracy TF (1991) Acquired tracheal stenosis in infants and children. J Thorac Cardiovasc Surg 102:29–35

45. Wright CG, Graham BB, Grillo HC, et al (2002) Pediatric tracheal surgery. Ann Thorac Surg 74:308–314

Chapter 27

Tracheomalacia in Children

27

Jean-Michel Triglia, Richard Nicollas and Stephane Roman

Core Messages

- Tracheomalacia usually presents in the 1st year of life: 60% by the age of 3 months.
- Commonly, the child with tracheomalacia has breathing difficulty, with some or all of the following: stridor, wheezing, recurrent chest infections, dyspnoea at rest, apnoeic episodes.
- Definitive diagnosis is by tracheobronchoscopy with spontaneous respiration, if possible. The diagnostic finding is of 50% collapse of the lumen of the trachea during expiration.
- Magnetic resonance imaging is the imaging method of choice.
- Tracheomalacia may be associated with other airway anomalies, such as laryngomalacia, tracheal cleft or stenosis and tracheo-oesophageal fistula (TOF).
- Primary tracheomalacia occurs when there is failure of the tracheal rings to fully develop. It may occur after premature birth and after prolonged tracheal intubation and ventilation. Severe cases may be part of a complex congenital malformation syndrome.
- Secondary tracheomalacia is related to extrinsic abnormalities such as oesophageal atresia and TOF, cardiovascular abnormalities compressing the trachea, and tumours in the neck and mediastinum.
- Mild forms of primary tracheomalacia may be managed conservatively. Aortopexy is used for severe localised tracheomalacia affecting the distal trachea. Stents have been used, but are technically difficult to manage and have well-described complications. Biphasic positive airway pressure during spontaneous respiration is an effective alternative treatment.
- Tracheomalacia secondary to oesophageal abnormalities may respond to medical treatment and control of gastro-oesophageal reflux. Aortopexy is needed in severe cases.
- Secondary tracheomalacia from external vascular compression is treated by dealing with the cause of compression; however, after relief of the compression, the trachea may take months or years to achieve adequate rigidity.

Contents

Introduction

Tracheomalacia is a condition that is characterised by weakness of the cartilages supporting the trachea. It is usually suspected when endoscopy shows tracheal collapse with greater than 50% tracheal obstruction during expiration (Benjamin 1984). Two anomalies account for these findings: weakness of the tracheal wall resulting from reduction of the ratio between the cartilaginous rings and posterior transverse muscle, and hypotonia of the posterior transverse muscle, resulting in forward ballooning, especially during expiration. Tracheomalacia can be classified as primary and secondary. In secondary tracheomalacia, lesions are usually limited to one segment, whereas primary tracheomalacia (tracheal dyskinesia) extends for the entire length of the airway (see Table 27.1).

In everyday clinical practice, otolaryngologists are frequently called on to evaluate noisy respiration or dyspnoea for which tracheomalacia is a possible aetiology. Diagnosis of tracheomalacia depends on interpretation of a variety of findings including: (1) occurrence of characteristic clinical symptoms in relation to age, (2) detection of compatible radiological features, using standard techniques such as plain anterior and lateral chest x-rays and barium swallow studies, and (3) outcome of thorough

Table 27.1 Classification of tracheomalacia

*Primary tracheomalacia
Tracheal dyskinesia (inadequate development of tracheal rings)
*Secondary tracheomalacia (extrinsic causes)
Oesophageal atresia with or without tracheo-oesophageal fistula
Compression by cardiovascular structures
Complete rings (double aortic arch, Neuhauser anomaly)
Incomplete rings (innominate artery, retro-oesophageal right subclavian artery, aberrant left pulmonary artery)
Compression by cardiac structures (dilatation of the pulmonary arteries and/or left atrium)
Compression by cervical and mediastinal tumours

endoscopic examination of the trachea, bronchi and oesophagus. Management of tracheomalacia also requires the combined skills of a multidisciplinary team including paediatricians, radiologists, cardiothoracic surgeons and otolaryngologists.

Clinical Manifestations

The clinical manifestations of tracheomalacia usually appear during the 1st year of life. The delay before appearance is 3 months in 60% of cases and between 3 and 12 months in the remaining 40%. Later occurrence is sometimes observed during respiratory tract infection. The exact nature, intensity and timing of symptoms depend on the location, length, extent and cause of the tracheal narrowing. The most common clinical manifestations of tracheomalacia involve breathing difficulties with abnormal breathing noises such as stridor or wheezing, recurrent bronchitis, chronic cough, acute apnoea associated with blue spells, dyspnoea at rest and with hyperextension of the head and neck.

The natural course of tracheomalacia is characterised by recurrent respiratory problems. Symptoms usually resolve on their own before 2 years of age (McNamara and Crabbe 2004) and endoscopically detectable expiratory collapse may disappear completely, regardless of its initial severity. Prognosis also depends on whether there are associated abnormalities and on the anatomic cause of tracheal collapse.

Investigations

Endoscopy is the definitive diagnostic procedure. It should begin by careful fibre-scopic inspection of the supraglottic and glottic area without anaesthesia. This inspection should be followed by tracheobronchoscopy and oesophagoscopy under general anaesthesia, with spontaneous breathing whenever possible. Tracheobronchoscopy identifies the extent of tracheal collapse and allows planning of subsequent management. Based on the length of the lesion and its position in relation to the sides of the trachea and to the carina, as determined by endoscopy, it is often possible to assess the aetiology (see Fig. 27.1). Oesophagoscopy is a useful adjunct to tracheobronchoscopy to detect the presence of vascular anomalies located behind the oesophagus or between the trachea and oesophagus. Endoscopic examination also allows the detection of associated airway abnormalities such as laryngomalacia, tracheal cleft, tracheal stenosis and tracheo-oesophageal fistula (TOF).

Lateral chest x-rays and barium swallow studies can sometimes be carried out before endoscopy in order to facilitate diagnosis. However, further radiological assessment will be needed after endoscopy either to confirm the diagnosis in difficult cases, such as vascular rings, or to prepare for surgical treatment. Arteriography has been supplanted by digital subtraction angiography or magnetic resonance imaging (MRI), which are now the routine investigations (Faust et al. 2002; Triglia et al. 1994). In addition to being non-invasive, MRI is the procedure of choice to assess the degree of airway compression, to study the relationship between the airways and the cardiovascular structures, and to identify the underlying abnormality.

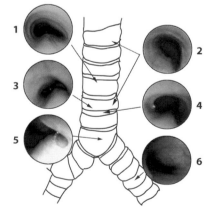

Fig. 27.1 Endoscopic views showing six different causes of extrinsic tracheal compression. *1* Innominate artery, *2* neuroblastoma (tumour compression), *3* double aortic arch, *4* Neuhauser anomaly, *5* aberrant left pulmonary artery, *6* left atrium

27

Aetiology of Tracheomalacia

Primary Tracheomalacia

Primary tracheomalacia, or tracheal dyskinesia, results from excessive expiratory reduction of the tracheal calibre, causing respiratory compromise and limiting the effectiveness of coughing in clearing secretions. Many aspects of the aetiology of primary tracheomalacia remain unclear. Isolated tracheal dyskinesia is often observed in association with premature birth and delayed neuronal maturation. It has been attributed to an intrinsic abnormality of the cartilage, resulting in failure of the tracheal rings to develop completely. Severe tracheal dyskinesia is generally part of a more complex congenital malformation syndrome such as Larsen syndrome, dyschondroplasia and median line syndrome. According to Waillo and Emery (1980), the occurrence of a symptom-free interval between birth and initial symptoms suggests that tracheomalacia is acquired. Many such cases are observed in children who have undergone long-term endotracheal intubation or tracheostomy. It can be speculated that deterioration of the fibro-cartilaginous components of the tracheal wall is induced by metaplasia due to chronic inflammation. Prolonged ventilation and gastro-oesophageal reflux could be exacerbating factors.

Management depends upon the severity of symptoms. Mild forms of tracheomalacia can be managed using appropriate conservative measures including chest physiotherapy, treatment of gastro-oesophageal reflux and prophylactic antimicrobial therapy. For severe localised tracheomalacia affecting the distal trachea, aortopexy appears to be the treatment of choice. The goal of aortopexy is to relieve airway compression by suspending the aortic arch from the undersurface of the sternum. For severe generalised tracheomalacia or tracheomalacia involving the upper airway, tracheostomy is necessary to support the airway until the trachea achieves the necessary rigidity. Placement of indwelling endotracheal stents demands great technical experience on the part of the practitioner (Furman et al. 1999). Both self-expanding or balloon-expandable stents can be used. A frequent and serious complication of stenting is airway obstruction due to the formation of granulation tissue. Another drawback of stenting is that the devices are difficult to reposition and remove. In most cases, aortopexy remains conceptually simple and safer in comparison with stenting (Valerie et al. 2005). However, this could change in the future with the introduction of biodegradable stents, which would avoid the need for removal and might prevent the formation of granulation tissue (Sewall et al. 2003). Another alternative to surgical treatment is spontaneous ventilation with biphasic positive airway pressure (BIPAP) to limit airway collapse by maintaining continuous positive airway pressure (Essouri et al. 2005).

Secondary Tracheomalacia

Secondary tracheomalacia is due to abnormalities outside the trachea such as oesophageal atresia with or without TOF, vascular or cardiac malformations and mediastinal masses.

Oesophageal Atresia and TOF

Tracheomalacia has been reported in more than 60% of cases of oesophageal atresia (Benjamin et al. 1976; Briganti et al. 2005; Triglia et al. 1994). It can involve the entire length or only one segment of the trachea. As it is generally a component of a congenital malformation syndrome, tracheomalacia is considered as a congenital disorder (Benjamin et al. 1976). In this regard, it is similar to tracheal dyskinesia. Numerous studies on infants with oesophageal atresia have confirmed the existence of malformations involving not only tracheal rings, but also the posterior transverse muscle. Wailoo and Emery (1979) described two defects: enlargement of the cartilaginous rings, producing a half-circle shape instead of the typical horseshoe shape, and an increase in the width of the posterior transverse muscle, resulting in forward ballooning of the posterior tracheal wall. The result of these two defects is to increase the internal tracheal circumference, leading to collapse of the lumen. The ratio between the cartilaginous rings and posterior transverse muscle decreases from 4:1 in normal children to 3:2 or 3:1 in children with oesophageal atresia. The weakened trachea is subject to compression from behind by a dilated oesophagus, or from the front by the innominate artery or aortic arch. Recent experimental studies showed that a teratogenic process could lead to oesophageal atresia by disrupting the structure of the tracheal cartilage (Pole et al. 2001)

Respiratory manifestations include reflux apnoea, which may occur during feeding or after meals. Recurrent lower airway infection has also been observed. Medical treatment can be used in milder cases. In severe forms, aortopexy can prevent collapse of the tracheal lumen, but better results can be obtained in combination with fundoplication to treat associated gastro-oesophageal reflux (Nasr et al. 2005).

Tracheal Compression due to Cardiovascular Malformations

Malformations resulting in compression of the trachea by cardiovascular structures are rare. Tracheomalacia caused by such malformations is classified as secondary and is located at the site of extrinsic compression. The goal of management is to relieve external compression. However, relief of compression following surgery does not lead to immediate resolution of symptoms. Several months and even years may be necessary for the trachea to achieve adequate rigidity.

Vascular rings have been classified as complete (encircling) or incomplete (non-encircling) (Triglia et al. 1999). They account for 38% of vessel-related airway compression. Complete forms include double aortic arch (DAA), Neuhauser anomaly (right aortic arch with a left ligamentum arteriosum) and their variants. These lesions are present at birth. Stridor and dyspnoea are the most prominent symptoms and worsen during feeding. The frequency of dysphagia, apnoeic episodes and respiratory infection increases with age. Endoscopy reveals pulsatile compression of the left anterolateral and right posterolateral sides of the distal trachea, which in some cases is associated with compression of the right main-stem bronchus. Barium swallow shows indentation on the right and, to a lesser degree, left wall on anterior–posterior view and severe posterior compression on lateral views. MRI confirms diagnosis and allows differentiation between DAA and Neuhauser anomaly. Surgical reconstruction is mandatory. In case of DAA, division of the smaller of the two arches (usually on the left), with division of the ligamentum arteriosum relieves tracheal obstruction. In case of Neuhauser anomaly, treatment consists of division of the ligamentum arteriosum.

Incomplete vascular rings include anomalies of the innominate artery and aortic arch, right retro-oesophageal subclavian arteries (lusoria) and aberrant left pulmonary arteries.

In patients with innominate artery compression syndrome (36% of vessel-related airway compression), tracheobronchoscopic examination usually reveals pulsatile compression of the right anterolateral side of the distal trachea. Pushing the bronchoscope against the compressed zone causes a decrease in the right radial and temporal pulse. In most cases, symptoms gradually regress and disappear within a few months to years. In severe forms, MRI allows accurate location of the innominate artery prior to aortopexy to correct tracheal collapse (Triglia et al. 1994).

Compression due to a retro-oesophageal right subclavian artery accounts for 17% of vessel-related airway compression. It is not usually associated with respiratory symptoms. Dysphagia is the most common presenting symptom and may require surgical treatment in severe cases. Diagnosis can be suspected by barium swallow study and confirmed by oesophagoscopy, revealing compression of the posterior side of the distal oesophagus.

Aberrant left pulmonary artery syndrome (3% of vessel-related airway compressions) is a rare anomaly that is present from birth and produces severe respiratory distress. The left pulmonary artery originates from the proximal segment of the right pulmonary artery and passes between the oesophagus and the trachea. A barium swallow study reveals an indentation on the anterior wall of the oesophagus above the carina. Surgical correction with reimplantation of the pulmonary artery is required. Management of this malformation must include measures to detect and, if necessary, correct associated tracheal stenosis.

Compression due to intracardiac defects usually involves the left main bronchus. The underlying mechanism is related to dilatation of the pulmonary arteries and/or left atrium. Any cardiac disease causing left-to-right shunting can lead to this type of compression. The most common presenting symptoms are recurrent respiratory infection, bronchial atelectasis, and obstructive emphysema. Bronchoscopy reveals compression of the anterior and lower walls of the left main bronchus.

Tracheal Compression due to Cervical and Mediastinal Tumours

Tracheomalacia due to extrinsic tumour compression comprises a heterogeneous group including congenital, benign and malignant tumours (see Chapter 12), requiring careful evaluation by computed tomography and MRI.

Teratoma is the most common benign anterior mediastinal tumour. It is usually present at birth and leads to severe respiratory distress. Surgical treatment is required. Cystic lymphangioma is a dysembryoplasia of the lymphatic system. Clinical manifestations appear during the newborn period in 50% of cases and before the age of 2 years in 90% of cases. Rapid growth of the tumour during an infectious episode or intracystic bleeding can lead to acute respiratory distress. Tracheal compression is often associated with involvement of the larynx, oropharynx and tongue.

Bronchogenic cysts are the most common benign tumours of the middle mediastinum. They are the result of supernumerary tracheal budding and correspond to an advanced form of tracheal diverticulum if the cyst loses contact with the trachea. Bronchogenic cysts can vary in size from a few millimetres to several centimetres. After an asymptomatic phase, rapid expansion due to intracystic bleeding can lead to acute respiratory distress. Endoscopic examination reveals smooth, nonpulsatile compression of the trachea. Surgical treatment is required.

Malignant tumours usually cause respiratory and systemic manifestations with nerve and vein compression and haematological disorders. Hodgkin and non-Hodgkin lymphomas are the most common malignant tumours of the anterior and middle mediastinum. Rhabdomyosarcomas are tumours of the middle mediastinum. Neuroblastomas are the most common malignant tumours of the posterior mediastinum, often occurring before the age of 2 years.

Summary for the Clinician

- The clinical manifestations of tracheomalacia are mainly respiratory and usually appear during the 1st year of life. Tracheobronchoscopy with spontaneous ventilation shows collapse of the trachea with more than 50% obstruction of the lumen during expiration, and allows differentiation between primary tracheomalacia (tracheal dyskinesia) and secondary tracheomalacia. Moderate forms of primary tracheomalacia respond well to conservative treatment including physiotherapy. For severe forms, BIPAP can prevent tracheal collapse during expiration and is a good alternative to surgical treatment. Most cases of secondary tracheomalacia are due to extrinsic compression by cardiovascular structures and mediastinal tumours. The goal of management is to relieve extrinsic compression.

References

1. Benjamin B, Cohen D, Glasson M (1976) Tracheomalacia in association with congenital tracheo-oesophageal fistula. Surgery 79:504–508
2. Benjamin B (1984) Tracheomalacia in infants and children. Ann Otol Rhinol Laryngol 93:438–432
3. Briganti V, Oriolo L, Buffa V, et al (2005) Tracheomalacia in oesophageal atresia: morphological considerations by endoscopic and CT study. Eur J Cardiothorac Surg 28:11–15
4. Essouri S, Nicot F, Clement A, et al (2005) Noninvasive positive pressure ventilation in infants with upper airway obstruction: comparison of continuous and bi-level positive pressure. Intensive Care Med 31:574–580
5. Faust RA, Rimell FL, Remley KB (2002) Magnetic resonance imaging for evaluation of focal tracheomalacia: innominate artery compression syndrome. Int J Pediatr Otorhinolaryngol 65:27–33
6. Furman RH, Backer CL, Dunham ME, Donaldson, et al (1999) The use of balloon-expandable metallic stents in the treatment of pediatric tracheomalacia and bronchomalacia. Arch Otolaryngol Head Neck Surg 125:203–207
7. McNamara VM, Crabbe DC (2004) Tracheomalacia. Paediatr Respir Rev 5:147–154
8. Nasr A, Eian SH, Gerstle JT (2005) Infants with repaired esophageal atresia and distal tracheoesophageal fistula with severe respiratory distress: is it tracheomalacia, reflux, or both? Pediatr Surg 40:901–903
9. Pole RJ, Qi BQ, Beasley SW (2001) Abnormalities of the tracheal cartilage in the rat fetus with tracheo-oesophageal fistula or tracheal agenesis. Pediatr Surg Int 17:25–28
10. Sewall GK, Warner T, Connor NP (2003) Comparison of resorbable poly-L-lactic acid-polyglycolic acid and internal Palmaz stents for the surgical correction of severe tracheomalacia. Ann Otol Rhinol Laryngol 112:515–521
11. Triglia JM, Guys JM, Louis-Borrione C (1994) Tracheomalacia caused by arterial compression in esophageal atresia. Ann Otol Rhinol Laryngol 103:516–521
12. Triglia JM, Nicollas R, Roman S, et al (1999) Tracheal compression due to blood vessel or cardiac birth defects. Ann Pediatr 46:87–93
13. Valerie E, Durrant AC, Forte V, et al (2005) A decade of using intraluminal tracheal/bronchial stents in the management of tracheomalacia and/or bronchomalacia: is it better than aortopexy? J Pediatr Surg 40:904–947
14. Wailoo M, Emery JL (1980) The trachea in children with respiratory diseases including children presenting as cot deaths. Arch Dis Child 55:199–203
15. Wailoo M, Emery JL (1979) The trachea in children with tracheo-oesophageal fistula. Histopathology 3:329–338

Tracheostomy: an Ancient Life Saver Due for Retirement, or Vital Aid in Modern Airway Surgery?

28

Hans L. J. Hoeve

Core Messages

- Nowadays, the most important indications for a tracheotomy are chronic airway obstruction and long-term ventilation.
- A vertical tracheal incision is preferred to the excision of a window or a Björk flap because of the risk of a tracheal stenosis.
- Infants and children with a tracheostomy need constant observation and monitoring.
- Children with a tracheostomy can be safely managed at home, provided the parents have been fully trained, the necessary equipment is present and immediate contact with the hospital is guaranteed.
- Unsuccessful decannulation necessitates endoscopic evaluation of the airway, especially the suprastomal region.

Contents

Introduction

In this chapter, the following are discussed: the changing indications for tracheotomy, the changing nature of the population of children with a tracheotomy, alternatives to a tracheotomy, the surgical technique and its complications, home care of a child with a tracheostomy, and how to decannulate a child.

Definitions

Tracheotomy refers to the operation meant to create direct access to the trachea, whereas a tracheostomy is the opening in the trachea (tracheotomy is cutting into the trachea; tracheostomy is the formation of a stoma). Often these terms are used interchangeably.

Indications

Indications for tracheotomy have changed more during the last five decades than during the many centuries following its first description. The major indication for a tracheotomy until halfway through the previous century was acute airway obstruction by infections, such as diphtheria, laryngotracheobronchitis, epiglottitis, bacterial tracheitis or by an aspirated foreign body. (Arcand and Granger 1988; Carter and Benjamin 1983; Crysdale et al. 1988; MacRae et al. 1984). With the introduction of vaccination programs in the developed world, diseases such as diphtheria, and later epiglottitis, have virtually disappeared.

Improvements in anaesthesia and in airway endoscopy equipment have allowed physicians to visualise the airway. This has enabled them to introduce safely an orotracheal tube or remove a foreign body from the larynx or more distal airways. Laryngeal intubation became an attractive alternative for tracheotomy. Intubated children could be looked after safely, and even artificially ventilated if necessary, in intensive care units. The enormous progress in medicine in general, and in paediatric intensive care in particular, so beneficial to children suffering from an infectious airway obstruction, had unforeseen benefit for other groups of children. Premature infants with respiratory distress syndrome, infants with craniofacial malformations (and airway obstruction), or infants with complex congenital disorders, could now often be treated and survive, although some with severe complications. Children with neuromuscular or respiratory diseases were treated with long-term assisted ventilation. Many of these infants were intubated, but needed a tracheotomy to prevent or treat laryngeal damage caused by the tube.

During the last two decades, tracheotomies have been performed on younger children. Sixty-three percent of the children in a study by Ang et al. (2005) and 44–63% in a literature study by Kremer et al. (2002) were less than 1 year old at the time of their tracheotomy.

The average duration of a tracheostomy is nowadays expressed in years, compared with a few weeks in the 1960s and 1970s (Palmer et al. 1995; Wetmore et al. 1999).

The great effect that changes in medical and surgical therapy had on the indications for tracheotomy is less apparent in the numbers of operations. Some authors report a decrease, others an increase in numbers (Arcand and Granger 1998; Crysdale et al. 1988; Palmer et al. 1995).

The most recent study of a rather small group of children mentions assisted ventilation as the most important (54%) indication for a tracheotomy. Chronic airway obstruction, such as bilateral vocal cord paralysis, craniofacial malformation, laryngeal or tracheal stenosis and tumours, constituted 40% of the indications. The remaining 6% of the patients needed a tracheotomy for pulmonary toilet (Ang et al. 2005).

The tracheotomy has evolved from an urgent solution to an acute airway obstruction into a procedure contributing to the treatment of a chronic disorder. The most frequent present indications for a tracheotomy are presented in Table 28.1.

Table 28.1 Indications for tracheotomy

Airway obstruction	Craniofacial malformation
	Acquired laryngeal stenosis (intubation)
	Bilateral vocal cord paralysis
	Lymphangioma
	Congenital laryngeal stenosis
	Tracheomalacia
	Laryngotracheo-oesophageal cleft
Artificial ventilation	Respiratory distress syndrome
	Neuromuscular disease
	Central nervous system disorder ("Ondine's curse")
Pulmonary toilet	Chronic aspiration in neurologic disorders

Alternatives to Tracheotomy

Intubation has replaced the tracheostomy for acute infectious airway obstruction. Epiglottitis, viral laryngotracheitis and pharyngeal abscess are managed with intubation instead of a tracheotomy. Children in whom the airway has to be secured for a short period after maxillofacial surgery are treated with intubation rather than with a tracheotomy.

Premature babies on artificial ventilation are often intubated for longer periods. They are thought to tolerate intubation better than older infants and children, who should undergo tracheotomy if intubation would last more than a few weeks. Nevertheless, premature babies all too often develop laryngeal injury from intubation, which could have been prevented by an early tracheotomy. It may be that in prolonged artificial ventilation, the scales have tipped too much towards intubation. Premature infants and older children on prolonged intubation may develop laryngeal oedema and granulation tissue, which may impede extubation. Various treatment options are available to manage this condition: prolonged intubation and endoscopic treatment, application of mitomycin, anterior cricoid split and single-stage laryngoplasty. If such a treatment is successful, which is certainly not always the case, a tracheotomy can be avoided. Even for an experienced endoscopist, it is difficult to decide under which circumstances laryngeal injury will heal without leaving too much scar tissue, and when to settle for a tracheotomy.

Obstructive sleep apnoea syndrome is seen frequently in children with a craniofacial malformation. Recently introduced surgical techniques such as distraction osteogenesis of the mandible or the midface may help to relieve the airway obstruction. These children are operated at an earlier age, thereby avoiding the need for a (long-term) tracheostomy in several cases. Other treatment modalities are a nasopharyngeal airway, continuous positive airway pressure, hyoid suspension or tongue-lip adhesion.

The fibre-optic bronchoscope has become an indispensable tool to aid in the intubation of children with micrognathia or macroglossia, as seen in craniofacial syndromes or in mucopolysaccharidosis.

The Technique of Tracheotomy

The classic tracheotomy begins with a vertical or horizontal skin incision. The vertical incision, which allows the tracheostomy tube to find a neutral position in the tracheal lumen, seems to have lost ground to the horizontal incision, which leaves a better scar. The trachea is entered through a vertical incision of two tracheal rings (usually the second and third, or third and fourth). Usually, the trachea is incised vertically, without excision of the cartilage. A horizontal incision between tracheal rings has the same advantage, but is not much used. An inferiorly based flap (the Björk flap) is advocated by some because it facilitates reinsertion of an accidentally dislodged tracheostomy tube.

A frequent serious complication, especially in growing children, is tracheomalacia or stenosis at the tracheostomy site when the tracheostomy is no longer needed (Kremer et al. 2002). For this reason, the creation of a tracheal window is generally avoided, because of the loss of cartilage support and subsequent stenosis or malacia. MacRae et al. (1984) report, in a study of 93 children, no difference in complications after various tracheal incisions (vertical, horizontal and excision of a window), but the follow-up period is not clear and the mortality rate (22.5%) high.

Fry et al. (1985), in their often-cited study on young, growing ferrets, report on the frequency of complications after three different incisions: an inferiorly based flap, a vertical incision and a 90° tilted H. The tracheas that were vertically incised had a lower air flow resistance than the tracheas with an H incision or a flap.

Maturation of the tracheostomy canal, by stitching the edges of the tracheal incision to the vertically incised skin after removal of subcutaneous fat, is common practice in several hospitals and in various countries. It promotes rapid wound healing and provides an easy access to the tracheal lumen if the tube is dislodged during the first post-operative days. A disadvantage could be the more frequent occurrence of a tracheocutaneous fistula.

The starplasty, described by Koltai (1998), is intended to produce an epithelium-lined tracheostomy immediately after the procedure. Both the skin and the trachea are incised crosswise, the skin at an angle of 45° to the trachea. The tracheal flaps are stitched to the skin flaps. This technique facilitates insertion of the tube, prevents subcutaneous emphysema and should diminish infection of the tracheostomy and even tracheal stenosis.

In adult patients, the classic tracheotomy has been partly replaced by the percutaneous techniques introduced by Ciaglia et al. in 1985. This percutaneous dilatation technique requires the introduction of a catheter into the trachea, dilatation of the tissues and introduction of the tracheostomy tube. The procedure has been developed for adult patients and not for children. Several other authors warn against percutaneous techniques in children, because of the risk of missing the trachea, entering the oesophagus or development of a tracheal stenosis (Scott et al. 1998; Warren 2000).

For the moment, these blind techniques are ill advised in young children. The cartilage framework is still soft and pliable, and the trachea is not always easily palpated. Missing the trachea, puncturing the posterior wall, or entering the larynx, is certainly not excluded, even in experienced hands. Because general anaesthesia remains necessary, the percutaneous procedure does not seem to be faster or cheaper than a classic tracheotomy. Use of the rigid endoscope makes the procedure probably safer, but also more elaborate.

Complications

Complications occurring after a tracheotomy are listed in Table 28.2, divided into complications of the operation, complications related to the presence of a tracheostomy and complications that become manifest after decannulation. Complication rates of more than 50% or even 60% are reported (Kremer et al. 2002).

Complications of a Tracheotomy

During the operation, the anterior laryngeal or tracheal wall may be damaged, usually behind the thyroid isthmus. Other complications are haemorrhage, accidental decannulation and, rarely, damage of the posterior tracheal wall. In the post-operative period, pneumomediastinum, pneumothorax, subcutaneous emphysema, haemorrhage, wound infection, breakdown of the skin and occlusion or dislodgement of the tube may occur. All of these complications, with exception of those related to the tracheostomy tube, are directly related to the operation, and do not occur later.

Table 28.2 Complications associated with tracheotomy and tracheostomy. *PDT* Percutaneous dilatation technique

Complications of tracheotomy	Damage to anterior wall larynx or trachea
	Damage to posterior tracheal wall (PDT)
	Accidental decannulation
	Haemorrhage
	Subcutaneous emphysema
	Pneumothorax
	Pneumomediastinum
	Wound infection
Complications of tracheostomy	Granulations stoma, trachea
	Suprastomal tracheal collapse
	Infection stoma trachea, lower airways, pneumonia
	Tracheostomy tube obstruction
	Accidental decannulation
	Failure to reintroduce the tracheostomy tube
	Aspiration
	Retarded psychomotor development
	Speech retardation
Complications manifest after decannulation	Tracheomalacia at tracheostomy site
	Stenosis at the tracheostomy site
	Tracheocutaneous fistula

Complications of a Tracheostomy

The consequences of having a tracheostomy and a foreign body inserted into the airway are many. The functions of the upper airway, voice, conditioning the inspired air, and protection against infection, are largely lost. Furthermore, the tracheostomy tube itself has its effect on the canal and the trachea. Granulations and suprastomal collapse are the consequence of mechanical pressure by a foreign body in combination with infection. Pneumonia, lower-airway infections and tracheitis occur frequently because of loss of the protective function of the upper airway. Development of speech is possible in most children, but is often retarded, as the child has to learn to direct airflow through the larynx (Kaslon and Stein 1985). Aspiration is a rather frequently observed complication. It is often silent, but may become manifest when coloured secretions are suctioned from the tracheostomy tube after feeding. Insufficient closure of the laryngeal entrance may be caused by mechanical factors related to the tracheostomy (impeded mobility of the larynx by the presence of the tube) or to the reason for the tracheostomy, such as laryngeal injury after intubation, or a neurological disorder.

The most dramatic complication of a tracheostomy is obstruction by an occluded or dislodged tube. Despite adequate nursing care, training of caregivers and monitoring, the tracheostomy-related mortality is as high as 3.4% (Dutton et al. 1995). Causes are tube obstruction, accidental decannulation and haemorrhage.

Some complications of a tracheostomy will have consequences only after decannulation. Tracheomalacia at the tracheostomy site is, like tracheal stenosis, caused by several factors such as mechanical pressure of the tube, infection and excision of supporting cartilage. Several treatment options have been proposed for tracheomalacia: endotracheal intubation for a few days, excision of the tracheostomy canal and the suprastomal granuloma, stitching the proximal and distal tracheal rings together, reinforcing the anterior wall, suspending the anterior wall onto the sternum or the adjacent musculature, or a combination of these. The tracheal stenosis may be treated with partial resection or by grafting the anterior tracheal wall. The tracheocutaneous fistula, a frequent complication, is managed by surgical closure.

Types and Sizes of Tracheostomy Tube

The shape of a tracheostomy tube should be simple, as short as possible, but long enough not to become dislodged, well aligned with the tracheal lumen, and with an opening not directed towards the tracheal wall. The material of the tube has to be soft enough to follow the shape of the airway, but firm enough not to kink or collapse. Most tubes for children are made of PVC or silicone. The thickness of the material and the necessarily small diameters do not allow for use of an inner cannula in children. Metal tubes make the use of an inner cannula possible, but are uncomfortable. For this reason they are usually only used in combination with a stent. Virtually all tubes have a standard 13-mm anaesthetic adaptor to connect with a ventilation tube, an artificial nose or a speaking valve.

Some types of tracheostomy tubes are available with and without cuffs. Cuffs are rarely indicated in young children, and have the risk of damaging the tracheal wall. Fenestration of a tube allows for flow of expired air through the larynx, but has disadvantages: the suction

Table 28.3 Types of paediatric tracheostomy tube. *ID* Inner diameter, *OD* outer diameter

Bivona			Portex blue line			Shiley			Tracoe		
ID (mm)	OD (mm)	Length (mm)	ID (mm)	OD (mm)	Length (mm)	ID (mm)	OD (mm)	Length (mm)	ID (mm)	OD (mm)	Length (mm)
2.5	4.0	38							2.5	3.6	32
3.0	4.7	39	3.0	4.2	36	3.0	4.5	39	3.0	4.3	36
3.5	5.3	40	3.5	4.9	39	3.5	5.2	40	3.5	5.0	40
4.0	6.0	41	4.0	5.5	43	4.0	5.9	41	4.0	5.6	44
4.5	6.7	42	4.5	6.2	46	4.5	6.5	42	4.5	6.3	48
5.0	7.3	44	5.0	6.9	50	5.0	7.1	44	5.0	7.0	50
5.5	8.0	46				5.5	7.7	46	5.5	7.6	55
									6.0	8.4	62

Table 23.4 Types of neonatal tracheostomy tube

Bivona			Shiley			Tracoe		
ID (mm)	OD (mm)	Length (mm)	ID (mm)	OD (mm)	Length (mm)	ID (mm)	OD (mm)	Length (mm)
2.5	4.0	30				2.5	3.6	30
3.0	4.7	32	3.0	4.5	30	3.0	4.3	32
3.5	5.3	34	3.5	5.2	32	3.5	5.0	34
4.0	6.0	36	4.0	5.9	34	4.0	5.6	36
			4.5	6.5	36			

catheter stops at the fenestration, breaking or kinking of the tube, and granulation formation.

In Tables 28.3 and 28.4, the diameters and lengths of various types of tracheostomy tubes are shown. Some types of the smaller-sized tubes come in two lengths, the shorter length being used for premature babies.

Tracheostomy Care in the Hospital, an Institution or at Home

A patient with a tracheostomy is in constant danger of airway obstruction. Therefore, well-organised care in a hospital, in another institution or at home, is of vital importance. The American Thoracic Society has published a standard of care for the child with a tracheostomy (Anonymous 2000).

Although young children with a tracheostomy are often monitored with a cardiorespiratory or oxygen saturation monitor, the best monitoring is constant vigilance by a well-trained nurse, parent or other caregiver. Monitors often produce false alarms or will alarm late. Obstruction of the tube by dry secretions may be prevented by humidification of the air, suctioning and regular tube changes. Passive humidifiers (e.g. an "artificial nose") help by leading the air through a filter to maintain a moisturised and warm environment in the trachea and lower airways. Another device that may be used is a nebuliser.

Suctioning serves to remove secretions, but is also a check on the patency of the tube. The frequency of suctioning depends on the volume of secretions, and may vary from a few times to more than a hundred times a day (and night). The generally advised depth of suctioning is as far as the distal end of the tube; further may damage the mucosa.

There is little consensus on the frequency of tube changes. Weekly changes are advised in many institutions, but monthly changes are not uncommon. PVC tubes lose their plasticiser and harden over a few months.

They are best treated as disposables. Silicone tubes can be reused after cleaning and sterilisation. Metal tubes can be cleaned and sterilised virtually indefinitely.

The ties securing the tracheostomy tube around the neck become wet and have to be changed daily. They should be tight enough to prevent decannulation and loose enough not to damage the skin or lead to vascular obstruction. Velcro ties are very convenient, comfortable for the child and very easy to change. No data exist on the safety of normal ties versus Velcro.

Voice with a tracheostomy is only possible when air can pass through the larynx and upper airway. The tube should have a diameter small enough to allow passage of air around it or it has to be fenestrated. It may be occluded by a finger or, more conveniently, by a speaking valve. When the child is on a ventilator, development of speech is more complex. The child may vocalise using the exhaled air. Specially manufactured tracheostomy tubes that incorporate a valve to direct flow of gas above the inflated cuff towards the larynx are available for these patients. Alternative ways of communication are sign language, manual language devices or an electrolarynx.

The changed indication pattern of tracheotomy has created a population of children with a long-term tracheostomy. Home is a much better environment in which to grow up than an intensive care unit, provided that good nursing and medical care can be continued. The parents or other caregivers should be willing and able to care for the child, and the health team in the hospital has to be convinced that this is the case. This involves training and passing an assessment for the parents, a process that may last a few months. Parents need to understand the anatomy of the trachea and the pathology that was the indication for the tracheostomy. Of vital importance is what should be done in an emergency: obstruction or dislodgement of the tube. Parents need to be confident that they can change the tube under all conditions, and have to be well trained in resuscitation techniques. Good home care is a shared responsibility of parents and hospital. Easy communication between the two has to continue after discharge of the child from the hospital. An emergency kit has to be available wherever the child is. It contains extra tracheostomy tubes with ties, some tubes of smaller sizes, a suction pump, suction catheters, scissors and equipment for resuscitation and ventilation. A short description of the pathology and instructions on how to ventilate the child (not by the upper airway in case of an upper airway obstruction) may save the child's life. The contents of the kit need to be checked regularly.

Decannulation

Decannulation is considered if the original indication for the tracheostomy is no longer present, the airway is not obstructed and the child is in a good cardiopulmonary, neurological and general condition. Decannulation procedures vary considerably, and may include: capping the tube, downsizing the tube, endoscopy of the airway or combinations of these. Capping is first tried for short periods at home, and when successful, for longer periods during daytime with permanent observation. If capping is tolerated for at least 24 h, decannulation may follow. Downsizing is not necessary with this method. Signs of obstruction during capping may be caused by an airway obstruction, or by too large a tube. Downsizing the tube may help in differentiating between the two. If downsizing solves the problem of obstruction, decannulation may follow. However, this method may fail, especially in very young children. Smaller tubes have an increased risk of occlusion by dried secretions and a much higher airway resistance. Another disadvantage may be the narrowing of the tracheostomy canal, resulting in difficulty when reinserting the original size of tracheostomy tube. Fenestration is an alternative for downsizing. The size of the tube may remain the same, but disadvantages are the risk of development of granulation tissue, kinking of the tube and difficulty passing a suction catheter.

Endoscopic evaluation of the airway is essential in most infants and very useful in many older children. It provides information on the obstruction that may have been the indication for the tracheostomy, or on any obstruction caused by the tracheostomy, such as a suprastomal granuloma. It also gives an idea of the size of the lumen around the tube. In those cases when the capping unexpectedly fails, endoscopy may solve the problem.

How can we be sure that the child really tolerates capping the tube and can be decannulated safely? The Great Ormond Street protocol stresses the importance of observation in a hospital by a nurse (Kubba et al. 2004; Waddell et al. 1997). Monitoring and even polysomnography is advised by others (Gray et al. 1998).

A combination of observation and monitoring provides a good indication for the success of decannulation. Nevertheless, it is difficult to predict the effect of an air

way infection on an incompletely resolved obstruction. The severity of obstructive sleep apnoea syndrome varies considerably. Neither normal polysomnography with a capped tube, nor an endoscopy exclude later episodes with serious symptoms.

Tracheomalacia, which may have been the original indication for the tracheostomy, poses a problem if decannulation is considered. The effect of removing the tube that splints the trachea is hard to predict with endoscopy, and impossible with monitoring and a capped tube. In such a case, the clinical judgement of the attending physicians must prevail.

Some authors advocate combining endoscopy with removal of suprastomal granulation tissue, repair of suprastomal collapse and even excision of the lining and closure of the tracheostomy canal (Gray et al. 1998).

Summary for the Clinician

- The indications for tracheotomy have changed from relief of acute airway obstruction to the need for a permanent access to the airway for artificial ventilation or bypass of a chronic obstruction, often in young infants. This creates a group of children with a permanent tracheostomy who need special care for a long period, preferably at home.

References

1. Ang AH, Chua DY, Pang KP, et al (2005) Pediatric tracheotomies in an Asian population: the Singapore experience. Otolaryngol Head Neck Surg 133:246–250
2. Anonymous (2000) Care of the child with a chronic tracheostomy. Am J Respir Crit Care Med 161:297–308
3. Arcand P, Granger J (1988) Pediatric tracheostomies: changing trends. J Otolaryngol 17:121–124
4. Carter P, Benjamin B (1983) Ten-year review of pediatric tracheotomy. Ann Otol Rhinol Laryngol 92:398–400
5. Ciaglia P, Firsching R, Syniec C (1985) Elective percutaneous dilatational tracheostomy. A new simple bedside procedure; preliminary report. Chest 87:715–719
6. Crysdale WS, Feldman RI, Naiti K (1988) Tracheotomies: a 10-year experience in 319 children. Ann Otol Rhinol Laryngol 97:439–443
7. Dutton JM, Palmer PM, McCulloch TM, et al (1995) Mortality in the pediatric patient with tracheotomy. Head Neck 17:403–408
8. Fry TL, Jones RO, Fischer ND, et al (1985) Comparisons of tracheostomy incisions in a pediatric model. Ann Otol Rhinol Laryngol 94:450–453

9. Gray RF, Todd NW, Jacobs IN (1998) Tracheostomy decannulation in children: approaches and techniques. Laryngoscope 108:8–12

10. Kaslon KW, Stein RE (1985) Chronic pediatric tracheotomy: assessment and implications for habilitation of voice, speech and language in young children. Int J Pediatr Otorhinolaryngol 9:165–171

11. Koltai PJ (1998) Starplasty: a new technique of pediatric tracheotomy. Arch Otolaryngol Head Neck Surg 124:1105–1111

12. Kremer B, Botos-Kremer AI, Eckel HE et al (2002) Indications, complications, and surgical techniques for pediatric tracheostomies – an update. J Pediatr Surg 37:1556–1562

13. Kubba H, Cooke J, Hartley B (2004) Can we develop a protocol for the safe decannulation of tracheostomies in children less than 18 months old? Int J Pediatr Otorhinolaryngol 68:935–937

14. MacRae DL, Rae RE, Heeneman H (1984) Pediatric tracheotomy. J Otolaryngol 13:309–311

15. Palmer PM, Dutton JM, McCulloch TM, et al (1995) Trends in the use of tracheotomy in the pediatric patient: the Iowa experience. Head Neck 17:328–333

16. Scott CJ, Darowski M, Crabbe DC (1998) Complications of percutaneous dilatational tracheostomy in children. Anaesthesia 53:477–480

17. Waddell A, Appleford R, Dunning C, et al (1997) The Great Ormond Street protocol for ward decannulation of children with tracheostomy: increasing safety and decreasing cost. Int J Pediatr Otorhinolaryngol 39:111–118

18. Warren WH (2000) Percutaneous dilatational tracheostomy: a note of caution. Crit Care Med 28:1664–1665

19. Wetmore RF, Marsh RR, Thompson ME, et al (1999) Pediatric tracheostomy: a changing procedure? Ann Otol Rhinol Laryngol 108:695–699

Recurrent Respiratory Papillomatosis

29

Brian J. Wiatrak

Core Messages

- Recurrent respiratory papillomatosis (RRP) is a disease of viral origin that occurs in both pediatric and adult populations.
- Its symptoms, primarily hoarseness and manifestations of airway obstruction, are due to human papilloma virus infection of the laryngotracheal airway and the development of exophytic growths that alter airflow.
- RRP is the most common benign laryngeal tumor to occur in children and the second most frequent cause (after vocal cord nodules) of chronic hoarseness (Wiatrak et al. 2004).
- RRP has no known cure, and it can cause significant morbidity.

Contents

Introduction

Recurrent respiratory papillomatosis (RRP) is a disease of viral origin that occurs in both pediatric and adult populations. Its symptoms, primarily hoarseness and manifestations of airway obstruction, are due to human papilloma virus (HPV) infection of the laryngotracheal airway and the development of exophytic growths that alter airflow. RRP is the most common benign laryngeal tumor to occur in children and the second most frequent cause (after vocal cord nodules) of chronic hoarseness (Wiatrak et al. 2004). RRP has no known cure, and it can cause significant morbidity.

RRP poses a significant clinical challenge for the otolaryngologist. The natural course of the disease is unpredictable. In some patients, lesions spontaneously regress with time. In other patients, however, the disease takes a more aggressive course and may involve the distal trachea and, rarely, the pulmonary airways. In these more aggressive cases, lesions must often be debulked surgically in the operating room, but they usually recur, sometimes at frequent intervals. In the most severe cases, chronic bronchopulmonary obstruction may result in respiratory failure and possibly death. Malignant degeneration may also occur in long-standing cases. Fortunately, these are very rare outcomes.

Historical Perspective

One of the first published reports of papillomatous growths in the larynx, noted at autopsy, was by the North American otolaryngologist Horace Green (Green 1846), who used the term "cauliflower excrescence" to describe polypoid lesions he had seen in the larynges of two patients. British laryngologist Mackenzie coined the term "papillomata" and presented surgical drawings of these lesions (Mackenzie 1880). Chevalier Jackson devoted significant attention to papillomata of the larynx in children in his 1922 textbook (Jackson 1922), describing indications for less aggressive or more aggressive treatment based on initial response. Ullmann (1923) confirmed the infectious nature of papillomatosis.

Hajek (1956) reported the first confirmed case of vertical, intrapartum transmission of RRP to a child from a mother infected with vaginal condylomata. In 1973, HPV was identified as the DNA viral agent responsible for the development of laryngeal papillomatosis (Boyle et al. 1973), and it was subsequently confirmed that this was the same virus identified in condylomata accuminata, suggesting the common infectious agent for both of these diseases. In the early 1990s, the American Society of Pediatric Otolaryngology (ASPO) and the Centers for Disease Control formed the Pediatric RRP Task Force to better track active cases of RRP in the United States as a means to estimate the true incidence, prevalence, and social impact of this disease in children (Armstrong et al. 1999). The goals of the Task Force are: (1) to develop an endoscopic staging system, (2) to facilitate multicenter clinical trials, and (3) to publish practice guidelines (Derkay 2001).

In recent years, significant new knowledge has been gained regarding the molecular biological and immunologic basis of RRP, and new surgical techniques have led to improved outcomes. New adjunctive medical treatments have also been reported. Despite these recent advances, RRP continues to have a significant impact on the quality of life of patients and their families (Lindman et al. 2005). In addition to the emotional burden, RRP has a high economic cost: this rare chronic disease has been estimated to cost the United States US$150 million dollars annually (Derkay 1995).

Pathogenesis of RRP in Children

Molecular hybridization analysis has determined that HPV types 6 and 11 (HPV-6 and HPV-11, respectively) are

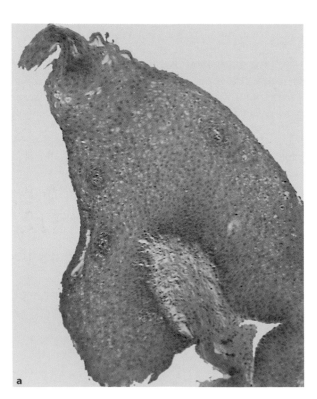
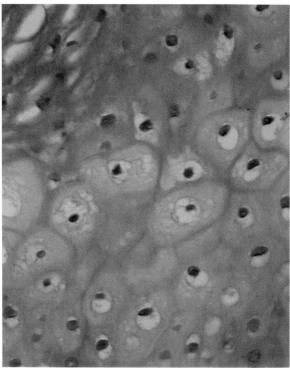

Fig. 29.1 a Light microscopic appearance of laryngeal squamous papilloma showing characteristic polypoid growth and small fibrovascular core containing a few lymphocytes (hematoxylin and eosin stain, H&E, magnification ×33). **b** Light microscopic appearance of papillomas with prominent koilocytes [keratinocytes with irregular nuclear size and shape and perinuclear cytoplasmic clearing (nuclear halos) H&E, magnification ×132]

the primary agents responsible for RRP. HPV is a double-stranded DNA virion in an icosahedral-shaped viral capsid with a diameter of 55 nm (Wiatrak et al. 2004). Of the 90 known subtypes of HPV, subtypes 16 and 18 are rarely identified in RRP patients, except in cases of malignant degeneration. Cutaneous warts are typically caused by HPV-2 and HPV-3, although a child with skin warts due to HPV-11 has been reported (Brown and Wiatrak 2002).

All species of HPV have a specific tropism for squamous epithelial tissue. HPV DNA integrates in the basal epithelial layer within epithelial transition zones in the airway, most often at the junction of squamous and ciliated epithelium. There it proliferates and stimulates the growth of overlying epithelial layers, resulting in papilloma formation. The viral protein capsid is assembled in the upper differentiated epithelial cells.

Histologically, the papillomas appear as exophytic projections of the keratinized stratified squamous epithelium overlying a fibrovascular core (Fig. 29.1). The viral etiology of the lesions is suggested by the presence of koilocytes (vacuolated cells with clear cytoplasmic inclusions; Wiatrak et al. 2004). There may be epithelial maturation abnormalities, including dyskeratosis, parakeratosis, and hyperplasia of the basement membrane. Interestingly, HPV DNA has also been identified in adjacent normal-appearing epithelial tissue in patients with RRP (Pignatari et al. 1992).

Papillomas typically arise within the larynx, specifically the true vocal cords, the false vocal cords, the subglottis, and the laryngeal surface of the epiglottis (Kashima et al. 1993), although they may spread to extralaryngotracheal sites such as the tonsils, palate, nasal cavity, pharynx, and esophagus. Lesions may be relatively flat and sessile, but even small growths on the vocal folds may cause significant vocal symptoms. Lesions arising in the supraglottic airway may become quite large before causing any symptoms of airway obstruction. Esophageal papillomas may be completely asymptomatic until they cause obstruction (Fig. 29.2).

Juvenile-onset RRP tends to be more aggressive than adult-onset disease. In addition, HPV DNA appears to have the ability to "colonize" mucosa and, after remaining dormant for up to many years, to activate host genes to replicate viral DNA and cause exacerbation many years after remission (Derkay and Darrow 2006; Wiatrak et al. 2004). Other factors that may be associated with the accelerated epithelial growth seen in RRP include the HPV effect on increasing levels of expression of epidermal growth factor receptor and interaction with p53 or other tumor-suppressor genes, inhibiting their normal

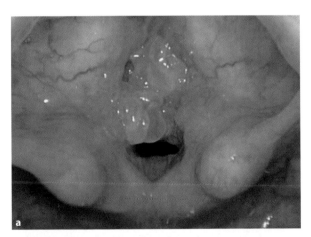

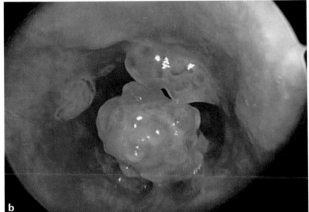

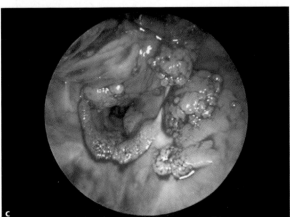

Fig. 29.2 **a** Near-complete airway obstruction by papillomas involving the glottic and supraglottic levels. **b** Obstructive papillomas in the mid-tracheal region. **c** Recurrent respiratory papillomatosis (RRP) involving the cricopharyngeal region and the upper esophagus

functioning and leading to deregulation of "checks" on cell proliferation. The viral genome itself consists of three primary regions: an upstream regulatory region and early (E) and late (L) regions. The E genes regulate oncogenes that are responsible for replication of the viral genome, interaction with host cell intermediate filaments, and transforming activities. The L region genes encode for the viral structural proteins (Aaltonen et al. 2002).

Research is now under way to elucidate the role of the host immune system in the pathogenesis of RRP. Both humoral and cellular immune responses may be compromised in pediatric patients with symptoms of RRP. Those with impaired immunocompetence, for example due to human immunodeficiency virus infection or receiving immunosuppressive drugs subsequent to organ transplantation, may develop RRP (Shah et al. 1998). There is emerging evidence that cytokines (such as interleukin-2, interleukin-4, and interleukin-10) and the expression of major histocompatibility complex antigens play roles in the altered function of cell-mediated immunity in patients with RRP (Derkay and Darrow 2006).

Epidemiology

The incidence of RRP in the United States is 4.3 per 100,000 children and 1.8 per 100,000 adults, with 2300 new cases diagnosed per year (Derkay 1995). A Danish study found an incidence of 3.8 cases of laryngeal papillomatosis per 100,000 (Derkay 2001).

In children, more aggressive disease is associated with earlier diagnosis. In the United States, children younger than 3 years at diagnosis of RRP were 3.6 times more likely to require more than four surgical endoscopic procedures for debulking of papillomas and 2.1 times more likely to have two or more anatomically separate laryngotracheal sites involved than those whose disease was not diagnosed until after their fourth birthday (Armstrong et al. 1999). More aggressive disease is also associated with infection by HPV-11 rather than HPV-6 (Rabah et al. 2001; Rimell et al. 1997; Wiatrak et al. 2004).

Most RRP in children is believed to result from transmission of HPV from the mother to the child as the baby passes through an HPV-infected birth canal. One study reported overt condyloma in more than 50% of mothers who give birth to children with RRP (Haleden and Majmudar 1986). Another study found that about 75% of children with RRP are first-born and most were delivered vaginally (Wiatrak et al. 2004). HPV infection in women typically manifests as condylomata acuminata ("warts") involving the cervix, vulva, and other anogenital sites. In support of this proposed mechanism of transmission, the most common genital HPV viral subtypes are 6 and 11, the same as the subtypes that cause RRP in children.

It is important to note, however, that although a high proportion of children with RRP were born to mothers with HPV cervical infection, only a small portion of children exposed to genital condylomata at birth actually develop RRP (Tenti 1999). Clearly, factors such as host immunity, genetics, and volume of virus to which the child was exposed play a role. In this regard, Buchinsky and colleagues (Buchinsky et al. 2004) demonstrated that susceptibility to RRP may be mediated by several host genes, such as those coding for major histocompatibility complex, cytokines, interleukins, and growth factors. Another study found an association between polymorphisms in transporter-associated with antigen presentation 1 (TAP1) protein and increased severity of HPV infection in those with RRP (Vambutas et al. 2000).

Although vaginal delivery to a mother with genital HPV infection is a risk factor for RRP, the role of Caesarean section in the prevention of RRP is controversial. HPV DNA has been recovered in umbilical cord blood from infants delivered to mothers with HPV infection, and it has been identified in amniotic fluid obtained from infected mothers (Wiatrak et al. 2004). In addition, RRP has been reported, although rarely, in children born by Caesarean section to mothers with HPV cervical infection (Shah et al. 1986). Most authorities do not endorse prophylactic Caesarean section in cases of maternal HPV infection in the absence of other indications for Caesarean section (Kosko and Derkay 1996).

Diagnosis and Staging of RRP in Children

Typically, juvenile RRP presents as progressive, chronic hoarseness and symptoms of airway obstruction. Early symptoms such as chronic cough may be misdiagnosed as asthma, croup, bronchitis, or other airway problems common in children. Later symptoms may include recurrent pneumonia, failure to thrive, dyspnea, or dysphagia (Derkay and Darrow 2006). In severe cases, aphonia and respiratory distress may occur. Symptoms have typically progressed for some time, in some cases as long as 1 year or more, before diagnosis.

For diagnosis of RRP, it is essential to obtain a comprehensive medical history, including the time of onset of symptoms, prior airway trauma, previous history of endotracheal intubation, and specific characteristics of the voice or cry. A history of progressive inspiratory or biphasic stridor suggests an expanding lesion of the glottis or subglottis. In infants, the possibility of a congenital airway anomaly such as vocal cord paralysis, subglottic hemangioma, or subglottic stenosis should be explored by flexible fiber-optic laryngoscopy and radiologic studies. A definitive diagnosis of RRP requires endoscopic evaluation with a rigid laryngoscope and bronchoscopy with biopsy sampling of visible lesions, followed by histopathology examination and viral typing. If HPV is found, the child's parents should be questioned in detail about a maternal or paternal history of genital condylomata.

Staging of RRP in children helps track progression of the patient's disease and facilitates communications with other physicians, although no staging system has been uniformly adopted by clinicians and researchers. A staging system used for the past 15 years by the author (Wiatrak et al. 2004) is shown in Fig. 29.3. In this staging system, the severity of disease at each point in time is determined by totaling the scores for disease severity at various specific anatomic sites in the airway. Several other staging systems have also been described (Derkay et al. 1998; Kashima et al. 1985).

Disease Progression and Complications

Tracheal disease has been reported in 26% of children with RRP (Wiatrak et al. 2004), but distal bronchopulmonary involvement occurred in less than 5% of children. Bronchopulmonary disease may manifest as recurrent pneumonia, bronchiectasis, or cystic pulmonary masses noted on chest radiographs and computed tomography (CT) scans. Chronic tracheal and bronchopulmonary disease may eventually lead to distal airway obstruction with resulting atelectasis, cystic pulmonary degeneration,

Date of Surgery.......   Name.....
Adjuvant Therapy.......   M.R.#
       Initiation date.......
SYMPTOMS
     Voice quality   Normal......
                         Mild Hoarseness.....
                         Severe Hoarseness......
                         Aphonic.......
     Airway   No obstruction........
                         Mild Obstruction.......
                         Severe obstruction.........

SEVERITY RATING	
1+	Mild
2+	Moderate
3+	Severe

LARYNX
     Epiglottis
          Lingual Surface.......
          Laryngeal Surface.......
     Aryepiglottic Folds   Right.......   Left.......
     False Vocal Cords   Right.......   Left........
     True Vocal Cords   Right.......   Left........
     Anterior Commissure........
     Posterior Glottis...........
     Subglottis..........
     Other......

PAPILLOMA STAGING SHEET

TRACHEA
     Upper 1/3   Anterior......   Posterior........
     Middle 1/3   Anterior.......   Posterior.......
     Lower 1/3   Anterior......   Posterior........
     Bronchi   Right.........   Left...........
     Tracheostomy Stoma......   TOTAL SCORE ....

OTHER
     Nose.......   Oesophagus......   TOTAL SCORE _____
     Palate......   Lungs Right......
                         Left......
     Pharynx......   Other.......

Fig. 29.3 RRP lesion staging sheet (Wiatrak et al. 2004)

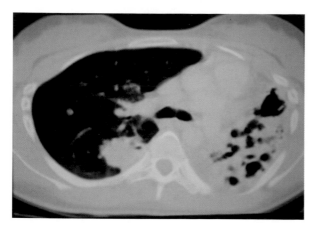

Fig. 29.4 Computed tomography scan (coronal) at the level of the chest shows widespread bronchopulmonary disease (*white areas*)

and postobstructive infections requiring frequent hospitalizations for antibiotic therapy. Serial CT scans of the chest may be helpful in monitoring the progression of disease (Fig. 29.4).

The data regarding viral subtype as a risk factor for distal tracheal spread of RRP are mixed. In two series of patients, HPV-11 was associated with greater tendency for distal spread than HPV-6 (Rabah et al. 2001; Wiatrak et al. 2004), but in another series there was no significant difference in tracheal spread between viral subtypes (Gabbott et al. 1997). Furthermore, others report greater disease severity in children with HPV-6 infection (Padayachee and Prescott 1993).

Although rare, malignant transformation may occur in children or adults with long-standing RRP. Malignant degeneration in children usually occurs in the lung parenchyma or distal bronchopulmonary tree. In contrast, malignant degeneration in cases of adult-onset RRP occurs more commonly within the larynx. The risk of malignancy is higher in those with certain viral subtypes, namely HPV-16 and HPV-18. In addition, patients who have other predisposing factors (i.e., prior history of radiation or cigarette smoking) are at greater risk of malignancy. Lesions should be biopsy sampled at every surgical intervention and examined histologically for any evidence of malignant changes. The prognosis after diagnosis of malignant degeneration in children is universally poor (Solomon et al. 1985).

Managing RRP in Children

Patients presenting with severe respiratory distress may require a tracheotomy. Some patients requiring tracheotomy may have concurrent tracheal disease at the time of presentation; however, on many occasions tracheotomy is performed simply to relieve obstruction of laryngeal papillomatosis. Once the larynx has been debulked and airway patency restored, the tracheotomy may be reversed. It has been reported that tracheotomy may increase the risk of distal tracheal spread of RRP (Cole et al. 1989; Rimell et al. 1997; Shapiro et al. 1996). It is unclear whether the tracheotomy itself predisposes the tracheal mucosa to papillomatous spread, or if the necessity for tracheotomy implies more severe disease. Although research has not yet provided a definitive answer to this question, tracheotomy should be reserved for cases in which it is absolutely necessary and decannulation should be considered as soon as possible.

Typically, young patients diagnosed with RRP require more surgical interventions for debulking papillomas to relieve airway obstruction than do older patients (Derkay 2001; Wiatrak et al. 2004). Although there is variability from one patient to the next, it has been shown that at least half of all RRP patients require ten or more surgical procedures. Approximately 7% of children with RRP require more than 100 operations to maintain airway patency (Derkay 2001).

Spontaneous remission of RRP may occur, but this is unpredictable and highly variable. Endocrine, immunologic, or hormonal influences may lead to remission around puberty; however, some children never enter remission. Papillomas may recur after long periods of remission. Children whose disease is in remission still have HPV DNA in biopsy specimens from normal-appearing mucosa (Steinberg et al. 1988). Pregnancy has been associated with severe exacerbations of RRP, and in one reported case led to death by airway obstruction (Helmrich et al. 1992).

Principles of Surgical Management

Because there is no known medical cure for RRP, the mainstay of therapy is endoscopic debridement and debulking of lesions to improve airway patency, improve voice quality, decrease overall tumor burden, and prevent the distal spread of disease while preserving normal structures. Although various surgical modalities may be used to manage RRP, overaggressive use of any technique may lead to complications such as glottic or subglottic stenosis, or laryngeal webbing. It may be preferable to leave small lesions in areas such as the anterior commissure, rather than risking stenosis or webbing by excessive resection of tissue.

The frequency of surgical intervention varies. Some patients experience more frequent periods of aggressive growth of papillomas and thus must undergo more frequent surgical debulking. Long-term, close follow up is required for all children with RRP. Often, the course of disease, and thus the projected time to the next debulking operation, will become apparent in the first 6 months after diagnosis. However, increased disease activity, heralded by worsening voice quality or airway obstruction, may lead to reoperation in a shorter time period.

Anesthesia/Airway Management Techniques

Various anesthetic/airway management techniques may be utilized for surgical debulking of RRP lesions. Therefore, it is crucial that the otolaryngologist discuss anesthetic management issues with the anesthesia team in detail before the start of surgery. The goal is to provide a safe and secure airway during anesthesia, while allowing the surgeon an unobstructed view of the laryngotracheal airway. The techniques most frequently used are spontaneous ventilation, intermittent apnea, and jet ventilation.

Spontaneous Ventilation Technique

With a spontaneous ventilation technique, the patient undergoes induction of anesthesia without neuromuscular paralysis, and anesthetic gasses are typically insufflated through a side port of the laryngoscope or through an endotracheal tube that has been placed in the pharynx. The larynx may be anesthetized by spraying a local anesthetic onto the larynx under direct visualization. The patient continues to breathe under his/her own efforts during the procedure.

Intermittent Apnea Technique

With the intermittent apnea technique, the patient is well oxygenated and then temporarily extubated. The patient is reintubated when he/she shows signs of oxygen desaturation. This cycle continues until adequate debulking of the papillomas has been achieved.

Jet Ventilation Technique

Another anesthesia/airway management technique that may be used for debulking RRP lesions is jet ventilation. However, there is a theoretical risk that HPV particles could be carried into the distal airway with this technique. In addition, jet ventilation poses risks of pneumothorax and pneumomediastinum.

Endoscopy Techniques

Once the patient has been anesthetized, direct laryngoscopy and bronchoscopy are performed with Hopkins Rod lens telescopes and bronchoscopes (Karl Storz En-

doscopy-America). Video-endoscopic documentation is usually performed as well as still digital imaging, which can be utilized for patient education or academic purposes. A pediatric tracheotomy tray must be available in case an airway emergency occurs.

After the extent of disease has been determined by laryngoscopy and bronchoscopy, the patient undergoes suspension microlaryngoscopy, typically utilizing a Lindholm suspension laryngoscope (Karl Storz Endoscopy-America). If the intermittent apnea technique is to be utilized, the patient is then intubated endotracheally for ventilation before suspension occurs. Lesions should always be biopsy sampled before being debulked.

Laser Techniques

Until recently, the most common technique for debulking papillomas was to evaporate lesions using a CO_2 laser coupled with a micromanipulator, under observation through an operating microscope with a 400-mm lens. Light energy from the CO_2 laser is absorbed by water in affected tissues; energy absorption causes tissue to superheat, resulting in controlled destruction of the papillomas and cauterization of the tissue surfaces. Cottonoids soaked in a vasoconstrictor agent may be helpful to control any bleeding that cannot be cauterized with the laser. A small amount of thermal energy is dissipated from the surgical site to surrounding tissues, with minimal effect. However, if overaggressive tissue destruction is performed, stenosis or webbing may occur. Although HPV DNA has been demonstrated to be present in the CO_2 laser plume (smoke), no case of RRP transmission to operating room staff has been reported (Abramson et al. 1990). Nevertheless, a smoke evacuator should be used during laser excision of RRP lesions. In addition, precautions must be taken to prevent a laser fire.

A potassium titanyl phosphate laser is another option. With this type of laser, energy is transmitted through a thin, flexible glass fiber that can be passed through the suction port of a bronchoscope or through a specially designed fiber-optic hand-piece.

The feasibility and safety of the flash-pump dye laser has been demonstrated in the literature (Bower et al. 1998; McMillan et al. 1998). A major advantage of this technique is that it requires only local anesthesia and thus could be performed in the office. Many adult patients are good candidates for this technique. However, most pediatric patients would not be able to cooperate during such a procedure performed under local anesthesia.

Microdebridement

Microdebrider blades have been designed with a very small, protected oscillating blade coupled to a suction

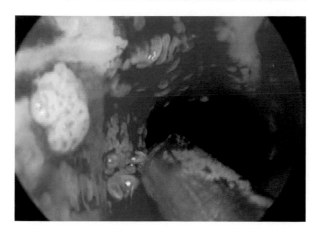

Fig. 29.5 View of tracheal airway through Hopkins rod telescope showing microdebrider, used to debulk papillomas (*white patches*) that are impairing airflow

port, which allows for delicate dissection of laryngotracheal papillomas. Recent studies have demonstrated potential advantages of the microdebrider versus the CO_2 laser for debulking RRP lesions. These include shorter operating time, less pain, less expense, and no risk of laser fire (Myer et al. 1999; Pasquale et al. 2003). A recent survey of the ASPO membership determined that for removal of papillomas, the microdebrider technique is now favored over the CO_2 laser or cold-steel microdissection techniques (Derkay and Darrow 2006).

Another advantage of the microdebrider is its ability to debulk tracheal disease. While the patient is in suspension microlaryngoscopy, a Hopkins rod lens telescope may be passed through the suspension laryngoscope for visualization, while simultaneously passing the microdebrider to debulk the tracheal lesions (Fig. 29.5). For pediatric patients, microdebrider blades are available that may be able to reach as far as the level of the carina.

Other reported surgical techniques include argon plasma laser coagulation and endolaryngeal microsurgery for excision of glottic papillomas (Schraff et al. 2004).

Adjuvant Medical Therapy

No current treatment has proved effective in complete eradication of HPV from affected tissues in patients with RRP. Nevertheless, for the 20% of patients in whom HPV cannot be eradicated by surgery alone, adjuvant medical therapy may help (Wiatrak et al. 2004). Indications for the use of adjuvant medical therapy include the following: need for four or more surgical procedures in a year, distal tracheal or pulmonary disease, or rapid regrowth of papillomas resulting in airway compromise.

Treatments that have been reported but that have not demonstrated clear benefit include radium implants, radiation therapy, chemical or electric fulguration, escharotics, the application of calcined magnesium, celandine, estrogen, formaldehyde, podophyllin, and hydrocortisone (Wiatrak et al. 2004). Medical treatments currently being used include antiviral agents, antiproliferative agents, and immune system agents. Specific agents include indol-3 carbinol (I3C), α-interferon, cidofovir, photodynamic therapy, and viral agents such as heat-shock protein (Hsp).

Indol-3 Carbinol

I3C is a dietary supplement that is derived from cruciferous vegetables (cabbage, broccoli, and cauliflower). It is broken down by stomach acid to glucobracin and diidolymethane. Endoplex, a condensed form of I3C that forms naturally in an acidic environment, tends to be more absorbable and has a more stable shelf life compared to I3C. I3C and other estrogen metabolites have slowed the progression of papillomatous disease in some cases, particularly cases of laryngeal papillomatosis (Rosen et al. 1998). I3C may be used in combination therapy with other agents, if necessary.

Alpha Interferon

The α-interferons are glycoproteins that are produced by leukocytes in response to a variety of stimuli, including viral infection. Interferons stimulate host immunologic defenses to block replication of viral RNA and DNA, and alter cell membranes to make them less susceptible to viral penetration. Interferon α-2A treatment is initiated at 5 million units per square meter of body surface area, administered by subcutaneous injection, twice a day, for 28 days, followed by a reduced dose 3 days a week for at least 6 months. If an adequate response is obtained, or if side effects develop, the dosage can be decreased to 3 million units per square meter of body surface area, administered three times per week. Common side effects of interferon include fever, generalized flu-like symptoms, chills, headaches, myalgias, and nausea. Chronic reactions to interferon may also occur. These include decrease in the child's growth rate, elevation of liver transaminase levels, leucopenia, spastic diplegia, and febrile seizures (Derkay and Darrow 2006). It appears that interferon produced by recombinant DNA techniques may result in fewer side effects and is associated with a better treatment efficacy.

Cidofovir

Cidofovir (Vistide) is a cytosine nucleotide analog that suppresses DNA replication by selective inhibition of viral DNA synthesis (Wiatrak et al. 2004). Cidofovir has been approved by the United States Food and Drug Administration for the treatment of cytomegalovirus retinitis in individuals with autoimmune deficiency syndrome. The drug also has a broad spectrum of antiviral activity and is effective against other DNA viruses, including herpes virus, adenovirus, and HPV. Cidofovir prepared as a topical gel has demonstrated efficacy in the treatment of condylomata acuminata (Wiatrak et al. 2004), although no topical preparation is available for use in the airway. Cidofovir is typically delivered by intralaryngeal injection at the sites of papillomatous involvement at the time of endoscopic debulking. The therapy has been reported to have positive effects in several case series (14 of 17 adults with laryngeal RRP, Snoeck et al. 1998; several of 10 children, Pransky et al. 2000; 3 of 11 children, Shirley and Wiatrak 2004; an 8-year-old child, Van Valckenborgh et al. 2001), but no controlled clinical trials have been reported. In addition, animal trials have indicated the drug may have nephrotoxic and carcinogenic effects (Derkay and Darrow 2006), so cidofovir should be used cautiously and only in the most severe cases (Inglis 2005).

Photodynamic Therapy

Photodynamic therapy with the photosensitizing drug dihematoporphyrin ether (DHE) has been used for RRP. DHE is administered intravenously and tends to concentrate within papillomatous tissue to a greater degree than in the surrounding tissue. The papillomatous tissue is destroyed after photoactivation of DHE with an argon-pump dye laser. The side effects of photodynamic therapy can be quite severe, including photosensitivity that may manifest as skin blistering, ocular discomfort, or skin erythema. Although short-term results appeared promising, recent studies indicate that the long-term efficacy is no better than other adjuvant medical therapies (Shikowitz et al. 2005).

Other Agents

Oral agents such as acyclovir, *cis*-retinoic acid (Accutane), and ribaviran, and injection of mumps vaccine into RRP lesions in laryngeal sites, have been tried. None has demonstrated long-term benefit.

Investigational Agents

Modulation of the immune system with Hsp E7, a recombinant fusion protein derived from Hsp65 from *Mycobacterium bovus* (BCG) and E7 protein from HPV-16, is currently under development for the treatment of HPV-related diseases in adults and in children. This immune-system modulator is injected subcutaneously every 30 days, which results in stimulation of a cell-mediated immune response to HPV. A recent multi-institutional study demonstrated the safety and potential efficacy of this treatment modality. More multi-institutional, controlled studies are planned (Derkay et al. 2005).

There is hope that a vaccine against HPV could be effective in treating RRP in addition to preventing HPV infection. A vaccine against HPV-16 has been approved after a large-scale, multi-institutional study demonstrated significant efficacy in preventing cervical neoplasia due to HPV (Poland et al. 2005). Recently, the FDA approved usage of a quadrivalent HPV vaccine which is active against HPV types 6, 11, 16 and 18. Although there is no known effect on RRP patients if they are directly vaccinated, it is possible that the vaccine may decrease the prevalence of HPV disease in women and subsequently reduce the risk and incidence of RRP in children.

Voice Outcome

This subject is discussed in detail in Chapter 6.

Summary for the Clinician

- RRP is a rare, but unpredictable and difficult to manage disease that can lead to severe respiratory problems in children and has the potential for malignant transformation. Current treatment consists of surgical debridement of symptomatic lesions, and medical therapies to augment surgery in severe cases. New techniques have been developed, including use of a microdebrider or pulse-dye laser therapy, to improve the results of surgery for this often intractable disease. Recurring symptoms and repeated surgical procedures to manage this disease take a heavy toll on children and their families in terms of missed school days, psychological distress and issues with self-esteem, and financial concerns. Healthcare professionals and organizations such as the RRP Foundation (www.rrpf.org) can be very important in providing the information and support patients and families need to manage this condition. There is also hope that immune modulators and HPV vaccines for women may prove helpful in decreasing the incidence of RRP. Ongoing and future research related to the immunologic and genetic aspects of RRP and to new treatment modalities will hopefully lead to improved outcomes.

References

1. Aaltonen LM, Rihkanen H, Vaheri A (2002) Human papillomavirus in the larynx. Laryngoscope 112:700–707
2. Abramson AL, DiLorenzo TP, Steinberg BM (1990) Is papillomavirus detectable in the plume of laser-treated laryngeal papilloma? Arch Otolaryngol Head Neck Surg 116:604–607
3. Armstrong LR, Derkay CS, Reeves WC (1999) Initial results from the national registry for juvenile-onset recurrent respiratory papillomatosis. RRP Task Force. Arch Otolaryngol Head Neck Surg 125:3–8
4. Bower CM, Waner M, Flock S, et al (1998) Flash pump dye laser treatment of laryngeal papillomas. Ann Otol Rhinol Laryngol 107:1001–1005
5. Boyle WF, Riggs JL, Oshiro LS, et al (1973) Electron microscopic identification of papova virus in laryngeal papilloma. Laryngoscope 83:1102–1108
6. Brown L, Wiatrak B (2002) Concurrent respiratory and cutaneous papillomatosis with human papillomavirus type 11. Otolaryngol Head Neck Surg 127:465–466
7. Buchinsky FJ, Derkay CS, Leal SM, et al (2004) Multicenter initiative seeking critical genes in respiratory papillomatosis. Laryngoscope 114:349–357
8. Cole RR, Myer CM III, Cotton RT (1989) Tracheotomy in children with recurrent respiratory papillomatosis. Head Neck 11:226–230
9. Derkay CS (1995) Task force on recurrent respiratory papillomas. A preliminary report. Arch Otolaryngol Head Neck Surg 121:1386–1391
10. Derkay CS (2001) Recurrent respiratory papillomatosis. Laryngoscope 111:57–69
11. Derkay CS, Darrow DH (2006) Recurrent respiratory papillomatosis. Ann Otol Rhinol Laryngol 115:1–11
12. Derkay CS, Malis DJ, Zalzal G, et al (1998) A staging system for assessing severity of disease and response to therapy in recurrent respiratory papillomatosis. Laryngoscope 108:935–937
13. Derkay CS, Smith RJ, McClay J, et al (2005) HspE7 treatment of pediatric recurrent respiratory papillomatosis: final results of an open-label trial. Ann Otol Rhinol Laryngol 114:730–737
14. Gabbott M, Cossart YE, Kan A, et al (1997) Human papillomavirus and host variables as predictors of clinical course in patients with juvenile-onset recurrent respiratory papillomatosis. J Clin Microbiol 35:3098–3103
15. Green H (1846) A treatise on diseases of the air passages: comprising an inquiry into the history, pathology, causes and treatment of those affections of the throat called bronchitis, chronic laryngitis, clergyman's sore throat. Wiley and Putnam, New York
16. Hajek EF (1956) Contribution to the aetiology of laryngeal papilloma in children. J Laryngol Otol 70:166–168
17. Haleden C, Majmudar B (1986) The relationship between juvenile laryngeal papillomatosis and maternal condylomata acuminate. J Reprod Med 318:804–807
18. Helmrich G, Stubbs TM, Stoerker J (1992) Fatal maternal laryngeal papillomatosis in pregnancy: a case report [corrected][erratum appears in Am J Obstet Gynecol 166:1313]. Am J Obstet Gynecol 166:524–525
19. Inglis AF Jr (2005) Cidofovir and the black box warning [Comment. Editorial]. Ann Otol Rhinol Laryngol 114:834–835
20. Jackson C (1922) Benign growths in the larynx. In: Jackson C (ed) Bronchoscopy and Esophagoscopy. A Manual of Peroral Endoscopy and Laryngeal Surgery. WB Saunders, Philadelphia, PA, pp 203–208
21. Kashima HK and the Papilloma Study Group (1985) Scoring system to assess severity and course in recurrent respiratory papillomatosis. In: Howley PM Broker T (ed) Papillomaviruses: Molecular and Clinical Aspects. Alan R. Liss, New York, pp 125–135
22. Kashima H, Mounts P, Leventhal B, et al (1993) Sites of predilection in recurrent respiratory papillomatosis. Ann Otol Rhinol Laryngol 102:580–583
23. Kosko JR, Derkay CS (1996) Role of cesarean section in prevention of recurrent respiratory papillomatosis – is there one? Int J Pediatr Otorhinolaryngol 35:31–38
24. Lindman JP, Lewis LS, Accortt N, et al (2005) Use of the Pediatric Quality of Life Inventory to assess the health-related quality of life in children with recurrent respiratory papillomatosis. Ann Otol Rhinol Laryngol 114:499–503
25. Mackenzie M (1880) Non-malignant tumors of the larynx. diseases of the pharynx, larynx, and trachea. William Wood, New York, pp 218–243
26. McMillan K, Shapshay SM, McGilligan JA, et al (1998) A 585-nanometer pulsed dye laser treatment of laryngeal papillomas: preliminary report. Laryngoscope 108:968–972
27. Myer CM III, Willging JP, McMurray S, et al (1999) Use of a laryngeal micro resector system. Laryngoscope 109:1165–1166
28. Padayachee A, Prescott CA (1993) Relationship between the clinical course and HPV typing of recurrent laryngeal papillomatosis. The Red Cross War Memorial Children's Hospital experience 1982–1988. Int J Pediatr Otorhinolaryngol 26:141–147
29. Pasquale K, Wiatrak B, Woolley A, et al (2003) Microdebrider versus CO_2 laser removal of recurrent respiratory papillomas: a prospective analysis. Laryngoscope 113:139–143
30. Pignatari S, Smith EM, Gray SD, et al (1992) Detection of human papillomavirus infection in diseased and nondiseased sites of the respiratory tract in recurrent respiratory papillomatosis patients by DNA hybridization. Ann Otol Rhinol Laryngol 101:408–412
31. Poland GA, Jacobson RM, Koutsky LA, et al (2005) Immunogenicity and reactogenicity of a novel vaccine for human papillomavirus 16: a 2-year randomized controlled clinical trial. Mayo Clin Proc 80:601–610
32. Pransky SM, Brewster DF, Magit AE, et al (2000) Clinical update on 10 children treated with intralesional cidofovir injections for severe recurrent respiratory papillomatosis. Arch Otolaryngol Head Neck Surg 126:1239–1243

33. Rabah R, Lancaster WD, Thomas R, et al (2001) Human papillomavirus-11-associated recurrent respiratory papillomatosis is more aggressive than human papillomavirus-6-associated disease. Pediatr Develop Pathol 4 :68–72

34. Rimell FL, Shoemaker DL, Pou AM, et al (1997) Pediatric respiratory papillomatosis: prognostic role of viral typing and cofactors. Laryngoscope 107:915–918

35. Rosen CA, Woodson GE, Thompson JW, et al (1998) Preliminary results of the use of indole-3-carbinol for recurrent respiratory papillomatosis. Otolaryngol Head Neck Surg 118:810–815

36. Schraff S, Derkay CS, Burke B, et al (2004) American Society of Pediatric Otolaryngology members' experience with recurrent respiratory papillomatosis and the use of adjuvant therapy. Arch Otolaryngol Head Neck Surg 130:1039–1042

37. Shah K, Kashima H, Polk BF, et al (1986) Rarity of cesarean delivery in cases of juvenile-onset respiratory papillomatosis. Obstet Gynecol 68:795–799

38. Shah KV, Stern WF, Shah FK, et al (1998) Risk factors for juvenile onset recurrent respiratory papillomatosis. Pediatr Infect Dis J 17:372–376

39. Shapiro AM, Rimell FL, Shoemaker D, et al (1996) Tracheotomy in children with juvenile-onset recurrent respiratory papillomatosis: the Children's Hospital of Pittsburgh experience. Ann Otol Rhinol Laryngol 105:1–5

40. Shikowitz MJ, Abramson AL, Steinberg BM, et al (2005) Clinical trial of photodynamic therapy with meso-tetra (hydroxyphenyl) chlorin for respiratory papillomatosis. Arch Otolaryngol Head Neck Surg 131:99–105

41. Shirley WP, Wiatrak B (2004) Is cidofovir a useful adjunctive therapy for recurrent respiratory papillomatosis in children? Int J Pediatr Otorhinolaryngol 68:413–418

42. Snoeck R, Wellens W, Desloovere C, et al (1998) Treatment of severe laryngeal papillomatosis with intralesional injections of cidofovir [(S)-1-(3-hydroxy-2-phosphonylmethoxypropyl)cytosine]. J Med Virol 54:219–225

43. Solomon D, Smith RR, Kashima HK, et al (1985) Malignant transformation in non-irradiated recurrent respiratory papillomatosis. Laryngoscope 95:900–904

44. Steinberg BM, Gallagher T, Stoler M, et al (1988) Persistence and expression of human papillomavirus during interferon therapy. Arch Otolaryngol Head Neck Surg 114:27–32

45. Tenti P (1999) Perinatal transmission of human papillomavirus from gravidas with latent infections. Obstet Gynecol 93:475–479

46. Ullmann EV (1923) On the etiology of laryngeal papilloma. Acta Otolaryngol 5:317–374

47. Vambutas A, Bonagura VR, Steinberg BM (2000) Altered expression of TAP-1 and major histocompatibility complex class I in laryngeal papillomatosis: correlation of TAP-1 with disease. Clin Diagn Lab Immunol 7:79–85

48. Van Valckenborgh I, Wellens W, De Boeck K, et al (2001) Systemic cidofovir in papillomatosis. Clin Infect Dis 32: E62–E64

49. Wiatrak BJ, Wiatrak DW, Broker TR, et al (2004) Recurrent respiratory papillomatosis: a longitudinal study comparing severity associated with human papilloma viral types 6 and 11 and other risk factors in a large pediatric population. Laryngoscope 114:1–23

Chapter 30

Pharynx and Oesophagus

David Rawat and Mike Thomson

30

Core Messages

■ The upper aerodigestive tract, which consists of the nose, mouth, pharynx, larynx and oesophagus, allows for the passage of air and food. These structures form one of the most complex neuromuscular systems of the body, providing the structural and dynamic components for swallowing, respiration, and speech.

■ Pathological processes in the paediatric oesophagus have received a disproportionately small amount of attention until recently, when appreciation of their pathophysiology and clinical importance has been highlighted. In this chapter, we outline the relationship and interactions between pharyngeal and oesophageal function and dysfunction.

■ Disorders of the upper gastrointestinal tract frequently involve interactions between the oropharynx and the oesophagus.

■ Aerodigestive tract disorders are associated with multiple aetiologies including anatomic or structural defects, neurologic deficits and some systemic and complex medical conditions.

■ This chapter highlights some of the interactions between the pharynx and oesophagus, with particular focus on gastro-oesophageal reflux, one of the most common conditions related to the upper gastrointestinal tract, and which can have an impact on supra-oesophageal function.

Contents

Introduction

The upper aerodigestive tract, which consists of the nose, mouth, pharynx, larynx and oesophagus, allows for the passage of air and food. These structures form one of the most complex neuromuscular systems of the body, providing the structural and dynamic components for swallowing, respiration and speech.

Pathological processes in the paediatric oesophagus have received a disproportionately small amount of attention until recently, when appreciation of their pathophysiology and clinical importance has been highlighted. In this chapter, we shall outline the relationship and interactions between pharyngeal and oesophageal function and dysfunction. Disorders of the upper gastrointestinal tract (GIT) frequently involve interactions between the oropharynx and the oesophagus. Aerodigestive tract disorders are associated with multiple aetiologies, including anatomic or structural defects, neurologic deficits and some systemic and complex medical conditions. This chapter will highlight some of the interactions between the pharynx and oesophagus, with particular focus on gastro-oesophageal reflux (GOR), one of the most common conditions related to the upper GIT, and which can have an impact on supra-oesophageal function.

30

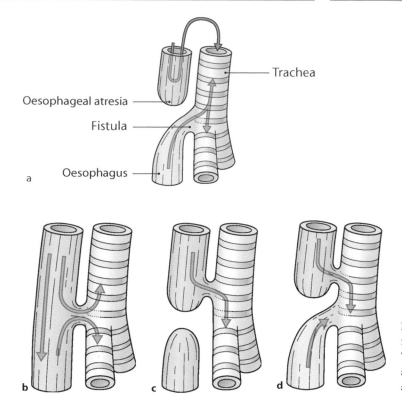

Fig. 30.1a–d Types of tracheo-oesophageal fistula (TOF). **a** Oesophageal atresia with distal TOF. **b** Isolated, H-shaped TOF. **c** Oesophageal atresia with proximal TOF. **d** Separate proximal and distal TOFs

An abnormal communication, or fistula, connecting the trachea and oesophagus can occur (1 in every 2500 births) due to incomplete division of the trachea and digestive portion of the foregut during the 4th and 5th weeks of foetal life (Fig. 30.1, and see Chapter 22). Oesophageal atresia probably develops from lack of deviation of the tracheo-oesophageal septum in a posterior direction, although isolated (very rare) oesophageal atresia can develop from failure of re-canalisation of the oesophagus in the embryonic period. Congenital stenosis of the oesophagus can occur in any area, but it is usually present in the distal third as a web or band, or as a long segment of the oesophagus with a very narrow lumen; again this is due to failure of re-canalisation of the oesophagus in the embryonic period, by the 8th week of development. Occasionally, a short oesophagus may occur, with a portion of the stomach displaced through the diaphragm as a hiatus hernia. Equally, diverticuli, duplication cysts and other anatomical abnormalities arise due to lack of correct embryonic development, usually of the proximal oesophagus.

The oesophagus has four narrow areas, which may be relevant to endoscopists, but are usually easily traversed: (1) at the oropharyngeal junction, (2) where it is crossed by the aortic arch, (3) where it is crossed by the left main bronchus and finally (4) when it traverses the diaphragm (Fig. 30.2). Other anatomical relationships can be seen in these figures. Emerging from the right crus of the diaphragm slightly left of the midline in older children, like

adults, there is a short intra-abdominal portion. This is absent in infants, which is important in explaining the

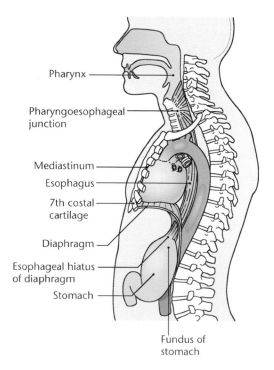

Fig. 30.2 Sagittal section of head and neck, thorax and abdomen

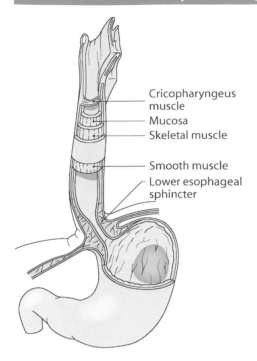

Cricopharyngeus muscle
Mucosa
Skeletal muscle
Smooth muscle
Lower esophageal sphincter

Fig. 30.3 Diagram showing tissue layers of oesophagus, the upper and lower sphincters, the stomach and the diaphragm

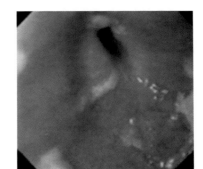

Fig. 30.4 Benign oesophageal stricture

ease with which GOR occurs. The intra-abdominal portion is normally exposed to the relatively higher pressure of the abdominal cavity compared to the lower, and during inspiration, negative pressure within the thoracic cavity. This acts as an important "physiological sphincter" in preventing reflux (Fig. 30.3). It is also clear that the position of the insertion of the oesophagus into the stomach may be a contributory factor in infants for GOR. In adults and older children, the insertion is much more oblique than in infants, in whom it is comparatively straight.

Ontogeny of Oesophageal Motor Function

The components required to produce mature oesophageal motor function are: (1) an integrated enteric and autonomic neural system, (2) the inherent rhythmicity of smooth muscle and (3) the initial propagation of the peristaltic wave by the coordination of striated muscle (Fig. 30.4). The previously simplistic understanding of the interaction between the excitatory parasympathetic cholinergic pathways, mediated by the vagal nerve, and the inhibitory sympathetic adrenergic control, in controlling oesophageal and intestinal smooth muscle activity via the submucosal and myenteric plexi, has had to be adapted in the light of a recent understanding of the complex processes at work in gut movement. These include the identification of a network of complex intrinsic innervation within the gut. The intrinsic nerves of the submucosal

and myenteric plexi are now known to be non-adrenergic non-cholinergic fibres that contain a wide variety of neurotransmitters and are not solely involved with transmitting autonomic signals (Fig. 30.5).

It should be mentioned that the central nervous system may play a part in overall oesophageal motility, as demonstrated by the disruption of normal oesophageal peristalsis that occurs in neonates with the peri-partum cerebral insults that result in cerebral palsy.

Swallowing in the Normal Infant and Child

The process of swallowing consists of four phases for liquids and solids alike: oral preparatory, oral, pharyngeal and oesophageal. We will consider only the latter two here.

The Pharyngeal Phase

Pharyngeal swallows are initiated in an ordered, sequential pattern in response to stimulation, by food, of the medullary swallowing centre via cranial nerves V, IX and X. In the older child or adult, the upper pharynx and the soft palate close against the posterior pharynx as the food bolus is propelled by the tongue into the pharynx, sealing the nasal cavity. Closure of the larynx protects the airway. Simultaneously, there is complete and automatic closure of the cords, and elevation of the larynx brings the epiglottis down over the glottis. This deflects the bolus laterally and posteriorly towards the upper oesophageal sphincter (UOS). The UOS opens and peristaltic contractions of the pharyngeal constrictor muscles drive the bolus through the pharynx, past the displaced, closed larynx, and into the oesophagus.

The other major function of the laryngopharyngeal space is in eliciting a protective cough reflex precipitated by several vagally mediated receptors that detect the presence of potentially damaging noxious stimuli and cause laryngeal closure and a cough. This phenomenon is becoming increasingly important to gastroenterologists with the recent appreciation of the pathological importance of

Oesophageal Acid/Pepsin Clearance, LOS Relaxation, and GORD

30

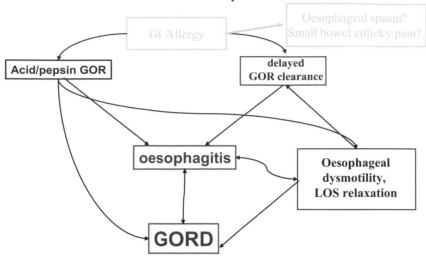

Fig. 30.5 Inter-relationships of gastro-oesophageal reflux disease (GORD). *LOS* Lower oesophageal sphincter, *GI* gastrointestinal, *GOR* gastro-oesophageal reflux

laryngopharyngeal reflux from the stomach in symptoms such as recurrent cough, hoarseness and dysphonia. An elevated resting pressure of the cricopharyngeal muscle is necessary to prevent pharyngeal penetration of the retrograde oesophageal bolus. A normal pharyngeal swallow includes complete bolus transport through the pharynx and the cricopharyngeus.

Anatomic abnormalities, including laryngeal clefts and other laryngeal deformities, can result in dysphagia and aspiration. Myopathies, central nervous system abnormalities, tumour masses or foreign bodies, oesophageal peristaltic disorders or inflammatory disorders all can disrupt the pharyngeal phase of swallowing. Infants and children with tachypnoea often have difficulty dissociating swallowing from inspiration, making feeding difficult.

Coordination of the oral and pharyngeal phases of swallowing is essential for preventing aspiration. Early overflow of the food bolus into the pharynx before respiration ceases and the swallow is initiated may allow food to be aspirated during inspiration. An unrelaxed UOS results in pooling of food in the piriform sinus. This food overflows into the airway when the larynx descends after a swallow sequence and inspiration begins.

The Oesophageal Phase

The oesophagus is a conduit between the pharynx and the stomach, with the muscular UOS and lower oesophageal sphincter (LOS) at either end. The UOS relaxes during swallowing to allow the food bolus to enter the oesopha-

gus. Peristaltic contractions propel the bolus down into the stomach. Oesophageal primary peristalsis involves an orderly and progressive series of contractions that begin in the pharynx and advance towards the stomach. The process of peristalsis moves the bolus through the oesophagus and ends when the food passes the LOS. This entire process takes between seven and ten seconds in adults. The LOS relaxation occurs within 2 s of the act of swallowing and lasts 8–10 s, allowing food into the stomach. Propagation of the peristaltic wave depends on the intrinsic myenteric plexus and the vagal afferents.

An oesophageal phase promptly follows each separate pharyngeal phase of the swallow when there is a definite time delay between swallows. However, an immediate and complete inhibition of the oesophageal phase is noted when a second pharyngeal swallow occurs while the bolus remains in the striated muscle segment (see Fig. 30.3) of the oesophagus. If the bolus from the first swallow is in the smooth muscle segment when the second swallow occurs, the initial bolus will progress for several seconds before dissipating. In contrast, the original swallow can alter the amplitude and velocity of subsequent swallows for as long as 10 s, depending on the bolus size. A series of rapid swallows results in an inactive eosophageal body and LOS relaxation. The final swallow in the series will be followed by a solitary normal peristaltic wave that clears the oesophagus.

Abnormal peristalsis, inflammation, mechanical obstruction due to oesophageal atresia, oesophageal narrowing such as in congenital stenosis, strictures, webs, vascular rings, tumours or foreign bodies may all result in dysphagia in infants and children (Fig. 30.6).

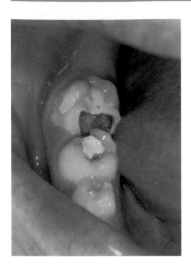

Fig. 30.6 GORD-related tooth enamel erosion

Oesophageal Sphincter Physiology

Relaxation of the LOS and UOS occurs during swallowing as well as in other situations. Secondary peristalsis that originates in the oesophagus rather than in the oropharynx includes a relaxation of the LOS, which allows oesophageal material to be propelled into the stomach. The LOS and UOS both relax to vent the stomach then the oesophagus retrogradely during belching or vomiting. The relaxation of the LOS is similar to inappropriate transient LOS relaxation (TLOSR). It is considered inappropriate because it is not associated with swallowing. Although other mechanisms have been proposed, normal individuals apparently increase the rate of TLOSRs postprandially due to gastric distension, particularly in the lesser curvature. The LOS relaxations are accompanied by relaxation of the crural diaphragm, which abolishes the pressure at the gasto-oesophageal junction.

Sphincter Dysfunction

UOS or LOS dysfunction may interfere with the customary direction of bolus flow and may signal the presence of other problems or pathology. These problems can result from disorders in tone or poor coordination of the sphincter movements in relation to bolus flow. Transient relaxation of the UOS and LOS are potential factors underlying pathologic GOR. Videoflouroscopic findings have demonstrated cricopharyngeal prominence in children with histories of GOR. Significant prominence of the UOS or failure of the UOS to relax (achalasia) can interfere with the bolus passage. Cricopharyngeal dysfunction may be the first diagnostic indicator of brainstem compression resulting from Chiari malformations. Achalasia, a rare congenital condition unrelated to GOR can affect both the UOS and LOS.

Other factors that affect clearance are posture–gravity interactions, volume, size, and contents of meal, for example breast milk, defective peristalsis of the oesophagus, gastric emptying and increasingly noxious refluxate.

Mucosal Immunology and Inflammation

From the immunological standpoint, the oesophagus is relatively quiescent in the non-pathologic state. It has no Brunner's glands or Peyer's patches involved in antigen recognition, but if the epithelial barrier is breached, then immunological functions can occur. Equally, in the pathological state induced by T-cell mediated allergy in the small bowel, homing of inflammatory cells to the oesophagus can occur without any luminal or epithelial damage.

Acid, particularly when combined with pepsin, which is still active up to around pH 5.5–6, is known to cause severe oesophagitis in animals and humans. Even a 24-week gestation infant in an intensive care setting has the ability to lower intra-gastric pH below 2. Pepsin plays a critical role in the oesophagitis associated with acidic, and possibly non-acidic refluxate – animal work has shown that in dogs and rabbits, infusion of HCl alone caused no damage, but that in combination with low concentrations of pepsin at pH<2, severe oesophagitis resulted. Proteolysis may allow deeper penetration of harmful refluxate, and the simple notion that acid causes epithelial damage must therefore be questioned in favour of a more complex interplay of several noxious stimuli in the pathogenesis of reflux oesophagitis in infants and children (Fig. 30.7).

There is recent evidence that oesophagitis is becoming a more common presentation of infant food allergy within the developed world, and that it may be induced by a variety of antigens in addition to cow's milk. Many affected infants have become sensitised while exclusively breast-fed, and a defect in oral tolerance for low doses of allergen has been postulated as the underlying cause.

Oesophageal mucosal eosinophilia has been described in both suspected cow's-milk-associated and primary reflux oesophagitis, as well as in other conditions such as primary eosinophilic oesophagitis. Some have suggested an active role for eosinophils in the inflammatory process of oesophagitis, and have supported this with the observation of activation of the eosinophils detected by electron microscopy.

Gastro-Oesophageal Reflux

GOR is defined as the involuntary passage into the oesophagus of gastric contents, the nature of which may vary: saliva, ingested foods and drinks, gastric secretions or pancreatic or biliary secretions (duodenogastric reflux). Over the past decade GOR disease (GORD) has

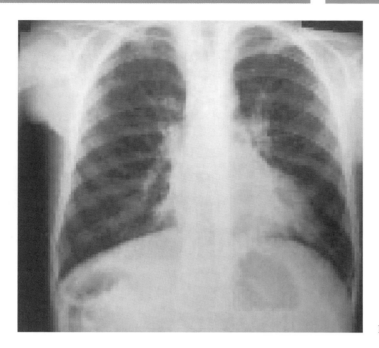

Fig. 30.7 Chest x-ray showing aspiration effects

formed a major part of paediatric gastroenterological practice and has subsequently received renewed interest and exposure. This is in part due to the refinement in existing techniques of investigation, such as endoscopy in younger infants; but also due to development of more physiologically appropriate techniques such as intraluminal impedance. In addition, advances in the field of mucosal immunology have yielded a clearer understanding of the pathophysiology and clinical importance of paediatric GOR.

GOR is most commonly seen in infants and is largely functional, usually resolving spontaneously without clinical significance. When associated with significant

clinical complications such as anaemia, faltering growth, excessive irritability, respiratory events such as apnoea, bronchoconstriction, hoarseness, near-miss sudden infant death syndrome or other events such as torticollis and infant pseudoconvulsions, GOR is generally labelled as GORD. It occurs less frequently in older children; however, in this group it is less likely to resolve and classically follows a pattern similar to that seen in adult GORD. GOR in older children may become pathological when it causes classical symptoms such as heartburn, oesophagitis and respiratory disease. A shift in clinical opinion has led to recognition that GOR in children is in fact a complex disease that may be a major cause of non-specific symptoms with extra-intestinal manifestations: respiratory, otolaryngeal, oral and even neurological. Atypical symptoms including those emanating from the upper respiratory tract (stridor, wheezing, coughing, hiccoughs), the laryngopharyngeal region (hoarseness, dysphonia), the tubotympanic region (otalgia, otitis) and even the teeth (dental erosions) have been described (Fig. 30.8).

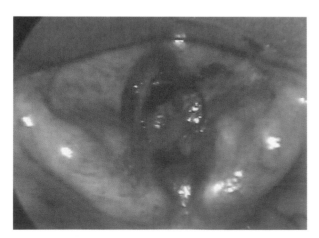

Fig. 30.8 Severe laryngeal oedema from reflux

Pathophysiology of GOR

There are many proposed hypotheses to explain the pathophysiological mechanisms of GOR and oesophagitis. The oesophagogastric pressure gradient is maintained by the LOS, a specialised, tonically contracting region of the distal oesophagus that functions as a physiological valve. Low basal LOS pressure and spontaneous transient relaxations of the LOS not associated with a corresponding oesophageal peristaltic wave are possible mechanisms. Complications and GORD may result from reflux when there is delayed clearance of refluxate, especially when this is particularly noxious, when respiratory function is compromised, if regurgitation results in significant calorific loss or when specific neurobehavioral symptoms are evident. Other causative factors include cow's milk protein intolerance or allergy, which may account for anywhere between 18 and 80% of all cases of GOR in infancy. It is becoming clear that a complex interaction exists between allergic upper GIT dysmotility, LOS relaxation and the neurohumoral mechanisms controlling smooth muscle tonic contraction at the LOS. In other words, cow's milk protein may cause the LOS to relax inappropriately, allowing GOR to occur.

GOR-Related Apparent Life-Threatening Events and Sudden Infant Death Syndrome

GOR may provoke apnoea when the gastric contents reach the pharynx, possibly by the stimulation of laryngopharyngeal chemoreceptors. In paediatrics, GOR is considered to be one of the reasons for apparent life-threatening events (ALTE) and sudden infant death syndrome (SIDS). Indeed, histopathological and pH-metry investigations have shown that approximately 47% of infants with ALTE experience GOR, and approximately 10% of the victims of SIDS had apnoea caused by GOR (Herbst 1978; Orenstein and Orenstein 1988).

GOR and Asthma

Symptoms of GOR in children with asthma have been reported with a prevalence ranging from 25 to 75%. Aspiration of refluxate may directly aggravate airway inflammation and reactivity. Improvement of respiratory function has been described in infants and older children with or without atopy following a variety of medical antireflux therapies.

A trial of vigorous, prolonged medical therapy for GOR is recommended for children when symptoms of asthma and GORD (e.g. heartburn, regurgitation) coexist, and in infants and toddlers with chronic vomiting or regurgitation and recurrent episodes of cough and wheezing.

Recurrent Pneumonia

Several reports have shown an association between GOR and recurrent pneumonia (Chen et al. 1991; Euler et al 1979). Most reported paediatric studies on GOR and recurrent pneumonia have been described in children with

neurological disabilities and abnormalities of the upper GI tract. It is therefore difficult to estimate the incidence of GOR and recurrent pneumonia in otherwise normal children, but clinical experience would indicate this to be rare.

Upper Airway Symptoms

Airway symptoms such as hoarseness, stridor, chronic cough, dysphonia and globus sensation are recognised associations with GOR (Curran et al 1995; Fitzgerald et al 1991; Ing et al. 1991). Gastropharyngolaryngeal reflux was more prevalent in a small study of children with recurrent laryngotracheitis compared to control patients (Contencin and Narcy 1992). An increased frequency of daytime GOR events in children with hoarseness has been suggested in one series (Gumpert et al 1998). Halstead (1999) suggested that GOR either contributes to the pathogenesis of subglottic stenosis or compromises surgical results, while another case series noted increased pharyngeal reflux in children with laryngomalacia (Matthews et al 1999). An uncontrolled case series describes an improvement in a variety of upper-airway symptoms in children following treatment of GOR with a variety of therapies (Conley et al. 1995). There is, however, no evidence from randomised placebo-controlled treatment trials to support these data.

Significant associations were found between the presence of histologic oesophagitis and recurrent croup, cough, stridor, laryngomalacia, suglottic stenosis, posterior glottic erythema and posterior erythema (Yellon 2000). GORD may have a causal role in voice disorders. Investigation of GOR in children with stridor, laryngomalacia and laryngitis should be considered when there is failure of the usual treatment. Although there are several studies describing the presence of GOR in children with either chronic or recurrent laryngeal symptoms, there remains a lack of uniform interpretation of laryngeal findings.

Chronic Tubotympanic Disorders

The association between ear problems and GORD remains uncertain. GOR has been suggested as a potential cause of recurrent sinus disease, pharyngitis and otitis media. Tolia and Zeng (2001) found no significant association between GORD and otitis media, when endoscopic biopsy was used to make the diagnosis. However, a study by Rozmanic et al. (2002) reported that pathologic GORD was detected, using either dual-level or distal oesophageal pH probes, in 15 of 27 children with secretory or recurrent otitis media. More recently, Tasker et al. (2002) suggested that reflux of gastric juice could be a major cause of glue ear in children. They analysed middle-ear effusion fluid for the presence of pepsin (which can only have come from the stomach by reflux) at the time of grommet insertion, and found it to be present in 83% of cases. This elegant study supports further the association between GOR and tubotympanic disorders.

Diagnostic Options

Oesophageal pH monitoring has gained general acceptance as the method for assessment of GOR in children, and until recently has been regarded as the investigation technique of first choice in infants and children with unusual presentations of GOR disease such as apnoea and recurrent respiratory disease. However, pH measurements cannot detect GOR in the pH range 4.0–7.0, as this is close to the normal oesophageal pH (Grill 1992; Vandenplas et al 1992). For this reason, pH-metry also misses many episodes of post-prandial reflux in young infants because of neutralisation of gastric contents by milk formula for 1–2 h after a meal. Currently available pH-independent techniques for the study of reflux include ultrasound, aspiration scintigraphy, fluoroscopy and bilirubin monitoring.

Intraluminal Impedance

A new, pH-independent, intraluminal oesophageal impedance technique, which relies on the higher conductivity of a liquid bolus compared with oesophageal muscular wall or air, has been validated in adults (Fig. 30.9). When used in infants with GOR who had simultaneous pH measurement for prolonged periods, intraluminal oesophageal impedance showed that 73% of all GOR occurs during or in the first 2 h after feeding. This GOR is pH neutral, and therefore will be missed by pH-metry. Seventy-five percent of GOR extends proximally as far as the pharynx, and this has broad implications for the study of GOR-associated respiratory phenomena and symptoms caused by gastrolaryngopharyngeal reflux (Skopnik et al. 1996). Wenzl et al. (2001) re-examined the temporal association between infant apnoea and reflux in a recent study and found, on the basis of impedance, a marked association between these two phenomena (Fig. 30.10). Approximately one-third of all documented apnoeas occurred in the 30 s before or after an impedance-identified reflux event, of which only 23% were acid-reflux events, hence the hypothesis that GOR may stimulate laryngeal receptors. Wenzl et al. (2001) suggest that forced respiratory effort with increased abdominothoracic pressure, as occurs during episodes of obstructive apnoea, can overcome LOS pressure and cause a reflux episode.

Using the impedance technique, episodes of GOR can be characterised by the level they reach in the oesophagus and by their duration. This is especially useful in the post-prandial period and in clinical situations of gastric hypoacidity. Simultaneous pH and impedance monitoring allows further categorisation of GOR episodes.

The impedance technique can be incorporated into other diagnostic systems, for example manometry (Cucchiara et al 1996; Gilger et al 1997) and sleep studies. Technical effort has now developed a portable recording device for mobile, outpatient impedance studies in all age groups.

Endoscopy and Biopsy Sampling

In general, oesophagogastroduodenoscopy (OGD) is not indicated for uncomplicated GOR. Infants with symptoms suggestive of oesophagitis (complicated GOR), such as haematemesis, anaemia, GOR-related feeding disturbance, failure to thrive and pronounced irritability, should be considered for OGD. Oesophageal biopsy should always complement OGD because correlation with macroscopic appearance is poor. The recent realisation that specific histological appearances may reflect specific causes or associated pathologies has reinforced this recommendation. A specific pattern of oesophageal eosinophilia has now been associated with cow's milk protein allergic oesophagitis. Intraepithelial T lymphocytes, and a variety of immunohistochemical markers have also been used to examine the oesophageal mucosa, including eotaxin, a recently described eosinophil-specific chemokine, and markers of T-cell lineage and activation (Butt et al. 2002; Garcia et al. 1996).

Oesophageal Dysmotility, Extrinsic Compression and Mechanical Obstruction

Oesophageal dysmotility may interfere with food or liquid passage form the oropharynx into the stomach. This condition is associated with anatomic changes resulting from surgery (e.g. tracheo-oesophageal fistula repair) or from oesophagitis associated with GOR. Extrinsic compression may interfere with bolus passage by narrowing the oesophageal lumen. Children with tracheostomy tubes or anatomic anomalies (e.g. vascular rings, tumours or masses) may be at higher risk of oesophageal impairment associated with external compression. Oesophageal function may be compromised by the presence of mechanical obstruction, such as a stricture or foreign body. Strictures are associated with scar tissue from surgery, complicated GORD, eosinophilic oesophagitis and ingestion of corrosive substances.

TW

Intraluminal impedance technique

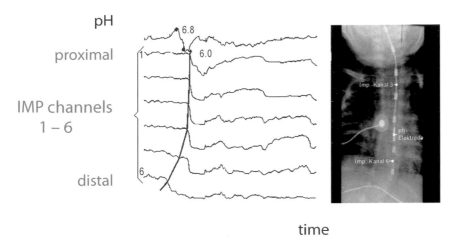

Skopnik et al. Gastroesophageal reflux in infants: Evaluation of
a new intraluminal technique. JPGN 1996,23:591-8

Fig. 30.9 Technique for measuring intraluminal impedance. The probe, with impedance channels, is shown on the chest x-ray

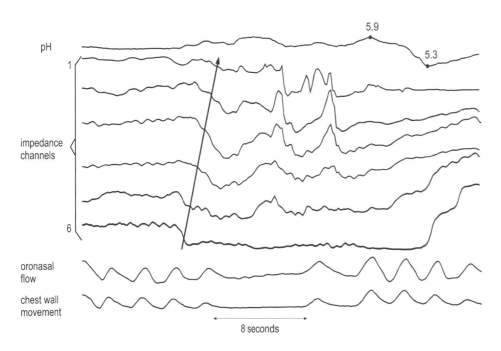

Fig. 30.10 Demonstrating the relationship between non-acid gastro-oesophageal reflux and central apnoea

Summary for the Clinician

- Until recently, GORD in children has been a relatively underdeveloped area of research and clinical understanding. It is now clear that GORD in children has many causative pathways. These may have complex interactions and extra-intestinal manifestations, and require equally complex diagnostic and therapeutic strategies. With new investigative techniques such as intraluminal impedance and ambulant motility recorders, a clearer understanding of the motility and the physiology of the oesophagus should allow us to link already suspected clinical hypotheses. Improved understanding of the complex immunology that lies behind inflammatory processes in the oesophagus is also an important focus of future research in children. These advances highlight the mutual interest that exists between paediatric gastroenterology and otorhinolaryngology, which should open the door to a vast area of mutually beneficial research.

References

1. Butt AM, Murch SH, Thomson MA, et al (2002) Upregulated eotaxin expression and T cell infiltration in the basal and papillary epithelium in cow's milk associated reflux oesophagitis. Arch Dis Child 87:124–130
2. Chen PH, Chang MH, Hsu SC (1991) Gastroesophageal reflux in children with chronic recurrent bronchopulmonary infection. J Pediatr Gastroenterol Nutr 13:16–22
3. Conley SF, Werlin SL, Beste DJ (1995) Proximal pH-metry for diagnosis of upper airway complications of gastroesophageal reflux. J Otolaryngol 24:295–298
4. Contencin P, Narcy P (1992) Gastropharyngeal reflux in infants and children. A pharyngeal pH monitoring study. Arch Otolaryngol Head Neck Surg 118:1028–1030
5. Cucchiara S, Campanozzi A, Greco L, et al (1996) Predictive value of oesophageal manometry and gastroesophageal pH monitoring for the responsiveness of reflux disease to medical therapy in children. Am J Gastroenterol 91:680–685
6. Curran AJ, Barry MK, Callanan V, et al (1995) A prospective study of acid reflux and globus pharyngeus using a modified symptom index. Clin Otolaryngol 20:552–554
7. Euler AR, Byrne WJ, Ament ME, et al (1979) Recurrent pulmonary disease in children: a complication of gastroesophageal reflux. Pediatrics 63:47–51
8. Fitzgerald JM, Allen CJ, Craven MA, et al (1991) Chronic cough and gastroesophageal reflux. Thorax 46:479–483
9. Garcia-Zepeda EA, Rothenberg ME, Ownbey RT, et al (1996) Human eotaxin is a specific chemoattractant for eosinophil cells and provides a new mechanism to explain tissue eosinophilia. Nat Med 2:449–456
10. Gilger MA, Boyle JT, Sonderheimer JM, et al (1997) Indications for pediatric manometry. Statement of the North American Society for Pediatric Gastroenterology and Nutrition (NASPGN). Pediatr Gastroenterol Nutr 24:616–618
11. Grill B (1992) Twenty-four hour oesophageal pH monitoring: what's the score? J Paediatr Gastroenterol Nutr 14:249–251
12. Gumpert L, Kalach N, Dupont C, et al (1998) Hoarseness and gastroesophageal reflux in children. J Laryngol Otol 1112:49–54
13. Halstead LA (1999) Gastroesophageal reflux: a critical factor in pediatric subglottic stenosis. Otolaryngol Head Neck Surg 120:683–688
14. Herbst JJ (1978) Gastroesophageal reflux in the "near miss" sudden infant death syndrome. J Paediatr 92:73–75
15. Ing AJ, Ngu MC, Breslin AB (1991) Chronic persistent cough and gastroesophageal reflux. Thorax 46:479–483
16. Matthews BL, Little JP, McGuirt WJ, et al (1999) Reflux in infants with laryngomalacia: results of 24-hour double-probe pH monitoring. Otolaryngol Head Neck Surg 120:860–864
17. Orenstein SR, Orenstein DM (1988) Gastroesophageal reflux and respiratory disease in children. J Paediatr 112:847–858
18. Rozmanic V, Velepic M, Ahel V, et al (2002) Prolonged oesophageal pH monitoring in the evaluation of gastroesophageal reflux in children with chronic tubotympanic disorders. J Pediatr Gastroenterol Nutr 34:278–280
19. Skopnik H, Silny J, Heiber O, et al (1996) Gastroesophageal reflux in infants: evaluation of a new intraluminal impedance technique. J Pediatr Gastroenterol Nutr 23:591–598
20. Tasker A, Dettmar PW, Pearson JP, et al (2002) Reflux of gastric juice in glue ear. Lancet 359:493
21. Tolia V, Zeng M (2001) Evaluation of gastroesophageal reflux disease in children with chronic ear, nose, throat and respiratory conditions. J Pediatr Gastroenterol Nutr 33: A92
22. Vandenplas Y, Belli D, Boige N, et al (1992) A standardised protocol for the methodology or oesophageal pH monitoring and interpretation of the data for the diagnosis of the gastroesophageal reflux. Society statement of a working group of the European Society of Paediatric Gastroenterology and Nutrition. J Paediatr Gastroenterol Nutr 14:467–471
23. Wenzl T, Schenke S, Peschgens T, et al (2001) Association of apnoea and non-acid gastroesophageal reflux in infants: investigations with the intraluminal impedance technique. Paediatr Pulmonol 31:144–149
24. Yellon RF, Coticchia J, Dixit S (2000) Esophageal biopsy for the diagnosis of gastroesophageal reflux-associated otolaryngologic problems in children. Am J Med 108:131S–138S

Chapter 31

Paediatric Thyroid Disease

Michael Kuo and Tim Barrett

Core Messages

- Thyroid disease in children is uncommon.
- In regions where iodine intake is adequate, the commonest cause of acquired paediatric thyroid dysfunction is autoimmune thyroid disease.
- Ultrasonography is the primary imaging modality for paediatric thyroid disease.
- Thyroid disease in children may be associated with certain syndromes, for example with sensorineural deafness in Pendred syndrome and with endocrine tumours in multiple endocrine neoplasia type 2 (MEN-2) syndrome.
- Affected children carrying the RET (rearranged before transcription) mutation in MEN-2A and MEN-2B require prophylactic surgical treatment before the ages of 5 years and 1 year, respectively.
- Thyroid malignancies in childhood are rare, accounting for <1% of all childhood malignancies; however, they should be treated aggressively to ensure an excellent long-term outcome.

Contents

Introduction

Thyroid disease is uncommon in children. The most commonly encountered surgical pathologies of the thyroid apparatus in children are thyroglossal duct cysts and fistulae. These and the management of ectopic thyroid tissue are discussed elsewhere (Chapter 19). This chapter reviews the embryology, anatomy and physiology of the thyroid gland, investigation of thyroid disease, functional thyroid diseases and thyroid neoplasia in the paediatric population. It assumes in the reader a knowledge of the management of adult thyroid disease.

Embryology, Physiology and Anatomy

Embryology

Understanding of the embryology of the thyroid gland forms the basis for the management of congenital thyroid anomalies as well as neoplasia in ectopic thyroid tissue. The thyroid gland originates from an endodermal thickening in the midline of the primitive pharynx anterior to the respiratory tract, which ultimately becomes the foramen caecum at the base of the tongue. This thyroid primordium forms a diverticulum, which plunges caudally as a result of elongation of the embryo and growth

31

of the median tongue bud, completing its journey by the 8th week of gestation, becoming solid and dividing in its final position as a bi-lobed structure straddling the cervical trachea. The hollow diverticulum degenerates at the same time, but persistence will result in the presence of a thyroglossal duct. During descent, the second-arch cartilages migrate ventrally to meet their opposite numbers and, with the third-arch cartilages, form the hyoid bone. If the thyroglossal duct persists, it will therefore be enveloped in the developing hyoid bone. Meanwhile, the endodermal thyroid primordium differentiates into thyroid follicles during the 11th week of gestation, and shortly after that colloid and thyroxine begin to be produced.

Physiology

The basic functional unit of the thyroid gland is the thyroid follicle, which is responsible for the synthesis and storage of thyroglobulin and its iodination to form thyroid hormones. These processes are under the control of the hypothalamo-pituitary-thyroid gland axis, by means of a classical hormone feedback loop. The end products are the biologically active thyroid hormones, which regulate the basal metabolic rate via metabolism of substrates, energy production and protein synthesis, and so affect every tissue and organ system in the body.

The thyroid gland both makes and stores thyroid hormones, and requires an adequate intake of iodide for its proper functioning. In Western Europe, a level of 200 µg per day is thought to be ideal, and dietary iodide is found in many foods, water and fortified foods such as some bread and table salt. Dietary iodide is almost completely absorbed from the gut and actively trapped by thyroid follicular cells. It is then modified by the enzyme thyroid peroxidase into hormonally inactive iodotyrosines (mono-iodotyrosine and di-iodotyrosine). The coupling of these iodinated tyrosines forms the biologically active iodothyronines T3 and T4. These are then bound into thyroglobulin, a large glycoprotein present in the follicular lumen as colloid, which acts as a store of thyroid hormone. T4 and T3 are released by proteolytic cleavage of thyroglobulin, under the influence of thyroid stimulating hormone (TSH), which is released from the anterior pituitary. T4 and T3 are transported in the circulation bound to thyroxine-binding globulin, so that only about 0.04% of T4 and 0.4% of T3 are in the unbound (free) state. T3 is by far the most metabolically active form of the hormone, and T4 is converted to T3, mainly in the target tissues, by de-iodinase enzymes. Both T4 and T3 are transported into cells by passive diffusion and specific thyroid hormone transporters, and act on thyroid hormone receptors on the nuclear membrane. The thyroid hormone receptor–thyroid hormone complex then interacts with the DNA sequence of the thyroid hormone response elements of target genes to enhance gene activation and protein production.

Thyroid hormone synthesis is regulated by a classic feedback control system: the hypothalamus secretes thyrotrophin releasing hormone (TRH), which stimulates the anterior pituitary to release TSH into the bloodstream. TSH stimulates the thyroid gland to release and synthesise T4 and, to a lesser extent, T3. T4 and T3 both feed back at the levels of the pituitary and hypothalamus to inhibit the release of TRH and TSH.

Anatomy

The thyroid is a bi-lobed gland, with the two lobes joined by an isthmus, which overlies the second to fourth tracheal rings and which may extend superiorly into a pyramidal lobe. The thyroid gland receives its blood supply from the superior thyroid artery, which arises from the external carotid, and from the inferior thyroid artery, a branch of the thyrocervical trunk, which arises from the subclavian artery. The superior and inferior thyroid arteries also provide the blood supply to the paired parathyroid glands on the posterolateral aspects of each thyroid lobe. The superior parathyroid glands are more constantly placed near to the cricothyroid joint, while the location of the inferior parathyroid glands is more variable. The venous drainage of the thyroid and parathyroid glands is through the superior and middle veins into the internal jugular vein and through the inferior thyroid vein into the brachiocephalic vein. The lymphatic drainage of the thyroid gland goes to the lateral cervical lymph nodes at levels III–V and the anterior cervical lymph nodes (level VI).

Of particular surgical anatomical importance in this area are the courses of the superior laryngeal nerves and the recurrent laryngeal nerves (RLNs). The superior laryngeal nerve is a mixed nerve, with its internal (sensory) branch supplying the supraglottic larynx and tongue base and its external (motor) branch supplying the cricothyroid muscle. Its close relationship to the superior thyroid pedicle puts the external branch in jeopardy during ligation of the superior thyroid vessels. Injury to this nerve causes a loss of tension in the vocal cord, which is clinically manifest as rapid fatigue of the voice and a failure to reach the higher vocal registers. The RLN supplies all of the other intrinsic muscles of the larynx apart from the cricothyroid. The right RLN loops around the right subclavian artery and the left RLN around the aortic arch. This asymmetry results in the left RLN travelling in a paratracheal course towards the larynx more tightly within the tracheo-oesophageal groove than the right RLN, which tends to have a more oblique final course towards the laryngeal entry point. The relationship between the RLN and the inferior thyroid artery is, unfortunately, variable, rendering the artery a poor guide to the location of the nerve.

There are two specific aspects of neck anatomy of which it is important to be aware in managing paediatric thyroid disease. The first is the thymus, which is a gland that is present in childhood, which gradually increases in size but ultimately dwindles and disappears after reaching maximal size at puberty. The thymus is a lobulated structure that may extend from the mediastinum into the neck, from the level of the fourth costal cartilage up to the inferior aspect of the thyroid gland. The surgeon needs to be aware of its anatomy when dissecting the inferior pole of the thyroid or carrying out a central compartment neck dissection.

The second is a persistent fourth branchial arch sinus. Acute anterior neck infection with abscess formation is an uncommon condition compared with that in the lateral neck. It is often associated with acute suppurative thyroiditis. The latter diagnosis, especially if recurrent, should always lead to the consideration of a persistent fourth branchial arch sinus. A persistent fourth branchial arch sinus starts in the pyriform fossa and extends posteroinferiorly behind the larynx into the superior mediastinum. Infection of this sinus can result in anterior neck infection or acute suppurative thyroiditis. The investigation of choice would be a contrast swallow examination, which may reveal the persistent sinus. Almost invariably, these occur on the left side, and definitive management can be achieved by open surgery or by endoscopic surgery to obliterate the sinus and close the opening of the sinus into the pyriform fossa.

Investigation of the Thyroid Gland

Thyroid Function Tests

The tests used to investigate thyroid dysfunction include hormone assays [TSH, free T4 (FT4) and free T3 (FT3)], and thyroid autoantibodies. Many labs routinely only offer the TSH assay; this is because TSH measurement in a blood sample by a sensitive immunometric assay provides the single most sensitive, specific and reliable test of thyroid status in both overt and subclinical primary thyroid disorders (Spencer et al. 1990). A normal reference range for TSH is typically 0.3–4.5 mU/l. Patients with TSH levels above 5.0 mU/l are at risk for primary hypothyroidism. TSH levels below 0.01 mU/l usually indicate hyperthyroidism. The main exception is in patients with hypothalamic/pituitary disorders, in whom TSH alone is not a reliable test.

Free (unbound) thyroid hormones (FT3, FT4) are the biologically active part of the total circulating thyroid pool, and there are several assay techniques that can be used to measure them. Normal ranges are dependant on the assay used, but are usually between 9 and 25 pmol/l for FT4 and 3.5–7.8 pmol/l for FT3. There are situations where the free hormone levels do not correlate with thyroid status: these include critically ill patients on Paediatric Intensive Care Units and patients receiving certain drugs, such as amiodarone, which interfere with hormone binding to the plasma binding proteins

Thyroglobulin is also present in the circulation and its measurement is useful for monitoring patients with differentiated thyroid papillary or follicular carcinoma. It is usually present at low levels of up to 30 pmol/l.

Thyroid Immunology

In the UK, where iodine intake is usually adequate, the commonest cause of acquired thyroid dysfunction is autoimmune thyroid disease. Almost all patients with autoimmune thyroid disease have antibodies to thyroid peroxidase at some point in the disease process, so this antibody is the most commonly measured. Antibodies that bind to TSH receptors on the thyroid gland and stimulate thyroid function (TSH receptor antibodies) result in autoimmune hyperthyroidism or Graves' disease. TSH receptor antibodies that bind the receptor without stimulating it, and thus block the receptor from being occupied by TSH, can be found in autoimmune hypothyroidism. Finally, antibodies to thyroglobulin are also detected in autoimmune thyroid disease.

The most clinically useful measure is of thyroid peroxidase antibodies, which are present in almost all patients with autoimmune thyroid disease. They may occasionally be detected in apparently healthy people, but usually their presence precedes the development of thyroid disorder. The measurement of thyroglobulin antibodies is mainly confined to the management of differentiated thyroid carcinoma. TSH receptor antibodies are useful to measure in pregnancy, as they are mainly of the IgG subclass and cross the placenta, so can predict neonates at risk for transient hyper- or hypothyroidism.

Genetic Testing

Genetic testing for inherited thyroid disorders is required in two situations. First, when thyroid dysfunction is present as part of a syndrome. Examples include multiple endocrine neoplasia (MEN) type 2 (thyroid cancer and phaeochromocytoma). This is a familial cancer syndrome caused by mutations in the *ret* (rearranged before transcription) proto-oncogene, for which genetic testing is available. Thyroid dysfunction can also be associated with sensorineural deafness in Pendred syndrome. Second, there are rare inherited disorders of thyroid development and dyshormonogenesis caused by mutations in

31

single genes. Clues to this include more than one affected child in a family, or parents who are related (Park and Chatterjee 2005).

Ultrasonography/Computed Tomography/ Magnetic Resonance Imaging

Ultrasonography is an effective method of assessing neck lesions. It is very well tolerated by children, making it the primary imaging modality for paediatric thyroid disease. In the assessment of children with thyroglossal duct cysts, it aids in diagnosis and planning by identifying the presence of normally placed thyroid lobes. In the assessment of solitary thyroid lesions, ultrasound effectively differentiates cystic from solid lesions. This is of value because cystic lesions are less likely to be malignant, although 50% of malignant lesions may have a cystic component. Ultrasonography can also accurately size nodules and allows them to be monitored by interval ultrasound scanning if a conservative management protocol is adopted. Ultrasonography is highly sensitive in the assessment of cervical lymphadenopathy, but in children with established thyroid malignancy, a staging magnetic resonance imaging (MRI) scan is recommended for its soft-tissue resolution and the avoidance of radiation.

Ultrasonography is widely used in the diagnosis and follow-up of thyroiditis. In acute and subacute (de Quervain's) thyroiditis, ultrasound and Doppler ultrasound findings correlate with the extent, form and phase of disease. The characteristic ultrasound appearances in chronic lymphocytic (Hashimoto's) thyroiditis makes ultrasound the investigation of choice, with sensitivity surpassing that of antibody testing (Pedersen et al. 2000).

Radionucleotide Scan

The role of radionucleotide scanning in thyroid disease diagnosis is now small because of the sensitivity of ultrasonography and because fine-needle aspiration cytology has largely superseded the functional evaluation of solitary thyroid nodules. In difficult cases, there is still a role for discriminating a functioning "hot" or "warm" nodule from a "cold" one in children with suppressed TSH, the latter being more likely to be malignant; but in established differentiated thyroid malignancy, the role of radionucleotide scanning is mainly in the detection of metastases and local recurrence.

Congenital hypothyroidism affects 1 in 3,000-6,000 live births in Europe and the USA. It is in the assessment of these children that radionucleotide scanning (^{99m}Tc pertechnetate or ^{123}Iodide) holds a key role. In children, it differentiates between a normal gland, one with no detectable activity, one with normal location but is abnormal in size, and ectopic thyroid tissue.

Fine-Needle Aspiration

Fine needle aspiration cytology (FNAC) is central to the diagnostic work-up of adults with thyroid pathology, because of its low morbidity, high sensitivity and high specificity. The main limitation of FNAC is its inability to distinguish follicular adenomas from follicular carcinomas, despite attempts at molecular characterisation of the cell aspirates. FNAC is an effective diagnostic tool in the paediatric population, but the willingness of children, despite topical local anaesthetic, to undergo the procedure without general anaesthesia is variable. In the authors' experience, few children under the age of 12 years will permit FNAC while awake.

Congenital Abnormalities

Thyroglossal Duct Cysts and Fistulae, and Ectopic Thyroid

This is discussed in Chapter 19.

Congenital Hypothyroidism

Congenital hypothyroidism occurs in about 1 in 4000 births, and before 1980 was a common and preventable cause of mental retardation. With the introduction of universal screening, almost all affected babies are detected in the neonatal period and treated with thyroxine. On a worldwide basis, the commonest cause is iodine deficiency; however this is rare in the UK, where the commonest cause is a defect in thyroid development leading to thyroid dysgenesis (80%) or dyshormonogenesis (20%).

In dysgenesis, the thyroid gland is either aplastic or fails to descend normally during embryological development. Dyshormonogenesis includes failure of the gland to synthesise normal thyroid hormone due to defects in the biosynthetic pathway of thyroxine, and may be associated with a goitre, the result of hyperplasia of the gland.

All newborn babies should be screened for congenital hypothyroidism by measurement of a blood spot TSH from a sample collected at 2–7 days after birth. This is done in the UK as part of the national neonatal screening programme. The sample should not be measured before 2 days of age because of the normal physiological TSH surge that occurs from 30 min after birth, falling again after 1–2 h. A TSH level above the cut-off is likely to indicate primary hypothyroidism. This neonatal screen will not detect secondary hypothyroidism due to hypothalamic and pituitary defects; these are much rarer and usually present with multiple hormone deficiencies.

Treatment should be initiated as soon as possible. It is not necessary to wait for further confirmatory tests such as radio-iodide scanning or ultrasound. If treatment is started promptly, a normal intellectual outcome can be expected in 85% of affected children.

Thyroid imaging (scintigraphy using technetium) is useful to provide information about the size and location of the thyroid gland, in combination with ultrasound scanning of the neck. There are rare instances when technetium scanning fails to show a gland that has been identified on ultrasound, because of defects in the sodium/iodide symporter (*NIS*) gene.

Syndromes Associated with Thyroid Abnormalities

Pendred syndrome is an autosomal recessive disorder that is characterised by a late-onset goitre and sensorineural deafness; it is thought to be the commonest form of syndromic deafness. Children with Pendred syndrome commonly have widened vestibular aqueducts and may also have incomplete partition of the cochlea (Mondini malformation). The thyroid dysfunction is often mild; children are often euthyroid, and they can present with a goitre in the second decade of life. Genetic testing is available for mutations in Pendrin, the Pendred Syndrome gene (see Chapter 7).

MEN syndromes result in endocrine tumours, as their name suggests. MEN-1 affects the parathyroid glands but not the thyroid. MEN-2A includes medullary thyroid carcinoma (MTC), phaeochromocytoma and primary hyperparathyroidism, and is often familial. MEN-2B is defined by MTC, phaeochromocytoma, marfanoid habitus, mucosal neuromas and intestinal ganglioneuromas. MTC affects about 1 in 40,000 people, while there are only about 500–1000 families with MEN-2 worldwide (Cocks 2005). Therefore, most cases of MTC in adults are sporadic, and only about 10% are related to MEN-2. However, when MTC develops in a child, it is likely to be related to MEN-2, and therefore appropriate investigations need to be undertaken. In MEN-2, C-cell hyperplasia develops early in life, and this is the basis for the pentagastrin stimulation test. This was an unpleasant test for children, and has been superseded by mutation testing for the *ret* proto-oncogene.

Functional Abnormalities of the Thyroid Gland

Hypothyroidism

Juvenile-onset hypothyroidism is commonly autoimmune and due to lymphocytic infiltration of the thyroid (Hashimoto's thyroiditis); this often presents with a goitre. Occasionally, children develop idiopathic or atrophic thyroiditis. In both situations, the presenting features include slow growth, a tendency to gain weight, the gradual development of a pale, puffy face, increased lethargy and sometimes a fall-off in school performance. The onset can be so insidious that the immediate family do not recognise the signs. The diagnosis is confirmed by the finding of a low FT4 and raised TSH. Thyroid peroxidase antibodies are positive in Hashimoto's thyroiditis. Treatment of acquired hypothyroidism is with thyroxine. This is given as tablets once a day with a low starting dose. The dose of thyroxine is gradually titrated until full replacement levels are reached. The outlook is excellent, but affected children will need hormone replacement for life.

Hyperthyroidism

Autoimmune hyperthyroidism is most commonly caused in the UK by Graves' disease. This is characterised by a diffusely enlarged thyroid gland, and usually, ophthalmopathy. The exact cause is unknown, but there is a familial predisposition, and females are affected more often than males. The effects include tachycardia, resting tremor, increased height velocity, heat intolerance, behaviour problems including restlessness and agitation, and a fall-off in school performance. Occasionally, the goitre can cause dysphagia or even tracheal compression. The diagnosis is confirmed by the finding of a raised FT4 and suppressed TSH. The first-line treatment in children is the use of antithyroid drugs such as thionamides (carbimazole), in combination with beta blockers to reduce the cardiac side effects. Most UK children are offered a "block and treat" regime, whereby the antithyroid drug is used to suppress thyroxine production completely, and thyroxine replacement is titrated against the thyroid function tests. This results in remission in the majority of children, but they have a tendency to relapse when treatment is withdrawn. The side effects of thionamides include itchy skin rashes; less commonly, agranulocytosis may occur in 1% of treated patients; this complication tends to occur early in the course of treatment, and presents with fever, sore throat and mouth ulcers. Patients and parents should be warned to seek medical help immediately if these complications develop. If thionamides are not tolerated, then propylthiouracil, the active metabolite of carbimazole, is an alternative.

Although most children achieve remission, a significant proportion relapse when treatment is withdrawn. Radio-iodine is a permanent treatment, although the long-term result is hypothyroidism. Despite the lack of evidence for long-term development of radiation-induced malignancy, radio-iodine is not usually offered to children. The more popular option in the UK is thyroidectomy. Patients need to be in remission before surgery, and the vascularity of the gland can be reduced by the addition of Lugol's iodine solution (0.1–0.3 ml 8 hourly) for 3–5 days immediately prior to surgery.

Neoplasms of the Thyroid Gland

Thyroid malignancies are extremely rare in childhood, accounting for 1% of all childhood malignancies and 5% of paediatric head and neck malignancies. Therefore, recommendations for their management are not based on evidence any more robust than level three. The principles governing the management of paediatric thyroid cancer are similar to those in adults, with certain special considerations that will be discussed. Previous irradiation of the neck (whether historical as in the management of adenotonsillar hypertrophy, therapeutic as in the management of head and neck malignancies or accidental as in the Chernobyl disaster) is an important aetiological factor. Chemotherapy for Hodgkin's disease is also a major factor, increasing the risk of thyroid cancer by 68-fold. An association between thyroid cancer and carotid body tumours, Gardner's syndrome and Cowden's disease is recognised, as is the special case of familial medullary thyroid cancer in the context of multiple endocrine neoplasia syndromes.

Approach to the Solitary Thyroid Nodule in Children

There are significant differences between adults and children in the behaviour of solitary thyroid nodules. The prevalence of solitary thyroid nodules in children is low (around 1% compared with 5% in adults). Very few patients with solitary thyroid nodules actually present to the clinician. However, of the small minority that do present to an endocrinologist or surgeon, 1 in 20 adults turn out to have a malignancy, while for children the proportion is 1 in 3. Differentiated thyroid cancers tend to be advanced at presentation in children, yet they have an excellent prognosis if managed appropriately. Therefore, a meticulous diagnostic work up is essential in children with solitary thyroid nodules, and while the algorithm is similar to that in adults, there are certain specific emphases. Bearing in mind the aetiological factors in paediatric thyroid cancer, obtaining an accurate past medical history and family history is of particular importance. In the absence of dysphonia or a high suspicion of malignancy, elective assessment of vocal fold function is probably unnecessary. Few children will tolerate indirect laryngoscopy but where indicated, they may tolerate the introduction of the new, ultrafine (2 mm) fibre-optic nasendoscopes with topical anaesthesia. The relatively high risk of malignancy in a solitary thyroid nodule in children requires the prolonged follow-up of children with equivocal cytology, inadequate sampling (Thy1) or benign cytology (Thy2) with serial ultrasonography. The risk of malignancy also tends to reduce the threshold for recommendation of diagnostic lobectomy in children with Thy3 (indeterminate, follicular) and Thy4 (indeter-

minate, suspicious of malignancy) cytology, although the parent and, if appropriate, the child or adolescent, needs to be involved in the thought process underlying such recommendations. Approximately two-thirds of solitary thyroid nodules in children are follicular adenomas (Hung 1999).

Sporadic Differentiated Thyroid Cancer

Thyroid malignancies in the paediatric age group tend to be well-differentiated, with papillary thyroid carcinomas predominating. Careful staging of children with cytologically or histologically proven disease is crucial, as children tend to present with advanced disease. A combination of ultrasonography and MRI scanning is recommended for the assessment of regional metastases in the neck, while computed tomography scanning is preferred for exclusion of intrathoracic metastases.

The choices in the management of thyroid cancer are complicated in children by the anatomy, the presence of the thymus gland and the difficulties of managing hypoparathyroidism in a growing child. The surgical options for management of the primary site are total thyroidectomy, near-total thyroidectomy and thyroid lobectomy. There is little evidence that near-total thyroidectomy reduces the risk of injury to the RLN and of hypoparathyroidism, and therefore the choice is largely between total thyroidectomy or thyroid lobectomy. The high incidence of regional and distant metastases, with the need for diagnostic thyroglobulin monitoring, diagnostic ^{123}I scanning and, if indicated, adjuvant radio-iodine treatment, inclines the surgeon towards total thyroidectomy. Total thyroidectomy is also associated with improved long-term disease-free survival, with one study showing a recurrence rate of 57% in patients with lobectomy compared with 14% in those with more extensive surgery (Welch Dinauer et al. 1999). However, although relatively infrequent (0–17%), permanent hypoparathyroidism is extremely difficult to manage in the growing child. Management requires calcium and vitamin D supplements with dose titration against regular serum calcium measurements.

There is no indication for elective dissection of the N0 neck in differentiated non-medullary paediatric thyroid cancer. In children with node-positive disease, 90% will have involvement of the pre-tracheal and paratracheal lymph nodes. Therefore, surgical treatment must include a complete central compartment (level VI) dissection. This is often complicated by the presence of the thymus in smaller children. There is no place for selective "node-picking" in the treatment of thyroid cervical metastases in children, which should be treated by a selective neck dissection (levels II–VI).

The use of adjuvant radioactive iodine ablation in children with non-metastatic differentiated thyroid cancer is controversial. A post-operative diagnostic radioactive iodine uptake scan may detect otherwise subclinical pulmonary metastases in 20% of paediatric patients, particularly in those with papillary carcinoma (Farahati et al. 1997). The extensive literature on the safety and efficacy of radioactive iodine ablation in thyroid cancer treatment does not give data specific to the paediatric age group. While it is almost universally offered to adult patients, the decision as to whether to offer adjuvant radioactive iodine to a child must be made on an individual basis, taking into consideration the tumour factors and the diagnostic uptake scan, because of the increased risks from irradiation in childhood (Mazzaferri 1997).

Despite a tendency towards advanced stage at diagnosis, a high incidence of metastatic disease and poor histological features, differentiated thyroid cancer is associated with an excellent prognosis. A retrospective review of 112 patients at the MD Anderson Cancer Center, with a mean follow-up period of 25 years, showed a 100% 10-year survival and a 93% disease-specific survival overall, with those succumbing to thyroid cancer doing so at more than 26 years from initial diagnosis (Vassilopoulou-Sellin et al. 1998). Therefore, children with differentiated thyroid cancer treated aggressively surgically, and with radioactive iodine ablation if indicated, should expect an excellent chance of long-term disease-free survival if surveillance is carried out for life.

MTC and the Management of the Thyroid in MEN-2

MTC arises from the parafollicular C-cells. These cells have a neuroendocrine origin and produce calcitonin, which plays a role in calcium homeostasis. Their anatomical distribution near the upper and middle third of the thyroid lobes raises the index of suspicion of a MTC in nodules in that anatomical location as well as presenting a challenge to the surgeon by their proximity to the RLN as it enters the cricothyroid membrane.

MTC comprises 10% of paediatric thyroid cancers. The overwhelming proportion of paediatric medullary carcinomas are familial, occurring within the autosomal dominant MEN-2A (90%), MEN-2B (5%) or familial MTC syndrome (5%). Diagnosis of MTC makes genetic testing mandatory (above). If a *ret* mutation is detected, all potentially affected family members should be screened for the mutation. The timing of prophylactic surgery for affected individuals depends on the specific *ret* mutation. Affected MEN-2A patients should undergo prophylactic total thyroidectomy before the age of 5 years, while affected MEN-2B patients should undergo prophylactic total thyroidectomy with elective central compartment dissection before the age of 1 year (Machens et al. 2003). Timely prophylactic thyroidectomy prevents the development of MTC, which is the commonest cause of death in patients with MEN-2 (Skinner et al. 2005).

The treatment of MTC is by total thyroidectomy and elective central compartment neck dissection. Sixty percent of patients with tumours larger than 2 cm exhibit cervical metastases, and these patients should also have an ipsilateral selective neck dissection in addition to central compartment dissection. There is no role for radioiodine treatment in MTC, and while adjuvant external beam radiotherapy has been shown to reduce recurrence in high-risk patients, its role in children is uncertain. Monitoring of recurrence is achieved by serial calcitonin measurements. Although medullary thyroid cancer is considered one of the less favourable histological subtypes, long-term outcome in MTC is excellent, with those showing biochemical (calcitonin) cure predicted to have a 97.7% 10-year survival (Modigliani et al. 1998).

Summary for the Clinician

- Thyroid disease is uncommon in children, but occurs with sufficient frequency and in the context of syndromes that paediatric otolaryngologist should have a practical awareness of their management. The management of thyroid malignancy in children requires close multidisciplinary cooperation to ensure a good long-term outcome despite a tendency towards advanced disease stage at presentation.

References

1. Cocks HC (2005) A review of the evidence base for the management of thyroid disease. Clin Otolaryngol 30:500–510

2. Farahati J, Bucksy P, Parlowsky T, et al (1997) Characteristics of differentiated thyroid carcinoma in children and adolescents with respect to age, gender, and histology. Cancer 80:2156–2162

3. Hung W (1999) Solitary thyroid nodules in 93 children and adolescents: a 35-years experience. Horm Res 52:15–18

4. Machens A, Niccoli-Sire P, Hoegel J, et al (2003) Early malignant progression of hereditary medullary thyroid cancer. N Engl J Med 349:1517–1525

5. Mazzaferri EL (1997) Thyroid remnant 131I ablation for papillary and follicular thyroid carcinoma. Thyroid 7:265–271

6. Modigliani E, Cohen R, Campos JM, et al (1998) Prognostic factors for survival and for biochemical cure in medullary thyroid carcinoma: results in 899 patients. The GETC Study Group. Groupe d'etude des tumeurs a calcitonine. Clin Endocrinol (Oxf) 4:265–273

31

7. Park SM, Chatterjee VK (2005) Genetics of congenital hypothyroidism. J Med Genet 42:379–389

8. Pedersen OM, Aardal NP, Larssen TB, et al (2000) The value of ultrasonography in predicting autoimmune thyroid disease. Thyroid 10:251–259

9. Skinner MA, Moley JA, Dilley WG, et al (2005) Prophylactic thyroidectomy in multiple endocrine neoplasia type 2A. N Engl J Med 353:1105–1113

10. Spencer CA, Lopresti JS, Patel A, et al (1990) Applications of a new chemiluminometric thyrotropin assay to subnormal measurement. J Clin Endocrinol Metab 70:453–460

11. Vassilopoulou-Sellin R, Goepfert H, Raney B, et al (1998) Differentiated thyroid cancer in children and adolescents: clinical outcome and mortality after long-term follow-up. Head Neck 20:549–555

12. Welch Dinauer CA, Tuttle RM, Robie DK, et al (1999) Extensive surgery improves recurrence-free survival for children and young patients with class I papillary thyroid carcinoma. J Pediatr Surg 34:1799–1804

Chapter 32

Nasal Foreign Bodies, Epistaxis and Nasal Trauma

32

Sean Carrie

- A nasal foreign body should be suspected in all cases of unilateral childhood rhinorrhoea.
- Button batteries should be removed from the nose urgently.
- Most childhood epistaxes are self-limiting.
- Nasal fractures are uncommon before adolescence.

Contents

Introduction

This chapter covers the common childhood conditions of nasal foreign bodies, epistaxis and nasal trauma. In general, patients with these conditions can be managed in the outpatient setting without requirement for follow up.

Foreign Bodies

Types

Foreign bodies may be exogenous, both animate and inanimate, or endogenous in the form of a concretion or rhinolith (Walby 1997).

Presentation

Foreign bodies (Fig. 32.1) are most commonly inserted into the nose by children from the age of 18 months to 4 years. The presentation is classically a unilateral malodorous rhinorrhoea; however, it is likely that most foreign bodies inserted into the nose are either witnessed by an adult, or noted soon thereafter. Alternatively, the child itself may report the misdemeanour! A unilateral rhinitis should alert the physician to the possibility of a foreign body. Vegetable matter is likely to cause early mucosal irritation, and although inert material is initially well tolerated, granulation tissue does gradually develop causing an intense local reaction, possibly associated with

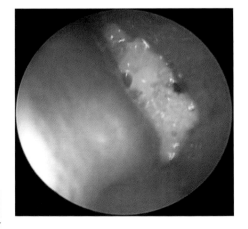

Fig. 32.1 Piece of foam plastic in the right nostril of a child

the erosion of bone. Particular note should be made of button batteries, the contents of which can cause extreme irritation producing chemical burns, with risk of nasal septal perforation.

Signs and Symptoms

Nasal obstruction, foetor, unilateral rhinorrhoea and unilateral bleeding are the main symptoms of nasal foreign bodies. Although antibiotic treatment is likely to relieve the patient's symptoms temporarily, it is only upon complete removal of the foreign body that the symptoms abate. The main potential complication with an intranasal foreign body is the risk of aspiration. This is not a common occurrence, although the proportion of aspirated foreign bodies in the larynx, pharynx or tracheobronchial tree is unknown.

Management

The assessment and removal of foreign bodies is undoubtedly best performed by individuals with experience. Most can be removed atraumatically in the outpatient setting. In selected cases, including the very young, or agitated child, or in those children with behavioural problems, a general anaesthetic may be required.

Once the decision has been made to remove the foreign body the child should be held firmly by the parent. The child's legs are held between the parent's crossed legs, an arm is placed around the torso and the upper limbs and the child's head is held steady. Wrapping a small child up in a blanket to assist immobilisation and the assistance of a paediatric nurse are often extremely helpful.

A topical nasal decongestant may assist visualisation and removal of the foreign body, although this may cause distress to the younger child. Using a head light for illumination, secretions can be gently removed from the child's nasal vestibule with a micro sucker. The author's preference for removal of inert foreign bodies such as beads is a right-angled wax hook, placing the hook behind the foreign body to deliver it from the nose. Friable foreign bodies should be removed piecemeal with crocodile aural forceps or microsuction. If the child becomes excessively distressed, the procedure should be performed with the aid of a general anaesthetic with endotracheal intubation and nasal decongestion. Rigid nasal endoscopy should be performed to ensure that both nostrils and the post-nasal space are free of foreign material. If an object is not identified, careful assessment of the oropharynx and hypopharynx should be made to ensure the foreign body has not slipped further into the upper aerodigestive tract.

Rhinolith

The aetiology of rhinoliths is unclear, but they are considered to result from the presence of a long-standing intranasal foreign body. Over time, the foreign body becomes a nidus for the deposition of calcium, magnesium, phosphate and carbonate and becomes encrusted by minerals. Initially symptomless, they become symptomatic as they increase in size, presenting with nasal obstruction or unilateral rhinorrhoea. Diagnosis is based on examination with a probe revealing a hard or gritty lesion, which may be partially mobile. Diagnosis can be confirmed by computerised tomography, which may reveal erosion of the floor of the nasal cavity and extension into the antrum. Pernasal removal may be achieved under general anaesthesia, in a piecemeal fashion if necessary. In cases where the rhinolith is particularly large, a lateral rhinotomy approach may be necessary.

Epistaxis

Epistaxes in childhood are generally repeated, short-lasting and self-limiting. However, they are a cause of significant distress to children and their parents and result in significant morbidity and hospital referral.

Prevalence

Epistaxis may occur at any age, but is rare under the age of 2 years, with a peak frequency between the ages of 3 and 8 years. In most cases the condition is self-limiting, but those cases that are prolonged or frequent may require hospital treatment.

Blood Supply to the Nose

The blood supply to the nose is derived from both the internal and external carotid arteries. The internal carotid artery supplies the superior nasal cavity by means of the ophthalmic artery, through its anterior and posterior ethmoidal branches. The sphenopalatine artery, a branch of the internal maxillary artery, which is derived from the external carotid artery, provides the main blood supply to the nasal cavities. The sphenopalatine artery enters the nose through the sphenopalatine foramen in the lateral nasal wall at the posterior end of the middle turbinate. It divides into a variable number of branches, which supply most of the nasal septum and lateral nasal wall. Branches of the facial artery also contribute blood flow to the anterior part of the nasal vestibule and septum. Kiesselbach's plexus (Little's area, Fig. 32.2), a confluence of arterial blood supply from several vessels on the anterior nasal

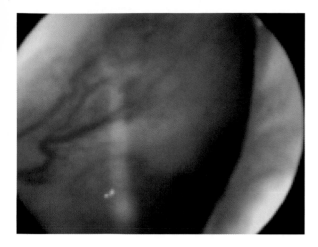

Fig. 32.2 Endoscopic view of Little's area on left side of nasal septum

septum is the commonest site of epistaxis in childhood. The mucosa at this point is relatively thin and exposed to the desiccating effect of inspired dry air.

Aetiology

Trauma

Nasal vestibulitis is associated with crusting, inflammation, fissuring and discomfort in children. This may encourage digital trauma to the nasal vestibule and septum, resulting in epistaxis, although no identifiable cause is found in the majority of childhood epistaxes. Nunez et al. (1990) identified an increased incidence of epistaxis in all ages during the colder winter months in northern climates. A decrease in humidity both at home and in the work place may also be associated with a greater incidence. Other common factors associated with childhood epistaxis include upper respiratory tract infections, allergic rhinitis and nasal foreign bodies. Table 32.1 lists the common primary causes of epistaxis.

Assessment and Management

Management of a child with epistaxis is underpinned by demonstrating an appropriate attitude of concern towards the child and the child's family. In a quiet and reassuring environment, an initial assessment of the degree of blood loss should be made. It is unusual for children presenting with epistaxis to require resuscitation, but facilities and expertise must be available if this is necessary. Initially, the child or parent pinches the nostrils at the tip of the nose, as digital compression is an excellent

first-aid measure. A careful history is taken to determine the frequency and severity of epistaxis and to establish that there is no evidence of an underlying systemic disease. Once the confidence of the child is gained, a careful inspection of the nose is made. Blood clots in the anterior nares can be removed with microsuction or a cotton pledget. The fresh blood or a clot usually overlies the bleeding point on the nasal septum and the source of the bleeding is thus easily identified. If a bleeding point cannot be identified, the nose can be topically anaesthetised with cophenylcaine and in older children examined with a rigid, or flexible endoscope. Although unusual, it may be necessary to examine a child's nose under general anaesthesia if initial measures to arrest bleeding are unsuccessful. Acute epistaxes in childhood normally cease spontaneously or with direct digital pressure by the time the child reaches the hospital. Conventionally, the child with active epistaxis is treated with chemical cautery to the bleeding vessels using a silver nitrate stick. This procedure can be performed under local or general anaesthesia and can be repeated if necessary. Care must be taken to avoid excessive cautery and it is unwise to cauterise both sides of the nasal septum at the same session, which may lead to the formation of a nasal septal perforation. Rarely, anterior epistaxes fail to be controlled by direct pressure or chemical cautery, and tamponade with a nasal pack becomes necessary. Nasal sponge tampons (Merocel) are particularly effective and once hydrated, should be left in situ for 24–48 h. The patient should be admitted to hospital for rest and observation. Arterial ligation for

Table 32.1 Aetiology of epistaxes in childhood

Trauma	Digital trauma (nose picking)
	Nasal fracture
Inflammation	Viral
	Bacterial
	Vestibulitis
	Foreign body
	Pyogenic granuloma
	Allergic
Haematological	Platelet defects (e.g. idiopathic thrombocytopenia)
	Purpura/leukaemia
	Drug induced (aspirin)
	Coagulation defects (e.g. haemophilia)
Neoplastic	Nasopharyngeal angiofibroma
	Haemangioma
Vascular abnormalities	Hereditary haemorrhagic telangiectasia

refractory epistaxis is rarely required in children. Endoscopic ligation of the ipsilateral sphenopalatine artery as it exits from the sphenopalatine foramen is well recognised and an accepted treatment for adult epistaxis. There are few reports of this technique in childhood, suggesting such invasive treatments are rarely required. Obviously, endoscopic techniques are technically more challenging because of the smaller anatomy in childhood.

The management of acute, recurrent, self-limiting epistaxis in childhood remains controversial. Ruddy et al. (1991) compared a topical antiseptic nasal barrier cream (Naseptin) with silver nitrate cautery to prominent vessels with no statistical difference in the frequency of recurrent epistaxis with either treatment. Kubba et al. (2001) compared the effectiveness of Naseptin with no treatment in a prospective trial and described a significant short-term benefit with the use of antiseptic cream. Loughran et al. (2004) compared petroleum jelly (Vaseline) with no treatment and found no improvement in the treatment group. Unfortunately, all three studies were of short-term interventions, and the effectiveness of each modality on the patient with recurrent and episodic bleeds is unclear (Burton and Doree 2005).

Nasal Trauma

Nasal fractures are by far the commonest facial fractures among children. The true incidence of these fractures is difficult to ascertain as many are not referred on to ENT services.

The nose of a child is very different anatomically from that of an adult. First, the nose in childhood has less projection from the facial plane and is less likely to

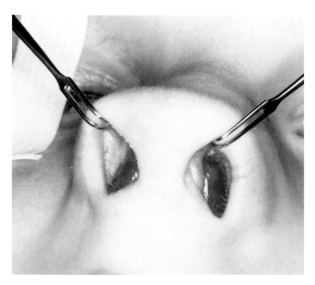

Fig. 32.3 Nasal septal haematoma

suffer injury. Secondly, the soft tissues and cartilages are sufficiently compliant to allow considerable deformation without permanent injury. The nasal septum is, however, at risk of injury with the formation of a septal haematoma, (Fig. 32.3). Untreated, this may result in a thickened fibrotic septum or even abscess formation, loss of cartilage and a saddle deformity of the nasal dorsum.

Assessment

Nasal fractures produce symptoms of facial swelling, pain, nasal obstruction and epistaxes. Examination should focus on the degree of cosmetic and functional impairment. It is important to perform a complete examination of the full facial skeleton to avoid missing occult fractures of the zygoma, maxilla and, in particular, coincidental orbito-ethmoidal fractures. The nasal pyramid is variably cartilaginous with soft nasal bones and, therefore, greenstick fractures are not uncommon. Splaying of the nasal bones over the frontal process of the maxilla is more common in childhood, compared to the C-shaped deformities seen in adulthood. Nasal fractures in infancy are extremely uncommon; only from the age of 6 years are children more susceptible to bony fractures. Intranasal examination will demonstrate the degree of septal displacement and the presence of a septal haematoma. Although unlikely, a high index of suspicion for a cerebrospinal fluid leak should be maintained. A diagnosis of nasal fracture is made by clinical assessment; plain radiographs have no role in the management.

Management

The majority of children presenting with nasal trauma do not have an underlying fracture to either the bony or cartilaginous structures, although the degree of subcutaneous swelling may make this assessment difficult. If there is any doubt, the child should be reviewed 4–5 days later when external swelling has subsided. Most nasal fractures are not associated with significant displacement and, therefore, no specific therapy is required. Definitive management, under general anaesthetic, is required if there is functional or cosmetic deformity.

Displaced fractures are manipulated by bimanual external pressure, normally with good cosmetic result. Cartilaginous deformities respond poorly to manipulation and in most cases further treatment is delayed until after puberty to avoid interrupting the expected nasal growth potential. More severe injuries to the septum should be treated by a limited septoplasty, preserving as much cartilage as possible.

A septal haematoma requires urgent surgical treatment to avoid the complications previously noted. Under general anaesthesia, the haematoma is evacuated through a hemitransfixion incision. The haematoma is often bilateral and the quadrilateral cartilage may be incised to drain the opposite side of the septum. Once the haematoma has been evacuated, the septal mucosa should be reapproximated with a through-and-through 4-0 Vicryl suture on a Keith needle. Although not strictly necessary, the nasal cavities are packed with dressings for 48 hours post-operatively. Treatment with a broad spectrum antibiotic for 5 days is instituted.

Summary for the Clinician

- This chapter has dealt with some of the most common everyday ENT problems occurring in children. It is relatively common for children to put foreign objects into their noses. Unless the event is witnessed, unilateral nasal discharge is the main physical sign. Batteries are the most dangerous objects, with a high risk of septal perforation and alteration of nasal growth. Skill is often required to remove a foreign body with the minimum of trauma, making sure that it does not slip back and into the pharynx or larynx, and remembering that more than one object may have been inserted by the child. Epistaxis is usually self-limiting and can be controlled in the short-term with antibacterial creams. Displaced fractures of the nasal bones are relatively uncommon after trauma, but are relatively easy to reposition.

References

1. Burton MJ, Doree CJ (2004) Interventions for recurrent idiopathic epistaxis (nosebleeds) in children. Cochrane Database Syst Rev 1:CD004461
2. Kubba H, McAndie C, Botma M, et al (2001) A prospective, single-blind, randomised controlled trial of antiseptic cream for recurrent epistaxes in children. Clin Otolaryngol 26:465–468
3. Loughran S, Spinou E, Clements WA, et al (2004) A prospective, single-blind randomised controlled trial of petroleum jelly/Vaseline for recurrent paediatric epistaxis. Clin Otolaryngol 29:266–299
4. Nunez DA, McClymont LG, Evans RA (1990) Epistaxis: a study of the relationship with weather. Clin Otolaryngol 15:49–51
5. Ruddy J, Proops DW, Pearman K, et al (1991) Management of epistaxis in childhood. International J Paediatr Otolaryngol 21:139–142
6. Walby PA (1997) Foreign bodies in the ear or nose. In: Adams DA, Cinnamond MJ (eds) Scott-Brown's Otolaryngology, Vol. 6, Chapter 14, pp 3–6

Chapter 33

Management of Choanal Atresia

33

Patrick Froehlich and Sonia Ayari-Khalfallah

Core Messages

- Bilateral choanal atresia constitutes a neonatal emergency.
- Bilateral choanal atresia is much rarer than unilateral atresia; when it occurs it is often part of the CHARGE (coloboma of the eye, heart defects, atresia of the choanae, retardation of growth and/or development, genital and/or urinary abnormalities, and ear abnormalities and deafness) syndrome.
- The features of CHARGE and other polymalformation syndromes should be looked for, with referral to paediatricians and geneticists as part of the management.
- Choanal atresia is twice as common in girls as in boys.
- Ninety percent of cases involve bony obstruction; 10% are entirely membranous.
- Computed tomography should be performed if surgery is contemplated.
- Most cases can be dealt with using an endonasal approach.
- Bilateral cases should be operated on during the 1st week of life.
- Unilateral cases may be operated on at 1 year of age; however, some authors recommend delaying surgery until the child is 3 or 4 years old.
- Cutting and diamond burs are generally used to perforate the bony atresia plate, controlling the procedure with a view from the nasopharynx.
- Lasers may also play a part in surgery. Mitomycin C may be used with the aim of preventing restenosis.
- The use of post-operative stents in common for neonates. In older children, not all surgeons use stents.
- There is a recognised restenosis rate: authors report the need for between 1.5 and 3 operations per child.

Contents

Introduction

Choanal atresia, a malformation in which the nasal fossae do not open onto the aerodigestive pathway, was first described as early as 1755, by Roederer. A variety of corrective surgical approaches, transmaxillary, transseptal, transpalatine and sublabial intranasal, have been developed over the subsequent 250 years. Surgical management has recently made significant progress, thanks to developments in endonasal surgery.

Anatomical and Physiological Background

The malformation, which prevents communication between the nasal fossa and rhinopharynx, is complex and goes beyond the mere choana itself, to involve the posterior half of the fossa, with excess bone both from the lateral wall, constituted by the pterygoid apophysis, and of a malformed and enlarged vomer, as well as of the floor of the nasal cavity. The obstruction most often consists of bone, but may also include a membranous component; in 10% of cases the obstruction is entirely membranous. Choanal atresia is rarely bilateral, usually in that case featuring as part of a polymalformation syndrome, commonly the CHARGE (coloboma of the eye, heart defects, atresia of the choanae, retardation of growth and/or development, genital and/or urinary abnormalities, and ear abnormalities and deafness) association (see Chapter 8).

No embryological theory accounts fully for this malformation. One of the most recent suggestions is that disturbed neural-crest-cell migration in neurocristopathy could be implicated (Garabédian and Ducroz 1996).

33

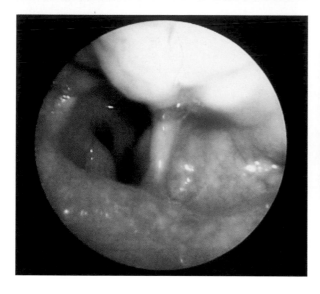

Fig. 33.1 Endoscopic view of unilateral choanal atresia

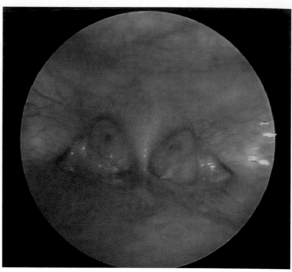

Fig. 33.2 Endoscopic view of bilateral choanal atresia

Clinical Presentation

Choanal atresia occurs in 1 in 8000 live births and affects girls twice as commonly as boys. Unilateral choanal atresia may be diagnosed during routine neonatal nasal catheter screening, but may escape notice if the probe rolls up in the nasal fossa. In that event, atresia may then be suspected when there is unilateral nasal obstruction associated with very thick unilateral mucous rhinorrhea (the main alternative differential diagnosis is a foreign body), with endoscopy confirming the choanal obstruction (Figs. 33.1 and 33.2).

Bilateral choanal atresia presents classically in the neonatal period as an airway emergency, since neonates lack the capacity for mouth breathing. The airway needs to be secured using a neonatal airway or an adapted nipple from a feeding bottle. These must be taped securely to the infant. Unless there are other medical problems that need prior management, definitive surgery should take place in the 1st week after delivery.

After clinical examination, a computed tomography scan should be performed if surgery is being envisaged, to specify the degree and site of bony obstruction and that of membranous obstruction (Fig. 33.3).

Cross-disciplinary assessment follows local assessment, to check for any polymalformation syndrome, and notably that of CHARGE. Polymalformation syndromes are found mainly in the case of bilateral choanal atresia, although they are occasionally associated with unilateral occurrence.

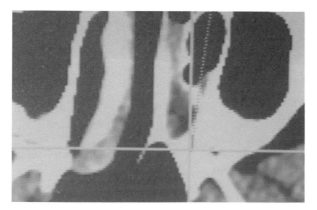

Fig. 33.3 Axial computed tomography scan showing left bony choanal atresia. Atresia in this case is mainly due to excess bone of the pterygoid ala

Management is by Surgery

The aim is to ensure good and post-operatively stable choanal patency. In the neonate with bilateral atresia, the intranasal approach is necessary and should take place in the 1st week of life. After the age of 5 years, both the intranasal or the transpalatal approach are feasible.

Intranasal Approach

Advances in intranasal surgical equipment for use with children since the 1990s have enabled an approach via the natural intranasal pathway. In the neonate, a 2.7-mm straight telescope is used to visualise the atretic area and operative field. This can often be replaced during the procedure by a larger, 4-mm telescope. The risk of post-operative stenosis is higher in the neonate, but when it occurs it is not usually bilateral or complete; this allows the infant to maintain an adequate airway until revision surgery takes place after 6 or 12 months, when access is easier and an acceptable long-term result obtained.

After careful decongestion, with topical or infiltrated adrenaline (epinephrine) or phenylephrine, various tools may be used to open the choana. The CO_2 laser has proved effective on purely membranous atresia, as has simple perforation using a metal probe such as a urethral sound. However, most atresias tend to be predominantly bony. Cutting and diamond burs may be used to perforate the bony atresia plate and then widen the aperture. It may be helpful to obtain a view from the nasopharynx using a mirror or flexible fibre-optic telescope, during this widening procedure. The potassium titanyl phosphate laser has also been used (Kubba et al. 2004); its use often needs to be supplemented by burring to remove residual bone. Posterior vomer dissection – previously controversial because of fears of compromising nasal growth – is now common practice. Mitomycin C may be applied to the choana at the end of surgery (Prasad et al. 2002). The aim is to limit the risk of post-operative re-closure.

Some authors leave a choanal stent and others do not: its usefulness in preventing restenosis is currently under debate. Most surgeons continue to prefer stenting for neonates.

Transplatine Approach

This is the classic approach to choanal atresia. A posteriorly based palatal flap is raised. The opening is made by drilling anteriorly from the posterior margin of the hard palate. The excess bone causing the obstruction is removed by gradual drilling from the lower edge of the choana. A stent is left across the choana for between 2 and 12 weeks.

This approach provides no direct view of the choana, and requires cutting and detaching healthy palatine mucosa. It has therefore gradually come to be replaced by an endonasal approach, using a more natural pathway. A transpalatine approach, however, can still be indicated when endonasal surgery is technically unfeasible or has encountered failure.

Indications and Timing of Surgery

As mentioned earlier, bilateral choanal atresia represents an emergency and must be dealt with in the 1st week of life. For unilateral choanal atresia, the main issue, with regard to indications, is age at surgery. Surgery may be indicated during the first months of life when (rarely) unilateral obstruction is badly tolerated, particularly when there is obstructive sleep apnoea. If tolerance of unilat-

eral atresia is clinically acceptable, the surgeon can wait until anaesthesia-related risks reach acceptable levels, at around the age of 1 year, and the endonasal approach becomes easier to perform. Some authors have recommended waiting until the age of 3 or even 5 years for the sake of greater technical facility and less risk of restenosis (Ayari et al. 2004). Certain cases of atresia go unoperated until adulthood, but tend to continue to cause functional disturbance.

Contraindications

There are no real contraindications to choanal atresia surgery, except for anaesthesia-related risks in case of associated malformation – mainly severe cardiac malformation.

Risks and Side Effects

The main risk is restenosis, with reports of a mean of 1.5 to 3 operations per patient (Postec et al. 2002; Samadi et al. 2003; Van Den Abbeele et al. 2003). Restenosis tends to begin early, within the first 3 post-operative months. The various improvements being made to the endonasal approach seek to reduce this risk, mainly by means of posterior vomer dissection and mitomycin C application, which both serve to limit but not eliminate the risk. A second or third intervention may be needed. How to schedule these and choose between endonasal and transpalatine approaches are issues currently under debate. At the present time, the problem of restenosis remains to be solved (Triglia et al. 2003).

Summary for the Clinician

- Bilateral choanal atresia is a neonatal emergency. The neonate's airway must be secured at once and definitive surgery planned as soon as possible. The surgical approach to unilateral choanal atresia has progressed in the direction of mini-invasive endonasal surgery. The risk of restenosis has fallen, but is still present.

References

1. Ayari S, Abedipour D, Bossard D, Froehlich P (2004) CT-assisted surgery in choanal atresia. Acta Otolaryngol 124:1–3

2. Garabédian EN, Ducroz V (1996) Imperforations choanales. In: Garabédian EN, Bobin S, Monteil J-P, Triglia J-M (eds) ORL de l'enfant. Flammarion (Médecine-Sciences), Paris, pp 127–131

3. Kubba H, Bennett A, Bailey CM (2004) An update on choanal atresia surgery at great Ormond street hospital for children: preliminary results with mitomycin C and the KTP laser. Int J Pediatr Otorhinolaryngol 68:939–945

4. Postec F, Bossard D, Disant F, Froehlich P (2002) Computer-assisted navigation system in pediatric intranasal surgery. Arch Otolaryngol Head Neck Surg 128:797–800

5. Prasad M, Ward RF, April MM, Bent JP, Froehlich P (2002) Topical mitomycin as an adjunct to choanal atresia repair. Arch Otolaryngol Head Neck Surg 128:398–400

6. Samadi DS, Shah UK, Handler SD (2003) Choanal atresia: a twenty-year review of medical comorbidities and surgical outcomes. Laryngoscope 113:254–258

7. Triglia JM, Nicollas R, Roman S, Paris J (2003) Choanal atresia: therapeutic management and results in a series of 58 children. Rev Laryngol Otol Rhinol (Bord) 124:139–143

8. Van Den Abbeele T, François M, Narcy P (2002) Transnasal endoscopic treatment of choanal atresia without prolonged stenting. Arch Otolaryngol Head Neck Surg 128:936–940

33

Allergic Rhinitis

Alexander N. Greiner

Core Messages

- Allergic rhinitis (AR) may affect up to 40% of children; peak incidence occurs during early adolescence.
- AR is only one manifestation of systemic allergic inflammation and is often seen in association with otitis media with effusion, rhinosinusitis, allergic conjunctivitis, asthma, atopic dermatitis and food allergies.
- New AR classification guidelines focus on quality of life, which should be a principal consideration in the evaluation and treatment of AR.
- Even though sometimes difficult to implement, allergen avoidance remains one of the guiding principles of treatment.
- Nasal congestion is the most bothersome symptom of AR and is usually not adequately addressed by treatment with an antihistamine alone.
- Older antihistamines often cause sleep disturbance and a reduction in intellectual and motor performance, and thus their use should be discouraged.
- Intranasal corticosteroids remain the single most effective class of medications for treating AR.

Contents

Introduction

Allergic rhinitis (AR) is a prevalent, yet underappreciated, inflammatory condition of the nasal mucosa, characterized by pruritus, sneezing, rhinorrhea, and nasal congestion. It is mediated by early- and late-phase hypersensitivity responses to indoor and outdoor environmental allergens. AR affects a large portion of children in the developed world. Both basic science and epidemiological studies have demonstrated that AR is part of a systemic inflammatory process and is associated with other inflammatory conditions of the mucous membranes. These include otitis media with effusion, rhinosinusitis, allergic conjunctivitis (AC), and asthma. The ARIA guidelines (Allergic Rhinitis and its Impact on Asthma) have provided a pragmatic, stepwise approach to treating AR. Allergen avoidance remains one of the guiding principles of treatment, although it may sometimes be difficult to implement. While there is an ever-increasing armamentarium of pharmacotherapeutic agents available to the clinician, intranasal corticosteroids remain the single most effective class of medications for treating AR.

Epidemiology

AR affects a large portion of the pediatric population in the developed world. Physician-diagnosed AR in this population has been reported in as many as 42% (Wright et al. 1994). Older children have a higher prevalence of AR than younger ones, with a peak occurring in children aged 13–14 years. Approximately 80% of individuals diagnosed as having AR develop symptoms before the age of 20 years (Skoner 2001). While boys are more likely than girls to be afflicted with AR, this tendency tends to reverse in puberty, so that equal numbers are affected in adulthood. AR and other conditions mimicking AR are listed in Table 34.1. These should be considered when children present with nasal congestion, sneezing, itching of the nose and anterior rhinorrhea and/or postnasal drainage.

Table 34.1 Differential diagnosis of rhinorrhea and nasal obstruction in children. *CT* computerized tomography, *ASA* acetylsalicylic acid (aspirin), *NSAIDs* nonsteroidal anti-inflammatory drugs

34

Allergic rhinitis:
– Seasonal, perennial, or perennial with seasonal exacerbations

Nonallergic rhinitis

Mechanical obstruction/structural factors:
– Septal deviation. Can compound nasal obstruction.
– Foreign body. Unilateral purulent nasal discharge is the usual manifestation of a foreign body and resolves after removal.
– Adenoidal hypertrophy.
– Hypertrophic turbinates.
– Nasal tumors.
– Choanal atresia or stenosis. Bilateral choanal atresia must be diagnosed early in life, but unilateral choanal atresia or stenosis can go unnoticed for several years. Easily diagnosed by nasal endoscopy and axial CT of the midfacial skeleton.

Infectious rhinitis/rhinosinusitis:
– Bacterial, viral or fungal

Perennial (vasomotor, idiopathic):
Probably not as common in children, especially younger ones, as in adults. Frequent symptoms of profuse, clear rhinorrhea and nasal congestion without correlation to specific allergen exposure or signs of atopy.
Often triggered by environmental triggers:
– Cold air induced. Nasal congestion and rhinorrhea upon exposure to cold, windy weather. Occurs in both allergic and nonallergic individuals.
– Odors
– Barometric pressure

Nonallergic rhinitis with eosinophilia syndrome:
Most often seen in adults. Characterized by eosinophilia on nasal smears in the absence of specific allergic antibodies.

Reflex induced:
– Gustatory rhinitis: Vagally mediated, copious, watery rhinorrhea occurring immediately after food ingestion, particularly hot and spicy foods.
– Chemical or irritant induced
– Postural reflexes: Many different postural reflexes exist-a commonly encountered reflex involves ipsilateral nasal congestion when supine or prone with the head turned to one side.
– Nasal cycle: refers to the unilateral nasal congestion that cycles from one side to another over time in normal individuals.

Drug-induced rhinitis:
– Oral contraceptives.
– Antihypertensives: hydralazine, β-adrenergic blockers.
– ASA and other NSAIDs (with or without ASA triad/Samter's syndrome: rhinosinusitis, nasal polyps, asthma; usually adults only).
– Topical decongestants (rhinitis medicamentosa).

Table 34.1 *(Continued)* Differential diagnosis of rhinorrhea and nasal obstruction in children. *CT* computerized tomography, *ASA* acetylsalicylic acid (aspirin), *NSAIDs* nonsteroidal anti-inflammatory drugs

Hormonally induced:
– Hypothyroidism.
– Pregnancy.
– Menstrual cycle.
– Exercise.
Miscellaneous:
– Cerebrospinal rhinorrhea (usually presents with unilateral, clear rhinorrhea).

Etiology of AR

Atopy is the abnormal tendency to develop specific IgE in response to innocuous and ubiquitous environmental allergens. Atopic diseases include allergic rhinoconjunctivitis, asthma, atopic dermatitis and food allergies. Atopy has been linked to multiple genetic loci, including those on chromosomes 2, 5, 6, 7, 11, 13, 16, and 20. Therefore, a family history represents a major risk factor for AR. In one study, development of atopic disease in the absence of parental family history was only present in 13%, whereas if one patient or sibling was atopic, the risk increased to 29%. This risk increased to 50% if both parents were atopic and 72% if both parents had the same atopic manifestation.

Other risk factors linked to the development of AR include ethnicity other than Caucasian, higher socioeconomic status, environmental pollution, birth during a pollen season, lack of older siblings, late entry into daycare, heavy maternal smoking during the 1st year of life, exposure to indoor allergens such as animal dander and dust mites, higher serum IgE levels (>100 IU/ml before age 6 years), the presence of positive allergen skin-prick tests, and early introduction of foods or formula. Multiple studies have also found that early environmental exposure to various infectious agents such as hepatitis A, mycobacterium, *Toxoplasma gondii,* and lipopolysaccharides, a compound found in Gram-negative bacteria, protects against development of atopy (Von Mutius and Martinez 2003).

AR and its Associated Conditions and Comorbidities

There has been increased understanding that AR is part of a systemic inflammatory process rather than an isolated local disease. As such, it is closely linked to other inflammatory diseases affecting the respiratory mucous membranes such as asthma, rhinosinusitis, otitis media with effusion, and AC. Epidemiological evidence has repeatedly and consistently demonstrated the coexistence of rhinitis and asthma. Nasal symptoms have been noted in up to 80% of the asthmatic population (Leynaert et al. 1999). Conversely, asthma is more frequent among children with AR, as evidenced by a longitudinal North American study, which found that a personal history of asthma represented the single most significant risk factor for having physician-diagnosed AR (odds ratio 4.06, 95% confidence interval: 2.06–7.9; Wright et al. 1994).

There is also considerable epidemiological evidence to support the linkage between sinus disease and AR. Studies have noted that 25–30% of patients with acute sinusitis have AR, as do 40–67% of patients with unilateral chronic sinusitis and up to 80% with chronic bilateral sinusitis. In acute rhinosinusitis, the putative mechanism by which AR predisposes to sinusitis is via nasal inflammation resulting in nasal congestion and obstruction of the ostia, which connect the sinuses to the nasal cavity. Decreased ventilation of the mucosa in the sinus cavity leads to ciliary dysfunction, transudation of fluids, and stagnation of mucus, thereby promoting the growth of bacterial pathogens. Chronic rhinosinusitis is an inflammatory disorder likely due to multiple factors and with different phenotypes (see Chapter 35). The two most commonly recognized forms of chronic rhinosinusitis are characterized by either eosinophilic or neutrophilic infiltration. Some appear to share the same underlying immune mechanism as other atopic disorders, including AR. While intriguing, the proposed mechanisms that most chronic inflammatory sinus disease is driven by an abnormal response to inhaled ubiquitous fungal material (Shin et al. 2004), is unlikely with recent large-scale, double-blind, placebo-controlled studies of antifungal douching proving negative (Ebbens et al. personal communication).

AC is characterized by ocular itching, swelling, and discharge that may be clear or, less commonly, may resemble "string-cheese" or beeswax. Eye symptoms are common in sufferers of AR, especially among those sensitized to pollen and animal dander. While eye symptoms are often overlooked, they may overshadow the nasal symptoms and represent the major reason for referral. While perennial AC is the second most common form of AC after seasonal conjunctivitis, one needs to pay special attention to two more severe forms of AC not uncommon to the atopic population: vernal and atopic keratoconjunctivitis. These atopic eye diseases are potentially sight threatening and should be managed in cooperation with an ophthalmologist.

Quality of Life

Until recently, the focus on AR and its treatment has revolved around symptoms and symptom improvement rather than on how well being or quality of life (QOL) is affected. While AR causes bothersome practical problems such as the need to rub the eyes and nose, drip, and cough as well as carry tissues and medications, it is now understood that AR may affect well being in other ways. For example, children may have problems at school due to learning impairment secondary to distraction, fatigue, poor sleep, or irritability. In the United States alone, children miss approximately 2 million school days per year because of symptoms of AR. They may also be unable to take part in family or social events such as hiking, playing with pets, or engaging in sports. These numerous limitations may result in emotional disturbances that manifest as anger, sadness, frustration, and withdrawal (Meltzer 2001).

Using the SF-36 health survey, a generic instrument focusing on sleep, work and school performance, family functioning, and social relationships, it was noted that perennial AR impaired the health-related QOL (HRQL) to a similar degree as asthma, which has long been recognized as having a significant impact on QOL. In a study of 2084 adolescents 13–14 years of age, those with physician-diagnosed AR or rhinitis-like symptoms were more likely than those without rhinitis to report sleep loss, have limited activity, and lack self-satisfaction (Arrighi et al. 1996).

While generic instruments allow for the comparison of the impact of unrelated diseases on QOL, they lack specificity, and thus frequently fail to identify clinically important variables. Based on this new paradigm, questionnaires have been devised and validated to better determine the impact of AR on an individual's health. These HRQL instruments measure a series of variables that focus on issues most relevant to the disorder under study and more sensitively measure the full impact of AR and its treatment on QOL. They include the rhinoconjunctivitis QOL questionnaire and its age-specific adaptations – the adolescent rhinoconjunctivitis quality of life questionnaire (ages 12–17 years) and the pediatric rhinoconjunctivitis quality of life questionnaire (ages 6–12 years). It is likely that these instruments will be used increasingly in the literature, especially as an outcome variable in clinical trials.

Classification

Traditionally, AR has been classified as seasonal or perennial, depending on whether an individual was sensitized to cyclic pollens or year-round allergens such as dust mites, pets, cockroaches, and molds. This classification scheme has proven to be artificial and often inconsistent since, depending somewhat on the locale, allergic sensitization to multiple seasonal allergens can result in year-round disease and, conversely, allergic sensitization to "perennial" allergens such as animal dander can result in symptoms during only a limited period of time. Furthermore, molds, varying with the species and geographical climate, can function as seasonal and/or perennial allergens.

Recent global guidelines for classification and treatment of AR (ARIA) have led to the definition of allergic nasal disease as being intermittent or persistent, and mild or moderate-severe (see Fig. 34.1; Bousquet et al. 2001). Intermittent rhinitis is defined on the basis of symptoms that are present for less than 4 days per week or less than 4 weeks. If symptoms are present for more than 4 days per week and are present for more than 4 weeks, the rhinitis is defined as persistent. Mild symptoms do not affect sleep, impair daily activities, sports and leisure, interfere with work or school, and are not considered troublesome. Conversely, moderate–severe symptoms result in abnormal sleep, impair daily activities, sports and leisure, impair work and school activities, and are considered troublesome. The diagnosis of AR may be made presumptively based on the types of symptoms and the history of allergen triggers. However, confirmation

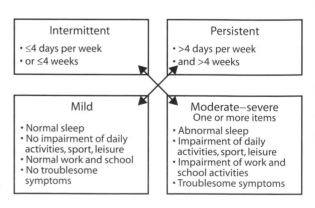

Fig. 34.1 Classification of allergic rhinitis according to Allergic Rhinitis and its Impact on Asthma (ARIA) guidelines (from Bousquet et al. 2001)

of the diagnosis requires documentation of specific IgE reactivity. Appropriate determination of allergen sensitivity via skin-prick testing or the radioallergosorbent test (RAST) can not only help in diagnosing AR, but provides information that can direct interventions with specific environmental control measures. Specific IgE analysis via RAST is slower and less cost-effective than skin-prick testing, but it is useful in patients with dermatographism or for those unable to discontinue antihistamine therapy. While current second- and third-generation RAST assays produce more quantifiable and reproducible measurements of IgE than ever before, skin testing remains a more sensitive tool in the hands of an experienced physician or nurse and for now continues to be the gold standard for the detection of allergen-specific IgE (Hamilton et al. 2004).

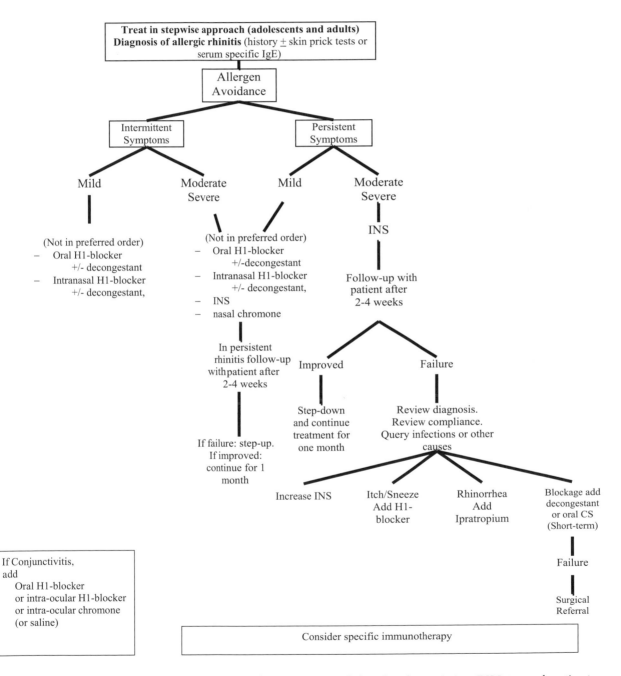

Fig. 34.2 Stepwise treatment of allergic rhinitis. Adapted from Bousquet et al. (2003) with permission. *INS* Intranasal corticosteroids, *CS* corticosteriod

Treatment Modalities

Environmental Control Measures

The ARIA guidelines have provided a pragmatic, stepwise approach to treatment of AR (see Fig. 34.2). As noted, the choice of the various modalities of treatment available depends on the perceived severity of symptoms as well as whether symptoms are persistent.

Allergen avoidance is one of the guiding principles of treatment. However, it often proves impractical and difficult to implement, and may not be effective when used alone. Individuals sensitive to pollen may need to minimize time spent outdoor during times of high pollen counts. Environmental measures to minimize indoor pollen exposure include keeping the windows of homes and cars closed, especially in the evening when pollen descends as the air cools, and if available, employing an air conditioner in the recycling /indoor mode.

For individuals allergic to dust mite, proposed measures include encasing mattresses, pillows, and quilts/duvets in impermeable covers as well as washing all bedding weekly on a hot cycle (55–60°C; 131-140°F) to reduce dust mite allergen levels and live dust mites (Arrighi et al. 1996). Of interest, a recent study looking at the addition of impermeable bed covers in AR did not show any additional benefits over nonimpermeable covers (Terreehorst et al. 2003). While some acaricides such as disodium octaborate tetrahydrate can lower the number of live dust mite in carpets, it remains unknown whether this translates into symptom amelioration. House dust mites are sensitive to humidity and thus growth should be suppressible with sufficient dehumidification. However, a recent randomized controlled trial in the UK showed that dehumidifiers did not have a major effect on house dust mite counts or allergen levels (Hyndman et al. 2000).

Individuals allergic to cats and dogs have few effective ways to reduce their exposure to pet allergens short of ridding themselves of the animals. Although weekly washing can reduce allergens, clinical studies have not shown a clear benefit on rhinitis. Similarly, HEPA filters did not lead to symptom improvement in cat-sensitized individuals with AR in a placebo-controlled study (Wood et al. 1998).

Cockroach infestation is associated with AR and asthma, especially in the inner city. Control measures are based on eliminating suitable environments and restricting access by sealing, caulking, and controlling the food supply as well as using chemical control and traps (Arrighi et al. 1996). While cockroach extermination by professionals may reduce allergen levels by 80–90%, no studies have evaluated the clinical significance of this reduction. Reinfestation from adjacent apartments is a frequent problem and thus extermination efforts will likely need to be repeated and extended beyond the affected home.

Molds are ubiquitous both indoors and outdoors. Mold-allergic individuals should carefully inspect their home for mould damage, paying special attention to the more humid areas of the house. When indoor levels of a specific mold are significantly greater than outdoor levels, mold damage is likely present. Localized growth may be removed with a dilute bleach solution. More extensive damage may require more aggressive measures, such as replacing the affected surface. Controlled clinical studies showing that these measures effectively reduce the suffering from rhinitis have not been undertaken.

Overview of Pharmacological Treatment

A detailed algorithm to treating AR is presented in Fig. 34.2. With mild intermittent AR, suggested initial pharmacological therapy consists of an oral H1-blocker, an intranasal H1-blocker, and/or an oral decongestant. If intermittent disease is moderate or severe, intranasal corticosteroids provide an alternative to the aforementioned pharmacological agents. Persistent mild AR is treated in the same manner as moderate or severe intermittent AR. If symptoms are persistent and moderate or severe, intranasal corticosteroids should be the first class of medications employed. Investigation into the presence of AC should also take place, since appropriate therapy with oral H1-blockers, intraocular H1-blockers or intraocular chromones will need to be integrated into a comprehensive therapeutic approach. With all grades of severity, appropriate follow-up should take place in a reasonable amount of time and therapy stepped up or stepped down, as indicated.

H1-Antihistamines

Oral H1-antihistamines are an established first-line pharmacotherapy for the treatment of mild pediatric and adult AR. Oral antihistamines available in the UK are listed in Table 34.2 according to age. They act by stabilizing the H1-receptor on smooth muscle cells, nerve endings, and glandular cells, leading to a reduction in sneezing, rhinorrhea, and itching of the nose, palate and eyes. However, they only have a modest effect on nasal congestion. While oral H1 receptor antagonists reduce conjunctival itching, redness, and tearing, they are less effective than topical agents in this class. Tolerance to the clinical effects of H1-antihistamines has not been shown to occur.

Oral H1-antihistamines are commonly separated into two classes: first or second generation. First-generation antihistamines available in the UK include brompheniramine maleate, hydroxyzine hydrochloride, chlorpheniramine maleate, diphenhydramine, clemastine, alimemazine tartrate, cyproheptadine hydrochloride, and promethazine hydrochloride. The first-generation AHs are often referred to as "sedating," a term used to denote both drowsiness as well as a reduction in intellectual and motor performance. Sedating H1-antihistamines can lead to behavioral changes, ranging from hyperactivity to drowsiness to cognitive impairments and reduction of academic performance (Vuurman et al. 1996) Even though dosing for first-generation H1-antihistamines is often undertaken several times a day, the terminal elimination of first-generation AH half-life varies from 9.2 to 27.9 h (Simons 2003), thus leading to potential daytime deficits even when administered only at bedtime. One study suggested that tolerance can develop to the sedating properties of diphenhydramine (Richardson et al. 2002).

Second-generation oral H1-antihistamines have largely replaced the older antihistamines because of their greater specificity for the H1 receptor, lower likelihood of crossing the blood–brain barrier, and relative lack of anticholinergic and central nervous system effects. Except for fexofenadine, all second-generation H1-antihistamines have the potential to cause increased sedation when used at more than the recommended dose. Cetirizine and acrivastine may cause an increased incidence of sedation at recommended doses. Occasionally, paradoxical hyperactivity occurs in children given antihistamines.

Currently, azelastine (Rhinolast) is the only intranasal antihistamine available in the UK after the discontinuation of levocabastine (Livostin) in 2005. This agent appears to have mechanisms of therapeutic action in addition to its H1 receptor effect. These include interference with the vasoactive neuropeptide substance P and inhibition of leukotriene B4 and C4 production. Azelastine has demonstrated efficacy in both seasonal and vasomo-

Table 34.2 Oral antihistamines licensed in the UK according to age

Age	Generic (brand) name	Formulation	Recommended dose (pediatric/≥12 years)
First-generation H1 antihistamines			
Birth onwards	Brompheniramine maleate (Dimotane)	Tablets 4 mg, 8 mg,* 12 mg* Syrup 2 mg/5 ml	0.5 mg/kg/day in four divided doses (max 6 mg/24 h for ages 2–6 years; 12 mg/24 h for ages 6–12 years) / 4 mg qid or 8–12 mg bid*
>6 months	Hydroxyine (Atarax)	Capsules 10 mg, 25 mg, 50 mg Syrup 10 mg/5 ml	25–50 mg tid or od (hs)/50–100 mg qid
>1 year	Chlorpheniramine (Piriton)	Tablets 4 mg, 8 mg*, 12 mg* Syrup 2.5 mg/5 ml Parenteral solution 10 mg/ml	1–2 mg tid to qid/8–12 mg bid*
>1 year	Clemastine (Tavegil)	Tablets 1 mg Syrup 0.5 mg/5 ml	0.5 mg bid/1 mg bid
>2 years	Alimemazine tartrate (Vallergan)	Tablets 10 mg Syrup 7.5 mg/5 ml	2.5–5 mg tid
>2 years	Cyproheptadine hydrochloride (Periactin)	Tablets 4 mg Syrup 2 mg/5 ml	2–4 mg bid to tid/4–20 mg od
>2 years	Promethazine hydrochloride (Phenergan)	Tablets 25 mg Syrup 6.25 mg/5 ml Parenteral solution 25 mg/ml	6.25–12.5 mg tid/25 mg tid
>12 years	Diphenhydramine (Benadryl)	Capsules 25 or 50 mg Elixir 12.5 mg/ 5 ml Syrup 6.25 mg/5 ml Parenteral solution 50 mg/ml	6.25–25 mg od/ 25–50 mg tid

*Extended release

Table 34.2 *(Continued)* Oral antihistamines licensed in the UK according to age

Age	Generic (brand) name	Formulation	Recommended dose (pediatric/≥12 years)
Formulations and dosages of representative H1 antihistamines			
Second-generation oral H1 antihistamines			
>1 year	Desloratadine (Neoclarityn)	Tablets 5 mg Syrup 2.5 mg/5ml	1–2.5 mg od/ 5 mg od
>2 years	Loratadine (Loratadine)	Tablets 10 mg Rapidly disintegrating tablets (Reditabs) 10 mg Syrup 5 mg/5 ml	2.5–5 mg od/ 10 mg od
>2 years	Cetirizine hydrochloride (Cetirizine)	Tablets 10 mg Syrup 5 mg/5 ml	2.5–5 mg od/ 5–10 mg od
>6 years	Fexofenadine hydrochloride (Telfast)	Tablets 30 mg, 60 mg, 120 mg, 180 mg Syrup 6 mg/1 ml	30 mg bid/ 60 mg bid or 180 mg od
>6 years	Levocetrizine dihydrochroride (Xyzal)		
>12 years	Mizolastine (Mizollen)		

34

tor rhinitis. While some studies have shown a decrease in nasal congestion, others have not been able to confirm this. Dose-ranging trials have shown an onset of action within 3 h after initial dosing and persistence of efficacy over a 12-h interval. The most common side effects at the recommended dose of two sprays per nostril twice a day in children over 12 years are bitter taste (19.7% vs. 0.6% placebo) and sedation (11.5 vs. 5.4% placebo).

Intranasal Corticosteroids

Intranasal corticosteroids represent the single most effective class of medications for AR and improve all nasal symptoms including nasal congestion, rhinorrhea, itching, and sneezing. The comprehensive clinical effects of INS are based on a broad mechanism of action, which includes proinflammatory gene product downregulation or, less commonly, anti-inflammatory gene upregulation.

Currently available intranasal corticosteroids in the UK are listed in Table 34.3 according to age. Although intranasal corticosteroids may vary with regard to their sensory attributes (such as taste and/or smell) and thus patient acceptance and adherence, there do not appear to be any clear clinically relevant differences in efficacy among them (Corren 1999).

The reported side effects include nasal burning and stinging, dryness, and epistaxis. These can occur in 5–10% of patients. Local atrophy, such as occurs with dermatological high-potency corticosteroids, was not observed in year-long studies with fluticasone and mometasone. In terms of systemic side effects, laboratory evaluations of the hypothalamic-pituitary-adrenal axis by multiple means have shown minimal or lack of suppression except for betamethasone (betnesol), which has caused Cushing's syndrome in children. By implication, dexamethasone, the other first-generation corticosteroid, may have similar properties. Linear growth has not been shown to be affected by the administration of budesonide, fluticasone, and mometasone at recommended doses, as evidenced in several long-term studies.

Decongestants

Vasoconstrictors exist in both topical and oral form. Topical applied vasoconstrictor sympathomimetic agents belong to the catecholamine (e.g., phenylephrine) or imidazoline family (e.g., ozymetazoline), while oral vasoconstricting agents are primarily catecholamines (phenylephrine and pseudoephedrine). These agents exert their effect via the alpha1 and alpha2 adrenoreceptors present

Table 34.3 Nasal corticosteroids licensed for use in the UK according to age

Age	Drug	Product name	Volume (µl)	Phenyl EtOH/ Fragrance	Starting dose pediatric/ ≥12 years
>4 years	Fluticasone proprionate	Flixonase	95	+	1/nost od/ 2/nost od
>5 years	Flunisolide	Syntaris	120	–	2/nost bid/ 2/nost bid
>5 years	Dexamethasone isonicotinate and tramazoline (topical decongestant)	Dexa-rhinaspray duo	20 + 120		1/nost bid/tid
>6 years	Mometasone Furoate	Nasonex	100	–	1/nost od/ 2/nost od
>6 years	Triamcinolone acetonide	Nasacort	130	–	1/nost od/ 2/nost od
>6 years	Beclomethasone diproprionate	Beconase	50	–	1/nost od/ 2/nost od
>12 years	Budesonide	Rhinocort	50	–	1/nost od/ 2/nost od

on nasal capacitance vessels, which are responsible for mucosal swelling and associated nasal congestion. The reduction in blood flow to the nasal vasculature after administration leads to increased nasal patency in 5–10 min when used topically or 30 min when used orally. Nasal decongestion may last up to 8–12 h with topical and 24 h with extended-release oral decongestants. Symptoms of rhinitis other than nasal congestion are not affected, and thus monotherapy with vasoconstrictors has a limited role in the treatment of AR.

The adverse affects of topical nasal decongestants include nasal burning, stinging, dryness, and less commonly, mucosal ulceration. Tolerance and rebound congestion can occur when these agents are used for longer than 1 week, and can culminate in rhinitis medicamentosa. Adverse affects of oral decongestants include central nervous stimulation such as insomnia, which may occur in up to one-third of people, hyperactivity, nervousness, anxiety, and tremors, as well as dry mouth, tachycardia, palpitations, and increases in blood pressure.

Cromolyn

Cromolyns inhibit the degranulation of sensitized mast cells, thereby blocking the release of inflammatory mediators. Cromolyn (Rynacrom) is indicated for both seasonal and perennial AR. The onset of relief appears during the 1st week of treatment, and symptoms often continue to improve as the medication is continued over the subsequent weeks. The 4% intranasal solution is recommended for children ages 2 years and older. The frequency of dosing may lead to adherence problems given the need to initially instill the solution four times daily. However, once symptoms are under control, a less frequent dosing regimen may suffice for adequate symptom control. Topical adverse effects such as sneezing, nasal irritation and unpleasant taste are uncommon and cromolyn is poorly absorbed systemically and, therefore, has an excellent safety record. Tolerance to the effects of cromolyn has not been described.

Antileukotrienes

Cysteinyl-leukotrienes (cys-LTs) are potent lipid mediators derived from the enzymatic action on nuclear membrane phospholipids. These inflammatory molecules appear to play an important role in both upper and lower airway inflammation. Nasal challenge with LTD4 in normal human subjects can lead to a significant increase in nasal mucosal blood flow and nasal airway resistance (Bisgaard et al. 1986). However, leukotrienes do not appear to stimulate the sensory nerves present in the nasal mucosa, and thus probably do not contribute significantly to nasal itching or sneezing (Fujita et al. 1999). Blockage of the LTs can be accomplished by either inhibition of synthesis via 5-lipoxygenase (5-LO) inhibitors or by receptor blockade of the cys-LT1 receptor via cys-LT receptor antagonists. Zileuton has been the only drug approved for human use that blocks the 5-LO pathway, but is currently not available in the UK. Currently available receptor antagonists in the UK include montelukast (Singulair) and zafirlukast (Accolate). In general, antileukotriene drugs are well-tolerated.

Montelukast has been the most extensively studied antileukotriene in AR and it has shown clinical efficacy in both seasonal and perennial AR. It is indicated in children with perennial AR as young as 6 months and children with seasonal AR aged 2 years and over. Leukotriene antagonists do not appear to be more effective than nonsedating antihistamines and are less effective than intranasal corticosteroids in the treatment of AR. Nonetheless, antileukotrienes may be an attractive alternative in individuals with concomitant mild persistent asthma and intermittent AR.

Omalizumab (Anti-IgE)

Omalizumab represents one of the more exciting recent developments in the treatment of atopic diseases and is probably only the first of several monoclonal antibodies aimed at modulating allergic inflammation. Unfortunately, at present, it is expensive for routine treatment of AR and is indicated primarily in the treatment of severe asthma. Omalizumab is a "humanized" monoclonal antibody that effectively hinders the interaction between IgEs and the high-affinity IgE receptor present on mast cells, basophils, and dendritic cells. After initial dosing, free IgE concentrations decline in a rapid dose-dependent fashion by 97–99%. Omalizumab has been shown to be effective in both allergen-challenge studies and randomized, double-blind, placebo-controlled studies evaluating seasonal and perennial AR.

Allergen Immunotherapy

Immunotherapy (IT) is the only treatment modality to alter the natural history of allergic disease. While popular in many parts of the world, it has yet to gain broad-based acceptance in the UK. IT involves the repeated administration of increasing doses of individually selected allergens to induce immunologic tolerance. Over the last few years, the quantity of allergen necessary to lead to substantial clinical improvement and immunologic changes has been elucidated for many of the major standardized allergens (Joint Task Force on Practice Parameters 2003). Several placebo-controlled, double-blind studies have shown the clinical efficacy of vaccination with allergy extracts. Furthermore, in patients receiving grass allergen vaccinations for a period of 3–4 years, approximately 50% of patients continued to derive clinical benefits 3 years after IT had been discontinued. Prolonged clinical benefits correlate with persistent changes in immunity and allergic inflammation. Recently, it has been noted that specific IT to birch and/or grass in children aged 6–14 years who were not otherwise sensitized to other allergens, led to a markedly reduced risk (Odd's ratio = 2.52; $p<0.05$) of being newly diagnosed with asthma during the 3 years of receiving allergy vaccines (Möller et al. 2002).

IT is most commonly reserved for patients not responding to pharmacotherapy or those either unwilling to take or unable to tolerate medications. Patients need to understand the principles and risks of IT prior to its commencement. First, improvement requires several months of vaccinations. It is generally accepted that a 1-year trial will determine who will and will not respond to IT. Second, adverse reactions occur in both local and systemic form. Local reactions are characterized by swelling after injections and may last for days. Systemic reactions range from mild to fatal. The risk of a fatal reaction after receiving an allergy vaccine is estimated to be 1 in 2 to 2.5 million. It is unclear how many fatal reactions are due to human error. In the UK, allergen IT is administered only to patients with a clearly defined allergen sensitivity who do not suffer from poorly controlled asthma. It has to be undertaken by trained personnel with full cardiorespiratory resuscitatory facilities to hand, and the patient must be observed for 1 h after the injection at each visit. Oral IT, primarily sublingual/swallow, is gaining in popularity in parts of Europe. It is efficacious, although possibly less so than traditional, subcutaneous IT, but appears safer with the need for observation by trained personnel only for the first dose and for 1 h afterwards.

Other Treatment Modalities

Short bursts of oral corticosteroids (3–7 days) may be necessary to treat severe AR and decrease turbinate swelling sufficient to allow the effective administration of topical agents. Nasal irrigation with saline may be a helpful adjunct in the treatment of AR. Nasal irrigation usually involves the administration of several ounces of isotonic or hypertonic saline via an appropriate device, such as a large-volume or bulb syringe, Netti Pot, turkey baster, or water-pick coupled to a nasal adaptor. Isotonic saline can be created at home by adding half a teaspoon of salt to 8 ounces (240 cm^3) of water.

For refractory rhinorrhea, intranasal ipratropium bromide (Atrovent) 0.03% or 0.06% may also be an option. This anticholinergic agent has a rapid onset of action and can be used several times daily. Side effects are usually limited to local irritation.

Summary for the Clinician

- AR is a very common condition affecting children of all ages, but peaking in the early teenage years. Those afflicted with AR often suffer from associated inflammatory conditions of the mucosa such as AC, rhinosinusitis, asthma, otitis media with effusion, and other atopic conditions such as eczema and food allergies. Lack of treatment or treatment with suboptimal therapy may result in reduced QOL and compromise productivity at school. While a diagnostic trial of pharmacotherapy may be employed for clinically diagnosed AR, confirmation of the diagnosis requires documentation of specific IgE reactivity. This has the added benefit of guiding the implementation of environmental controls, which at times may significantly ameliorate the symptoms of AR. Many different classes of medications are now available and have been shown to be effective and safe in a large number of well-designed, double-blind, placebo-controlled clinical trials. Intranasal corticosteroids are safe when used at recommended doses and most effectively treat all symptoms of AR. Second-generation antihistamines represent a first-line treatment modality that is most appropriately employed in children with milder and more seasonal disease. Some of the first-generation antihistamines have been associated with increased sedation. Only IT with increasing doses of individually targeted allergens results in sustained changes of the immune system.

References

1. Arrighi HM, Cook CK, Redding GJ (1996) The prevalence and impact of allergic rhinitis among teenagers. J Allergy Clin Immunol 94:430

2. Bisgaard H, Olsson P, Bende M (1986) Effect of leukotriene D4 on nasal mucosal blood flow, nasal airway resistance and nasal secretions in humans. Clin Allergy 16:289–297

3. Bousquet J, van Cauwenberge PB, Khaltaev N, et al (2001) Allergic rhinitis and its impact on asthma. ARIA workshop report. J Allergy Clin Immunol 108:S147

4. Bousquet J, van Cauwenberge PB, Khaltaev N (2003) Allergic rhinitis and its impact on asthma. ARIA – executive summary. Allergy 57:841–855

5. Corren J (1999) Intranasal corticosteroids for allergic rhinitis: how do different agents compare? J Allergy Clin Immunol 104:S144–149

6. Fujita M, Yonetomi Y, Shimouchi K, et al (1999) Involvement of cysteinyl leukotrienes in biphasic increase of nasal airway resistance of antigen-induced rhinitis in guinea pigs. Eur J Pharmacol 369:349–356

7. Hamilton RG, Franklin Adkinson N Jr (2004) In vitro assays for the diagnosis of IgE-mediated disorders. J Allergy Clin Immunol 114:213–225

8. Hyndman SJ, Vickers LM, Htut T, et al (2000) A randomized trial of dehumidification in the control of house dust mite. Clin Exp Allergy 30:1172–1180

9. Joint Task Force on Practice Parameters (2003) Allergen immunotherapy: a practice parameter. American Academy of Allergy, Asthma and Immunology. American College of Allergy, Asthma and Immunology. Ann Allergy Asthma Immunol 90:1–40

10. Leynaert B, Bousquet J, Neukirch C, et al (1999) Perennial rhinitis: an independent risk factor for asthma in nonatopic subjects: results from the European Community Respiratory Health Survey. J Allergy Clin Immunol 104:301–304

11. Meltzer EO (2001) Quality of life in adults and children with allergic rhinitis. J Allergy Clin Immunol 108:S45–53

12. Möller C, Dreborg S, Ferdousi HA, et al (2002) Pollen immunotherapy reduces the development of asthma in children with seasonal rhinoconjunctivitis. J Allergy Clin Immunol 109:251–256

13. Richardson GS, Roehrs TA, Rosenthal L, et al (2002) Tolerance to daytime sedative effects of H1 antihistamines. J Clin Psychopharmacol 5:511–515

14. Shin SH, Ponikau JU, Sherris DA, et al (2004) Chronic rhinosinusitis: an enhanced immune response to ubiquitous airborne fungi. J Allergy Clin Immunol 111:1369–1375

15. Simons FER (2003) H$_1$-Antihistamines. In: Adkinson NF Jr, Yunginger JW, Busse WW, et al (eds) Middleton's Allergy: Principles and Practice, 6th edn. Mosby, Philadelphia, pp 834–869

16. Skoner DP (2001) Allergic rhinitis: definition, epidemiology, pathophysiology, detection, and diagnosis. J Allergy Clin Immunol 108:S2–8

17. Terreehorst I, Hak E, Oosting AJ, et al (2003) Evaluation of impermeable covers for bedding in patients with allergic rhinitis. N Engl J Med 349:237–246

18. Von Mutius E, Martinez FD (2003) Natural history, development, and prevention of allergic disease in childhood. In: Adkinson NF Jr, Yunginger JW, Busse WW, et al (eds) Middleton's Allergy: Principles and Practice, 4th edn. Mosby, St Louis, pp 1169–1174

19. Vuurman EF, van Veggel LM, Sanders RL, et al (1996) Effects of semprex-D and diphenhydramine on learning in young adults with seasonal allergic rhinitis. Ann Allergy Asthma Immunol 76:247–252

20. Wood RA, Johnson EF, Van Natta ML, et al (1998) A placebo-controlled trial of a HEPA air cleaner in the treatment of cat allergy. Am J Respir Crit Care Med 158:115–120

21. Wright AL, Holberg CJ, Martinez FD, et al (1994) Epidemiology of physician-diagnosed allergic rhinitis in childhood. Pediatrics 94:895–901

Useful websites of allergy societies

www.allergyuk.org
www.bsaci.org
www.eaaci.org
www.theucbinstituteofallergy.com

34

Chapter 35

Rhinosinusitis in Children

35

Peter A. R. Clement

Core Messages

- Rhinosinusitis is common in childhood; 45% of unselected magnetic resonance imaging scans are abnormal, 100% of those in children with purulent rhinorrhoea.
- Childhood rhinosinusitis differs from adult rhinosinusitis in that it is more extensive, often relates to immunoincompetence and tends to resolve spontaneously.
- Underlying disease should be sought in persistent or severe rhinosinusitis: this includes cystic fibrosis, primary ciliary dyskinesia and immunoglobulin deficiencies.
- Many children do not require treatment, and very few need surgery.
- Acute rhinosinusitis can spread locally to involve the orbit or central nervous system.
- Visual loss or nausea and vomiting accompanied by signs of sinusitis are rhinologic emergencies.
- In a child with an extradural haematoma and no history of head trauma, sinusitis must be excluded.

Contents

Introduction

Rhinitis and sinusitis usually coexist and are concurrent in most individuals. Therefore, rhinosinusitis is a more appropriate term. The clinical definition of rhinosinusitis in children is an inflammation of the nose and paranasal sinuses, characterised by nasal blockage (congestion, discharge) and one or more of these signs and symptoms (i.e. anterior/posterior secretions, or post-nasal drip, facial pain or pressure, and reduction or loss of smell).

35

Management of sinusitis in children is a controversial issue among ENT specialists. It was often assumed that a young child did not have any paranasal sinuses and therefore the paediatric runny nose was mostly due to rhinitis or adenoid hyperplasia. Since the introduction of better imaging techniques, such as computed tomography (CT) and magnetic resonance imaging (MRI), it has been demonstrated that chronic nasal complaints in children are mostly accompanied by extensive inflammation of the sinus mucosa. In fact, infection of the upper respiratory tract (URTI) is the commonest organic disease of the child seen by the primary care physician.

Morphogenesis, Epidemiology and Pathophysiology

In general, the sinuses are established in pre-natal life, with the shape of each sinus being regular in appearance and somewhat "globular" (Anon et al. 1996). The maxillary sinus extends to a depth of about 7 mm, is 3 mm wide and 7 mm high. The overall growth of the sinuses is slow the first 6 years of life. In the newborn, two or three ethmoid cells are found bilaterally. The growth of the ethmoid air cell complex through childhood is a process of development of thick-walled cavities into finished delicate spaces. The sphenoid sinuses are also present in the neonate. Each sphenoid sinus is 4 mm wide and 2 mm high. Originally, the frontal sinuses are not present but they gradually develop from the anterior ethmoidal cells into the cranium. When the upper edge of the air cells (cupola) reaches the same level as the roof of the orbit, it is termed a frontal sinus, a situation that appears around the age of 5 years. When a child reaches the age of 7–8 years, the floor of the maxillary sinus already occupies the same level as the nasal floor.

Gordts et al. (1997) showed that in a non-ENT population (n=100), the prevalence of abnormal signs on MRI images was as high as 45%. This prevalence increased in the presence of a history of nasal obstruction to 50–80%

when bilateral mucosal swelling of the inferior turbinates was present on rhinoscopy, and to 100% in the presence of purulent secretions.

Unfortunately, most studies in the paediatric ENT literature deal with patient populations (children with nasal complaints who are already attending outpatient clinics). Very few prospective studies are available and practically no documentation exists on the natural history of the disease.

The first prospective epidemiologic and long-term longitudinal study was performed by Maresh and Washburn (1940). It was started in 1925 and the authors followed 100 healthy children from birth to maturity, looking at history and performing physical examination and routine posteroanterior radiographs of the paranasal sinuses four times a year. It was noted that there existed a relatively constant percentage of "pathologic" antra (30%) in the films taken between 1 and 6 years of age. From 6 to 12 years, this percentage dropped steadily to approximately 15%. The authors noted that variations in size of the sinuses occur frequently, without any demonstrable relation to the amount or frequency of infections. When there was a recent URTI, less than 50% showed clear sinuses. Tonsillectomy had no demonstrable effect on the radiographic appearance of the sinuses. The decrease in the prevalence of sinusitis in older children was also confirmed by Van Buchem (1992) in patient populations.

Another very extensive prospective study was performed by Bagetsch et al. (1980), who followed the total paediatric population (24,000 children) in Rostock (Germany) for 1 year. Eighty-four percent aged between 0 and 2 years, 74% of those between 4 and 6 years, and 80% of those over 7 years had one or more episodes of URTI in that period. In the 0- to 5-year olds, 72% of those in daycare centres had one or more episodes of URTI compared to 27% of those staying at home. Of the 84% of children aged 1–3 years (n=4103), 32% suffered from rhinopharyngitis. The peak of the disease occurred in the months November to February.

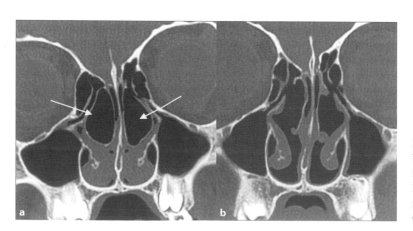

Fig. 35.1 a Hyperinflated concha media bullosa in a 10-year-old girl, resulting in medical therapy resistant rhinitis. Pre-operative coronal computed tomography (CT) scan. **b** Post-operative coronal CT-scan

These epidemiologic studies yield important information regarding the relevant factors influencing the prevalence of rhinosinusitis in children:

1. There exists a clear-cut decrease in the prevalence of rhinosinusitis after 6–8 years of age. This is the natural history of the disease in children.
2. In temperate climates there is a definite increase in the occurrence of rhinosinusitis in children during the autumn and wintertime.
3. There is a dramatic increase in the prevalence of chronic or recurrent rhinosinusitis among younger children who attend day-care centres compared to children staying at home.

Although viruses are not commonly recovered from sinus aspirates (Wald 2003), most authors agree that viral infections are the trigger to rhinosinusitis, and colds are much more frequent in children (range from 6–21/year) compared to adults (range 2–3/year).

In an MRI study of 60 children (mean age 5–7 years) with symptoms of uncomplicated URTI for an average of 6 days, Kristo et al. (2003) found abnormalities in the maxillary and ethmoidal sinuses in 60%, abnormalities in the sphenoidal in 35% and in the frontal sinuses in 18%. The MRI scores correlated significantly with symptom scores, especially nasal obstruction, nasal discharge and fever. In 26 children with major abnormalities in the first MRI, these findings subsequently (after 2 weeks) improved significantly, showing that these abnormalities of a URTI do not warrant antimicrobial medication.

The time course (i.e. clinical symptoms) of most simple URTIs is 5–6 days (Wald 2003). Therefore, persistence of respiratory symptoms beyond 10–19 days without improvement suggests the presence of acute bacterial sinusitis. The following three key elements are important in the normal physiology of the paranasal sinuses: the patency of the ostia, the function of the ciliary apparatus and the quality of the secretions. Once the ventilation and drainage of the sinuses is impaired, the sinusitis cycle will be initiated: congestion leads to more stagnation and thickening of secretions, impaired patency of the ostium results in oxygen resorption, a drop of local pH and metabolic changes develop and mucociliary transport is impaired, creating an ideal medium for bacteria, leading to more inflammation and more ostial blockage (Westrin 1994).

The factors predisposing to ostial obstruction can be divided into those that cause mucosal swelling and those related to mechanical obstruction. Mucosal swelling is mostly induced by URTI, but can be caused by systemic diseases such as cystic fibrosis, allergy, immune disorders and primary ciliary dyskinesia. Local insults such as pollution, facial trauma, swimming and/or diving (barotrauma) can contribute to poor ostial drainage and ventilation. Sometimes, hyperinflated anatomical structures (ethmoidal "emphysema", "black halo" image on CT scan, hyperinflated anatomic variations and ethmoidal cells; Fig. 35.1) can lead to persistent obstruction of narrow ethmoidal passages (tight spots) of the ostiomeatal complex. The most common mechanical factors in children, however, are choanal atresia, adenoid hyperplasia, extreme anatomical variations of the septum and lateral nasal wall (more common in the older child: Van der Veken et al. 1992; Tables 35.1 and 35.2), foreign bodies and tumours (juvenile angiofibroma) or pseudotumours (polyps, antrachoanal polyp, meningoencephalocoeles).

Bacterial infection contributes considerably to the ongoing inflammation. Despite the massive use of antibiotics for the last 40 years, the pathogenic microflora found in antral washings in children has not shown a shift (Clement et al. 1998). Over the years *Haemophilus influenzae* and *Streptococcus pneumoniae* have frequently been isolated in paediatric sinusitis (60%), especially during acute and recurrent sinusitis. The most common *H. influenzae* strain recovered from the sinuses is the non-typable *H. influenzae* (Wald 2003). *Moraxella catarrhalis* is beta-lactamase positive in 85% of cases, and is frequently found in combination with *H. influenzae* and *S. pneumoniae*. In

Table 35.1 Presence of anatomical variations (percentage) in children with chronic nasal complaints

Age group (years)	n=196	Septal deviation	Concha media bullosa	Concha superior bullosa	"Haller" cell
3–4	38	16	0	0	0
5–6	46	37	8	0	3
7–8	42	55	4	2	2
9–10	21	48	2	0	2
11–12	20	65	15	0	10
13–14	29	72	20	3	3

Table 35.2 Prevalence of involvement (percentage) of individual sinuses in children with chronic nasal complaints

Age group (years)	n (total=196)	Max	Involved sinus		
			Anterior ethmoidal	Posterior ethmoidal	Sphenoidal
3–4	38	63	53	34	29
5–6	46	39	24	24	13
7–8	42	52	38	26	26
9–10	21	33	14	14	19
11–12	20	45	20	5	10
13–14	29	65	10	3	0

this combination, they render the other microorganisms penicillin resistant (McLeod 1995), forming the "infernal trio" of Nord (1988). Multiple isolates are fairly common. Wald (2003) found anaerobes mixed with aerobes in 26% of cases. Some authors stress the importance of Gram-negative enteric bacteria (Bolger 1994 i.e. *Pseudomonas aeroginosa* and *Proteus mirabilis*, and of anaerobes (Brook 1981 i.e. *Peptostreptococcus* and *Bacteroides* (especially in chronic sinusitis).

Antral punctures are now rarely performed, but in children (Orobello et al. 1991) there is a good correlation between the maxillary sinus aspirates and the middle meatal specimen (83%). Gordts et al. (1999) compared the middle meatal bacteriology of 50 children who underwent minor ENT surgery, with a group of 50 children submitted to minor non-ENT surgical procedures. Again *H. influenzae*, *M. catarrhalis* and *S. pneumoniae* were the most cultivated organisms, not only in the ENT group (68, 50 and 60%, respectively), but also in the control group (40, 34 and 50%, respectively). On semi-quantitative analysis, however, richer colonies were obtained from the ENT group. This important finding means that in the younger child, these three organisms are frequently present as commensal flora, without triggering symptoms. However, during URTI the cultures become richer, and symptoms appear. Furthermore, it seems that there exists a significant difference (Table 35.3) between the commensal flora of adults and children.

Not only is the commensal flora different from the adult, but also the pathophysiology of chronic sinusitis in adults and children differs. Sanders et al. (1995) suspected that children with recurrent upper and lower respiratory infections may have a defective antibody response to polysaccharide antigens, while having normal serum immunoglobulins and normal antibody responses to protein antigens. In young children this may simply represent a physiological delay in the maturation of the

immune system (Pabst and Kreth 1980). It is known that the development of antibodies to polysaccharides of encapsulated bacteria such as *S. pneumoniae* in early life is much slower than to proteins. Defence against polysaccharide-encapsulated bacteria via immune globulin G subclasses 2 and 4 may not reach adult levels until the age of 10 years (Oxelius 1979). Besides the transient maturational delay, however, there may be a permanent selective impaired response to polysaccharide antigens in patients with recurrent URTI.

Finally, in a comparative histopathologic study of children and adults with chronic sinusitis, Chan et al. (2004) found that the sinus mucosa in children had less of the eosinophilic inflammation, basement membrane thickening and mucus gland hyperplasia, that are characteristic of adult chronic rhinosinusitis.

Nasal polyposis is rare in children with chronic rhinosinusitis (except in cystic fibrosis), as is chronic eosinophilic rhinosinusitis. Finally, chronic rhinosinusitis in the younger child is more extensive than in the adolescent, and anatomical variations are rare. All these observations show that the pathophysiology of chronic sinusitis in adults and children is different (Table 35.3).

Classification and Definitions

The classification of paediatric rhinosinusitis is based on the findings of the consensus meeting in Brussels (Clement et al. 1998).

Acute Rhinosinusitis

This is an infection of the sinuses initiated mostly by viral infection, in which complete resolution of symptoms (judged on clinical basis only) without intermittent URTI

Table 35.3 Differences between paediatric and adult chronic rhinosinusitis

	Young children	Adults
Commensal microflora		
Coagulase-negative staphylococci	30%	35%
Staphylococcus aureus	20%	8%
Haemophilus influenzae	40%	0%
Moraxella catarrhalis	24%	0%
Streptococcus pneumoniae	50%	26%
Corynebacterium species	52%	23%
Streptococcus viridans	30%	4%
Immunity	Immature Defective response to polysaccharide antigens (IgG2, IgA)	Mature
History	Self-limiting in time (improves after the age of 6–8 years)	No history of spontaneous improvement after certain age
Histology	Mainly neutrophilic disease, less basement membrane thickening and mucus gland hyperplasia	Mainly eosinophilic disease
Endoscopy	Polyps = rare, except in cystic fibrosis	Polyps = frequent
CT scan	Younger child more diffuse sinusitis involving all sinuses	Sphenoid and posterior ethmoid sinuses less often involved

Table 35.4 Symptoms and signs of acute rhinosinusitis in children

Non-severe	Severe
Rhinorrhoea (of any quality: thick, coloured)	Purulent rhinorrhoea (thick, opaque)
Nasal congestion	Nasal congestion
Headache, facial pain	Headache, nasal pain
Irritability (variable)	Peri-orbital oedema (variable)
Cough	High fever (≥39°C)

may take up to 12 weeks. It can be subdivided into severe and non-severe (Table 35.4).

According to the guidelines of the American Academy of Pediatrics Subcommittee (SMS/CQIAAP; 2001), acute bacterial rhinosinusitis (ABRS) is an infection of the paranasal sinuses, lasting less than 30 days, in which symptoms resolve completely. ABRS should be considered after a viral URTI, when the symptoms worsen after 5 days, are present for longer than 10 days, or are out of proportion to those seen with most viral infections. Recurrent acute sinusitis involves episodes of bacterial infection of the paranasal sinuses, separated by intervals during which the patient is asymptomatic. For the SMS/CQIAAP guideline, these episodes last less than 30 days and are separated by intervals of at least 10 days.

Chronic Rhinosinusitis

In children this is defined as a non-severe sinus infection with low-grade symptoms, present for longer than 12 weeks. Acute bacterial sinusitis may be superimposed on chronic rhinosinusitis: antimicrobials only resolve the additional acute symptoms.

The members of the Brussels consensus meeting noted that medical treatment such as antibiotics and nasal steroids may modify symptoms and signs of acute and chronic sinusitis, and consequently it is sometimes difficult to differentiate infectious rhinosinusitis from allergic sinusitis in a child on clinical grounds alone.

To classify sinusitis completely, one should note:
1. Which sinus or sinuses are involved (i.e. frontal, ethmoidal, sphenoidal, maxillary).
2. Which side is involved (i.e. left, right or bilateral).
3. Which microorganism is involved (if known): bacterial, fungal or viral.
4. Is the sinusitis complicated (i.e. mucocoele, orbital or intracranial)?
5. Is there a concomitant disease (e.g. diabetes, immune suppression)?

Diagnosis

Presenting Symptoms of Rhinosinusitis in Children

According to Clement (1998), the presenting symptoms of rhinosinusitis in children are:
1. Rhinorrhoea (71–80%; all forms).
2. Cough (50–80%; all forms).
3. Fever (50–60%; acute sinusitis).
4. Pain (29–33%; acute sinusitis).
5. Nasal obstruction (70–100%; chronic sinusitis).
6. Mouth breathing (70–100%; chronic sinusitis).
7. Ear complaints (recurrent purulent otitis media or otitis media with effusion in 40–68%; chronic sinusitis).

Wald (2003) stresses that two common clinical developments should alert a clinician: (1) signs and symptoms of a cold that persist beyond 10 days (any nasal discharge, daytime cough worsening at night) and (2) a cold that seems more severe than usual (high fever, copious purulent discharge, peri-orbital oedema and pain).

Clinical Examination

Physical examination of a child's nose is often extremely difficult, and only limited rhinoscopy is tolerated. The examination may be accomplished by simply lifting the tip of the nose upwards (young children have wide noses with round nostrils, allowing easy examination of the condition of the inferior turbinates). Another convenient method is the use of an otoscope. Usually, the nasal and pharyngeal mucosa appears erythematous, with yellow to greenish purulent rhinorrhoea of varying viscosity. Lymphoid hyperplasia of the tonsils, adenoids and parapharyngeal wall may also be observed. The cervical lymph nodes may be moderately enlarged and slightly tender.

Anterior rhinoscopy remains the first step, but is inadequate by itself. Endoscopy with a 2.7-mm rigid endoscope in the younger child and a 4-mm one in the older child is more useful then a fibroscopy, not only for the diagnosis, but also for the exclusion of other conditions, such as the presence of polyps, foreign bodies, tumours and septal deviations (Cools and Clement 1991). In the younger child, general anaesthesia is necessary to perform a thorough nasal endoscopy. Moreover, it allows direct sampling of middle meatus flora.

Microbiology

Microbiological assessment is usually not necessary in children with uncomplicated acute or chronic sinusitis. The indications for microbiology are: (1) severe illness or toxic child, (2) acute illness in a child not improving with medical therapy within 48–72 h, (3) an immune-compromised child and (4) the presence of suppurative (intra-orbital, intracranial) complications (orbital cellulitis excepted).

Because antral puncture in a child needs general anaesthesia, it is rarely performed and as the correlation between antral specimen and middle meatal specimen is good (83%), most clinicians will prefer the latter (Orobello et al. 1992). Quantification of bacterial growth can also help to distinguish contamination from real infection, and isolates should be considered positive when a type of bacteria is present in a quantity of at least 10,000 colonies/ml (Wald 2003).

Imaging

Imaging is not necessary to confirm the diagnosis of rhinosinusitis in children. The increase in thickness of both the soft tissue and the bony vault of the palate in children under 10 years of age limits the clinical usefulness of transillumination in the younger age group. Plain x-rays are insensitive and are of limited use for diagnosis or to guide surgery. The marginal benefits are insufficient to justify the exposure to radiation (Lusk et al. 1989).

CT scanning remains the imaging methodology of choice because of its ability to resolve both bone and soft tissue, with a good visualisation of the ostiomeatal complex. The indications for CT scanning in a child are the same as those given previously for a microbiology specimen with one extra indication, which is if surgery is being considered after failure of medical therapy.

Additional Investigations

In the presence of recalcitrant rhinosinusitis, underlying conditions must be considered.

Respiratory Allergy

This is perhaps the most important systemic disease that predisposes to sinus infections. In a CT scan study, Iwens and Clement (1994) found signs of mucosal inflammation in 61% of atopic children. Therefore in children with chronic rhinosinusitis and with suggestive history (asthma, eczema) and/or physical examination findings (allergic salute, watery rhinorrhoea, nasal blockage, sneezing, boggy turbinate), allergic assessment (skin prick, nasal smear, radioimmunosorbent test, radioallergosorbent test or trial treatment) should be performed for patients who continue to have clinical difficulties despite avoidance and simple pharmacological measures.

Immune Deficiency

All young children have a physiologic immune deficiency, which resolves around the age of 7–10 years (see Chapter 10). Recurrent and chronic sinusitis are the most common clinical presentations of common variable immune deficiencies (Polmar 1992).

Signs of Primary Immune Deficiency

The signs of primary immune deficiency are:
1. Eight or more new ear infections within 1 year.
2. Two or more serious sinus infections within 1 year.
3. Two or more months of antibiotics with little effect.
4. Two or more bouts of pneumonia within 1 year.
5. Failure of an infant to gain weight or grow normally.
6. Recurrent deep skin or organ abscesses.
7. Persistent thrush in the mouth or elsewhere on the skin after age 1 year.
8. Need for intravenous antibiotics to clear infections.
9. Two or more deep-seated infections.
10. A family history of immune deficiency.

The first-line investigations for patients with recurrent otolaryngological infections should be microbial sampling for culture, full blood count with differential white cell count, immunoglobulins and vaccine-specific IgG (tetanus toxoid, pneumococcus, *H. influenzae* type B). Further tests and therapy require help from an immunologist.

Cystic Fibrosis

This is discussed in detail in Chapter 11.

Primary Ciliary Dyskinesia

This is discussed in detail in Chapter 11.

Gastro-Oesophageal Reflux

The parallel existence of gastro-oesophageal reflux disease (GORD) with upper-airway inflammation and the ensuing problems of intractable sinusitis and otitis has been observed and suggests a causal relationship. Otolaryngologists should be suspicious of GORD in children complaining of chronic nasal discharge and obstruction combined with chronic cough, hoarseness and stridulous respiration. The endoscopic appearance of the laryngeal and tracheal areas are of considerable importance in conjunction with oesophageal examination, in determining potential relationship between GORD and otolaryngologic abnormalities. Barbero (1996) found 1 or more of the following endoscopic signs in 17 patients: cobblestoning of the mucosa of the laryngopharynx, inflammation of the upper respiratory tract, sinus involvement, rhinorrhoea, subglottic stenosis, velopharyngeal insufficiency, pharyngotracheitis and tracheomalacia. The diagnosis may be confirmed by 24-h pH or, preferably, impedance monitoring. When these are unavailable, a therapeutic trial may be helpful (see also Chapter 30).

Mechanical Obstruction

Mechanical obstruction of the nasal cavity, congenital as well as acquired (antrochoanal polyp, adenoid hyperplasia, nasogastric tube, foreign body, nasal trauma, lacrimal cyst, stenosis of the pyriform aperture, choanal atresia) can also induce chronic rhinosinusitis in infants or children. The most common polyp in children without any systemic disease is the antrochoanal polyp (Fig. 35.2). This solitary polyp originates mostly from the maxillary sinus, but also from the sphenoidal sinus or from the inferior turbinate. Among benign tumours, haemangiomas and tumours of neural derivation are the next most common. Gliomas are present at a very early age (2–6 weeks), exhibiting a reddish-bluish mass, and can induce stertor when the nasal passage is completely blocked.

Miscellaneous

Sinusitis occurs more frequently in certain ethnic groups (American Indian, Eskimo), in children with congenital velopharyngeal insufficiency without overt submucosal cleft palate and in 44% of children with cleft palate. Down syndrome, cyanotic heart disease and hypothyroidism can also predispose to sinusitis.

Some rare conditions include atelectasis of the maxillary sinus with eventual enophthalmus, and isolated turbinitis. Atelectasis of the maxillary sinus with eventual enophthalmus is a collapse of the maxillary sinus due to complete lack of ventilation. The CT shows an uncinate process that is plastered against the orbital wall (Fig. 35.3).

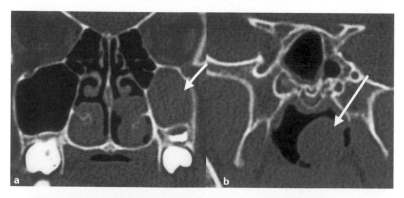

Fig. 35.2a,b Coronal CT scan in a 7-year-old child. Classic image of antrachoanal polyp. Note the soft-tissue mass in the left maxillary sinus (**a** *white arrow*) and choanal polyp in the nasopharynx (**b** *white arrow*)

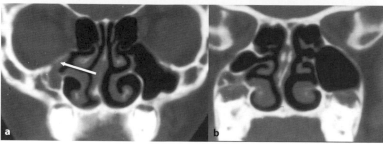

Fig. 35.3a,b Coronal CT scans of a 6-year-old child with atelectasis of the right maxillary sinus. Note the uncinate process plastered against the orbital wall (**a** *white arrow*)

Isolated turbinitis comprises isolated infection of one or both inferior turbinates resulting in a ballooning of this turbinate and the presence of purulent secretions on the floor of the nasal cavity. The CT scan confirms the ballooning of the inferior turbinate and shows no signs of sinusitis whatsoever (Fig. 35.4).

Therapeutic Management

Evidence-based schemes for therapy in children with acute and chronic rhinosinusitis are shown in Figs. 35.5 and 35.6.

Medical Treatment

The initial treatment of sinusitis consists of eradication of microorganisms with appropriate antibiotics and symp-

tomatic relief with decongestants, analgesics, anti-inflammatory drugs and antipyretics.

Antimicrobial Therapy

Acute Bacterial Rhinosinusitis

Patients with acute bacterial sinusitis who are treated with an appropriate antimicrobial agent respond promptly with reduction in nasal discharge and improvement of cough (Wald 2003). Not all children with acute rhinosinusitis need antimicrobials. According to the members of the consensus panel (Clement et al. 1998), indications for antibiotic therapy are:

1. A severe illness or toxic condition in a child with suspected or proven suppurative complication. Intravenous administration of an appropriate agent is recommended. The antibiotic selected should be effective

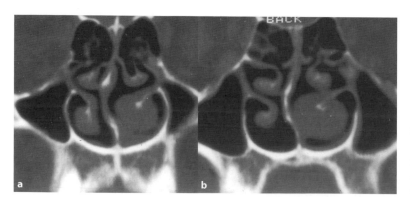

Fig. 35.4a, b Coronal CT scan of a 10-year-old child with ballooning of the inferior turbinate on the left side and presence of pus on the nasal floor, without any signs of sinusitis

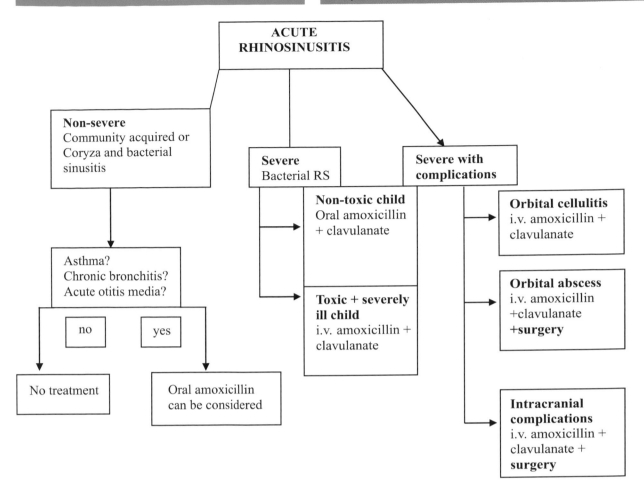

Fig. 35.5 Decisional algorithm: evidence-based scheme for therapy in children with acute rhinosinusitis

against the penicillin-resistant *S. pneumoniae*, beta-lactamase-producing *H. influenzae* and *M. catarrhalis*.

2. Severe acute rhinosinusitis: in ambulatory patients for whom oral therapy is appropriate, an agent should be selected that is resistant to the action of beta-lactamase enzymes (amoxicillin-potassium clavunate or a second-generation cephalosporin such as cefuroxime axetil).

3. Non-severe acute rhinosinusitis: only in a child with protracted symptoms to whom antibiotics can be given on an individual basis (e.g. presence of asthma, chronic bronchitis, acute otitis media). In those children for whom antibiotic therapy is preferred, amoxicillin (45 mg/kg/day, doubled if under 2 years or with risk factors for resistance) is appropriate. If the patient's condition has not improved within 72 h, a change of antibiotic to an agent effective against the resistant organism prevalent in the community should be considered.

Patients with a penicillin allergy should receive a suitable alternative antibiotic such as azithromycin or clarithromycin as first-line therapy.

Chronic Rhinosinusitis

Antibiotic therapy is not indicated in the young child (less than 6–8 years of age) with a runny purulent nose who is healthy and active. This condition is mostly due to an immature immune system – it could be regarded as a self-limiting disease – and antibiotics will only relieve the symptoms of purulent rhinorrhoea temporarily. Frequent administration will only enhance antimicrobial resistance and does not reduce the development of empyema (van Buchem et al. 1992). Otten and Grote (1988) performed a long-term follow-up of children with maxillary sinusitis treated in four different ways (antibiotics, antral lavage, combination of two previous regimens and placebo) and were not able to demonstrate any difference in therapeutic effect.

Antibiotics are indicated in children with chronic rhinosinusitis with frequent acute infective exacerbations. Again, amoxicillin with or without clavulanic acid is the first choice. If there is no response within 5–7 days, the antibiotic should be changed. If there is again no response within 5–7 days, a specimen of sinus secretions should be

35

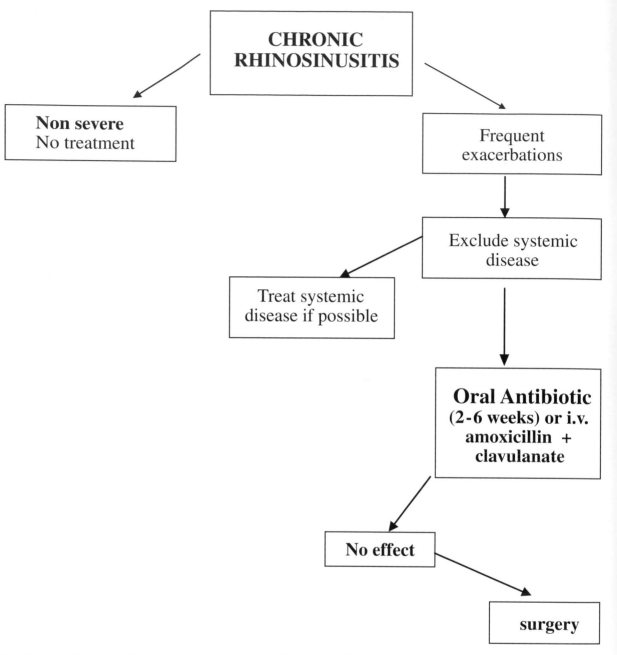

Fig. 35.6 Decisional algorithm: evidence-based scheme for therapy in children with chronic rhinosinusitis

obtained for culture, or a non-infectious condition could be considered (see "Additional Investigations" above). If, however, the patient responds rather slowly, a longer course (up to 3 months) can be prescribed.

Additional Medical Therapy

Decongestants

Most authors prefer topical alpha-2-agonists (xylo- and oxymetazoline) in appropriate concentrations depending on the age of the child. Careful dosage is important when treating an infant and young children, to prevent toxic manifestations. The ratio of the area of nasal mucosa to body weight is an important factor in infants. It is three times as high as in the neonate as in the adult, and twice as high in children age 2–3 years. Care should be taken to use the decongestant for no longer than 1 week, because they also decrease the local blood flow, have some ciliotoxic effects and involve a potential rebound. On the other hand, they give rapid relief of the symptom of nasal blockage. Oral decongestants are less appropriate because of their side effects and contraindications.

Other treatments that offer some decongestant effect include the use of humidifiers and/or inhalation of moist heat.

Oral or Topical Mucolytics

Oral or topical mucolytics such as guaifenesin and acetylcysteine have never been proved to be efficacious in sinus disease.

Analgesics and Antipyretics

These have some effect on pain and elevated temperature.

Antihistamines

Antihistamines are ineffective in the treatment of common cold and sinusitis. They reduce coexisting allergic symptoms of running, itching and sneezing. Preference should be given to newer molecules without cardiotoxic, sedative or anticholinergic effects.

Topical Steroids

These are indicated when allergy is involved. To minimalise the effect on childhood growth, the least bio-available topical steroid should be preferred (i.e. mometasone, fluticasone; Scadding 2003).

Saline Nose Drops, Sprays and Nasal Douches

Saline nose drops, sprays and nasal douches using a bulb syringe or lavage are popular with paediatricians. As long as the saline is isotonic and at body temperature, it can help in eliminating nasal secretions and inducing some decongestion of the mucosa. Some authors also use saltwater-buffered hypertonic saline nasal irrigations in young children.

Most children with proven (GERD) will show improvement of sinus disease after treatment for gastro-oesophageal reflux, and not infrequently, surgery can be avoided. Treatment consists of ranitidine and cisapride for mild cases and omeprazole and cisapride for more serious cases, (mean duration of therapy 8.2 months). Nisson fundoplasty is reserved for refractory cases (Bothwell et al. 1999).

Intravenous gamma globulins are only useful when a gamma-globulin deficiency has been demonstrated. Pneumococcal polysaccharide polyvalent vaccines are limited in their usefulness for children because of their inability to induce a protective antibody response in children younger than 2 years of age and lack of immunologic memory. In contrast, pneumococcal protein conjugate vaccines induce presumptive protective responses in infants younger than 6 months, and immunologic memory further enhances responses after booster doses are given (Overturf 2002). The decrease in the overall incidence of acute otitis media in children after vaccination with conjugate pneumococcal vaccine has been minimal. A possible explanation for this apparent lack of efficacy is replacement of the common pneumococcal serotype (covered by the vaccine) with other serotypes and other species such as *H. influenzae* (Zacharisen and Casper 2005).

Surgical Treatment

Adenoidectomy

Adenoidectomy has been recommended by many authors for different indications, for example recurrent sinusitis with adenoiditis as the source of recurrent infections or adenoid hyperplasia with almost total nasal obstruction by an adenoid pad, resulting in stasis of secretions. The author did not find any significant correlation between the size of the adenoids and the presence of purulent secretions in the middle meatus on fibroscopic examination of 420 children between the age of 1 and 7 years, while there existed a strong correlation between the size of the adenoid and the complaints of mouth breathing ($p<0.001$) and snoring ($p<0.001$). Thus, one can state categorically that in a case of sinusitis when signs of nasal obstruction, snoring and speech defects are prominent, adenoidectomy should be considered.

Many authors are not certain of the benefit of adenoidectomy on sinusitis and note that the effect of adenoidectomy is not well documented, and has not been proven statistically.

Antral Lavage, Nasal Antral Window

It has been demonstrated that the benefits of antral lavage in children are not long lasting. Lund (1990) demonstrated that, particularly in children under the age of 16 years, there occurs a high rate of closure of antral windows. She concluded that the inferior meatus in children in smaller than in adults, making it impossible to create an adequate-sized antrostomy.

Endoscopic Sinus Surgery

A Caldwell-Luc operation is contraindicated in children as it can cause damage to unerupted teeth. Since the introduction of the endoscope, sinus surgery is now pos-

35

sible in children via an endonasal approach. Most controversies relate to the indications for functional endoscopic sinus surgery (FESS) in children. During the Brussels consensus meeting (Clement 1998), an international agreement was reached concerning the indications for FESS in children.

Absolute Indications

Absolute indications for FESS include:
1. Complete nasal obstruction because of massive nasal polyposis or medialisation of the lateral nasal wall in cystic fibrosis.
2. Orbital abscess.
3. Intracranial complications.
4. Antrachoanal polyp.
5. Mucocoeles or mucopyocoeles.
6. Fungal sinusitis.

Possible Indications

FESS in children should be the exception. Children with chronic sinusitis and frequent exacerbations that persist despite optimal medical therapy and after exclusion of any systemic disease, will benefit from endoscopic sinus surgery; here, surgery is a reasonable alternative to continuous medical treatment. Optimal treatment includes several weeks of adequate antibiotics (oral) or a course of intravenous antibiotics with treatment of any concomitant systematic disease.

Surgery for chronic sinusitis is mostly limited to a partial ethmoidectomy, including removal of the uncinate process, with or without middle meatal antrostomy, and opening of the bulla. In other cases, the extent of the surgery depends on the disease: a complete sphenoidectomy is preferred in children with cystic fibrosis and massive polyposis.

Lusk and Muntz (1990) found a success rate of 88% in 24 children who had only one procedure. There was a 24% improvement in purulent rhinorrhoea, 33% in fever and 13% in cough. A meta-analysis performed by Herbert and Bent (1998) focussing on the number of children per study, length of follow-up, prospective versus retrospective, separation or exclusion of patients with significant underlying disease, showed in eight published articles (n=832 patients) positive outcome rates ranging from 88 to 92%. The average combined follow-up was 3.7 years. They concluded that FESS is a safe and effective treatment for chronic rhinosinusitis that is refractory to medical treatment.

No influence of FESS on facial growth could be demonstrated, using qualitative anthromorphic analysis of 12 facial measurements with a 13-year follow-up or an encephalographic measurement of 10 different parameters

in adults with cystic fibrosis who underwent complete spheno-ethmoidectomy before the second growth spurt in childhood.

Complications of Rhinosinusitis

Osteomyelitis of the Maxilla

A special condition that needs to be differentiated from acute sinusitis is acute osteomyelitis of the maxilla in the infant (from a few days to 2 years of age), which is now a rare condition. It is a staphylococcal infection of an unerupted tooth and the surrounding bone. The swelling is usually considerably more extensive than in sinusitis and involves the cheek, the hard palate and the eyelids. Appropriate intravenous antibiotic therapy is indicated.

Odontogenic Sinusitis

Peri-apical abscess or persistent disease of the upper teeth may extend into the sinus cavity and cause maxillary sinusitis. The incidence of odontogenic sinusitis in children is unknown, but is probably significant, particularly in adolescents. Treatment consists of drainage of the dental abscess and operative closure of the ora-antral fistula (Wald 2003).

Orbital and Intracranial Complications

There exist no exact figures on the prevalence of these, but it is estimated that in adults, orbital or intracranial complications can occur in 0.8–0.01% of sinusitis cases. The majority are complications of chronic rhinosinusitis (80%).

Paediatric intracranial complications (Herrmann et al. 2006) are more common in adolescents (mostly over 14 years of age) and the distribution is as follows: 56% subdural abscess, 44% epidural, 19% cerebral abscess, 19% meningitis (13% isolated and 6% in combination with another intracranial complication).

The spread of the infection can be local, with direct extension of the infection via a natural dehiscence or weakness of the surrounding bone (lamina orbitalis, os lacrimale, infra-orbital canal, dental roots) or spread via venous channels or lymphatics.

Pott's Puffy Tumour

Pott's puffy tumour (Figs. 35.7 and 35.8) is a subperiostial abscess, sometimes accompanied by skin break down, and formed from bacterial spread of frontal sinusitis via venous channels through the outer table of the skull. The microbiology mostly shows aerobes (alpha and beta haemolytic streptococci, staphylococci, enterococci) and anaerobes (*Bacteroides*). Therapy consists of sinus surgery resulting in adequate drainage of the involved sinus and also drainage of the abscess (puncture).

Osteomyelitis of the Posterior Wall

Osteomyelitis of the posterior wall (the most predominant organisms are *Fusobacterium*, bacteroides species and anaerobic streptococci) will lead via the valveless veins of Breshet or via bone erosion to intracranial complications such as meningitis, epidural abscess, subdural abscess or empyema, venous sinus thrombosis and brain abscess. These complications are more frequent in children and young adolescents, and in patients with depressed immune function, than in adults.

Meningitis (Leptomeningitis)

Symptoms are neck stiffness, vomiting, fever, mild headache and subtle changes of consciousness. The diagnosis is confirmed by a spinal tap, which shows leukocytosis, increase in protein levels and decrease in glucose level. A CT or MRI is needed to exclude a space-occupying lesion and increased intracranial pressure before lumbar puncture is considered. Symptoms of increased intracranial pressure are: bradycardia, pupil oedema (which takes some time to develop), stiff neck, hyper-

tension, nausea, vomiting, decreased consciousness and, finally, dilated pupils (an ominous sign suggesting transtentorial herniation).

Epidural Abscess

Symptoms are: dull headache, spiking fever, normal cerebrospinal fluid CSF (Fig. 35.9).

Subdural Abscess or Empyema

Symptoms are: fever (toxic patient), intense headache and meningeal signs (Fig. 35.9). Sometimes there may be a fulminant progression leading to nuchal rigidity, altered consciousness, hemiparesis, seizures, focal neurologic changes and papilloedema. The CSF is cloudy with leucocytes, but negative culture and no bacteria. Organisms found in abscesses are most commonly *Staphylococcus* and *Strepcococci*, Gram-negative bacteria such as *Escherichia coli*, *Pseudomonas*, *Proteus* and many anaerobes.

Brain Abscess

This can be multiple, mostly frontal. The mortality rate is still 20–30% and morbidity includes post-survival seizures (30–50%). Symptoms are: lack of neurologic signs

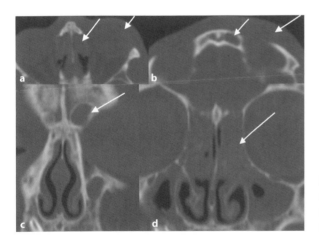

Fig. 35.7a–d Axial CT scan (bony window settings) showing symmetric proptosis and subperiosteal abscess of the forehead ("Pott's puffy tumour", **a**, **b**) and coronal CT scans showing bilateral pansinusitis (**c**, **d**)

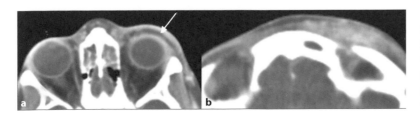

Fig. 35.8a,b Same patient as shown in Fig. 35.5. Axial CT scans, soft-tissue window settings. **a** Orbital cellulitis with symmetric proptosis. **b** Subperiosteal abscess of the forehead "Pott's puffy tumour"

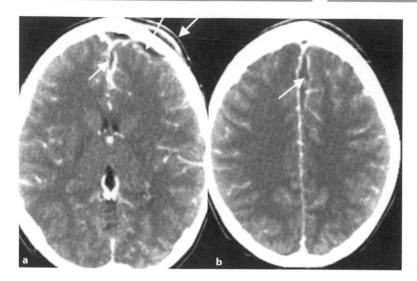

Fig. 35.9a,b Axial CT scans of the brain with contrast of the same patient as shown in Figs. 35.5 and 35.6 (Pott's puffy tumour) with subperiostal abscess of the forehead (epidural, subdural and sagittal abscesses are shown by *white arrows*)

in the frontal lobe, mental dullness (60% altered level of consciousness), lethargy and headache, and cranial nerve palsies in 26%. Germs are *St. aureus*, *St. epidermitis*, *S. pneumoniae* and *S. intermedius*, beta-haemolytic streptococci groups F and C, and anaerobic streptococci.

An axial CT scan with contrast is needed to visualise an intracranial abscess, and an MRI-venogram to exclude venous sinus thrombosis (Fig. 35.10). Nausea and vomiting accompanied by signs of sinusitis are a rhinologic emergency.

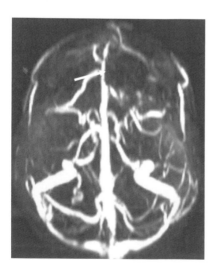

Fig. 35.10 Magnetic resonance imaging axial venogram impression on the sagittal sinus (*white arrow*) because of the sagittal abscess; there are no signs of thrombosis

Extradural Haematoma

Spontaneous extradural haematoma secondary to sinusitis is extremely rare (Griffiths et al. 2002). The diagnosis should be considered when signs of frontal sinusitis are present with symptoms such as severe headache, diminished consciousness and elevated temperature. There is an elevated white blood cell count and raised C-reactive protein. No history of head injury is available and there are no signs of external trauma. The extradural haematoma and sinusitis are confirmed by CT scan. If the patient is not treated in time (drainage of epidural haematoma and involved sinuses) death may follow. Haematoma may be the result of spread of the infection through diploic vascular channels, resulting in blood vessel rupture, or of granulation tissue eroding the bone and causing spontaneous extradural haematoma (Fig. 35.11). Mostly the organisms involved are: *Streptococcus*, *St. aureus*, *H. influenzae* and *Pseudomonas*. In a child with an extradural haematoma and no history of head trauma, sinusitis must be excluded.

Orbital Complications

These are the most common complications and occur mainly in children. The bacteria are *H. influenzae*, and *Streptococcus* and *Staphylococcus* species. The most widely accepted classification of orbital complications is Chandler's:

1. Pre-septal cellulitis: characterised by oedema of the eyelids without tenderness, visual loss or limitation of ocular motility (Figs. 35.12 and 35.13).
2. Orbital cellulitis without abscess formation: characterised by diffuse oedema of the peri-ocular adipose tissues (Fig. 35.14).

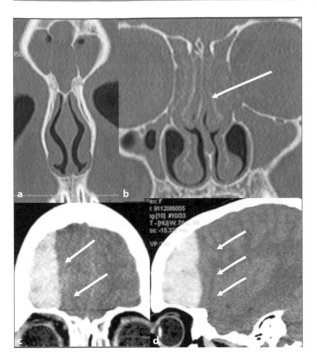

Fig. 35.11a–d A 14-year-old girl with a history of severe headache and recent common cold, and no head trauma. Culture of haematoma and middle meatus were positive for *Streptococcus*. **a**, **b** Coronal CT scan, bone window, bilateral pansinusitis; the *arrow* points to a septal deviation to the right. Note the paradoxically bent turbinate and very narrow, poorly drained frontal recess. Coronal (**c**) and sagittal (**d**) CT scan (soft tissue window + contrast) shows a huge right-sided extradural haematoma

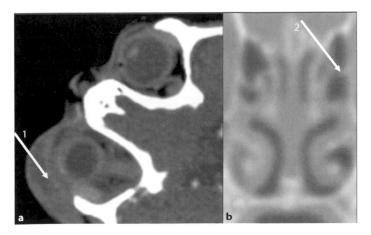

Fig. 35.12 A 16-month-old girl with recent Varicella, developing a pre-septal orbital abscess that needed surgical drainage due to scratch lesions with superinfections

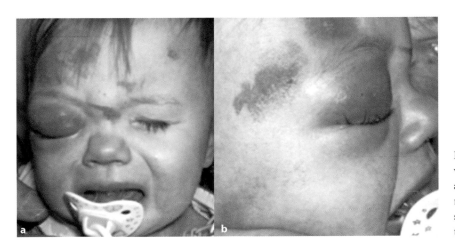

Fig. 35.13a, b Same patient as shown in Fig. 35.10. **a** Axial CT-scan showing pre-septal abscess. **b** Coronal CT scan. There are no signs of sinusitis

3. Orbital cellulitis with subperiostal abscess and displacement of the globe which, if severe, may limit

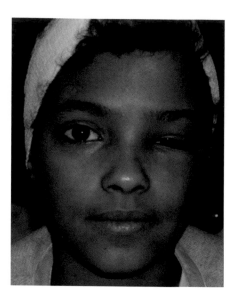

Fig. 35.14 A 10-year-old girl with bilateral pansinusitis and orbital cellulitis, reacting well on intravenous antibiotics (amoxicillin and clavulanic acid). After 4 days she suddenly experienced nausea, vomiting and headache

extra-ocular movement and be associated with visual loss (Figs. 35.15 and 35.16)

4. Orbital cellulitis with intraperiosteal abscess: the displacement of the globe is severe, with obvious limitation of extraocular movement and visual loss due to optic neuropathy in up to 13% of the cases.

5. Cavernous sinus thrombosis: the mortality rate varies from 10 to 27%. The visual deficit may be permanent in 50% of the cases. Sometimes the ophthalmologic and maxillary branches of the trigeminal nerve are involved, leading to hypo-aesthesia and paraesthesia of the cornea, skin and mucosa of the eye. An important sign is the sudden bilateral development of the disease. Spread of the infection can lead to multiple venous thromboses of other dural sinuses. An emergency CT with contrast and MRI venogram is indicated. Organisms are mostly *St. aureus*, *S. pneumoniae* and the aerobic and anaerobic streptococci.

Subperiostal and retrobulbar abscess will lead to a compressive optic neuropathy (Lusk et al. 1992) from pressure on the nerve, its dural sheath and vascular supply. This can be accompanied by a relative pupillary defect or "Marcus Gunn" pupil. This symptom is determined by the "swinging flashlight" test. The compressed nerve fails to transmit the light impulses as readily as the normal nerve, resulting in a small amount of papillary dilatation when the flashlight is moved from the normal eye to the abnormal eye.

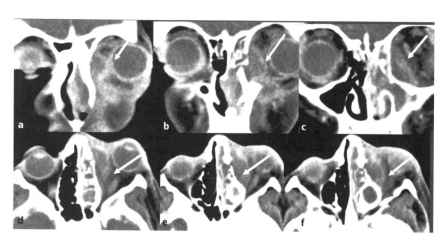

Fig. 35.15a–f CT scans of a 12-year-old child with subperiostal orbital abscess (window settings for soft tissue). **a–c** Coronal scans showing a huge abscess displacing the eyeball (*white arrows*), resulting in an asymmetrical proptosis. **d–f** Axial scans

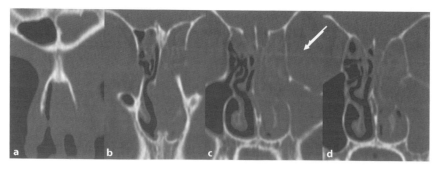

Fig. 35.16a–d Coronal CT-scan of the same patient as shown in Fig. 35.15. Pansinusitis of the left side. The bone window setting does not show the huge abscess very well

Differentiation between orbital cellulitis and subperiostal abscess may be possible on clinical grounds: orbital cellulitis leads to a symmetric proptosis and symmetric limitation of ocular motility. A subperiostal abscess should be suspected when orbital cellulitis progresses rapidly or fails to respond to intravenous antibiotics and there is "asymmetric proptosis", with the eye displaced away from the abscess and asymmetric limitation of eye movements.

However, using clinical signs will lead to a correct staging only in 50% of the cases. CT scanning with MRI improves correct staging to 82%. Moreover, CT scanning is the best technique to differentiate a subperiostal from a retrobulbar abscess (Lusk et al. 1992).

The indications for a CT scan in a patient with an intra-orbital complication are :

1. The patient does not respond to intravenous antibiotics within 24 h.
2. When a subperiostal, periorbital abscess or cavernous sinus thrombosis is suspected, a CT scan is mandatory.
3. An MRI is indicated if frontal cerebritis, abscess or thrombosis of the intracranial sinuses is suspected.

Visual loss accompanied by sinusitis is a rhinologic emergency. Treatment of orbital complications depends on the staging. An orbital cellulitis needs to be treated with intravenous antibiotic therapy. A subset of children with a subperiostal abscess (younger than 5.1 years) with less restriction of ocular mobility can be managed medically. Mostly, however, a subperiostal abscess, periostal abscess and sinus cavernous thrombophlebitis need surgery.

An endoscopic approach allows a good drainage of the sinuses and the orbit. An ethmoidectomy is sometimes sufficient to drain a subperiostal abscess. Applying some pressure on the eyeball will drain the abscess. Often, the lamina orbitalis needs to be removed when drainage is not adequate during the surgery. In cases of a retrobulbar abscess, the periosteum needs to be incised. For intracranial complications, if the condition of the patient allows it, a complete endoscopic spheno-ethmoidectomy is needed, with good drainage of the frontal sinus. Of course the treatment of these complications needs to be discussed and decided in close collaboration with the dental surgeon, ophthalmologist and neurosurgeon.

Mucocoeles

Sometimes (rarely in children) a sinus or a compartment of a sinus can be filled with mucus due to a complete obstruction of the drainage pathway. This will be followed by an increase in pressure of the trapped mucus, resulting in flattening and deformation of the bony structures. The diagnosis is confirmed by CT scan (Figs. 35.17 and 35.18). The treatment consists of endoscopic drainage of the mucocoele. Cystic fibrosis should be excluded.

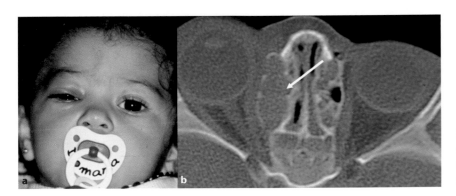

Fig. 35.17a,b A 1-year-old girl with cystic fibrosis. a orbital cellulitis. b axial CT scan shows mucocoele on the same side

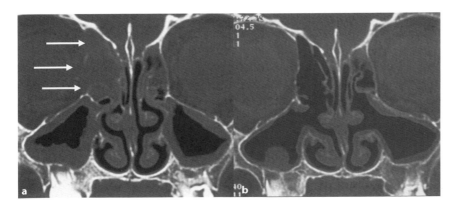

Fig. 35.18a,b A 7-year-old boy with mucocoele of right ethmoid. Pre-operative (a) and post-operative (b) coronal CT scans

Summary for the Clinician

- Paediatric rhinosinusitis is common and often follows a viral URTI with subsequent bacterial infection, usually by commensal organisms. Predisposing factors include immune deficiency, allergy, gastro-oesophageal reflux and pollution. It differs in many respects from the adult form, being more extensive, less eosinophilic (with polyps a rarity seen mainly in cystic fibrosis) and tending to spontaneous resolution. Microbiology and CT scans are rarely indicated, except in severe illness or a toxic child, acute illness in a child not improving with medical therapy within 48-72 hours or an immune-compromised child or in the presence of suppurative (intra-orbital, intracranial) complications. A CT scan may also be considered if surgery is contemplated in a child who has not improved on medical therapy. However, significant underlying disease such as cystic fibrosis, primary ciliary dyskinesia, hypogammaglobulinaemia, allergy and GERD should be excluded first.

- Medical therapy should be tried for children whose rhinosinusitis is interfering with their quality of life. This includes simple measures such as exclusion of tobacco smoke, douching and consideration of topical nasal corticosteroids and antibiotics. Surgery is rarely needed. As an abnormal CT scan is common, this alone is not an indication for operation.

- Rhinosinusitis can spread to local structures such as the eye and brain. Visual loss or nausea and vomiting accompanied by signs of sinusitis are rhinologic emergencies. In a child with an extradural haematoma and no history of head trauma, sinusitis must be excluded.

References

1. American Academy of Pediatrics, Subcommittee of Management of Sinusitis and Committee on Quality Improvement (2001) Clinical practice guideline: management of sinusitis. Pediatrics 108:798–808
2. Anon JB, Rontal M, Zinreich SJ (1996) Anatomy of the Paranasal Sinuses. Part 1. Pre- and Postnatal Morphogenesis of the Nose and Paranasal Sinuses. Thieme, New York, pp 3–11
3. Bagatsch K, Diesel K, Parthenheimer F, et al (1980) Morbiditätsanalyse der unspezifisch-infektbedingten akuten Erkrankungen der Respirationtraktes und der Mittelohrräume des kindesalterns in einen Ballungsgebiet mit modernen Wohnbedingungen. HNO Praxis 5:1–8
4. Barbero GJ (1996) Gastro-esophageal reflux and upper airway disease. Otolaryngol Clin North Am 29:27–38
5. Bolger WE (1994) Gram negative sinusitis: an emergency clinical entity. Am J Rhinol 8:279–283
6. Bothwell MR, Parsons DS, Talbot A, et al (1999) Outcome of reflux therapy in pediatric chronic sinusitis. Otolaryngol Head Neck Surg 121:255–262
7. Brook I (1981) Bacteriologic features of chronic sinusitis in children. JAMA 246:967–969
8. Chan KH, Abzug MJ, Coffinet L, et al (2004) Chronic rhinosinusitis in young children differs from adults: a histopathology study. J Pediatr 144:206–212
9. Clement PAR (1998) Management of sinusitis in infants and young children. In: Schaefer SD (ed) Rhinology and Sinus Disease – a Problem-Oriented Approach. Mosby, St. Louis, pp 105–134
10. Clement PAR, Bluestone CD, Gordts F, et al (1998) Management of rhinosinusitis in children. Consensus meeting, Brussels 1996. Arch Otolaryngol Head and Neck Surg 124:31–34
11. Cools GHE, Clement PAR (1991) The use of a rigid nasal endoscope in children, with special interest in the middle meatus. Acta Otolaryngol Belg 45:399–404
12. Gordts F, Clement PA, Destryker A, et al (1997) Prevalence of sinusitis signs on MRI in a non-ENT paediatric population. J Int Rhinol 35:154–157
13. Gordts F, Abu Nasser I, Clement PAR, et al (1999) Bacteriology of the middle meatus in children. Int J Pediatr Otorhinolaryngol 48:163–167
14. Griffiths SJ, Jatavallabhula NS, Mitchell RD (2002) Spontaneous extradural haematoma associated with craniofacial infections: case report and review of the literature. Br J Neurosurg 16:188–191
15. Hebert RL, Bent JP (1998) Meta-analysis of outcomes of pediatric functional endoscopic sinus surgery. Laryngoscope 108:796–799
16. Herrmann BW, Chung J, Eisenbeis JF, Forsen JW Jr, (2006) Intracranial complications of pediatric frontal rhinosinusitis. Am J Rhinol 20:320–324
17. Iwens P, Clement PAR (1994) Sinusitis in allergic patients. Rhinology 32:65–67
18. Kristo A, Uhari LM, Luotonen J, et al (2003) Paranasal sinus findings in children during respiratory infection evaluation with negative resonance imaging. Pediatrics 111:586–589
19. Lund VJ (1998) Inferior meatal antrostomy. Fundamental considerations of design and function. J Laryngol Otol Suppl 10:1–18
20. Lusk RP, Lazar R, Muntz HR (1989) The diagnosis and treatment of recurrent and chronic sinusitis in children. Pediatr Clin 36:1411–1421
21. Lusk RP, Muntz HR (1990) Endoscopic sinus surgery in children with chronic sinusitis: a pilot study. Laryngoscope 100: 654–658
22. Lusk RP, Tychsen L, Park TS (1992) Complications of sinusitis. In: Lusk RP (ed) Pediatric Sinusitis. Raven, New York, pp 127–146

23. Maresh MM, Washburn AH (1940) Paranasal sinuses from birth to late adolescence. Clinical and roentgengraphic evidence of infection. Am J Dis Child 60:841–861

24. McLeod DT (1995) Moraxella catarrhalis: its importance as a respiratory pathologic agent. Spectrum 38:1–4

25. Nord CE (1988) Efficacy of penicillin treatment in purulent maxillary sinusitis. A European multicentre trial. Infection 16:209–214

26. Orobello PW, Park RI, Belcher LJ, et al (1991) Microbiology of chronic sinusitis in children. Arch Otolaryngol Head Neck Surg 117:980–983

27. Otten FWA, Grote JJ (1988) Treatment of chronic maxillary sinusitis in children. Int J Pediatr Otorhinolaryngol 15:269–278

28. Overturf GD (2002) Pneumococcal vaccination in children. Semin Pediatr Infect Dis 13:155–164

29. Oxelius VA (1979) IgG subclass levels in infancy and childhood. Acta Pediatr Scand 68:23–27

30. Pabst HF, Kreth HW (1980) Ontogeny of the immune response as a basis of childhood disease. J Pediatr 97:519–534

31. Polmar SH (1992) Sinusitis and immune deficiency. In: Lusk RP (ed) Pediatric Sinusitis. Raven, New York, pp 53–58

32. Sanders LA, Rijkers GT, Tenbergen-Meekes AM, et al (1995) Immuno-globulin isotype-specific antibody responses to pneumococcal polysaccharide vaccine in a patient with recurrent bacterial respirator tract infections. Pediatr Res 37:812–819

33. Scadding GK (2003) Recent advances in the treatment of rhinitis and rhinosinusitis. Int J Pediatr Otorhinolaryngol 67:S201–S204

34. Van Buchem FL, Peeters MF, Knotnerus JA (1992) Maxillary sinusitis in children. Clin Otolaryngol 17:49–53

35. Van Der Veken PJ, Clement PAR, Buisseret TH, et al (1992) Age-related CT scan study of the incidence of sinusitis in children. Am J Rhinol 6:45–48

36. Wald ER (2003) Rhinitis and acute and chronic sinusitis. In: Bluestone CD, Stool SE, Alper CM (eds) Pediatric Otolaryngology, 4th edn. Saunders, Philadelphia, pp 995–1012

37. Westrin KM (1994) Pathogenesis of pediatric sinusitis. Am J Rhinol 8:291–292

38. Zacharison M, Casper R (2005) Pediatric sinusitis. Immunol Allergy Clin North Am 25:313–332

Chapter 36

Management of the Deaf Child

Kevin Patrick Gibbin

Core Messages

- Hearing impairment is the most prevalent congenital sensory deficit in the human population, with at least 1 in every 842 babies born in the UK with a permanent hearing loss or deafness detectable at birth.
- Otitis media with effusion (OME) is the single commonest cause of hearing loss in childhood; the presence of sensorineural deafness does not preclude the presence of OME and vice versa.
- Thirty percent of children with a severe to profound sensorineural hearing loss have other significant disabilities.
- Bacterial meningitis is the commonest cause of acquired, severe to profound sensorineural deafness in childhood.
- Auditory neuropathy and central auditory processing disorders are complex, hearing-related problems that should be considered.
- Risk factors for permanent childhood hearing impairment include: low birth weight, prematurity and associated prolonged admission to neonatal intensive care, positive family history of hearing impairment in childhood, and craniofacial anomalies.
- Universal neonatal screening should be the aim, with early diagnosis of hearing loss and early provision of hearing aids; significantly better language is achieved if children are aided before the age of 6 months.
- The team required to manage children with permanent hearing loss should be inclusive, including parents/carers, paediatric otologist and audiologist, paediatric physician, paediatric ophthalmologist, clinical geneticist, and teacher of the deaf.
- Voluntary groups, both local and national, provide great support to the families of deaf children.

Contents

Introduction

Management of any child with a hearing loss will depend on several factors including the age at which the child presents, the cause of the hearing loss and its degree. The most common cause of deafness in childhood, otitis media with effusion (OME), is the subject of a separate chapter and will not be referred to further in this chapter other than in the context of OME being superimposed on a sensorineural hearing loss. It is fundamental that the paediatric otologist involve other agencies, both medical and non-medical, in the management of patients in his or her care; these will include the paediatric audiologist, teacher of the deaf, geneticist, general medical paediatrician and developmental paediatrician. Large numbers of children with congenital deafness may also have visual difficulties and the paediatric ophthalmologist will also be a part of the team managing such children, partly to exclude visual problems, but also to manage those discovered. Some children with complex hearing disorders such as auditory neuropathy (auditory dysynchrony) or central auditory processing disorders (APD) may also need the involvement of the paediatric neurologist.

The impact of permanent childhood hearing impairment can be devastating; congenital hearing loss may lead to poor development of spoken language and this in turn can lead to poor literacy skills, poor educational achievement and subsequent poor income and socio-economic status.

In the UK there are about 20,000 children under 16 years of age who are moderately to profoundly deaf; about 12,000 of these were born deaf. An estimated 840 children are born in the every year in the UK with moderate to profound deafness.

Deafness in childhood may present in a variety of ways. It is to be hoped that all cases of congenital deafness will be detected at birth with the introduction of the Universal Neonatal Hearing Screening. Wales, Scotland and Northern Ireland are already screening all newborn children and it is anticipated that all newborns in England will be screened by 2006. All four countries have different protocols for screening. Information on neonatal hearing screening may be obtained from the website www.nhsp.info, which also has a separate area for parents, www.nhsp.info/nhsphomeparent.php

The paediatric otologist carries responsibility for all aspects of managing children with deafness, including investigating and diagnosing the cause of the loss as well as its treatment. The logistics of managing children with deafness depend on many factors including the age of the child at presentation or suspicion of the hearing loss, the degree of the deafness, the likely nature of the cause or aetiology of the loss, social and developmental background and whether there is any other concomitant or related pathology. The management of a baby with a profound congenital hearing loss, for example, will differ considerably from the management of an older child with deafness due to OME.

The role of the parents or carers is, of course, crucial in the management of the deaf child, and how the otologist approaches the parents with the diagnosis of their child's deafness may influence subsequent dealings; it is imperative to present a positive view of the child's hearing loss stressing what the child can hear as well as indicating what difficulties in hearing the child may have. It is fundamental in the management of the child to acknowledge the uncertainties parents may face at the time of diagnosis, having to adjust to the sudden change in their lives. The psychological impact of childhood hearing impairment should not be overlooked; the initial reaction of most parents to the diagnosis of deafness is one of denial, with a subsequent process of grieving. There may be other issues to address as the child grows up.

It is also important to stress the need for recognition of the child's other developmental needs, the parent/child relationship and the other medical and developmental problems the child may have; 30% of children with a severe to profound sensorineural hearing loss have other significant disabilities.

Cochlear implants have revolutionised both the approach to and management of the child with a profound hearing loss, but have also raised ethical issues, acknowledging that some deaf children may be born into deaf families. The parents of these children may not recognise deafness as a disability requiring treatment and may opt for a signing approach to the development of communication skills for their child. Such children may still require otological support and it remains important that the paediatric otologist should engage with the families. The learning of signing does not preclude later cochlear implantation, and children who develop visual language are able to benefit from this modality of learning and use it to facilitate development of spoken language.

The role of the voluntary sector should not be overlooked, organisations such as the National Deaf Children's Society (NDCS; www.ndcs.org.uk) and the Royal National Institute for the Deaf (www.rnid.org.uk). The NDCS has produced a series of quality standards for the provision of paediatric audiology services and for cochlear implantation.

Aetiology and Pathology of Childhood Deafness

Deafness may be conductive or sensorineural or mixed; the most likely aetiology in individual cases is often dependent on the age of the child. Reference has already been made to the commonest cause of hearing loss in childhood, chronic non-infective middle ear disease, OME; it should be noted, however, that a diagnosis of OME does not preclude the presence of sensorineural deafness, nor the converse. This chapter will not cover issues related to OME, nor to causes of middle ear deafness other than syndromal ones.

Deafness in childhood may also be classified according to the timing of its onset in relation to birth: pre-natal, perinatal and post-natal. This may influence diagnostic and management strategies.

Pre-natal Causes

Pre-natal causes of deafness include genetic, syndromal and non-syndromal causes. Syndromic causes of deafness are covered in Chapter 8, noting that some syndromes may have a genetic basis. It should also be noted that syndromes affecting the ear may produce either a conductive or a sensorineural loss, or possibly both. Other causes include intrauterine infections such as cytomegalovirus (CMV), toxoplasmosis and rubella, intrauterine exposure to ototoxic and teratogenic agents (e.g. thalidomide) and other developmental anomalies.

Perinatal Causes

Perinatal causes include prematurity, low birth weight, hypoxia and jaundice.

Post-natal Causes

Post-natal acquired causes of deafness are many and varied and may cause either sensorineural deafness or conductive losses or both, again noting that the single commonest cause of deafness in childhood is OME. Postnatal causes of deafness include:

1. Bacterial meningitis: this is the commonest cause of acquired severe to profound sensorineural deafness in childhood (Martin 1982; Davis and Wood 1992; Fortnum and Davis 1997).
2. Infections – most commonly middle ear – acute and chronic otitis media, but also including CMV, with deafness the commonest sequela.
3. Complications of otitis media and OME
4. Viral labyrinthitis including measles and mumps
5. Immunisation
6. Genetic causes: examples of acquired sensorineural deafness in association with genetic abnormalities include Pendred's syndrome, which may be associated with large vestibular aqueduct

Progressive hearing loss may be a result of various factors including genetic ones, and mention has already been made of LVAS and its associated genetic conditions. Usher syndrome type III is also associated with progressive sensorineural deafness.

As well as presenting at birth sensorineural deafness due to CMV may also produce either delayed-onset deafness, or a fluctuating or progressive loss of hearing. CMV is the commonest intrauterine infection, affecting 0.2–2% of all live births, with sensorineural deafness as its commonest sequela. Ten percent of cases are overtly symptomatic at birth, approximately half going on to develop deafness, with bilateral severe or profound loss as the most likely outcome in those children who are symptomatic Any audiometric pattern of hearing loss may be seen and it has been suggested (Barbi 2003) that up to 30% of all childhood sensorineural hearing loss is due to CMV. The onset of deafness is delayed in about 40–50% of cases. There is a useful CMV Association website: http://mysite.freeserve.com/CMVsupport.

More recently, interest has developed regarding the effects on the development of the child of unilateral hearing loss, and a randomised controlled trial is currently being undertaken on providing amplification for these children. Hitherto it was felt that as long as a child has one ear with normal hearing there may be little need for concern provided that parents, carers and particularly teachers are aware of the deafness and use appropriate strategies. Similarly, the effect of more mild losses is now being studied and the results are awaited with interest.

Auditory neuropathy or auditory dysynchrony is a condition that has come to attention in recent years. First described by Worthington and Peters (1980), it is a complex condition in which there is evidence of cochlear outer hair cell function, demonstrated by the presence of either evoked otoacoustic emissions or cochlear microphonics. The characteristic finding is an absent or severely abnormal brainstem evoked potential that does not correspond to the patient's behavioural audiometric threshold. Patients with this condition have poor speech discrimination scores relative to their audiometric status. More detailed information may be obtained from Sininger and Starr (2001). Its aetiology is complex and includes anoxia, hyperbilirubinaemia, infections such as mumps, immune disorders such as Guillain-Barré syndrome and several genetic or syndromal conditions. The latter groups include Freidreich's ataxia, Charcot-Marie-Tooth syndrome and Stevens-Johnson syndrome, among others.

Another important group of conditions recently receiving attention is central Auditory Processing Disorder (APD) (Bamiou et al. 2001). In essence, children with APD appear to be uncertain about what they hear, in particular while listening to speech in background noise; they may be unable to understand rapid or degraded speech. The problems may also be associated with other global deficits such as memory disorders or attention deficit disorders. There may be problems with language, reading and spelling as well as difficulty in following oral instructions. Few cases of APD have an underlying neurological deficit, however they may be the occasional manifestation of a neurological problem, emphasising the need for full evaluation. Neurological conditions may include tumours, prematurity and low birth weight, meningitis, Lyme disease, head injury, metabolic disorders and cerebrovascular disorders. There may be some diagnostic overlap with attention deficit disorders, dyslexia and specific language impairment. In some children with learning disability, there may also be a central APD.

Epidemiology

Hearing impairment is the most prevalent congenital sensory deficit in the human population, with at least 1 in every 842 babies born in the UK with a permanent hearing loss or deafness detectable at birth (Davis 1993). Various statistics are quoted for prevalence rates of permanent childhood hearing impairment, most commonly in the region of 1–1.2 per 1000 live births with a hearing loss of at least 40 dB in the better ear. (See Davis et al. in McCormick 2004).

Fortnum and colleagues undertook a questionnaire based ascertainment study (Fortnum et al. 2001) of 26,000 notifications and identified deafness in (ascertained) 17,160 individual children. Prevalence rose from 0.91 (95% confidence interval, 95%CI, 0.85–0.98) for 3-year-olds to 1.65 (95%CI 1.62–1.68) for children aged 9–16 years. Adjustment for underascertainment increased estimates to 1.07 (95%CI 1.03–1.12) and 2.05 (95%CI 2.02–2.08). Comparison with previous studies showed that prevalence increases with age to a level higher than previously estimated.

Risk Factors for Hearing Loss in Children

Several risk factors for the presence of sensorineural hearing loss in children exists, and in the past these have contributed to the development of targeted neonatal hearing screening, and indeed screening later in childhood. The American Academy of Audiology Joint Committee on Infant Hearing (JCIH) has identified several risk factors, published initially in 1994, modified in 2000 (www.audiology.org), based on infants from birth to 28 days and those from 29 days to 2 years (see Tables 36.1 and 36.2). The JCIH also noted the risk of auditory neuropathy and other similar conditions.

Davis et al. (in McCormick 2004) concluded that the three major risk factors for hearing loss identifiable at or around birth are (1) admission to a neonatal intensive care unit for 48 h or longer, (2) positive family history of hearing impairment arising in childhood and (3) craniofacial abnormality. These factors may be cross-referenced to the pre- and perinatal causes of hearing loss already identified in this chapter. Individual elements can be identified, the major ones associated with low or very low birth weight. Sutton and Rowe (1997) have demonstrated that birth weight below 2500 g gave a raised risk with an odds ratio of 4.5, rising to 9.6 for weight below 1500 g. It should also be stressed that low birth weight is also commonly associated with other significant disability, a factor highlighted by Power and Li (2000) and Davis and Wood (1992), noting the presence of substantial other problems in 35% of children with hearing loss and 70% in those requiring neonatal intensive care; they also noted the 10-fold risk of hearing loss in graduates of neonatal intensive care units.

Identification of Hearing Loss

Screening – Targeted versus Universal

From the above discussion it may be argued that targeted screening will detect the majority of cases of permanent childhood hearing impairment. It remains the case, however, that the average age of diagnosis of hearing loss in infants and young children remains high both in the UK, with a mean age of prescription for aids of 40.1 months for a child with a loss of between 40 and 69 dB (Fortnum and Davis 1997), and in the USA, where the quoted average of diagnosis was 30 months (JCIH 2000). In light of studies published from Colorado (Yoshinago-Itano et al. 1998), it may be argued very readily that all children should be screened at birth, a position adopted by the JCIH and many others including Davis et al. (1997) in their report to the Department of Health of the UK Government. Universal hearing screening of newborns is now well established in the UK.

Current protocols for hearing screening centre on two main technologies, testing for otoacoustic emissions and

Table 36.1 Joint Committee on Infant Hearing (JCIH) risk factors: birth to 28 days

Family history of hereditary childhood sensorineural hearing loss
In utero infection
Craniofacial anomalies
Birth weight less than 1500 g
Hyperbilirubinaemia requiring exchange transfusion
Ototoxic drugs
Bacterial meningitis
Apgar scores 0–4 at 1 min; 0–6 at 5 min
Ventilation required for 5 days or more
Stigmata of a known syndrome associated with hearing loss

Table 36.2 JCIH risk factors: 29 days to 2 years. *OME* Otitis media with effusion

Parental concern regarding hearing, speech, language or developmental delay
Bacterial meningitis or other infection causing hearing loss
Head trauma with loss of consciousness or skull fracture
Stigmata of a known syndrome associated with hearing loss
Ototoxic drugs
Recurrent or persistent OME for at least 3 months

use of electric response audiometry, either separately or in combination. It is not the purpose of this chapter to discuss this further.

Early Childhood/Pre-school Programmes

It should be noted that the prevalence of permanent hearing loss increases with age (Fortnum et al. 2001), but also that middle-ear pathology accounts for the majority of cases of hearing loss in young children. Programmes therefore also need to be in place to detect these losses, and most children undergo further hearing screening on school entry.

Monitoring of Special Groups

Children with Down's syndrome typically demonstrate hearing loss due to OME, but may also have a sensorineural loss; in many centres these children are kept under active review by Paediatric departments, which liaise with local Otology/Audiology departments to ensure that any hearing loss is detected early.

Children with cleft palate are almost universally at risk of OME, and following the Clinical Standards Advisory Group (CSAG) report into the management of cleft lip and palate in the UK, almost all cleft units have a consultant otologist as a member of the team (see Chapter 16).

Post-Meningitis Screening

Meningitis remains a devastating disease and it is imperative that all children who recover should have their hearing assessed as soon as possible. One of the major concerns with hearing loss post-meningitis is that cochlear ossification may occur and impede surgical cochlear implantation; once the presence of deafness is established, recovery of hearing is rare (McCormick et al. 1993).

Reactive Testing

It remains axiomatic that if there is ever any doubt about a child's hearing, it should be assessed formally. Parents and carers including nursery and school teachers may raise such concerns; all should be heeded. Language delay, poor performance in school and general parental concerns should lead to audiometry to exclude hearing loss as a contributing factor.

Investigation

Clinical History Taking

A most important element in the diagnosis of the cause of deafness in any child with a demonstrated hearing loss is the history, although clearly other investigations may also prove highly important. The history should be targeted to three key areas, pre-natal including family history, perinatal and post-natal.

Family History

Clearly, a family history may be of great significance, but more especially a history of consanguinity should be sought, particularly in those of Asian extraction where this is more common.

Pre-Natal History

Pre-natal history should include whether the mother was exposed during pregnancy to any viral illness, particularly rubella, and whether there was a history of drug exposure, especially in the first trimester. Similarly, history of ABO compatibility and Rhesus disease should be established. Maternal endocrine disorders such as diabetes and hypothyroidism are other factors to be sought.

Perinatal History

As already noted, low birth weight, prematurity and need for neonatal intensive care are perhaps the single most important risk factors for deafness in any neonate or newly diagnosed young child with deafness. Other factors to be established include perinatal hypoxia, respiratory distress syndrome, hyperbilirubinaemia, sepsis and exposure to ototoxic drugs.

Post-Natal History

The single most important cause of post-natally acquired hearing loss in childhood is meningitis, almost exclusively bacterial. It should, however, be remembered that CMV and some congenital anomalies and genetic conditions can also be associated with either a progressive, fluctuating or sudden sensorineural hearing loss. Exposure to ototoxic medication should be inquired after, particularly to cytotoxic drugs used in childhood cancers, and also to aminoglycoside antibiotics. In the latter context, it should also be noted that there may be a genetic basis for the hearing loss as a result of maternal mitochondrial transmission; this is as a result of A15555G mitochondrial mutation.

Viral illness in childhood is rarely a cause of acquired hearing loss. In the past, mumps has been thought to be a likely cause of unilateral sensorineural deafness detected in children aged 3–6 years; however, in many cases there had been no audiometry to confirm previously normal hearing. Most of such cases are now considered more likely to have been congenital. Reports also exist of exposure to vaccines that have resulted in deafness.

There are many other factors that can result in acquired hearing loss and these are not particularly different from those in the adult population; they including trauma, noting also the relationship of the latter to possible enlarged vestibular aqueduct syndrome, in turn possibly linked to either Pendred's syndrome or BORS.

It is also important to establish a history of general developmental progress, including such factors of when the child started to talk and walk. The history of the development of spoken language is extremely important and may indicate whether the diagnosis of deafness in an older child represents a delayed diagnosis, or whether the

36

hearing loss is of delayed onset. Inquiry about walking may raise suspicion about balance disorders and hence a possible diagnosis of Usher syndrome.

Clinical Examination

A full clinical examination is essential, although the majority of children with congenital or acquired sensorineural hearing loss will show no related clinical abnormality. However, it should also be remembered that syndromic hearing loss may occur in up to 30% (Reardon 1992; Parving 1996) and the diagnosis may be suspected or even established as a result of full examination.

Clearly, otological examination is fundamental. Most congenital anomalies of the external ears will be apparent; middle ear anomalies may remain undiagnosed pending imaging and a formal tympanotomy, and of course anomalies of the inner ear will only be shown by diagnostic imaging (see Chapter 40). Other conditions that will be apparent from examination include the presence of craniofacial anomalies, pre-auricular pits and sinuses and branchial pits. Ocular abnormalities should be sought and an ophthalmological opinion should always be obtained, as 40–60% of deaf children have ophthalmic problems (Nikolopoulos et al. 2006), and this may have a major impact on the child's development of communication skills. Some causes of deafness such as CMV, rubella, Toxoplasmosis and many others may have associated ophthalmological disorders; Usher syndrome is a very important condition to diagnose due to concern over dual sensory deprivation. Examination of the eyes may lead directly to a diagnosis of Waardenburg's syndrome, with its characteristic dystopia canthorum/telecanthus and heterochromia iridis; in these cases, ophthalmological examination may also demonstrate heterochromia of the fundus. There are many other syndromes where ophthalmological examination may contribute to the diagnosis. These are listed in Nikolopoulos et al. (2006).

Special Investigations

These may be grouped into several different areas of further audiological investigation including objective testing of hearing, discussed below.

Haematology

TORCH (*Toxoplasma gondii*, other viruses, rubella, CMV and herpes simplex) screening is arguably the main blood test to be undertaken in a newly diagnosed neonate, screening for the presence of antibodies to toxoplasmosis, syphilis, rubella, CMV and *Herpesvirus hominis*. Maternal serology may also be important seeking raised

IgM to CMV in such cases. Although involving a disorder of thyroid metabolism, thyroid function studies are probably not helpful in establishing the diagnosis of Pendred's syndrome and the recommended perchlorate discharge test is rarely used. In older children with a fluctuating, sudden or progressive sensorineural loss, evidence of auto-immune disorders should be sought.

Disorders such as Alport's syndrome and BORS are associated with renal impairment and therefore both blood and urine examination should be undertaken, the latter looking for evidence of haematuria.

Electrocardiography

An extremely important test, necessary in all otherwise undiagnosed children with sensorineural hearing loss, is electrocardiography (ECG) to confirm the presence or otherwise of a prolonged Q–T interval, the cardiological feature of Jervell-Lange-Neilsen syndrome, an autosomal recessive disorder. It is particularly important, as many of these children with a profound hearing loss will submit to several general anaesthetics as part of their assessment for possible cochlear implantation. The cardiac abnormality is associated with syncope and sudden death. There may of course be other indications for ECG, including its use in children with rubella deafness, CMV, toxoplasmosis and velocardiofacial syndrome, among others.

Imaging

The use of radiological imaging, either computerised tomography or magnetic resonance imaging, in newly diagnosed neonates remains a debatable issue. Imaging remains a fundamental component of the work-up for possible cochlear implantation and there are several conditions when its use is diagnostic, including those associated with LVAS. Rarely will it alter early management, although the finding of abnormalities may subsequently guide the clinician and the geneticist towards the diagnosis. The essential role of urgent early imaging after meningitis, however, is dealt with below.

Other imaging includes possible renal ultrasound or scanning in cases of possible Alport's syndrome and BORS.

Medical Assessment

A formal general paediatric medical assessment is essential in all children newly diagnosed with sensorineural deafness, especially those diagnosed on neonatal screening, both in order to exclude systemic illness and to provide information towards the diagnosis. As already noted, up to 30% of children with severe to profound sensorineural hearing loss may have other significant developmental disability and will require the ongoing support of the paediatric physician.

Genetic disorders constitute a large percentage of the causes of otherwise unexplained sensorineural deafness in children; Parker et al. (2000) state that the majority of genetic hearing impairment is inherited in a recessive autosomal manner.

From the above, it is clear that a clinical geneticist is a member of the team managing any child with a newly diagnosed sensorineural hearing impairment, and may also be needed in some cases of conductive hearing loss in children. Of course the geneticist may not be required if the cause of the loss has already been diagnosed as a non-genetic one. Genetic and chromosomal studies will be undertaken by the geneticist and this is discussed in Chapter 7.

Bamiou et al. (2000) have provided a good review of the investigation of hearing loss in childhood.

Audiological Assessment

This is discussed in Chapter 37; also refer to McCormick (2004).

Treatment of Children with Hearing Loss

The single most important element in the treatment of any child with a hearing loss is clear, unambiguous and sensitive communication with the parents or carers; what is said during early contacts with them may colour relationships for long periods and it is essential that the professionals include the family, both immediate and extended, in the team caring for the child. This is particularly important in those cases where the loss has been diagnosed on the basis of hearing screening, especially in the neonatal period. The support for parents may take many forms including provision of relevant literature; that provided by the UK Neonatal Hearing Screening Programme is comprehensive, if voluminous, and it is the author's practice to ensure that it is provided to the parents in stages.

Local and national support groups play an essential and valued role in helping parents and may be accessed *inter alia* via the National Deaf Children's Society; information on this should be provided routinely to parents.

A major source of support for the child and family is that provided by the local Teacher of the Deaf Service, and the presence of a teacher of the deaf at initial consultations provides a clear link and ensures that common standards and objectives are agreed.

The aim of any treatment programme for deaf children is to ensure that appropriate and early (re)habilitation is provided (Yoshinago-Itano 1998). This will vary depending on the age of the child and the degree and nature of the loss; in almost all children with permanent loss this will include provision of appropriate, typically post-aural, hearing aid or aids. Such aids will be inappropriate, for example, if the cause of the loss is major developmental anomaly of the outer and middle ear; other methods involving the use of bone-conduction aids will be more relevant and, when the child is older, possibly bone-anchored hearing aids, to be addressed in Chapter 44.

Some children with conductive deafness may also benefit from the provision of hearing aids, and it is the author's practice to prescribe hearing aids for children with Down syndrome rather than recommend surgery for their OME.

As already discussed, the presence of sensorineural hearing loss does not preclude the development of OME and it is important that the otologist and others on the team remain alert to this possibility. It is the view of the author that it should be treated promptly as the additional handicap of an extra 30 dB deafness can be devastating to the child.

One other potential major benefit of early diagnosis of hearing loss is early referral for cochlear implantation, where relevant. Cochlear implantation has transformed the management and potential of children with the more severe and profound degrees of sensorineural deafness. Comparison may be made with early provision of hearing aids in considering early implantation. It remains important to give a child an adequate trial of acoustic hearing aids, but it is becoming increasingly apparent that implantation should ideally take place well before a congenitally deaf child's second birthday: this will be considered in Chapter 45, which deals with cochlear implants. Early implantation remains the ideal in those cases of deafness following meningitis, especially if there is any radiological evidence of osteoneogenesis.

Regular audiometry is required for all children with hearing loss to detect OME and also any possible progression of the loss, likely in conditions associated with enlarged vestibular aqueduct such as Pendred's and BORS.

Children with unilateral sensorineural or conductive deafness present their own special needs and it is important that parents and others are made aware of the implications of such losses, stressing the risks of lack of sound localisation as a general risk. The needs of the child in the classroom must also be clearly presented and advice about appropriate seating position in the classroom should be given. Suitable literature may be given to the parents and teachers stressing these points

36

Summary for the Clinician

- Deafness presents the single most prevalent sensory disability in childhood, with at least 1 in every 842 babies born with a permanent hearing loss detectable at birth. The management of the child will depend on a variety of factors, including the age at presentation/diagnosis, the cause and degree of the loss and any other associated disability. Thirty percent of children with severe to profound permanent hearing impairment will have other significant disability, and up to 60% may have ophthalmological problems, either as part of the cause of their hearing loss or due to refractive errors or other eye disease.

- Genetic factors account for a large percentage of causes of permanent childhood hearing impairment and may be syndromal or non-syndromal; the majority of genetic hearing impairment is inherited in an autosomal recessive manner. Deafness syndromes may include association with almost all other systems in the body.

- Low birth weight and prematurity with their associated conditions, and the need for neonatal intensive care present significant risk factors for congenital sensorineural deafness, birth weight below 2500 g carrying an odds ratio of 4.5, weight below 1500 g an odds ratio of 9.6. There is a tenfold risk of hearing loss in babies requiring neonatal intensive care. Other significant risk factors include the presence of craniofacial anomalies.

- Universal neonatal hearing screening should be the objective, as it has been well demonstrated that providing hearing aids to a child before the age of 6 months significantly improves the development of both receptive and expressive language.

- Bacterial meningitis is the commonest cause of acquired severe to profound sensorineural deafness in childhood. OME is the commonest cause of hearing loss in childhood. The presence of OME does not preclude the diagnosis of sensorineural deafness and vice versa.

- It is important that the team managing a child with permanent hearing impairment is inclusive and should recognise the intrinsic role and importance of the parents/carers as well as developmental and general paediatric needs, genetic causes of the loss, visual needs, educational needs of the child and many other factors. The otologist managing the child plays a fundamental role.

References

1. Bamiou DE, Macardle B, Bitner-Glindzicz M, et al T (2000) Aetiological investigation of hearing loss in childhood: a review. Clin Otolaryngol Allied Sci 25:98–106
2. Bamiou D, Musiek FE, Luxton LM (2001) Aetiology and clinical presentations of auditory presentation disorder – a review. Arch Dis Child 85:361–365
3. Barbi M (2003) A wider role for congenital cytomegalovirus infection in sensorineural hearing loss. J Paediatr Infect Dis 22:39–42
4. Chen A, Francis M, Ni L, Cremers CW, et al (1995) Phenotypic manifestations of branchio-oto-renal syndrome. Am J Med Genet 58:365–370
5. Cremers CWRJ, Bolder C, Admiraal RJC, et al (1998) Progressive sensorineural hearing loss and a widened vestibular aqueduct in Pendred syndrome. Arch Otolaryngol 124:501–505
6. Davis A (1993) The prevalence of deafness. In: Ballantyne J, Martin A, Martin M (eds) Deafness. Whurr, London, pp 1–11
7. Davis AC, Bamford J, Wilson I, et al (1997) A critical review of the role of neo-natal screening in the detection of congenital hearing impairment. Health Technol Assess 1:1–177
8. Davis A, Wood S (1992) The epidemiology of childhood hearing impairment: factors relevant to planning services. Br J Audiol 26:77–90
9. Davis A, Mencher G, Moorjani P (2004) An epidemiological perspective on childhood hearing impairment. In: McCormick B (ed) Paediatric Audiology 0–5 Years, 3rd edn. Whurr, London, pp 1–41
10. Fahy CP, Carney AS, Nikolopoulos KP, et al (2001) Cochlear implantation in children with large vestibular aqueduct syndrome and a review of the syndrome. Int J Pediatr Otolaryngol 59:207–215
11. Fortnum H, Davis A (1997) Epidemiology of permanent childhood hearing impairment in Trent Region, 1985–1993. Br J Audiol 31:409–446
12. Fortnum HM, Summerfield A Q, Marshall DH, et al (2001) Prevalence of permanent childhood hearing impairment in the United Kingdom and implications for universal neonatal hearing screening: questionnaire based ascertainment study BMJ 323:536–539
13. Jackler RK, De La Cruz A (1989) The large vestibular aqueduct syndrome. Laryngoscope 99:1238–1242
14. Joint Committee on Infant Hearing High Risk Register for Identification of Hearing Impairment (2000) Principles and Guidelines for Early Intervention Programs: Year 2000 Position Statement. www.audiology.org
15. McCormick B (ed) (2004) Paediatric Audiology 0–5 Years, 3rd edn. Whurr, London
16. McCormick B, Gibbin KP, Lutman ME, et al (1993) Late partial recovery from meningitic deafness after cochlear implantation; a case study. Am J Otol 14:610–612

17. Martin JAM (1982) Aetiological factors relating to childhood deafness in the European Community. Audiology 21:149–158

18. Nikolopoulos TP, Lioumi D, Stamataki S, et al (2006) Evidence-based overview of ophthalmic disorders in deaf children: a literature update. Otol Neurol 27:S1–S24

19. Parker MJ, Fortnum HJ, Young ID, et al(2000) Population-based genetic study of childhood hearing impairment in the Trent region of the United Kingdom. Audiology 39:226–231

20. Parving A (1996) Epidemiology of genetic hearing impairment. In: Martini A, Read A, Stephens D (eds) Genetics and Hearing Impairment. Whurr, London, pp 73–81

21. Power C, Li L (2000) Cohort study of birthweight, mortality and disability. BMJ 320:840–841

22. Reardon W (1992) Genetic deafness. J Med Genet 29:521–526

23. Sininger Y, Starr A (eds) (2001) Auditory Neuropathy. A New Perspective on Hearing Disorders. Singular, San Diego, California, USA

24. Sutton GJ, Rowe SJ (1997) Risk factors for childhood sensorineural hearing loss in the Oxford Region. Br J Audiol 31:39–54

25. Worthington DW, Peters J (1980) Quantifiable hearing and no ABR: paradox or error? Ear Hear 1:281–285

26. Yoshinago-Itano C, Sedey AL, Coulter DK, et al (1998) Language of early- and later-identified children with hearing loss. Pediatrics 102:1161–1171

Chapter 37

Audiometric Testing of Children

John Graham, Milanka Drenovak and William Hellier

Core Messages

- Universal screening using transient otoacoustic emission (TOAE) testing is now widely performed in neonates to identify those with a potential hearing loss, allowing early management of deafness.
- TOAE testing assesses cochlear outer hair cell function and can be used in all age groups for this purpose. It is an objective test and has a high sensitivity but relatively low specificity. Test failure requires further alternative investigation. It cannot identify retrocochlear causes of hearing loss.
- Auditory brainstem response testing assesses the auditory pathway from cochlea to cortex and can accurately predict the hearing threshold. It is an objective measurement and has a high sensitivity and specificity. It can be used to test anatomically normal and abnormal ears, and can be used in children with cochlear implants, but requires experience to identify the waveforms and has limited frequency specificity. It is a very useful tool in the further investigation of potential deafness in infants and children.
- Audiometric steady-state response testing investigates the brainstem response to auditory stimuli. It is a more recent development and requires further validation, but may offer rapid, accurate, frequency-specific assessment of hearing thresholds under a variety of test conditions.

- Tympanometry is a reliable objective test for examining the middle ear pressure in children. It can accurately predict the presence of a middle ear effusion or Eustachian tube dysfunction.
- Behavioural testing allows assessment of the entire auditory pathway and the cortical response to sound. Distraction testing from 6 to 18 months, and visual reinforcement audiometry from 6 months to 3 years tests a child's active head-turning response to noise. Behavioural testing is frequency specific and can be performed in the community, but requires the participation of the child, which may not be possible for medical or developmental reasons.
- Conditioned and speech audiometry are used to test children from the ages of 2–3 years. Play audiometry can accurately assess frequency-specific thresholds with appropriate conditioning. Verbal discrimination testing, such as the McCormick test, investigates recognition of speech. Both require a certain level of development and cooperation and may not be possible in children with neurological problems or learning difficulties.

Contents

Introduction

The assessment of hearing in children requires several different testing techniques to be available. The choice of test will depend upon the age of the child, his or her medical state and whether an objective or behavioural investigation is needed.

This chapter will describe briefly the range of hearing tests currently in use for children. The tests will be arranged according to the age at which they are used. The benefits and limitations of each test will be noted and the main usefulness of each test summarised. The tests to be described are shown in Fig. 37.1.

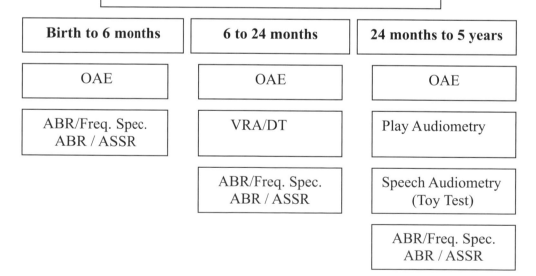

Fig. 37.1 The audiometric tests commonly performed on children of different ages. Note that these refer to children of normal developmental age. The tests will need to be modified in cases of developmental delay. *OAE* Otoacoustic emissions, *ABR* auditory brain response, *ASSR auditory steady-state response, VRA visual reinforcement audiometry, DT distraction test*

Neonatal Tests Used From Soon After Birth Until Six Months

Universal neonatal screening of hearing is now in use or is being introduced in most developed countries. This involves transient otoacoustic emission testing (TOAE; Kemp 1978).

Transient Otoacoustic Emission Testing

The automated version of this test is performed either in the maternity unit by specially trained midwives or nurses, or in the community by district nurses or midwives. A probe is inserted into the infant's external ear canal (EAC); an acoustic stimulus, consisting of broadband clicks, is applied to the ear through the probe, which also records the sounds remaining in the EAC. In the presence of normal or near-normal hearing (0–30 dB hearing level, dBHL), sound at a higher dB level than that originally introduced will be recorded after an interval of 5 ms. The response normally lasts about 15 ms. This amplified version of the original stimulus is produced by intact outer hair cells. Absence of the response means that the outer hair cells are not normal, indicating cochlear hearing loss. The response is averaged, recorded on the laptop computer and printed out. The test can normally be interpreted by eye, but normal values are provided and can be compared with values contained in the print-out (see Fig. 37.2). The TOAE response is only present in the presence of normal outer hair cell function in the cochlea. In almost all cases, a positive response means that the infant has normal or near-normal hearing. One exception is in the case of auditory neuropathy/dys-synchrony, usually following premature delivery with episodes of hypoxia, after severe neonatal jaundice or in the presence of mutations in the OTOF gene that interfere with inner hair cell synaptic transmission (see Chapter 7). Here, TOAEs are present, but other tests, including auditory brainstem responses (ABRs), are absent or grossly abnormal.

Benefits

- Automated, with little interpretation necessary.
- Not affected by sleep.
- High (97%) sensitivity.
- Rapid, and performed by nursing staff.
- Relatively inexpensive equipment.
- Objective.
- Allows early identification, and therefore early management, of deafness.

Limitations

- Identifies normal hearing only: failure does not give any estimate of the actual hearing threshold.
- Relatively low specificity: can fail with wax or debris in the EAC or middle ear effusion (otitis media with effusion: OME).
- Failures need further validation and threshold assessment by ABR.
- Not frequency specific.
- May be technically difficult in a crying infant and in a noisy environment. Best performed after a feed.
- TOAE responses may be present in cases of "auditory neuropathy".

Use

- Neonatal hearing screen, now universal for all neonates in the UK and other developed countries.
- Validation of normal hearing (with few exceptions above) at any age.
- An early, rapid test after meningitis. Can be performed even in an unconscious child.

Distortion Product Otoacoustic Emissions

Distortion product otoacoustic emissions (DPOAEs) are emissions produced when two pure tones, separated in frequency in the ratio of 1.22:1, are presented simultaneously. If, for example, the two frequencies are 1.6 kHz and 2 kHz, the maximum emission will be generated from the outer hair cells in the 1.3 kHz part of the cochlea. This test is therefore frequency specific and the DPOAEs are generated with hearing thresholds up to 60 dBHL from all parts of the basilar membrane. Usually, DPOAEs are recorded at between 500 Hz and 6 kHz. The test can therefore be used to provide some indication of hearing levels at different higher frequencies in neonates that fail TOAE screening. However, in practice, those infants who fail the TAOE screen will normally proceed straight to ABR testing.

Auditory Brainstem Response

The ABR was identified by Sohmer and Feinmesser and further refined by Jewitt and Willeston (1971). It records the averaged electrical response generated in the cochlear nerve, then the ipsilateral cochlear nucleus; the response then follows the classical ascending auditory pathway in the brainstem, with bilateral responses from the superior olivary complex, lateral lemniscus and inferior colliculus. Broad-band clicks, with alternating polarity, or occasionally frequency-specific tone bursts, are presented to

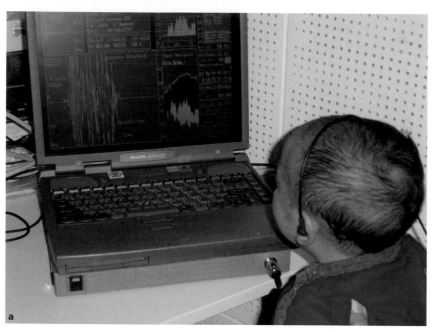

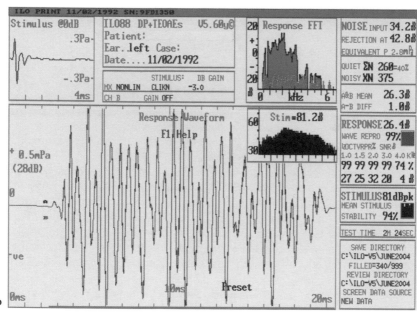

Fig. 37.2 a Test set-up for transient otoacoustic emissions in a child of 6 months. **b** TOAE response in a child with normal hearing

each ear separately. The clicks may be presented by headphones; however, insert earphones have the advantage of reducing the spread of sound to the contralateral ear, and so reduce the need for contralateral masking at higher intensities. The electric responses are recorded from scalp electrodes, taped to the child's forehead and behind the ears, averaged and then displayed on the screen of a laptop computer, then printed out. Masking of the contralateral ear may be required when there is a difference in threshold between the two ears of 50 dBHL or more. The test provides realistic threshold information for frequencies centred on 3 kHz for clicks. If tone-burst stimuli are used, more frequency-specific information between 500 Hz and 4 kHz can be obtained. It is extremely rare for a child with normal ABRs to have abnormal hearing; an exception is a child who may later be found to have a auditory processing disorder (APD) for speech. A typical series of ABR traces is shown in Fig. 37.3.

RIGHT EAR

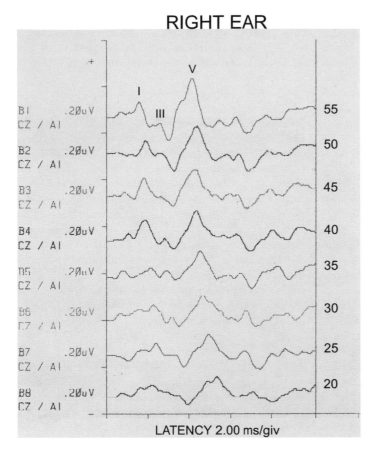

Fig. 37.3 Normal auditory brain responses, traced to 20 dB hearing level (dBHL) in a child with normal hearing

Benefits

- Accurate threshold measurement.
- Relatively rapid.
- Not affected by sleep, sedation or general anaesthesia.
- Can be performed by a specially trained nurse or midwife, but more commonly by an audiologist.
- High sensitivity and specificity (greater than 90% for both).
- Bone conduction (BC) ABR thresholds can also be obtained, for example in the presence of OME or congenital atresia and microtia.
- Automated scoring is also available (AABR).

Limitations

- More training of testers required than for TOAE.
- Depends on the state of the infant or child. Natural sleep is normally required, although can be performed under sedation or general anaesthetic, particularly with other procedures requiring anaesthesia.
- Requires an experienced tester to identify the waveform accurately.

- Not frequency specific; click-evoked responses identify thresholds centred around 3 kHz.

Use

- At birth, to validate TOAE and measure threshold of hearing.
- As a screening test for very low birth weight babies in neonatal intensive care, who are at risk from acquired deafness.
- Up to about 6 months, when hearing needs to be assessed, perhaps when neonatal screening was not performed.
- From to about 2 years of age, in natural sleep, to measure hearing in a child not giving clear responses to behavioural tests or who has learning difficulties or is difficult to test for any reason.
- After meningitis, even in an unconscious child.
- Special use in suspected "auditory neuropathy", when it can be used to detect abnormally large summating potentials, consisting of uninhibited and somewhat non-linear outer-hair-cell-generated cochlear microphonic responses (see Electrocochleography, below).

A special use of ABR is in children being assessed for cochlear implantation, when electrically evoked ABRs may either be recorded using a stimulating electrode placed against the round window membrane or, after implantation, using the implant itself as the stimulating agent. In this way the status of the afferent auditory pathway can be checked, together with the threshold of the cochlear nerve and the likely upper end of the range of tolerance for electrical stimulation.

Electrocochleography

Electrocochleography (ECochG; Portmann et al. 1967) was used in the past as a robust method of obtaining objective hearing thresholds in children who were hard to test by other methods. However, transtympanic ECochG in children requires a general anaesthetic and even extratympanic ECochG is technically difficult in children. As a threshold measurement it has largely been superseded by ABR testing.

Clicks or tone bursts are delivered by a loudspeaker and the response recorded by a transtympanic electrode or, in extratympanic recording, from a metal ball electrode placed in the anterior angle between the tympanic membrane and the EAC. A reference electrode is placed on the scalp behind the ear or on the ear lobe, with a ground electrode on the forehead in the midline. Clicks of alternating polarity are presented, allowing manipulation of the response by reversing the polarity of the signal obtained. Responses are detected from the outer hair cells (cochlear microphonic, CM: equivalent to the TOAE response) at stimulation levels above about 70 dBHL, and the compound action potential (CAP) of the cochlear nerve is detected about 1.6 ms after the onset of the CM and can be traced down to threshold level or to about 20 dBHL in a normally hearing ear.

Although no longer routinely used as a threshold measurement following the development of ABR, ECochG was used as an indicator of "auditory neuropathy/dyssynchrony" in infants whose hearing had been damaged by hypoxia or jaundice. Abnormally large CMs are obtained, comparable to the abnormally large TOAE found in this situation. These are linked to large, non-linear, direct current potentials with the same latency as the CM, and with no detectable CAP.

Benefits

- Robust assessment of peripheral hearing: cochlea and cochlear nerve function.
- Gives a clear indication of the presence of disturbances of peripheral hearing currently termed "auditory neuropathy/dys-synchrony".

Limitation

- Requires general anaesthesia in children and normally a medically qualified person to insert the needle electrode.

Behavioural Testing: Ages Six Months to Three Years

Behavioural testing uses the natural head-turning response of a child between the ages of 6 months and 2–3 years of developmental age to search for the origin of a sound. Sounds are presented to either ear at what is likely to be a suprathreshold level of 30 dBHL. The stimuli can be presented in "sound field" or using headphones or insert earphones. The child normally will turn his or her head to look for the origin of the sound; the frequency and intensity are recorded for each episode of stimulation; the test is dependent on the child having acquired head control.

Distraction Testing: Age Six to Eighteen Months

This was introduced as a method of assessing the auditory thresholds of children old enough to provide a reliable head-turning response, but too young for conditioned testing to be possible. The test is based on the distracting test described by Ewing and Ewing (1944); before the introduction of TOAE it formed the basis of universal hearing screening in the UK and elsewhere. In this situation it can be administered by nurses or local authority audiologists and used to screen the hearing of children at the age of about 9 months. It is also used widely in audiology clinics to measure hearing thresholds, although in many such clinics, visual reinforcement audiometry (VRA) has replaced distraction testing.

The test takes place in a "sound-field" environment. The child sits on the knee of the parent or carer, facing the first tester, who will attract the child's attention by an activity that is interesting enough to engage the child's attention but not too noisy or boisterous, and if possible avoiding prolonged eye contact with the child (Fig. 37.4). The second tester stands behind the parent, out of the child's visual field, and presents sound signals on one side or the other, at ear level, just out of the child's range of vision and at a distance of approximately 0.5 m. The head-turn response is confirmed by the first tester. Occasionally, a deviation of the child's eyes, rather than a head turn, is recorded as a positive response. Traditionally, familiar environmental sounds are used, the frequency range of which is known and whose sound levels are checked with a sound level meter after each positive

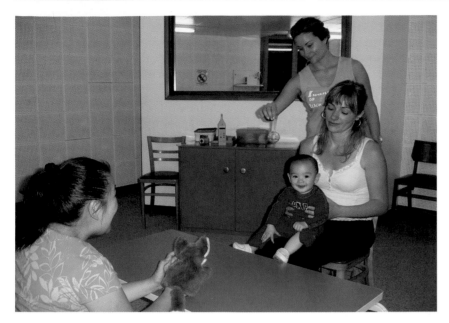

Fig. 37.4 Distraction testing. The child sits on his mother's lap. The first tester attracts the child's attention; the second tester presents the test sound 0.5 m from the child's ear and outside his range of vision. In this example, the test modality consists of the sound produced by a calibrated rattle

response. Test sounds include specially designed rattles (producing a narrow band sound of known frequency), a high-frequency hiss ("ss"), low-frequency voiced sound ("ba, ba"), sweet wrapping papers and rubbing a tea spoon around the inside rim of a china cup. Wooden xylophones can be used. High-intensity drum beats, tambourines and other loud sound generators may also be used to produce a startle response in apparently unresponsive children. Electronically generated sounds from portable equipment were introduced to provide frequency-specific warble tones or narrow-band stimuli. These have the advantage of providing more precise stimuli, although some children seem not to respond as reliably as they do to more familiar environmental sounds. During the test procedure it is important to include some episodes when no sound is presented, in order to check for false-positive responses. The sound levels presented should be monitored and checked using a sound level meter.

The reliability of distraction testing depends on the skill of the testers as well as the state of the child being tested. Children in an uncooperative mood, crying, sleepy, hyperactive or with other physical or developmental delays are hard to test using this method.

Benefits

- Inexpensive, quick, robust and relatively simple to administer by correctly trained staff in the community.
- Still has a place in specialist audiology clinics, though to some extent replaced by VRA.
- Frequency-specific.

Limitations

- Reliability relies on the training and skill of the testers.
- False positive responses may be wrongly interpreted as true ones.
- Depends on the state of child, who should not be sleepy or hyperactive.
- Depends on the developmental state of the child: earliest responses are obtainable at around 5–6 months. Responses more reliably expected at 6 months. A screening age of 9 months has been adopted for maximum likelihood of response.
- Responses may not be obtainable, or may appear at a relatively late age in children with learning difficulties.
- Special test procedures may be needed for children with physical disability.
- Depends on visual development. It may be of limited use in children with visual disorders.
- Although positive responses depend on head-turn towards the direction of the sound stimuli, it is not truly able to give thresholds for separate ears.
- Distraction testing has a lower sensitivity and specificity than VRA.
- Older children (over approximately 18 months) are too "sophisticated" for the test and are less willing to remain on a parent's lap.

Use

- Community screening and audiology clinics.
- Detects deafness acquired since neonatal screening, especially from OME. Also detects progressive sen-

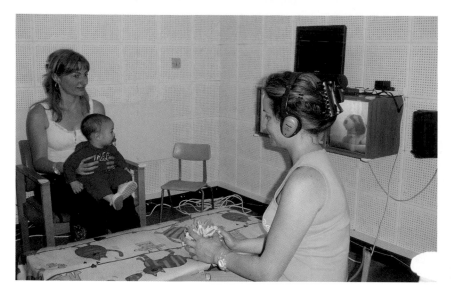

Fig. 37.5 Visual reinforcement audiometry (VRA). In this example, sound-field testing is taking place and insert microphones are not being used; the reinforcing object is a soft toy, illuminated in a glass-fronted box (seen behind the tester's head)

37

sorineural hearing loss when hearing may have been normal at birth.

- Detects congenital deafness missed at neonatal screening or in children who did not have neonatal screening.

Visual Reinforcement Audiometry: Age Six Months to Three Years

VRA is a more reliable variant of distraction testing. It requires more complex and expensive equipment, but is more accurate than distraction testing. As in the distraction test, the child sits on the knees of the parent, and the first tester attracts the child's attention from the front. The sound stimuli, however, are presented using an audiometer and delivered either from loudspeakers, positioned on either side of the child, or by headphones or "insert" earphones, sitting comfortably over or in the child's EACs, allowing the two ears to be tested separately. Masking of the contralateral ear can be performed if necessary. A bone vibrator can also be used to establish BC thresholds. The second tester sits behind the first tester, able to see the child's face, but out of sight of the child, if possible behind a one-way mirror, in communication with the first tester with a radio microphone and also able to hear sounds relayed from the test room.

Reinforcement of positive responses provides the child with a "reward", in the form of a visual display (Fig. 37.5). This may take the form of an illuminated moving toy in a glass-fronted box, activated by the second tester, or alternatively by an animated image on a television screen, such as many children are now accustomed to seeing in daily life. This reinforcement brings an element of conditioning to a mainly behavioural procedure, maintains the child's interest for longer and has been found to produce more accurate responses.

Benefits

- Comparable to distraction testing and covers the same ages, but with more reliable and accurate responses, and a longer attention span on behalf of the child.
- Ears can be tested separately using "inserts"; BC testing can be performed if required.

Limitations

- Same as for distraction testing, although since it is normally performed in a specialist audiology clinic, testers are better qualified and more skilled.
- Special test room with sound field, and special equipment both involve extra cost.

Use

- In specialist audiology clinics, to obtain more accurate thresholds of hearing.

Conditioned Audiometry: Two to Three Years and Upwards

Play Audiometry: Age Two to Three Years and Upwards

Also known as performance testing, play audiometry is possible once the child is old enough to respond to simple commands. This may be possible at the age of about 18 months in an alert, intelligent child, but is more generally used from the age of 2–3 years onwards.

In play audiometry, the tester provides the child with a simple, repetitive activity. This may be placing wooden,

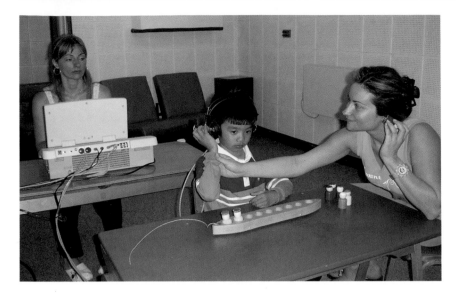

Fig. 37.6 Play audiometry. The child is conditioned to put the wooden sailor in place in the boat on hearing a pure tone delivered by headphones

cylindrical toy sailors in cylindrical holes in a wooden boat, dropping bricks into a box, or some comparable activity (Fig. 37.6). The child is first conditioned: taught to perform the action in response to a simple command, traditionally when the tester says "go". The child has to learn to wait for the command, then perform the action rapidly on receiving the command. Once the child has begun reliably to respond to the command, a sound signal, consisting of a pure tone, or preferably a frequency-modulated "warble" tone, is substituted for the verbal command. In fact, this progression from verbal command to sound stimulus may not be necessary in many cases, and sound stimuli may be used from the outset. This is an advantage when the child has been brought up to speak a different language from that used by the tester.

For young children, the test takes place in a sound-field environment, and the sound levels of each positive response are checked with a sound level meter. In this case, the responses are binaural. Older children may be persuaded to wear headphones or insert phones, allowing the ears to be tested separately. Masking of the contralateral ear in cases of unilateral hearing loss may be possible, depending on the age of the child. This will generally be at the age of 3 years and upwards. By the age of 5 years, most children should be able to cooperate with the standard pure-tone test procedure used for adults.

Benefits

- Rapid and relatively simple to perform in a cooperative child of appropriate age and with no other disability.
- Not language dependant. Most children understand the test procedure with minimal verbal instruction.
- Only one tester is required.

Limitations

- Depends on the cooperation of the child and on a certain level of development and intelligence.
- For children with learning difficulty or those with motor developmental delay, the test procedure may need technical modification.

Speech Audiometry: Age Two to Six Years and Upwards

This is a valuable additional form of test in children with an appropriate level of language development. The McCormick Toy Discrimination Test is a commonly used English version. In a sound-field environment a selection of 14 toys is placed in front of the child on a low table or on the floor. The toys are chosen to represent familiar objects that are likely to be included in the vocabulary of a child of this age and are monosyllabic. The names of each of the seven pairs of toys are matched to contain the same vowel sound: cup/duck, spoon/shoe, man/lamb, plate/plane, horse/fork, key/tree and house/cow.

The child and the tester sit facing each other (Fig. 37.7). The tester first establishes that the child knows the name of each toy, and is told to point to the toy when the tester names it. Occasionally, with a shy child, "eye pointing" can be used. The tester says "show me the (short pause)… cup", or "where is the … horse?", and the child should respond by pointing to the relevant toy. Having conditioned the child, the tester's mouth must be hidden, using some flat object, or a hand, to prevent lip reading, although lip reading may be allowed from time to time, to help reinforce the game or to demonstrate to a parent that the child may be relying on lip reading for better day to day communication. The tester then lowers his or her voice level to determine the quietest level at which the

37

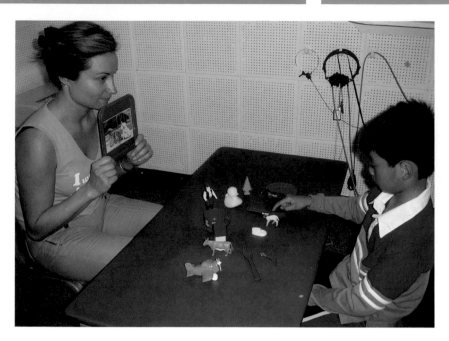

Fig. 37.7 The toy identification test. The child is asked to point to a toy named by the tester. In the automated version of the test (not shown here), the voice used to name the toys is recorded and delivered from a loudspeaker, with better control of sound levels

child correctly identifies at least four out of five requests (an 80% correct score). The sound level of each threshold response is checked with a sound level meter. A child with normal hearing will correctly identify the toys at a sound level of 35–40 dBA.

An automated version of the test is available in English, with the words produced from a recording and delivered by a loudspeaker. This allows better reproducibility and removes difficulties related to the accent or voice quality of the tester. The automated test is used to establish the level at which the child gives a 71% correct response rate.

The test is not, of course, a test of language, but does depend on a certain level of receptive language development. In a specialist audiology clinic, it is usual to have access to a speech and language therapist/pathologist to provide both an informal and formal assessment of the child's language and articulation.

Benefits

- Rapid and replicable assessment of speech perception thresholds.
- The test reproduces a situation of natural communication.
- Simple and inexpensive equipment is required.
- Non-intrusive to the child.
- Visual clues can be used for conditioning and reinforcement.
- An automated version is available.

Limitations

- Relies on cooperation and developmental age of the child.
- Not possible when child's own language is different from that of tester. Problems may also arise when the tester's accent is different from that of the child's parents and family.
- Not possible to test below 35–40 dBA using live voice; it may be difficult for the tester to monitor the voice level reliably.
- Inter- and intra-test variability in voice level and intelligibility, unless the automated version is used.

Other speech tests are available, for example the Manchester Picture Test, using picture cards. This is available using live or recorded voice. The child needs to score a minimum of 80% to pass at each level of loudness. The spondee test, asking older children to repeat two-syllable words from a printed list, is delivered with live voice, may also be useful and requires no special apparatus.

Cortical Electric Response Audiometry

This was the earliest form of electric response audiometry to be developed (Davis 1939). The "slow vertex" response arises in the primary and secondary auditory cortex in response to clicks or frequency-specific tone bursts presented to each ear separately. Three peaks: P1 (also known as Pb), N1 and P2 are recorded, with latencies, in adults and mature children, of 50–250 ms.

It has never been generally used as a test of hearing threshold in young children, as it depends very much on the conscious state of the test subject. It has a place in testing for non-organic hearing loss in older children and teenagers; it must be performed while the subject is awake and alert.

Recently, it has also been used in very young infants (Sharma et al. 2002) to measure the state of development of the central auditory pathways. In an infant aged 3–7 months with normal hearing, the P1 response occurs at 100–150 ms, rather than 50 ms. By the age of 5 years this shortens to the normal adult latency. In a deaf child, this latency fails to shorten, indicating the failure of the central auditory pathways to mature. If a young child with a moderate to severe hearing loss is successfully fitted with hearing aids, the latency can be made to shorten to normal levels (Purdy and Kelly 2001). Similarly, if a child with a severe to profound hearing loss is provided with a cochlear implant in the 1st year of life, a comparable shortening of P1 latency occurs, indicating the maturation of the central auditory pathways (Ponton et al. 1996).

Audiometric Steady-State Response

The auditory steady-state response (ASSR) is generated in the brainstem from the same sites that produce ABR waves II–V. However, rather than a series of waves representing responses generated in the brainstem by transient individual stimuli, it is a continuous, EEG-like electrical response to a continuous, modulated pure tone (Stapells et al. 2005).

The stimulus needed to produce ASSR is a frequency- or amplitude-modulated pure tone, in which the modulations occur at a rate of around 80–100/s (80–100 Hz). The frequencies of pure tone used for testing are between 250 Hz and 8 kHz.

The response consists of a continuous response that is phase-locked to, and therefore mirrors, the rate of modulation of the stimulus. It is recorded using scalp electrodes, averaged and automatically identified by computer software (Herdman et al. 2002; John and Picton 2000). It can be used at birth. It allows frequency-specific auditory thresholds to be measured between 20 and 120 dBHL, and responses to four different frequencies can be measured simultaneously from both ears at once (Fig. 37.8). It is stable during sleep, sedation and general anaesthesia.

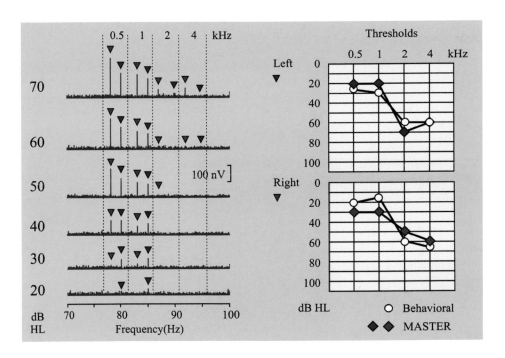

Fig. 37.8 The auditory steady-state response (ASSR). The averaged responses from both ears (separately) to four test frequencies (0.5, 1, 2 and 4 kHz) and following stimuli at 20–70 dB are the *vertical spikes* shown emerging from the background noise in the left half of the figure. The tester identifies these positive responses and places the *blue* and *red triangles* (corresponding to the left and right ears, respectively) over them. The scale at the bottom of the graph shows the different frequency modulation applied to each tone and to each ear. The test takes about 5 min to perform, allowing averages responses to be recorded from five to ten sweep stimuli. In the graphs on the right of the figure, the ASSR thresholds (*solid diamonds*) are compared with behavioural thresholds (*open circles*)

Benefits

- Rapid and replicable assessment of hearing thresholds (allows both ears to be tested simultaneously using four frequencies).
- Relatively short clinical testing time.
- Identifies frequency-specific thresholds between 250 Hz and 8 kHz at stimulus levels between 20 and 125 dBHL.
- More rapid and accurate than ABR in detecting frequency-specific thresholds. Better threshold detection above 90 dBHL than ABR.
- Can be used in sleep, sedation or anaesthesia.

Limitations

- Requires relatively good signal-to-noise ratio.
- ASSR is a relatively new test method and findings in infants with conductive and mixed conductive and sensorineural hearing loss and for BC stimuli have not yet been fully validated.
- The test stimulus is a group of continuous wavering tones. At high intensities there could be a risk of noise-induced hearing loss.

Use

- In specialist audiology clinics to obtain accurate and frequency specific thresholds of hearing.

Tympanometry and Acoustic Reflexes

Tympanometry has been used routinely since the 1970s as a clinical tool for assessing the middle-ear status of children (Fig. 37.9). It is a quick, non-invasive and objective procedure. A probe containing three tubes is inserted into the child's EAC. One tube delivers sound, usually a pure tone of 220 Hz, generated by a microphone. However, for infants younger than 4 months, a probe tone of 1 kHz produces more reliable results because of the physical properties of the EAC in young infants. The second tube measures the sound level in the EAC and the third tube is connected to a manometer, which alters and records the pressure in the EAC, between –300 and +200 daPa (mm H_2O).

The maximum transmission of sound from the probe through the tympanic membrane and ossicles (physical compliance, or "admittance") occurs when the tympanic membrane is in its normal position. Varying the pressure in the EAC moves the tympanic membrane inwards or outwards. Displacing the membrane in this way increases the stiffness of the membrane and ossicular chain, and so reduces the transmission of sound through the membrane and middle ear. The recording microphone in the second tube therefore records a higher level of residual EAC sound, since relatively little sound will have left the EAC to pass through the tympanic membrane and middle ear.

In the presence of a normal middle ear, with normal pressure, sweeping the EAC pressure between –300 daPa, 0 daPa and +200 daPa produces the typical tympanogram shown in Fig. 37.10, with low compliance at the lowest and highest EAC pressures and high compliance (a "peak")

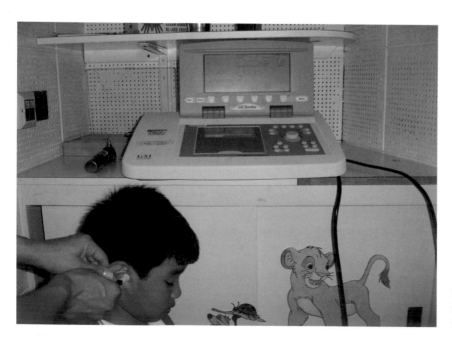

Fig. 37.9 A child undergoing tympanometry. The probe is being inserted into his right ear

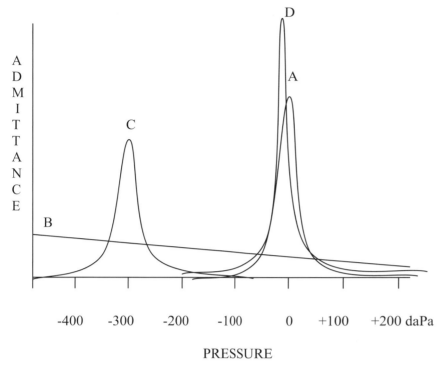

Fig. 37.10 A group of tympanograms; the *capital letters* refer to the Jerger classification (Jerger 1970), whereby type A is normal tympanogram, type B is flat and found in otitis media with effusion and when there is a defect in the tympanic membrane, type C is a peak, but occurring at a negative middle ear pressure and type D shows an abnormally high peak, suggesting hypermobility as a result of a weakened tympanic membrane or occasionally from ossicular discontinuity

where the EAC pressure is zero. If the middle-ear pressure is negative, this peak will be seen when the middle and external ear pressures are equal; the value of the EAC pressure at this point will be equal to the pressure in the middle ear. When the middle ear is full of fluid, middle ear effusion (OME), these pressure changes will have no effect on the transmission of sound through the middle ear, and no peak will be present: a flat tympanogram.

The stapedius reflex, a contraction of the stapedius muscle in the middle ear, occurs when a tone at or above about 70 dBHL is presented at 0.5, 1, 2 and 4 kHz. The stapedius reflex stiffens movements of the stapes and so produces a transient reduction of the sound passing through the tympanic membrane and middle ear. This is detected and recorded by the tympanometer. The presence of the reflex indicates normal middle ear function and, since the reflex arc passes through the cochlear nerve to the brainstem then outwards through the facial nerve to the stapedius muscle, the presence of the reflex following a tone of 70 dBHL indicates a mobile stapes, a functioning reflex arc and normal facial nerve function. The reflex is recorded in both ears following presentation of the stimulus to one ear. The response can therefore be recorded from the ipsilateral or contralateral ear.

Although many publications and reports use the Jerger tympanogram types, it may be easier simply to describe the findings of tympanometry in terms of the presence and size of the peak and the middle-ear pressure at which the peak occurs. The probe also measures the volume of the EAC. In a child, this is typically around 0.6 ml. A type

B, flat tympanogram may indicate OME; however, a type B tympanogram will also be observed if there is a perforation of the tympanic membrane (this can include the presence of a patent grommet or ventilation tube), but the volume recorded on the printout will include that of the middle ear cavity and will therefore be closer to 1.2 ml, rather than 0.6 ml. This is useful in establishing whether a ventilation tube is patent, as well as in detecting very small tympanic membrane perforations.

Special Situations

Children with learning difficulties require special consideration. In severe cases, objective hearing tests such as ABR are required, in natural sleep if possible, otherwise under sedation or general anaesthesia. Older children with suspected autism may also require objective testing, since they may not respond reliably to play and speech audiometry.

Children with microtia: if the microtia is bilateral, BC audiometry is required. In younger children, ABR using a BC stimulus is feasible, after careful calibration of the equipment.

Children with suspected auditory processing disorder (APD) may be referred for audiometric testing. Most test procedures are specialist tests of language and can only be applied to relatively old children; children with APD have normal pure-tone thresholds but poor ability to discriminate speech with background noise, and the P300 peak on cortical electric response audiometry is usually delayed.

The normal contralateral suppression of TOAE, with reduction of the size of the OAE response when noise is introduced into the opposite ear, does not occur.

Children using cochlear implants require some objective measurement of hearing thresholds. Electrically activated versions of CAP, ABR and steady-state response are available.

Summary for the Clinician

- The purpose of the audiological assessment of children is to identify accurately those with a hearing loss as early as possible, and so to try and minimise the disability caused by deafness. The assessment of hearing in children requires several different testing techniques to be available. The choice of test will depend upon the age of the child, his or her medical state and whether an objective or behavioural investigation is needed. The ideal test would provide an objective assessment of the entire hearing pathway, which is frequency specific, highly sensitive and specific, and provide robust and reliable results in a variety of settings with minimal staff training. No single test satisfies all of these demands. TOAE testing fulfils several of these criteria and is the ideal method for universal hearing screening of the neonatal population. However, it will only test cochlear function and there are always false failures that need further investigation. ABR testing is currently the gold standard for further assessment of children or of neonates with a high risk of hearing loss, but is time consuming and requires skilled staff for interpretation. ASSR testing may prove to offer more accurate, frequency-specific results than ABR, but is currently not widely available and more evaluation is needed.
- Distraction testing has traditionally been used in the community to screen for hearing loss at 8–9 months. This has largely been replaced by universal screening with TOAEs. However, behavioural testing remains important for the assessment of young children with hearing loss, especially as it tests the entire auditory pathway, including understanding of the relevance of the sound stimulus. Such behavioural methods should also detect hearing loss, for example from middle-ear effusion, appearing later in childhood.
- For a full account of audiological testing in children, the reader is recommended McCormick's Paediatric Audiology 0–5 Years (3rd edition, 2004).

References

1. Davis PA (1939) Effects of auditory stimuli on the waking human brain. J Neurophysiol 2:494–499
2. Ewing IR, Ewing AWG (1944) The ascertainment of deafness in infancy and early childhood. J Laryngol Otol 59:309–338
3. Herdman A, Lins O, Van Roon P, et al (2002) Intracerebral sources of human auditory steady-state responses. Brain Topogr 15:69–86
4. Jerger J (1970) Clinical experience with impedance audiometry. Arch Otolaryngol 92:311–324
5. Jewett DL, Williston JS (1971) Auditory-evoked far field responses averaged from the scalp of humans. Brain 94:681–696
6. John S, Picton W (2000). MASTER: a Windows program for recording multiple auditory steady-state responses. Comput Methods Programs Biomed 61:125–150
7. Kemp DT (1978) Stimulated acoustic emissions from within the human auditory system. J Acoust Soc Am 64:1386–1391
8. McCormick B (ed) (2004) Paediatric Audiology 0–5 Years, 3rd edn. Whurr, London
9. Ponton CW, Don M, Eggermont JJ, et al (1996) Auditory system plasticity in children after long periods of complete deafness. Neuroreport 8:61–65
10. Portmann M, Lebert G, Aran J-M (1967) Potentiels cochleares obtenus chez l'homme en dehors de toute intervention chirurgicale. Rev Laryngol 88:157–164
11. Purdy S, Kelly A (2001) Cortical auditory evoked potential testing in infants and young children. N Z Audiol Soc Bull 11:16–24
12. Sharma A, Dorman MF, Todd NW (2002) Early cochlear implantation in children allows normal development of central auditory pathways. Ann Otol Rhinol Laryngol 189:38–41
13. Stapells R, Herdman A, Small A, et al (2005). Current status of the auditory steady state responses for estimating an infant's audiogram. In: Seewald RC (ed) A Sound Foundation Through Early Amplification: Proceedings of an International Conference. Phonak, Chicago, pp 43–59

Otoplasty and Common Auricular Deformities

38

Werner J. Heppt

Core Messages

- The normal angle between the scalp covering the mastoid and helical rim averages 25–35°.
- In protruding ears, special moulding and dressings may have some benefit when applied in the first months after birth.
- Reduction of the conchal wall, remodelling of the antihelical and helical vault and trimming of the lobule are the most common surgical steps in pinnaplasty.
- As a rule, thick, stiff and unyielding cartilages and revision surgery require more invasive procedures than primary surgery on a weak and pliable cartilaginous framework.
- Corrections of the antihelix with underlying soft, pliable cartilage are best done using suture techniques. Stiff, unyielding cartilages and severe protrusion require additional cartilage weakening by anterior scoring, posterior incision or burring.
- Conchal hyperplasia is well addressed by the conchal setback technique, which may be supplemented by cartilage reduction and/or transection of the anterior helical ligaments.
- Correction of a prominent lobule may be achieved by mattress sutures to the concha, severing of the helical tail, trimming of the antitragus and resection of retrolobular skin and soft tissue.
- Cutting techniques are most suitable for revision surgery and severe primary deformities.
- In all traumatic lesions of the auricle, deeper injuries (ear canal, ear drum) have to be excluded.

Contents

Introduction

The auricle is often a point of fixation as well as one of the most eye-catching parts of the body. This may be the reason why the desire for an aesthetically shaped ear has developed in humans. Another reason might be that from ancient times, personality traits have been attributed to the shape of the auricle. Whereas Aristotle (384–322 BC) stated that persons with big ears have good memories and sagacity, nowadays this shape may be defined in some societies as a symbol of stupidity. Protruding ears are common. About one out of five children have them. Usually parents seek consultation for correction directly after birth or at the age of 4–5 years when children may begin to be teased by their peers. The next group of patients consists mainly of young ladies at puberty or between 20 and 25 years complaining about their limitations in hairstyling. Traumatic lesions are the second most common type of auricular deformity. They often result from fights, dog bites or accidents. Because many of the auricular lesions may result in disfigurement of the shape, an appropriate treatment plan has to be followed from the very beginning.

In the following, special emphasis is placed on both these types of common deformities, focussing on reliable surgical techniques as well as on conservative alternatives. See Chapter 39 for the epidemiology of microtia and management of severe congenital deformities of the ear.

Basics

Development of the Auricle

The development of the auricle commences in the 7th week during embryogenesis when six mesenchymal thickenings in the form of small hillocks (Fig. 38.1) appear on the dorsal margins of the first and second branchial arch (Davies 1987). For creation of the characteristic prominences and cavities, the hillocks of the second branchial arch are of paramount importance. They form the lobule, the antihelix and the dorsocaudal part of the helix. Only the tragus is created by the first hillock lying

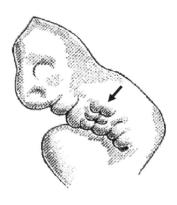

Fig. 38.1 The auricle develops from the six hillocks (*arrow*) of the first and second branchial arch

on the first branchial arch. While developing, the auricle shifts its position from ventrocaudal to dorsocranial corresponding to the movement of the jaw.

Minor malformations such as protruding ears are caused by disturbances between the 3rd and 7th month of development and mostly diagnosed at the age of 2 or 3 years when the proportions of the head and body have changed. Their genesis is considered multifactorial.

Clinical Anatomy

The position and shape of the auricle are characterised by various prominences and cavities (Fig. 38.2). These have a mild filtering effect on sounds entering the external ear canal, which contributes, to a slight degree, to directional hearing. Furthermore, in some societies, its appearance may have some irrational meaning in determining a person's beauty and intelligence.

The auricle is supported by a framework of elastic cartilage; only the lobule lacks cartilage and consists of firm trabecular subcutaneous tissue. The skin covering the auricle is thin and closely attached anteriorly, but thick and loose on the posterior surface. Superficial temporal and posterior auricular vessels provide the blood supply. Sensory innervation arises from branches of the facial, vagal, greater auricular and auriculotemporal nerves and the cervical plexus. Inner and outer ligaments attach the auricle to the head and keep the characteristic auricular shape. The auricular muscles are rudimentary and without clinical relevance, apart from their use for the postauricular muscle response.

The aesthetically normal auricle lies about one ear length posterior and lateral to the orbital rim, with its long axis tilted backwards by 10–15°. The top of the auricle is level with the eyebrow, and its width is about 60% of its height. According to anthropometric evaluation, the normal angle between the helical rim and the scalp covering the mastoid is 25–35°, and that between concha and scaphoid fossa is 80–90°. The angle between concha and scalp over the mastoid ranges from 45 to 90°. Ideally, the helical rim and antihelical contours are parallel, so that the helix is visible beyond the antihelix from the

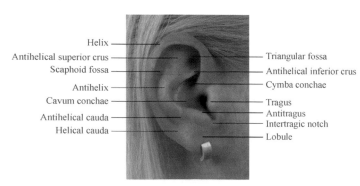

Fig. 38.2 Anatomy of the auricle

front. Posterior measurements from the helical rim to the scalp over the mastoid range between 10–12 mm at the superior pole and 16–18 mm at the middle and 20–22 mm at the lower part of the auricle depending on the shape of the skull. The difference between both auricles should be within 3 mm. Besides all morphometric measurements, the thickness and flexibility of the cartilage are of pivotal importance. Therefore, palpation is an essential diagnostic tool.

Classification of Congenital Deformities

At present, no universal classification of auricular deformities exists in the literature. The most accepted publications of Marx (1926), Tanzer (1977) and Weerda (1988) are based on embryology, degree and surgical approach. Protruding ears belong to the minor deformities, which are defined as first-degree dysplasias (Table 38.1).

Protruding Ears (Prominent Ears, Bat Ears)

Causes

There are no absolute rules for diagnosing ear protrusion. Most surgeons define it as when the helix–mastoid distance exceeds 2 cm at the midpoint of the ear and the angle between the mastoid and the outer helical rim reaches more than 40–45°. However, these measurements are only guidelines and vary according to the individual shape of the skull. The most important structural abnor-

Table 38.2 Characteristics of protruding ears

Underdeveloped or absent antihelical fold
Increased distance between the helical rim and scalp
Increased angle between the mastoid and helical rim
Overdeveloped concha with deep conchal wall
Protruding lobule

malities of the auricle that cause the appearance of protrusion are listed in Table 38.2.

Conservative Treatment Options

Minor deformities such as lop ears and protruding ears may be managed conservatively in the 1st months after birth. Pliability and auricular elasticity in neonates is supposed to be related mainly to the oestrogen level, which falls to the level of older children at the age of 6 weeks (Kenny et al. 1973). Therefore, the cartilage may be corrected to a certain degree early in life (Tan et al. 2003). Some authors recommend the application of Steri-strips (Fig. 38.3) with or without silicone splints placed into the scaphoid fossa; others describe custom-made silicone moulds made of dental compounds attached to the ear with methylmethacrylate glue and supported by tubular banding.

Table 38.1 Classification of congenital auricular deformities (Weerda 1988)

First-degree dysplasia	
Definition	Most structures of a normal auricle are recognisable, minor deformities are present
Deformities	Protruding ears, macrotia, cryptotia, satyr ear, Stahl's ear, coloboma, etc.
Surgery	Reconstruction without additional skin or cartilage
Second-degree dysplasia	
Definition	Some auricular structures recognisable
Deformities	Severe cup ear, mini ear deformity
Surgery	Partial reconstruction with skin and cartilage
Third-degree dysplasia	
Definition	No normal auricular structures recognisable, usually with atresia
Deformities	Unilateral or bilateral anotia
Surgery	Total reconstruction with skin and cartilage, or bone-anchored, silicone artificial pinna

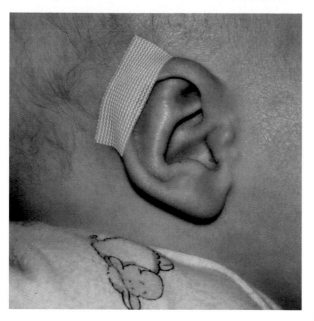

Fig. 38.3 Treatment of ear protrusion in a neonate using Steristrips

Conservative therapy should be started as early as possible. It should be applied constantly for 6–12 weeks depending on the extent of the deformity. Even with thorough parents, persistence and proper handling, however, the benefit is limited. Therefore, surgical procedures have been found to be the gold standard in the correction of protruding ears and other minor deformities.

Surgical Correction (Pinnaplasty)

Goals

The goals of aesthetic otoplasty are to produce a natural appearance, with symmetry and correct position. Restoration should result in smooth, regular lines without any sign of prior surgery. Sharp edges as well as an obliteration of the postauricular sulcus and of the access to the outer ear canal should be avoided. When viewed anteriorly, the helix should just be seen beyond the antihelical fold. As a rule of thumb, the normal auriculomastoid angle should be approximately 25–35°. The distance between the helical rim and the mastoid should range between 1 and 2 cm depending on the varying distance of the upper, middle and lower part of the auricle to the skull (see clinical anatomy, above). In general, a helix–mastoid distance of less than 1 cm should be avoided because of the resulting displeasing "pinned-back" look. Reconstruction is intended to restore certain abnormalities of the auricle rather than to achieve exact measurements. Reduction of the conchal wall, remodelling of the antihelical and helical vault and

trimming of the lobule are the most common surgical steps in the correction of protruding ears. To produce a good long-term result, the auricle's spring has to be released effectively. This is also true for the prevention of hypertrophic scars and keloids when trimming of excess retroauricular skin has been performed.

Choice of Appropriate Method

There is no single "right" technique that covers all varieties of ear protrusion. Otoplasty is an individualised procedure depending on the nature and localisation of the deformity as well as on the surgeon's experience. As a rule thick, stiff and unyielding cartilages and revision surgery require more invasive procedures than primary surgery on a weak and pliable cartilaginous framework.

Antihelix

The correction of an underdeveloped antihelix with underlying soft and pliable cartilage is best done using suture techniques. In all otoplasty procedures, the auricle's integrity must be particularly respected. Pleasing aesthetic results with smooth natural contours may be achieved using non-absorbable, braided threads via an open approach, according to Mustardé (1963; Fig. 38.4), or in a closed way, according to Kaye (1967) or Fritsch (1995; Fig. 38.5). The advantages of a suture technique are its simplicity, versatility and the low risk of early complications. Because the remaining spring of the cartilage can cause stretching of scars in the long term, however, suture

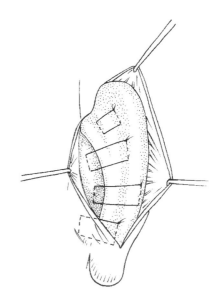

Fig. 38.4 Suture technique combined with posterior weakening of the cartilage using a diamond burr

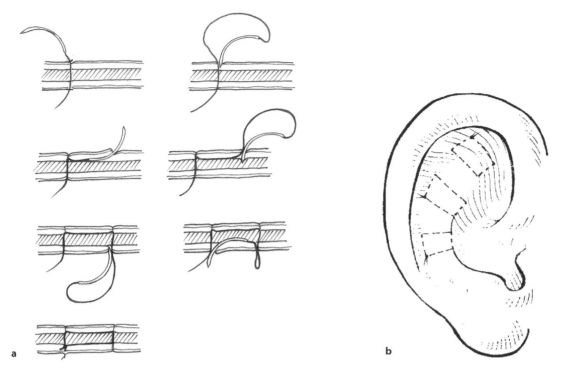

Fig. 38.5a,b Suture technique according to Kaye (1967) and Fritsch (1995). **a** Transcartilaginous mattress sutures are placed subcutaneously. **b** Sutures in place

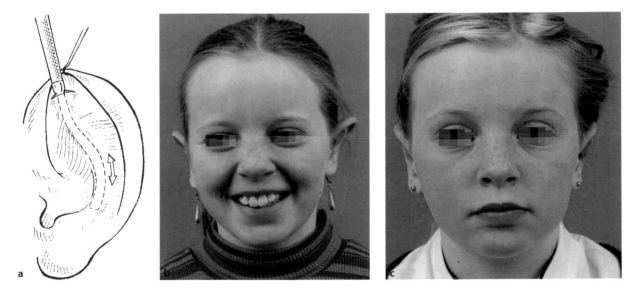

Fig. 38.6a–c Anterior scoring technique. **a** Surgical procedure. **b** Protrusion of the upper pole. **c** Six months after anterior scoring combined with retroauricular mattress sutures

techniques have a higher risk of relapse. Even late complications such as tearing of sutures through the cartilage or foreign-body reactions may give rise to unsatisfactory long-term results.

Major antihelical deformities with an underlying stiff, unyielding and thick cartilage require additional proce-

dures to suturing. The tendency of the auricle to slip back to the previous position is best reduced by the combination of scoring, burring and incision of the cartilage. The anterior scoring techniques described by Stenstroem (1963) and others are most appropriate, especially in severe protrusion of the upper pole (Fig. 38.6). They follow the findings of Gibson and Davis (1958), who showed that cartilage bends away from the scored surface. Thinning of the cartilage by a diamond burr from a posterior aspect is contrary to these findings, but also provides pleasing results when combined with adjusting mattress sutures (Heppt et al. 2001). This is true also for the Converse technique (Converse et al. 1955), which consists of suturing and posterior incisions of the cartilage without involvement of the anterior perichondrium (Fig. 38.7).

Conchal Hyperplasia, Increased Conchomastoid Angle

In ear protrusion caused by a conchal hyperplasia or an enlarged conchomastoid angle palpation and bending the pinna backwards determine the surgical procedure by providing information about the cartilaginous elasticity and traction forces of the anterior helical ligaments. Correction is done using a posterior approach. It usually consists

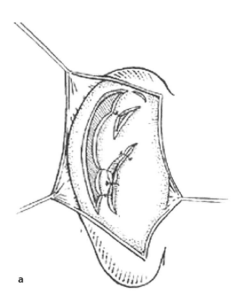

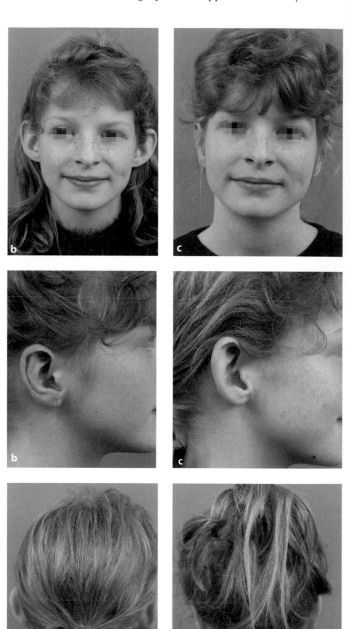

Fig. 38.7a–c Revisional surgery using the Converse technique. a Surgical procedure. b Preoperative view. c One year after surgery

of the removal of retroauricular soft tissue followed by a conchal setback technique using sutures between the conchal cartilage and the periosteum of the mastoid, as described by Furnas (1968). Excision of the conchal cartilage next to the outer ear canal and the anterior helical base, as well as severing of the anterior helical ligaments, are common procedures that may produce an additional setback of the auricle. These procedures release the cartilaginous spring and help to prevent obstruction of the outer ear canal. However, care must be taken to avoid injuring the superficial temporal vessels at the anterior helical base and obliterating the retroauricular sulcus. In severe hyperplasia of the conchal bowl, additional trimming of excess cartilage just below the antihelix is recommended.

Prominent Lobule

For the correction of a prominent lobule synthetic, slow absorbable mattress sutures placed between the lobule and the posterior cavum have found to be highly effective. Pulling the lobule medially may be helped by separation and trimming of the antitragus and the helical tail as well as by transection of fibrous attachments across the fissure between the antihelix and the cavum. If lobule malposition is caused by enlarged retrolobular soft tissue, skin and soft-tissue resection is needed in a dovetailed manner. However, this has to be done very carefully because of the higher risk for keloids in that area.

Severe Deformities, Revision Surgery

In revision surgery and severe primary deformities with strong unyielding cartilage, cutting techniques may be required to achieve pleasing and stable results (Walter 1977). Based on the finding that the separation of the cartilage into segments helps to minimise the tension within the cartilage, these methods help to reduce the recurrence rate markedly. Because the various incisions and excisions of cartilage can incur a higher risk of complications, however, these techniques should be restricted to experienced surgeons (Heppt 2004).

Operative Management

Timing

Otoplasty in protruding ears and other minor deformities is recommended by the age of 5–6 years to prevent psychological problems at school. At that time, the size of the auricle will have reached about 85–90% of the adult size. The cartilage of a child is relatively soft and easy for the surgeon to reshape.

Medical Consultation

The preoperative consultation should reveal the motivation and expectations related to ear correction. It is essential that not only the auricular deformity, but also the psychological situation is taken into consideration. To minimise surgical complications, information about the general medical history, with special regard to bleeding disorders, ingestion of drugs such as aspirin, allergic reactions and tendency for hypertrophic scarring and keloid formations is needed. Prior surgery, hair type and preferences of hairstyle are other factors influencing the preoperative planning. The patient or parents must have realistic expectations about what is surgically possible, as well as the potential risks of surgery. These include general surgical complications such as haematoma and infection, and risks that are specific to otoplasty: visible irregularities, scars, asymmetry, increased sensitivity to cold, disorders of sensation and the need for further surgery.

Peri- and Post-operative Care

In children, otoplasty is usually done under general anaesthesia as a day-case procedure. This changes around the age of 10–12 years when local anaesthesia with sedation starts to become feasible. The risk of post-operative infection may be minimised by the use of an intravenous single-shot antibiotic and by local dressing using antibiotic-impregnated cotton. For dressing and prevention of haematomas, dry cotton is placed into the curvatures and around the auricle, supported by a loose elastic hair band. Due to the risk of pressure necrosis, tight dressing has to be strictly avoided. The auricle has to be checked on the 1st day after surgery to inspect for haematoma formation and to ensure proper preservation of the auricular contours. A second, similar dressing is then reapplied for 5–6 days. An elastic hair band has to be employed for another 2–3 weeks, if possible all times, especially while asleep. Direct sun or cold should be avoided for about 2 months because the sensitivity of the auricle can be diminished; sport is not recommended for about 4 weeks. These periods of time are true for cutting and combined methods, but may be shortened in pure suture techniques.

Results

With selection of the appropriate technique and proper handling, otoplasty has been found to be highly effective for protruding ears. More than 90% of patients or parents are satisfied even when otoplasty results in a certain degree of overcorrection. The onset of early complications arising up to 14 days after surgery, including

38

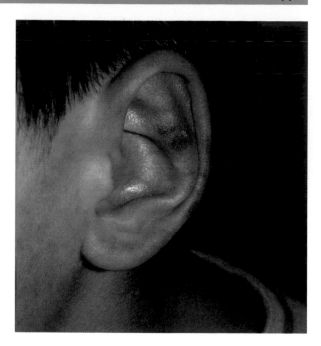

Fig. 38.8 Foreign body reaction due to non-absorbable threads after incisionless suture technique

haematoma, infection, allergic reaction to local materials, reaction to anaesthetics, pressure necrosis by tight dressing, paraesthesia, pain and hypersensitivity, is low. The risk of late complications depends primarily on the surgical method as well as on the surgeon's experience. According to the literature, the rate of relapse of auricular protrusion varies from 2 to 13%. On analysing the results, differences between certain procedures become evident. As a rule, the more invasive the technique, the less is the risk of recurrence. The lowest risk of relapse in the long term can be achieved by performing cutting or combined techniques, because these can release the auricle's spring most efficiently. However, the increased risk of other late complications such as overcorrection (telephone ear), cartilaginous irregularity, unpleasant scaring and keloids has to be taken into account. Due to the difficulties in revision of those complications, less invasive techniques should be preferred whenever possible, even when some permanent sutures might be visible from the posterior view and late foreign-body reactions may occur (Fig. 38.8).

Trauma

Owing to the exposed position of the auricle, traumatic lesions are common in childhood. Auricular avulsions, tearing out of earrings and human or animal dog bites are some common types of trauma. The treatment mo-

dality depends on the cause and the type of auricular injury. As every blunt and penetrating trauma may result in displeasing deformities, early examination and treatment is mandatory.

Abrasion

Superficial injuries of the epidermis (abrasion) usually heal without any scarring within a few weeks. The healing process may be supported by initial cleansing and topical application of antibiotic ointment. To prevent tattooing of the wound, any embedded foreign bodies must be removed meticulously.

Haematoma

Any trauma of the auricle may cause a haematoma between the perichondrium and the cartilage. Because the skin of the anterior surface is tightly attached to the underlying perichondrium and cartilage, even slight blunt trauma may lead to an injury of blood vessels within the perichondrium and to a detachment of both layers. This may be followed by cartilage necrosis and formation of new cartilage, creating a cauliflower appearance (Ohlsen et al. 1975). Thus haematomas have to be treated as early as possible. In general, simple puncture is not sufficient, as blood clots cannot be removed completely. Therefore, aseptic suction and curettage via a small local incision is required. Only in extended haematomas or in recurrence is it necessary to perform cartilage fenestration: removing cartilage in the area of the haematoma and allowing the anterior and posterior perichondrium to stick together, reduce the risk of recurrence. Local pressure after surgery applied by through-and-through mattress sutures tightened over bolsters and regular control of the dressing are essential to prevent the reaccumulation of fluid.

Laceration

In cases of lacerations with or without cartilage involvement, reapproximation of the wound is required. After proper preparation including aligning of the edges and removal of necrotic tissue, the skin is closed using 5-0 or 6-0 permanent sutures, and the cartilage with 4-0 absorbable sutures when needed. Complete or partial avulsions of the auricle are more challenging. As a rule, all separated parts of the auricle, even when the whole ear is torn, have to be repositioned, suturing all the different layers. Cartilaginous remnants may be stored in subcutaneous pockets adjacent to the wound area for repair at a second stage. Special reconstructive techniques using local flaps and cartilage grafts are needed for major primary defects.

Thermal Injuries, Frostbite

Due to the poor blood supply and the thin subcutaneous layer, the helical rim and the anterior surface of the auricle are predisposed to thermal trauma. Low temperature may lead to superficial or deep frostbite, especially in patients after otoplasty procedures, with loss of sensation or paraesthesia. Because thermal injuries may not only result in oedema and erythema, but in also blisters and necrosis, early treatment is important. The first-line therapy in frostbitten auricles consists of rewarming with warm, moist cotton swabs, a painful procedure that should be done under local anaesthesia and sedation. Small superficial blisters can be left to resorb spontaneously, whereas bigger ones have to be punctured aseptically. The local application of antibiotic-containing ointments protects against infection. Debridement and removal of necrosis as well as reconstruction should be carried out carefully in the late phase of wound healing, rather than in its initial stage. Following this treatment plan will provide acceptable results.

In all traumatic lesions of the auricle, deeper injuries (ear canal, ear drum) have to be excluded.

Summary for the Clinician

- In clinical practice, the most common auricular deformities patients seek treatment for are protruding ears and traumatic lesions. Correction of both has to meet the demand for a normal-sized, natural-looking ear with correct position in relation to other facial features.
- In protruding ears, the main structures to be addressed are the antihelix, the conchal wall and the lobule. Conservative treatment using moulding and special dressings may be of some benefit when applied early in life. Later, otoplasty procedures are the treatment of choice. The selection for the appropriate surgical technique depends on the type of the auricular deformity, the surgeon's experience and the characteristics of the cartilaginous framework. In general, suture techniques are best suited for a soft and pliable cartilage, whereas incision, scoring, burring and combined techniques for stiff, unyielding cartilages and for revision surgery.
- Early treatment is mandatory for traumatic lesions, to prevent infection and disfigurement of the auricle.

References

1. Converse JM, Nigro A, Wilson FA, et al (1955) A technique for surgical correction of lop ears. Plast Reconst Surg 15:411–418
2. Davies JE (1987) Surgical embryology. In: Davis JE (ed) Aesthetic and Reconstructive Otoplasty. Springer, New York, pp 93–125
3. Fritsch MH (1995) Incisionless otoplasty. Laryngoscope 105:1–11
4. Furnas DW (1968) Correction of prominent ears by conchamastoid sutures. Plast Reconstr Surg 42:189–193
5. Gibson T, Davis WB (1958) The distortion of autogenous cartilage grafts: its cause and prevention. Br J Plast Surg 10:257–264
6. Heppt W, Siegert R, Walter C, et al (2001) Otoplasty. Springer, Berlin
7. Heppt WJ (2004) The incision–excision technique in minor auricular deformities. Facial Plast Surg 20:287–292
8. Kaye BL (1967) A simplified method for correcting the prominent ear. Plast Reconstruct Surg 40:44–48
9. Kenny FM, Angsusingha K, Stinson D, et al (1973) Unconjugated estrogens in the perinatal period. Pediatr Res 7:826–831
10. Marx H (1926) Die Missbildungen des Ohres. In: Denker A, Kahler O (eds) Handbuch der Hals-Nasen-Ohrenheilkunde. Bd IV. Springer, Berlin, pp 131–152
11. Mustardé JC (1963) The correction of prominent ears by using simple mattress sutures. Br J Plast Surg 16:170–178
12. Ohlsen L, Skoog T, Sohn SA (1975) The pathogenesis of cauliflower ear. An experimental study in rabbits. Scand J Plast Reconstr Surg 9:34–39
13. Stenstroem SJ (1963) A "natural" technique for correction of congenitally prominent ears. Plast Reconstr Surg 32:509–518
14. Tan S, Wright A, Hemphill A, et al (2003) Correction of deformational auricular anomalies by moulding – results of a fast-track service. N Z Med J 116:1181–1185
15. Tanzer R (1977) Congenital deformities of the auricle. In: Converse JM (ed) Reconstructive Plastic Surgery. Saunders, Philadelphia, pp 1671–1719
16. Walter C (1977) Korrektur von Formfehlern der Ohrmuschel. Arch Otorhinolaryngol 202:203–228
17. Weerda H (1988) Classification of congenital deformities of the auricle. Facial Plast Surg 5:385–388

Diagnosis and Management Strategies in Congenital Middle and External Ear Anomalies

Frank Declau, Paul Van De Heyning and Cor Cremers

Core Messages

- Congenital anomalies of the middle ear, atresia of the external ear canal and microtia of the pinna often coexist in an individual child. It is rather uncommon for these to accompany malformations of the inner ear.
- Classification of congenital ossicular abnormalities, atresia and microtia is important, as it allows proper comparison of outcomes after treatment.
- All children found to have congenital atresia or microtia must be referred immediately for audiological assessment.
- In bilateral anomalies, amplification should be provided as early as possible after birth.
- In unilateral cases, additional help in the classroom may be needed; amplification should also be considered.
- Nearly 28% of children with aural atresia/microtia have other abnormalities. Paediatric and genetic assessment and counselling should form part of their overall management.
- Radiology is important:
  - to assess the degree of abnormality
  - to exclude cholesteatoma in cases of partial atresia
  - to assess the state of the middle ear and course of the facial nerve
  - to identify the rare concomitant inner ear anomalies.

- Surgery for ossicular malformations may be considered after the age of 10 years, but should only be undertaken by experienced surgeons. The parents should be advised of the potential risks to the facial nerve and of sensorineural deafness. Bone-anchored hearing aids (BAHA) should be mentioned as an alternative solution.
- Only 50% of children with atresia are considered potential candidates for surgical repair. Repair should take place after the age of 6 years and in experienced hands. BAHA should be offered as an alternative, and is also the best strategy for those who do not fit the criteria for surgery.
- Partial atresia with a bony stenotic canal diameter of 2 mm or less carries a 91% risk of cholesteatoma developing by the age of 12 years. Surgery is recommended in these cases.
- For microtia, total auricular reconstruction using autologous rib cartilage provides good results in the hands of an experienced surgeon, when a near-normal cosmetic appearance should result, and further maintenance is not required. An osseointegrated prosthesis is an alternative and is also available for cases of failed autologous reconstruction.

Contents

Introduction

The main types of congenital abnormality of the middle and external ear will be discussed in this chapter. In many cases, a single child may well have congenital malformations in two or three of the separate parts of the ear. It is relatively uncommon, however, for congenital problems in the middle and outer ear to be accompanied by parallel malformations in the inner ear (in about 8%), since this is formed in the embryo at a different period of intrauterine development. In discussing this group of congenital anomalies, there is still some variation in the use of descriptive terms. For this reason we begin with definitions of the terms to be used in this chapter.

Congenital middle ear anomalies may affect the dimensions of the middle ear cavity and one or more of the three ossicles. Congenital malformations of the external auditory canal (EAC) are described as atresia, and consist of absence or narrowing of the EAC. Microtia consists of malformation of the pinna and associated structures. Management of middle ear malformation, atresia and microtia, is one of the most challenging types of surgery faced by the reconstructive and ENT surgeon.

Epidemiology

In Europe, a prevalence of 1.07 in 10,000 births for microtia-anotia (M-A) was found in the period of 1980–2003. Health Department statistics of the City of New York for a 10-year period (1952–1962) showed that there was a rate of 1 in 5800 births (Jahrsdoerfer 1978). According to the Swedish Board of Welfare statistics, the frequency of isolated external ear and external ear canal malformations in 1980 amounted to 0.92 per 10,000 live births Variable prevalence rates can be due to variable registration as well as a lack of standardisation of definition and diagnosis.

Microtia can occur either as an isolated defect or in association with other defects. It occurs more often in right ears and males, especially in unilateral microtia. The occurrence in general is more often in Hispanics and Asians than blacks and whites. The cause of microtia is multifactorial. Fewer than 15% of the cases have a positive family history. Only in a minority of cases has a genetic or environmental cause been found; in these cases, microtia is usually part of a specific pattern of multiple congenital anomalies. For instance, microtia is an essential component of isotretinoin embryopathy, it is an important manifestation of thalidomide embryopathy, and can be part of prenatal alcohol syndrome or maternal diabetes embryopathy. Microtia occurs in association with several single gene disorders, such as Treacher Collins syndrome, or chromosomal syndromes, such as trisomy 18. M-A also occurs as part of seemingly non-random patterns of multiple defects, such as Goldenhar syndrome.

Congenital atresia has been reported in patients with chromosomal anomalies, especially terminal deletions starting at chromosome 18q23. Veltman et al. (2003) stated that atresia occurs in approximately 66% of all patients who have a terminal deletion of 18q. They reported a series of 20 patients with atresia, of whom 18 had microscopically visible 18q deletions. The extent and nature of the chromosome 18 deletions were studied in detail by array-based comparative genomic hybridisation. A critical region of 5 Mb on chromosome 18q22.3-q23 was deleted in all patients. Veltman et al. (2003) concluded that this region can be considered a candidate region for aural atresia.

Aural atresia is usually (70–85%) unilateral. The deformity on each side can vary in complexity. For unknown reasons, males outnumber females and the right ear is the ear more commonly involved (Okajima et al. 1996). There are no proper data on the prevalence or incidence of minor anomalies. The latter are syndromal in 25% of cases.

Table 39.1 HEAR classification for ossicular malformations (after Declau et al. 1999)

I: Isolated congenital stapes ankylosis
A. Footplate fixation
B. Stapes suprastructure fixation
II: Stapes ankylosis + another ossicular chain anomaly
A. Discontinuity of the chain
B. Epitympanic fixation
C. Tympanic fixation
III: Congenital anomaly of the ossicular chain but a mobile stapes footplate
A. Discontinuity of the chain
B. Epitympanic fixation
C. Tympanic fixation
IV: Congenital aplasia or severe dysplasia of the oval or round window: aplasia or dysplasia
VII nerve crossing oval window; persistent stapedial artery

Table 39.2 HEAR classification for congenital atresia of the external ear canal (after Declau et al. 1999)

Type I: mild: tympanic membrane is smaller in area than normal; various kinds of ossicular malformations may be present.
Type II: moderate: atretic plate; tympanic cavity is within normal limits
IIa: tympanic bone hypoplastic; course of the facial nerve usually normal
IIb: tympanic bone absent; abnormal course of the facial nerve
Type III: severe: no canal, and a severely hypoplastic tympanic cavity

Classification

Ossicular Malformation

The classification of the minor middle ear anomalies is modified after Teunissen and Cremers (1993; Table 39.1) and has been approved by the HEAR consensus group of the European Workgroup on Genetics of Hearing Impairment. This classification is based on the pre-operative findings and has direct impact on the reconstruction technique applied. This classification is not based on the degree of abnormality, but depends on the degree of fixation of the stapedial footplate or on the presence or absence of accompanying anomalies of the other ossicles.

Atresia Classification

The atresias are classified according a modification of the classification of Altmann (1955; Table 39.2). This classification is based on the degree of malformations present. Altmann (1955) was the first to propagate a histopathological classification according to the severity of the atresia. He divided his cases into three categories: mildly, moderately and severely malformed types; In mild cases (type I), the tympanic membrane is still present but smaller in area than normal. The tympanic bone is normal or reduced in diameter, with narrowing of the bony annulus. Type 1 atresia may be associated with various kinds of ossicular malformation. In moderate cases (type II), there is total or partial failure of the EAC to develop, with either an atresia plate or solid bone lying lateral to the middle ear cavity. The course of the facial nerve may be abnormal; the tympanic cavity is within normal limits. In severe cases (type III), there is no external canal and a severely hypoplastic tympanic cavity.

Marquet and Declau (1991) and Cremers et al. (1988) further subclassified the type II patients into types lla and llb, based on the surgical findings and functional outcome. This subdivision is included in Table 39.2 (Declau et al. 1997). Marquet and Declau (1991) based their subclassification of the moderate cases (type II) in Altmann's classification scheme on the course of the facial canal in its third segment, the morphology of the atretic plate, the presence or absence of a tympanic bone and the distance between glenoid cavity and the anterior surface of the mastoid. The surgical outcome was highly related to the proposed subclassification (Declau et al. 1997).

In type IIa, the course of the facial nerve is normal in its third segment. There is a total bony atresia over only a part of the length of the canal or the canal is partially aplastic and ends blindly with a fistula tract, sometimes leading to a rudimentary tympanic membrane (Fig. 39.1). The distance between glenoid cavity and mastoid is within normal limits.

In type IIb, the course of the facial nerve is situated more anteriorly in its third segment. There is total bony stenosis of the EAC (Fig. 39.2). The distance between glenoid cavity and mastoid is significantly diminished.

For radiological criteria, the scoring system defined by Jahrsdoerfer et al. (1992) is recommended.

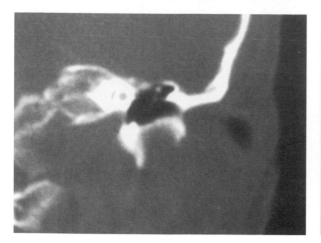

Fig 39.1 Coronal computed tomography (CT) view of atresia type IIa. Coronal view through the external auditory canal; incomplete bony closure by atretic plate formed by squamosal bone and malformed tympanic bone. Abnormal ossicular chain

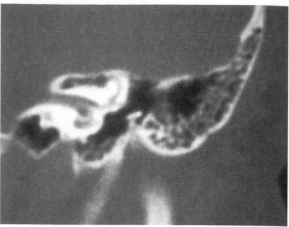

Fig 39.2 Coronal CT view of atresia type IIb. Absence of tympanic bone; bony closure by atretic plate formed by squamosal and petrous bone. Undeep hypotympanum and dysplastic ossicular chain fixed to the atretic plate

Microtia Classification

One widely adopted system assigns a grade from I to III based on the severity of the deformity. Grade I represents a pinna with all anatomic subunits present but abnormally shaped. Grade II represents a pinna with some recognisable subunits but rudimentary and malformed. Grade III includes the classic "peanut" ear (Fig. 39.3), which is severely deformed, with an inferior fibroadipose lobule and a nubbin of cartilage in the superior remnant.

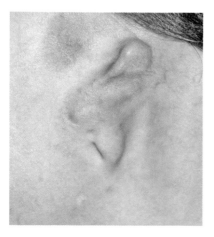

Fig 39.3 Typical aspect of microtia grade III which is often seen in combination with meatal atresia

Patient Evaluation

These congenital anomalies cause moderate to severe hearing loss and require early detection after birth. There needs to be accurate assessment of the hearing level within 3 months by auditory evoked potentials, using both air- and bone-conduction stimuli. In bilateral anomalies, amplification by air- or bone-conduction hearing aids within 6 months after birth is essential to avoid delays in speech or language development. According to current international opinion, infants whose permanent hearing impairment is diagnosed before the age of 3 months and who receive appropriate and consistent early intervention at an average of 2–3 months after identification of hearing loss, have significantly higher levels of receptive and expressive language, personal–social development, expressive and receptive vocabulary, general development, situation comprehension and vowel production (Yoshinaga-Itano et al. 1998; see also Chapter 36). Counselling is needed, not only to establish any hereditary pattern, but also to identify anomalies in other systems.

History and Physical Examination

Middle and external ear anomalies may be isolated or associated with other malformations. To determine a syndromal aetiology, a systematic physical examination and history are needed, not only in the craniofacial region, but also of other organ systems. The examiner should include questions on drug utilisation or toxic exposure during pregnancy and on any familial history of hearing impairment as well as auricular or other developmental craniofacial abnormalities. In addition to the aforementioned data, information regarding low birth weight, maternal intrauterine infections or trauma should be queried. If the patient is a young child, achievement of developmental milestones, such as speech and ambulation, are assessed through history and direct observation.

Of patients with aural atresia, 27.8% have concomitant abnormalities, whereas a well-defined syndrome can be found in 5.8%. In particular, the spine and genitourinary tract systems require careful evaluation. The calibre of the EAC should be graded as normal, stenotic, blindly ending or atretic. Patients with a stenotic or blindly ending external canal may escape diagnosis for years if the auricle is normal or only slightly deformed. There is no general agreement as to whether the degree of differentiation of the external ear correlates with the degree of malformation of the middle ear. Because the external ear develops embryologically earlier than the middle ear, it would be unlikely to find a normal middle ear in the presence of microtia, whereas a malformed middle ear can occur with a normal pinna (Jahrsdoerfer 1978). The face of the patient should be examined carefully to reveal any muscle weakness. It is rare to encounter a facial paresis or paralysis involving the entire hemiface, although there is occasionally involvement of the lower face or lip area. The most common anomaly of facial function is a congenital absence of the depressor anguli oris muscle. If surgery is planned, preoperative photographs are essential.

Audiometric Evaluation

According to the high-risk registry of the American Academy of Pediatrics, congenital aural atresia and microtia are identified as high-risk factors. The child's usable residual hearing and the need for amplification should be determined as soon as possible after birth. When congenital atresia or microtia is diagnosed in a neonate, the paediatrician must immediately refer the child to the ear surgeon for further audiological evaluation. Delay of testing or a wait-and-see strategy is not in the infant's best interest. In the vast majority of cases, sensorineural function is normal and the atresia of the external ear canal causes a 45–60 dB conductive hearing loss. If both ears are affected, early hearing-aid fitting is called for. If it seems that the atresia is unilateral, then the status of normal hearing in the opposite ear must be clearly established. Transient otoacoustic emission (TOAE) testing, if the contralateral ear canal and tympanic membrane appear normal, with auditory-evoked-brainstem-response technologies can be used as diagnostic tests for the hearing status. This testing will establish the presence of cochlear function and the overall degree of hearing loss, thus aiding determination of the type of auditory rehabilitation

needed. Adequacy of inner vestibular can also be assessed by a rotational or caloric response vestibular test.

Radiological Assessment

This is also discussed in Chapter 40. Axial and coronal computed tomography (CT) scans of the temporal bone are necessary in all patients with atresia as well as those with severe stenosis of the EAC. In the latter group, radiographic studies are important to examine for possible cholesteatoma formation. High-resolution, thin-cut (1.5 mm) imaging modalities form the standard for evaluation of congenital atresia and the status of the middle ear. CT scan also provides information on the position of the facial nerve. Special attention is focused on its relationship to the oval window (i.e. normally positioned or overhanging) and the position of its vertical segment. Anterior displacement of the vertical segment of the nerve restricts access to the middle ear space, reducing the chance for a successful hearing result after surgery and increasing the risk of facial nerve injury. Also, the extent and type of the atretic plate is examined as well as ossicular and inner ear development, and the pneumatisation of the middle ear and mastoid. Rarely, an abnormality of the horizontal semicircular canal or vestibule is seen. The latter finding suggests an abnormal communication between the perilymph and cerebrospinal fluid. In such cases, manipulation of the stapes should be avoided to avoid the potential complication of a cerebrospinal fluid gusher and loss of all remaining hearing. Three-dimensional CT may aid visualisation and has the ability plan surgical reconstruction, if this is contemplated. Also, stereolithographic model reconstruction from CT has been used for assessment and surgical planning in congenital aural atresia.

The CT scan may be obtained after birth or at the time of surgical repair. Although studies at an earlier age are rarely applicable to immediate rehabilitative plans, they may be important to establish the syndromal aetiology. Periodic CT scans are not necessary in patients with a completely atretic ear canal, given the rarity of cholesteatoma in that situation.

Medical Management

The otologic surgeon is usually alerted to the possibility of microtia or atresia by the obstetrician or paediatrician shortly after birth. Quite often the parents have some guilt about a particular incident or practice, and it is important to ascertain if this is the case so that these fears can be alleviated. During early infancy, the child should be evaluated in a complete and thorough fashion to determine the need for amplification. Genetic counselling is equally important to establish the aetiology and to rule out associated anomalies in other organ systems. During early childhood, it is important to survey both ears for the presence of otitis media. Especially in unilateral atresia cases, the normal ear should regularly be followed to exclude otitis media with effusion. If secretory otitis media is present, prompt medical or surgical therapy is needed. The atretic ear may also be involved and exhibit signs of acute otitis media. If the atretic ear is suspected of having an acute otitis media, prompt antibiotic treatment should be started to minimise the risk of complications such as coalescent mastoiditis or subdural abscess.

Minor deformities in ear shape may be overcome by early splinting or taping of a newborn child's ear. Such non-surgical treatment of microtia, involving a prosthetic device fixed with adhesives, is sometimes an alternative to surgical correction.

Unilateral Atresia

Medical intervention is not necessary in the infant discovered to have unilateral atresia. Paediatric audiometry should be performed to confirm that the child has normal hearing in the other ear. The parents are then reassured that speech, language and intellectual development will proceed normally. As the child enters school, preferential seating is advised, but rarely is a hearing aid recommended because of the poor acceptance by most children. In classrooms with unavoidable background noise, a sound field amplification system can be helpful. A trial with a hearing aid may be useful if speech and language development are delayed. Teenagers and adults often find the consequences of unilateral hearing loss from atresia to be a significant aggravation in social settings and at work, and may more readily accept a hearing aid. Conventional bone-conduction hearing aids are rarely helpful. If the canal is only stenotic, an air-conduction aid is preferred because of cosmetics, better sound localisation, broader frequency response and less sound distortion. Also, a contralateral routing of signal system mounted in a spectacle frame can be proposed in selected cases.

Bilateral Atresia

In infants with bilateral atresia, early amplification as early as the 3rd month of life is essential. Auditory training should begin at 6 months of age (Jahrsdoerfer 1978). The initial medical and audiological evaluations can be completed within the first few months of life, and a bone-conduction hearing aid fitted soon thereafter. With the latest addition to the bone-anchored hearing aid (BAHA) system, the BAHA Softband, even the youngest children can be provided with adequate amplification by bone conduction. The Softband is an elastic band with a

BAHA sound processor connected to a plastic snap connector disk sewn into the band. The band has a Velcro fastening, which enables it to be easily adjusted to fit the size of the baby's head. The results of this transcutaneous transmission are comparable with those of conventional bone conductors. In this application, the more powerful BAHA Classic is more appropriate than the BAHA Compact.

These children will remain deprived of bilateral speech "cues". However, there is experimental evidence that the auditory system is able to adapt in some way to binaural inputs even after childhood (van der Pouw et al. 1998).

Surgical Management

The accounts that follow, of surgical repair of congenital atresia of the EAC and of middle ear malformations, should be read in conjunction with the description of BAHAs and auricular prostheses given in Chapter 44.

Ossicular Malformation Surgery

In case of isolated ossicular malformations, the preoperative inclusion criteria are: (1) older than 10 years; (2) no intermittent periods of secretory otitis media; (2) tonal and speech audiogram performed as well as tympanometry with contralateral stapedial reflexes; (4) high-resolution CT scan performed.

The surgical results for ossicular malformations without atresia are quite good (Teunissen and Cremers 1993). With the exception of severe dysplasia or aplasia of the oval and/or round window, a post-operative air–bone gap of ≤20 dB was found in 72% of the operated cases. However, the risk of incurring a sensorineural hearing loss exists. This form of procedure should be performed by experienced surgeons, and parents and children should be carefully advised of potential risks to hearing and to the facial nerve.

Atresia Repair Surgery

Patients with atresia may be offered the choice between surgical correction and a BAHA. Atresia repair surgery should only be performed in carefully selected patients after a thorough investigation of all parameters involved. A proper selection based on stringent audiological and radiological criteria is obligatory. Preoperatively, a complete audiometric assessment is performed as well as a high-resolution CT scan of the temporal bones.

Since 1843, when Thomson published the first attempt of an operative treatment for congenital aural atresia, much work has been done to improve the surgical technique and many authors have published their techniques and results. Surgical management is aimed at obtaining functional hearing gain and establishing an auditory canal that is wide and stable enough for the application of hearing aids. Surgical correction is a one-stage procedure. However, revision surgery is often needed (25–50%: Jahrsdoerfer 1978).

Surgical Planning

Selection Criteria

Accurate preoperative assessment is essential in determining surgical candidacy, because only 50% of patients with aural atresia are candidates for repair (Jahrsdoerfer et al. 1992). Jahrsdoerfer et al. (1992) have developed a grading system (Table 39.3) based on preoperative temporal bone CT and auricular appearance, to aid in patient selection for surgical correction. In their system, there is a maximum score of 10 points. The total score aids in determining whether the patient will benefit from surgery to correct the hearing mechanism. A patient with a score of 5 or less is not a surgical candidate. This grading system correlates well with the degree of hearing improvement achieved, because 80% of patients with scores of 8 or higher have a post-operative speech reception threshold of 25 dB or less. Patients with syndromes involving craniofacial maldevelopment (Treacher Collins or hemifacial microsomia) are considered poor surgical candidates. In these and familiar syndromes, the middle ear is usually poorly developed and the surgical grade is often 5/10 (poor or marginal candidate) or worse.

Table 39.3 Selection criteria (after Jahrsdoerfer et al. 1992)

Parameter	Points
Stapes present	2
Oval window open	1
Middle ear space	1
Facial nerve	1
Malleus/incus complex	1
Mastoid pneumatisation	1
Incus–stapes connection	1
Round window	1
Appearance external ear	1
Total available points	10

Unilateral Versus Bilateral Atresia Repair

Although most otologic surgeons would consider atresia repair in bilateral cases, many are reluctant to operate on unilateral atresias. This reluctance is based on expectations of hearing recovery and the potential morbidity associated with the surgery (Fig. 39.4). In patients with unilateral aural atresia, the operated ear should compete against the good hearing threshold in the other normal ear. A patient with a unilateral congenital ear defect will only benefit materially from middle ear surgery if the hearing is sufficiently improved to provide binaural hearing. The patient with a unilateral conductive loss must be made to understand what he or she can expect from successful surgery. He or she will be able to hear stereo music, tell the direction of sound and will hear more readily in a situation where there is background noise; in a quiet room, on a one-to-one basis, little appreciable difference would be noted.

Evidence indicates that children with unilateral hearing loss from any cause are at risk for delayed language

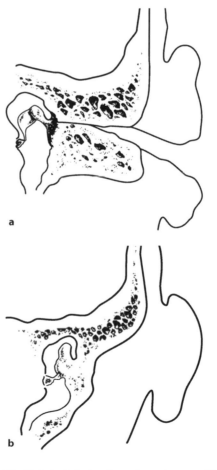

Fig 39.4 Artist's drawing of atresia types II a (**a**) and II b (**b**): coronal view

development, attention deficit and poor school performance. Speech recognition in patients after successful surgery for unilateral ear anomalies seems to be satisfactory, although poorer than those with normal ears. Dichotic listening tests have revealed a non-atretic ear advantage in post-operative unilateral atresia patients, suggesting a sensitive and critical period for aural development before the age of 5 years.

Patients with bilateral atresia present less of a surgical dilemma. The surgeon has to compare the suspected hearing improvement using surgery with the rehabilitation using a bone-conduction hearing aid (conventional or bone-anchored). The goal in these individuals is to restore sufficient hearing so that amplification is no longer needed. Therefore, the "better" (as determined on CT scan evaluation) ear is selected for the initial surgical procedure.

Timing of Surgery

Timing of surgical repair depends on whether unilateral or bilateral aural atresia is present. The vast majority of authors agree that surgery for bilateral atresia of the external meatus should not be carried out before the age of 5–6 years and they point out that surgical treatment of younger patients is justified only if complications such as cholesteatoma are present. By this time, accurate audiometric tests can be obtained, pneumatisation of the temporal bone is well advanced, and children are capable of co-operating with post-operative care. Although most surgeons are comfortable operating on the first ear of a child with bilateral atresia as he or she approaches school age, some are reluctant to recommend surgery at that age in unilateral cases. Delay until adulthood, when the patient can make his or her own decision, is then recommended.

Timing of Microtia Repair

According to Jahrsdoerfer (1978), what really matters is the co-operation and dialogue between plastic and otologic surgeon, and the willingness to integrate their ideas and surgical needs for the good of the patient.

It was originally believed that the atresia repair should precede the microtia repair. This was because it was thought that the opening in the mastoid could only be made precisely when the original position of the auricular remnant and of the temporomandibular joint was known. Furthermore, it was believed that there would be less manoeuvrability of the skin, and access to the middle ear would be limited. However, Aguilar and Jahrsdoerfer (1988) demonstrated that the auricular framework can be sufficiently manoeuvred to align the meatus and the new canal, and recommended that auricular reconstruction should be performed first in order to preserve the integrity of the blood supply.

Cholesteatoma

A patient with congenital aural atresia and chronic otorrhoea or cholesteatoma requires surgery for eradication of the disease to prevent further complications, regardless of the potential for hearing improvement. Should there be a draining fistula or trapped cholesteatoma, surgical intervention is warranted immediately. Congenital aural stenosis (canal opening of 4 mm or less), as compared to congenital aural atresia, carries a much greater risk of cholesteatoma.

A bony ear canal opening of 2 mm or less puts the patient at risk of cholesteatoma formation. According to studies, 91% of the ears with a stenosis of 2 mm or less have developed a cholesteatoma by the age of 12 years. Surgery is recommended for patients with stenosis of the external ear canal measuring 2 mm or less. The appropriate time is late childhood or early adolescence, before irreversible damage has occurred.

Surgical Techniques

There are three surgical approaches to the creation of a new EAC: the anterior, transmastoid and modified anterior approaches.

Anterior Approach

This method requires the removal of the atretic plate before the middle ear is reached. Dissection begins along the linea temporalis immediately posterior to the temporomandibular joint. The mastoid cells are not opened and the posterior wall of the EAC is preserved. The dura mater at the tegmen tympani superiorly and the glenoid fossa anteriorly are the key landmarks in this approach. These are followed medially through the atresia plate into the epitympanum, allowing the identification of the ossicles. This approach avoids injury to the variably located vertical portion of the facial nerve, as long as the dissection is carried out in an anterosuperior manner with entrance into the epitympanum prior to the exposure of the mesotympanum. The atretic plate is delicately removed with diamond burrs and curettes to avoid acoustic trauma to the inner ear from drill vibration. The abnormally located facial nerve is most commonly found in the inferoposterior portion of the atretic plate, lateral to the middle ear space.

Transmastoid Approach

This method employs a posterior approach to the middle ear and atretic plate. Dissection begins along the linea temporalis over the region of the mastoid cavity. The dura mater of the middle fossa, the sigmoid sinus and the sinodural angle are used as landmarks. Following these medially, the mastoid antrum is entered, allowing identification of the horizontal semicircular canal and atretic plate. If possible, the facial nerve should be identified. The atretic plate is removed, exposing the mesotympanum. The facial ridge is lowered, creating an open mastoid cavity. The cavity must be centred either on the lateral semicircular canal or on the stapes: the hypotympanum is usually never revealed

Modified Anterior Approach

This represents a combined method: first the mastoid at the antrum is opened to identify the short process of the incus. Then the bone immediately anterior of the mastoid is drilled away to obtain a new EAC, preserving an intact bony wall between the mastoid cavity and the newly formed canal. The approach can be compared with an intact canal wall procedure (Marquet and Declau 1991).

Surgical Results

Surgical results are difficult to compare because the selection criteria for surgery are quite divergent, leading to considerable differences in patient population. Moreover, every surgeon uses his or her own audiological criteria to define the operation as a surgical success. Although the kind of approach is readily defined, the surgical details differ considerably among different surgeons. To make meaningful comparisons of outcome, a consensus should be found on the criteria for audiological success. A successful operation can reasonably be defined as one that obviates the need for a hearing aid. Even for such a criterion, differences of interpretation can be found: Cremers et al. (1988) suggested an average hearing threshold level below 30–35 dB.

Even though the results of surgery in different centres are not really comparable, it seems obvious that the audiological results are not very encouraging in the more severe malformed atresia ears. The variability of hearing improvement depends on the severity of the malformation. Whether the aural atresia is unilateral or bilateral does not influence the results (Cremers and Teunissen 1991).

In the hands of the best surgeons, a mean hearing gain of only about 20–25 dB is attained in atresia type II (Altmann classification) and 30–35 dB in type I. The mean hearing gain with atresia repair surgery seems to be somewhat higher in less severely malformed ears. The more favourable cases also usually have a better preoperative hearing. As demonstrated on a Glasgow benefit plot (Browning et al. 1991; Fig. 39.5), the combination of these factors leads to the conclusion that atresia repair surgery should only be done in very selected patients after a thorough investigation of all parameters involved (e.g. age, anatomy, unilateral or bilateral, hearing status). Only the most favourable cases may sufficiently benefit from this kind of surgery.

Although some authors argue that the surgical results are only temporary and decline after some years, the long-term results of Cremers and Teunissen (1991) clearly demonstrate the stability of the acquired hearing results. The surgical results for ossicular malformations without atresia are quite good (Teunissen and Cremers 1993). With the exception of severe dysplasia or aplasia of the oval and/or round window, a post-operative air–bone gap of ≤20 dB was found in 72% of the operated cases.

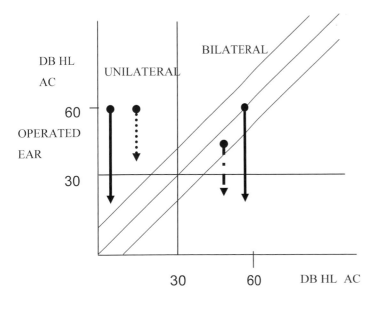

Fig 39.5 Glasgow Benefit plot for unilateral and bilateral aural atresias (after Declau et al. 1999). In this plot, surgical success for aural atresia has been defined as a post-operative hearing level below 30 dB HL. If the preoperative hearing level is around 60 dB HL, the surgical procedure will only be successful if the hearing gain is more than 30 dB. However, a hearing gain of only 20–25 dB is within realistic perspectives. The dotted arrow on the left represents a unilateral case with a functionally unsuccessful operation, while the dashed arrow on the right demonstrates a favourable bilateral case with an acceptable post-operative hearing gain

A meta-analysis of the surgical results of atresia surgery demonstrated a mean hearing gain of 20–25 dB in atresia type II and 30–35 dB in atresia type I (Declau et al. 1999). Surgical correction is only recommended if a post-operative hearing better than 25–30 dB can be predicted. The long-term results remain stable, with little change. Most frequently, the anterior approach is used to open the atretic plate. This type of surgery can be performed from the age of 5–6 years. In the literature, no agreement can be found on the surgery of unilateral cases: some surgeons will not operate on these cases, while others wait until the age of 18 years, so that the patients can decide for themselves. Patients with less favourable predicted outcomes should be helped by BAHAs.

Complications

The most common anatomical complications are chronic infection of the newly formed EAC and lateral displacement of the tympanic graft, canal and/or meatal stenosis. Anatomical complication rates of 20–60% are reported.

Functional complications are related to labyrinthine injury and facial nerve injury. High-frequency sensorineural hearing loss due to acoustic trauma is quite common, whereas accidental labyrinthine fenestration is rare. Despite anomalous positions of the facial nerve, injury to the nerve is rare, with most series reporting no injury or an infrequent transient paralysis. Facial nerve monitoring in surgery for congenital aural atresia is obligatory.

Bone Conduction Implant Surgery

The reader should also refer to Chapter 44 for more information on this topic. Based on the experience with dental implants, the idea of inserting titanium implants into the temporal bone for fixation of a hearing aid by bone conduction was developed by Tjellstrom (1990). The concept of direct bone conduction was introduced and is achieved by using a skin-penetrating coupling from an osseointegrated titanium implant in the mastoid bone to an impedance-matched transducer that the patients can apply and remove at will. Long-term results have been published from centres in Göteborg (Sweden), Nijmegen (The Netherlands) and Birmingham (UK).

The results of the BAHA show not only a hearing gain in the region of 89%, but also better comfort when compared to classical bone-conduction hearing aids. Also, speech discrimination and intelligibility scores are much better (Powell et al. 1996). Owing to the requirements concerning the thickness of the cortical bone and its composition, the age limit for implantation has been set around 2–3 years in most centres (Snik et al. 2005). In children, a two-stage procedure is performed under general anaesthesia: in the first stage the titanium fixtures are placed in the bone at the mastoid (usually 2). At least 3 months later, after osseointegration has taken place, the fixtures are liberated, and the implant can be loaded onto its pedestal 2 weeks later. Four different systems are now on the market: Divino, Classic 300, Compact and Cordelle II.

Total Auricular Reconstruction Surgery

Tanzer published a paper on the use of autogenous rib cartilage in reconstruction of the auricle in 1959 and brought in the new era of auricular reconstruction. Brent (1974) modified Tanzer's technique and has been treating patients with auricular malformation since the 1970s. Another popular technique based on a modification of Tanzer's technique was developed by Nagata (1993). He has been using his technique for treating microtia patients since the 1980s. Other modifications have been described by several authors, including Firmin (1998). Currently, the use of autogenous rib cartilage is still the gold standard for microtia reconstruction. However, many new techniques are being developed, including alloplastic implants, osseointegrated prostheses and tissue engineering.

Surgical Planning

The timing of microtia reconstruction has been much debated in the literature. Factors used to determine the most appropriate timing for auricular reconstruction include the age of external ear maturity, the availability of adequate rib cartilage and the psychological impact of the disease. At birth, the auricle is 66% of its adult size. By age 3 years, it is 85% of its adult size and by age 6 years, it is 95% of its adult size. Rib cartilage is rarely of sufficient size until the age of 5 or 6 years. Whilst the ideal age for rib cartilage harvesting is generally accepted to be 6 years, variations in the factors exist. Tanzer (1959) preferred children to be slightly younger at 5–6 years; Brent (1992) preferred patients to be 7–10 years old. Nagata starts his reconstruction at age 10 years and with a chest circumference of at least 60 cm, which can be confirmed with X-ray (Nagata 1993). This may be related to the relatively large volume of cartilage needed for using his technique for reconstruction. Bilateral microtia and atresia cases may be started at an earlier age, but, according to Brent (1992), beginning surgery prior to age 5.5 years creates technical handicaps and poor patient cooperation.

Surgical Techniques

Total auricular reconstruction has been described as a one- to six-stage procedure. The techniques of Brent

(1974) and Nagata (1993) will be discussed here. Currently, the two-stage technique is most frequently used.

In each of the approaches the basic elements are the same, although the timing and staging may differ. Each reconstruction involves three main elements. These elements are: (1) construction and placement of the costal cartilage framework; (2) rotation of the lobule, conchal excavation and tragal construction; (3) elevation of the helical rim.

Brent Technique (Brent 1974, 1992)

First Stage

This involves auricular framework fabrication using contralateral rib cartilage. A template is made by placing a piece of X-ray film against the normal ear in unilateral cases or the parent's ear in bilateral cases, and tracing all anatomic landmarks. The template is then made several millimetres smaller to accommodate for the thickness of the skin cover and overgrowth potential of the reconstructed ear. The contralateral sixth, seventh and eighth costal cartilages are usually harvested. The base of the framework is carved from the synchondrosis of the sixth and seventh rib cartilage. The helix is carved from the "floating" eighth rib cartilage. The helix is then sutured to the base with clear nylon suture. The fabricated framework is then positioned in a subcutaneous pocket through an incision at the posterior and inferior border of the vestige. An extra piece of cartilage is also banked either in a pocket posterior to where the framework is placed or underneath the chest incision to be used in the later stage for improved ear projection. Two small suction drains are placed and left for 5 days.

Second Stage

The second stage involves lobule transposition, which is performed several months after the stage I procedure. The lobule is mobilised as an inferiorly based tissue flap and rotated to receive the end of the framework. Unused lobule tissue is excised.

Third Stage

The third stage involves elevation of the auricular framework. An incision is made several millimetres from the margin of the rim. Dissection is carried over the capsule of the posterior surface of the constructed costal cartilage until the correct amount of projection is achieved. The banked piece of cartilage is placed between the framework and the mastoid to stabilise the ear position. A split-thickness skin graft is used to cover the back of the elevated cartilage framework.

Fourth Stage

To achieve tragus reconstruction, the fourth stage of this procedure, a composite skin/cartilage graft is taken from the anterolateral conchal surface of the normal ear in unilateral cases, or costal cartilage is used in bilateral cases. A J-shaped incision is made along the posterior tragal margin. The graft is placed through the incision and positioned so that it produces both projection of the tragus and cavitation of the retrotragal hollow. Soft tissue also is removed from the new concha to deepen the conchal bowl. The shadow of the neotragus imitates an EAC. Frontal symmetry is also addressed at this stage.

Recent Modifications

The most recent modification is to incorporate a small cartilage into the framework to create a tragus in stage 1. It is sutured to the inferior aspect of the framework to create an antitragus, then curved around and attached to the crus helix with a bridging mattress suture superiorly to create a tragus.

Nagata Technique (1993)

First Stage

This involves fabrication of the auricular framework, tragus reconstruction and lobule transposition. Ipsilateral costal cartilages of the sixth, seventh, eighth and ninth ribs are harvested. The base of the framework is carved from the synchondrosis of sixth and seventh ribs. The helix and crus helix are carved from the eighth rib. The ninth rib is used to construct the superior crus, the inferior crus, and the antihelix. The remaining structures are carved from residual cartilage pieces. The cartilage framework is assembled with fine-gauge wire suture. Most of the internal perichondrium is left intact to minimise anterior chest wall deformity. An incision is made at the anterior surface of the lobule. A 2-mm circular portion of the skin is removed at the end of the incision. A W-shaped incision is also made at the posterior lobule to divide the lobule into an anterior tragal flap and postero-anterior lobular skin flaps. A subcutaneous pocket is dissected through this incision. The central portion of the posterior skin flap is not elevated, to augment blood supply to the skin flap. The framework is then placed in the pocket. The posterior flap is then advanced to suture to anterior tragal flap and the lobule is transposed by assembling the flaps in the Z-plasty fashion. The small circular skin defect gives rise to the incisura intertragica. Bolsters are used to approximate skin flaps to the framework, and the bolsters are left in place for 2 weeks.

Second Stage

Framework elevation begins 6 months after the first stage; a crescent-shaped piece of cartilage is harvested from the fifth rib through the previous chest incision. An incision is made 5 mm posterior to the margin of the constructed costal cartilage. The framework is elevated and held in place by wedging the newly harvested cartilage into position. A temporoparietal fascia flap is elevated through a new scalp incision and tunnelled subcutaneously to cover the posterior surface of the cartilage graft and reconstructed auricle. The back of the framework is then covered with an ultra-delicate split-thickness skin graft harvested freehand from the occipital scalp.

Comparison of the Two Techniques

A major criticism on the technique of Brent is the number of stages required to achieve the final result. Also, the aesthetic result from the tragus reconstruction is not always satisfactory, as is the effacement of the postauricular sulcus causing decreased projection of the reconstructed ear. With the technique of Nagata, a better definition of the auricular contours is achieved as a result of the more elaborate fabrication of the framework (Somers 1998). However, manipulation of the perilobular flaps may compromise its vascularity and increases the risk of flap necrosis. Nagata's technique requires a considerable amount of cartilage, and a relatively high extrusion rate has been described, probably due to the use of wire sutures. The frontal symmetry is not addressed and the use of temporoparietal fascia in every case increases the risks of scalp scarring and temporal hair thinning, and makes it unavailable for future possible salvage of complications.

Other Techniques

Aguilar (1996) uses a five-stage protocol with the inclusion of atresia repair: stage one involves framework construction and placement; stage two involves lobule creation; stage three involves atresia repair; stage four involves tragal creation; stage five involves aurical elevation. Okajima et al. (1996) describes a three-stage protocol: stage one involves formation of the ear lobe, construction and placement of the framework; stage two is when transplanted costal cartilage is elevated with the skin; stage three involves tragus formation.

Results in Total Auricular Reconstruction

The appearance (shape, curve and size) of the reconstructed ear compared with the normal ear has been frequently used to indicate the success of the procedure.

Brent reported in 1992 on the results of 546 patients with microtia; depending on the degree of the malformation, a satisfaction rate of 83.3–100% was reported. Also the emotional benefit was highly significant, especially in the severely affected. Nagata (1993) reported an overall satisfaction rate of 64%. Okajima et al. (1996) had a 99% satisfaction rate after the third stage of the procedure. Only 20% of his patients reached this stage. Firmin (1998) found a "very good to good" outcome in 60% of 352 ears.

Complications in Total Auricular Reconstruction

These complications arise because the procedure is associated with technical difficulties. Overall, while the data are limited, it appears that complications at the ear site may arise in between 2 and 10% of patients. Aguilar (1996), who has reconstructed 63 ears, recommended that all plastic surgeons interested in auricle reconstructions should perform at least 10 reconstructions each year in order to maintain their expertise, as lack of experience is the main factor leading to patients having to undergo further restorative procedures.

Complications at the Donor Site

The immediate complications at the chest wall donor site include pneumothorax at the time of obtaining rib grafts. The delayed complications include anterior chest wall deformity and scarring. There are three main problems: (1) the incision site for cartilage harvesting can result in excessive scar length and post-operative discomfort for children, (2) the skin graft donor site, which is usually taken from the hip, can result in discomfort and anaesthesia, and (3) in occasional patients, there may be insufficient rib length to create a curled helix. The chest wall deformity was observed more often in younger children then in older children. The frequency of rib deformities was 20% when cartilages were harvested from patients older than 10 years of age, and 63% in patients younger than 10 years old. While early operation is recommended to reduce the adverse psychological impact on both patients and their parents, early surgery increases the risk of thoracic deformity. Nagata has recommended keeping the internal perichondrium intact to help prevent this problem.

Complications at the Graft Site

Early complications at the ear reconstruction site consist mainly of seromas and haematomas. Extrusion of the framework secondary to skin flap necrosis, and resorption of the framework have also been described. This event is caused by ischaemia of the overlying skin or of the transposed lobe (Furnas 1990). Pressure necrosis due to the patient sleeping on the reconstructed ear has been reported. The use of a tissue expander may provoke leakage, infection and extrusion of the expander. If the framework is exposed, early intervention with local skin and fascia flaps is usually used to salvage the reconstruction. The temporalis fascia is a potential salvage resource. Also, sutures placed too tightly or placement of the framework in a scarred, ischaemic bed may predispose to cartilage resorption. Other complications reported involve the inaccurate positioning of the ear, poorly designed cartilage framework and disruption of helix-baseplate attachment.

Late complications involve hypertrophic scars and keloids, more frequently seen in Afro-Caribbean children.

Prosthetic Auricular Reconstruction

This is discussed further in Chapter 44.

Indications

The osseointegrated anchoring device uses a titanium fixture to provide a direct structural connection between living bone and a load-carrying implant (Tjellström 1990). It was approved by the United States Food and Drug Administration to be used extra-orally in 1995. It has been used more frequently in Europe than in the USA. The three relative indications for prosthetic reconstruction are: (1) failed autogenous reconstruction, (2) significant soft-tissue and skeletal hypoplasia, and (3) a low or unfavourable hairline.

Even though prosthetic reconstruction usually involves less surgery, the prosthesis must be replaced every 2–5 years. In addition, the skin/implant interface is prone to irritation, therefore meticulous hygiene is necessary. Minor trauma may lead to infection. Finally, the prosthetic reconstruction precludes future autogenous reconstruction because all ear remnants and skin and soft tissue in the region are removed.

Results and Complications of Prosthetic Reconstruction

The Medical Services Advisory Committee Assessment report, published in 2000 (MSAC 2000), reviewed in a meta-analysis the results of the Branemark implant technique applied in prosthetic reconstruction. Only five reports discussed their clinical experience with the technique and the implants over a period of years. The studies involved only a few subjects and the reported information was not consistent between studies, making effective comparison difficult. Studies reported on the stability of the implants, skin conditions and levels of patient satisfaction. The complications with the fixtures are comparable with the BAHA technique. There seems to be no difference regarding satisfaction between microtia patients and craniofacial patients who received titanium implants. There were no adverse reactions at the insertion site of the fixtures in 89.6% of cases. In reviewing their clinical experience and patient feedback, the authors of the studies noted some advantages in using the Branemark bone-anchored technique over adhesive retention (an alternative of the Branemark technique in which the prosthesis is fixed by an adhesive, and is removed on a regular basis). Daily care, occasional loss, brittleness over time, colour difference and gradual discolouring were felt to be disadvantages (Somers 1998). As an advantage of the prosthetic implants, good reproduction of the pinna with minimal surgery was reported.

Granstrom et al. (1993) and Somers et al. (1998) compared total ear reconstructions with titanium implants. Granstrom et al. (1993) were disappointed with the results of surgical ear reconstruction as compared to the Branemark prostheses. Somers et al. (1998) pointed out that while the results of total ear reconstruction continue to improve and become more predictable, it is still a technique that is technically demanding, not always applicable to all types of ear deformities and not available everywhere. No daily care, no maintenance, no renewal and an "owned new ear" were felt to be major advantages of ear reconstruction as compared to implants.

Summary for the Clinician

- Aural atresia surgery is performed mostly to alleviate a patient's hearing disability and seldom to manage pathology. Surgical management is usually aimed at obtaining functional hearing gain. Assessing the real benefit from surgery is, unfortunately, much more complicated than we usually realise. Owing to the fact that aural atresia surgery is considered to be one of the most difficult forms of ear surgery, the less experienced surgeon may well consider the BAHA to be the best and most accessible solution for patients with aural atresia. This dilemma is reflected in the differences among surgical teams regarding selection criteria and the criteria for "surgical success". Review of the literature demonstrates large differences in the interpretation of this term. However, even in the hands of the best surgeons, a mean hearing gain of only 20–25 dB is attained in atresia type II and 30–35 dB in type I. The more favourable cases also usually have better preoperative hearing.

Therefore, atresia repair surgery is worthwhile if a proper patient selection is done using stringent audiological and radiographic criteria. A post-operative air–bone gap of less than 25–30 dB should be aimed for. The combination of these factors leads to the conclusion that atresia repair surgery should only be done in very selected patients after a thorough investigation of all parameters involved (e.g. age, anatomy, unilateral or bilateral, and hearing status); only the most favourable cases may sufficiently benefit from this kind of surgery. Less favourable patients should be helped with BAHAs, as this type of surgery does not interfere with the future use of new techniques. Total ear reconstruction using autogenous costal cartilage is the procedure of choice and has the advantage of creating a near-normal cosmetic appearance without ongoing maintenance. Although the success rate and benefits to patients' emotional well-being are satisfactory, it remains a complex surgical procedure with considerable complications at both the graft and donor sites. In less favourable patients, a prosthetic reconstruction with osseointegrated fixtures is a valuable alternative.

References

1. Aguilar EF (1996) Auricular reconstruction of congenital microtia (grade III) Laryngoscope 106:1–26

2. Aguilar EA III, Jahrsdoerfer RA (1988) The surgical repair of congenital microtia and atresia. Otolaryngol Head Neck Surg 98:600–606

3. Altmann F (1955) Congenital aural atresia of the ear in man and animals. Ann Otol Rhinol Laryngol 64:824–858

4. Brent B (1974) Ear reconstruction with an expansile framework of autogenous rib cartilage. Plast Reconstr Surg 53:619–628

5. Brent B (1992) Auricular repair with autogenous rib cartilage grafts: two decades of experience with 600 cases. Plast Reconstr Surg 90:355–374 discussion 375–376

6. Browning GG, Gatehouse S, Swan I (1991) The Glasgow benefit plot: a new method for reporting benefits from middle ear surgery. Laryngoscope 101:180–185

7. Cremers CW, Teunissen E (1991) The impact of a syndromal diagnosis on surgery for congenital minor ear anomalies. Int J Pediatr Otorhinolaryngol 22:59–74

8. Cremers CW, Teunissen E, Marres EH (1988) Classification of congenital aural atresia and results of reconstructive surgery. Adv Otorhinolaryngol 40:9–14

9. Declau F, Cremers C, Van de Heyning P (1999) Diagnosis and management strategies in congenital atresia of the external ear canal. Br J Audiol 33:313–327

10. Declau F, Offeciers F, Van de Heyning P (1997) Classification of the non-syndromal type of meatal atresia. In: Devranoglu I (ed) Proceedings of the XVth World Congress of Otorhinolaryngology Head and Neck Surgery: Panel Discussions, Istanbul, Turkey, pp 135–137

11. Firmin F (1998) Ear reconstruction in cases of typical microtia. Personal experience based on 352 microtic ear corrections. Scand J Plast Reconstr Hand Surg 32:35–47

12. Furnas DW (1990) Complications of surgery of the external ear. Clin Plast Surg 17:305–318

13. Granstrom G, Bergstrom K, Tjellstrom A (1993) The bone-anchored hearing aid and bone-anchored epithesis for congenital ear malformations. Otolaryngol Head Neck Surg 109:46–53

14. Jahrsdoerfer RA (1978) Congenital atresia of the ear. Laryngoscope 88:1–48

15. Jahrsdoerfer RA, Yeakley JW, Aguilar EA, Cole RR, Gray LC (1992) Grading system for the selection of patients with congenital aural atresia. Am J Otol 13:6–12

16. Marquet J, Declau F (1991) Considerations on the surgical treatment of congenital ear atresia. In: Ars B, Van Cauwenberghe P (eds) Middle Ear Structure, Organogenesis and Congenital Defects. Kugler, Amsterdam, pp 85–98

17. MSAC. Medical Services Advisory Committee Assessment report (March 2000) Total ear reconstruction. www.msac.gov.au/pdfs/reports/msac1024.pdf http://www.health.gov.au/haf/msac

18. Nagata S (1993) A new method of total reconstruction of the auricle for microtia. Plast Reconstr Surg 92:187–201

19. Okajima H, Takeichi Y, Umeda K, Baba S (1996) Clinical analysis of 592 patients with microtia. Acta Otolaryngol Suppl 525:18–24

20. Powell RH, Burrell SP, Cooper HR, Proops DW (1996) The Birmingham bone-anchored hearing aid programme: paediatric experience and results. J Laryngol Otol Suppl 21:21–29

21. Snik AF, Mylanus EA, Proops DW, Wolfaardt JF, Hodgetts WE, Somers T, Niparko JK, Wazen JJ, Sterkers O, Cremers CW, Tjellstrom A (2005) Consensus statements on the BAHA system: where do we stand at present? Ann Otol Rhinol Laryngol Suppl 195:2–12

22. Somers T, De Cubber J, Govaerts P, Offeciers FE (1998) Total auricular repair: bone anchored prosthesis or plastic reconstruction? Acta Otorhinolaryngol Belg 52:317–327

23. Tanzer RC (1959) Total reconstruction of the external ear. Plast Reconstr Surg 23:1–15

24. Teunissen E, Cremers CW (1993) Classification of congenital middle ear anomalies. Report on 144 ears. Ann Otol Rhinol Laryngol 102:606–612

25. Tjellstrom A (1990) Osseointegrated implants for replacement of absent or defective ears. Clin Plast Surg 17:355–366

26. Van der Pouw KT, Snik AF, Cremers CW (1998) Audiometric results of bilateral bone-anchored hearing aid application in patients with bilateral congenital aural atresia. Laryngoscope 108:548–553

39

27. Veltman JA, Jonkers Y, Nuijten I, Janssen I, van der Vliet W, Huys E, Vermeesch J, Van Buggenhout G, Fryns JP, Admiraal R, Terhal P, Lacombe D, van Kessel AG, Smeets D, Schoenmakers EF, van Ravenswaaij-Arts CM (2003) Definition of a critical region on chromosome 18 for congenital aural atresia by array CGH. Am J Hum Genet 72:1578–1584

28. Yoshinaga-Itano C, Sedey A, Coulter D, Mehl AL (1998) Language of early- and later-identified children with hearing loss. Pediatrics 102:1161–1171

Chapter 40

Imaging of the Deaf Child

Timothy J. Beale and Gitta Madani

40

Core Messages

After reading this chapter you should understand the following:

- The modalities used to image the deaf child and their respective advantages.
- Current imaging protocols.
- Normal computed tomography and magnetic resonance imaging anatomy.
- How to systematically review the images.
- Imaging algorithms for conductive, mixed and sensorineural hearing loss.
- The imaging features of a range of congenital and acquired causes of hearing loss.

This chapter may be read in conjunction with Chapters 7 (Genetics), 8 (Syndromes) and 43 (Chronic Otitis Media).

Contents

Part 1. A Radiological Overview of the Imaging of Children with Hearing Loss

Deafness is the most common sensory deficit, and more than 50% of all childhood deafness is due to hereditary disorders. The prevalence of permanent hearing impairment (>40 dB hearing threshold) is approximately 1.3 per 1000 children (Parker et al. 1999).

Computed tomography (CT) and magnetic resonance imaging (MRI) are the imaging modalities used in the assessment of deafness. Occasionally, ultrasound is used for renal screening and plain radiography for the assessment of cochlear implant positioning.

Key Points of CT Imaging

The advantages of CT include fast acquisition times and excellent detail of the bony and pneumatised structures of the ear. CT is preferred when there is middle or external ear malformation (Casselman et al. 2001). Bony dysplasias, such as otosclerosis and osteogenesis imperfecta, invariably have positive radiological findings and are best assessed on CT imaging (Weissman 1996). However, CT is poor at characterising soft tissue, assessing the eighth nerve and brainstem, and does not demonstrate the membranous labyrinth.

In summary, the advantages of CT are: fast acquisition, excellent detail of the bony and pneumatised structures of the ear, and multiplanar and three-dimensional reformatting capability. The disadvantages of CT are: the use of ionising radiation, it is poor at characterising soft tissue, it does not demonstrate the membranous labyrinth and it provides less detail of the central auditory pathways compared to MRI.

CT Imaging Protocols in Children

CT imaging protocols in children include:
1. Helical (spiral) scan.
2. Axial acquisition of a slice width equivalent (SW) of 0.5–1.0 mm reconstructed on an SW of 0.1–0.3 mm.
3. Axial–frontal scouting (to exclude tilt and allow for imaging at 10–15°; Swartz and Harnsberger 1997).
4. Bony algorithm and edge enhancement.
5. Avoidance of the lens of the eye.
6. Scan range from just inferior to the external auditory canal (EAC) to the roof of the petrous bone (i.e. the floor of the middle cranial fossa).
7. Reformatting in the coronal and sagittal planes.
8. Reviewing on broad window settings (width 4000, centre 700).
9. Reducing the dose (mAs) in children.

Multislice spiral acquisition enables excellent multiplanar reformatting, obviating the need to scan in a second plane.

Key Points of MRI

MRI provides good characterisation of the soft-tissue structures and is therefore the preferred technique for imaging the nerves and the brain. The advantages of MRI are: good visualisation of the membranous labyrinth, cranial nerves and central auditory pathway, and excellent soft-tissue characterisation. The disadvantages are: it is contraindicated with certain metallic implants and prostheses, it lacks bony detail, it involves longer scan times and the machine is more enclosed and poorly tolerated by claustrophobic patients.

MRI Protocols in Children

Imaging protocols vary. However, high resolution T2-weighted (T2W) imaging of the internal auditory meati (IAMs; demonstrating the intermediate-signal-intensity nerves against the high-signal-intensity cerebrospinal fluid) is essential. Recent advances involve the use of parallel surface coils (thus increasing the signal to noise ratio), a finer SW of 0.3 mm and a higher resolution scan matrix of 1024 (previously 256 and 512).

The MRI imaging protocol for our institution is as follows:
1. T2W three-dimensional fast/turbo spin echo of the IAMs; if a volume sequence is used then reformatting in any plane is possible.
2. Parasaggital images (if no volume sequence) perpendicular to the long axis of the IAC to visualise individual nerves.
3. T2W axial MRI of the head and, if this is abnormal, full head sequences: [fluid attenuation inversion recovery axial, T1-weighted (T1W) coronal and T2W sagittal].
4. Maximum-intensity projections and surface rendering for membranous labyrinth (optional but useful).
5. High-resolution T1W axial images through the IAMs, both pre- and post-gadolinium, are performed occasionally.

Recent advances in CT and MRI technology (smaller and multiple detectors are used in multislice helical CT, and superior coils and greater field strength are available for MRI) have resulted in reduced scan times and increased resolution of the images. More powerful software for post-processing algorithms have resulted in increased usage of maximum-intensity projection, surface rendering and three-dimensional reformatted images. Functional

MRI is increasingly available and, in particular, has been used to study pre-lingually deaf children.

Sedation

Protocols vary, but the following general rules apply:
1. Infants younger than 3 months can be scanned during natural sleep.
2. Those between 3 months and 5 years usually require general anaesthetic or sedation. Local protocols vary; take paediatric and anaesthetic advice.
3. Children older than 5 years usually require no sedation.

CT: Normal Cross-Sectional Anatomy

An example of normal anatomy of the inner ear and its associated nerves is shown in Fig. 40.1.

Systematic Review of CT Images

During the systematic review of any CT petrous temporal bone study, there are several questions to consider regarding the auricle, EAC, middle ear cleft and ossicles, inner ear, internal auditory canal (IAC), posterior fossa and petrous temporal bone.

Considerations regarding the auricle and EAC:
1. Shape of the auricle; is there microtia?
2. Is there atresia or stenosis of the EAC?

Considerations regarding the middle ear cleft and ossicles:
1. Is there an ossicular abnormality, in particular, is the stapes normal?
2. Is the path of the facial nerve normal?
3. What is the size of the middle ear cleft?
4. Is there normal petromastoid pneumatisation?

Considerations regarding the inner ear:
1. Are the oval and round windows normal, small or atretic?
2. Is there normal partitioning of the cochlea (with two and a half turns), is there evidence of hypoplasia/dysplasia, is there a normal bony plate between the cochlea and IAC?
3. Is the vestibule dysplastic?
4. Are the semicircular canals present/dysplastic?
5. Is the otic capsule of normal density?

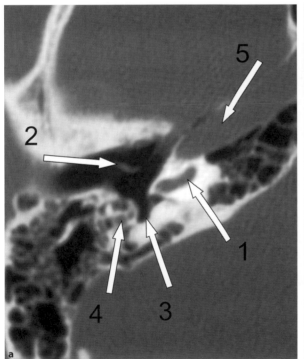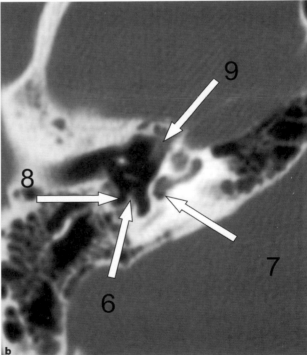

Fig. 40.1a–f Normal anatomy. Magnified axial computed tomography (CT) images of the right petrous temporal bone passing from inferior to superior: normal anatomy (see arrows). **a–c: a** 1 Basal turn of the cochlea, 2 handle of malleus, 3 sinus tympani, 4 facial nerve descending (mastoid segment), 5 horizontal intrapetrous internal carotid artery (ICA). **b** *see next page*

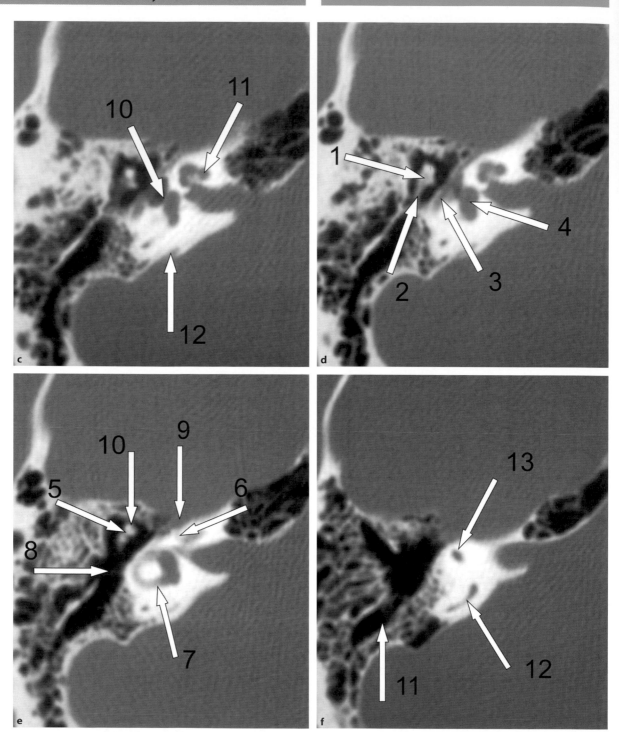

Fig. 40.1 *(Continued)* **b** *6* pyramidal eminence, *7* round window, *8* facial recess, *9* tensor tympani muscle. **c** *10* Oval window, *11* middle turn of cochlea, *12* vestibular aqueduct. **d–f: d** *1* Body of incus, *2* short process of incus, *3* facial nerve tympanic segment, *4* vestibule. **e** *5* Malleo-incudal joint, *6* facial nerve labyrinthine segment, *7* lateral semicircular canal (SCC), *8* aditus ad antrum, *9* geniculate ganglion, *10* head of malleus. **f** *11* Mastoid antrum, *12* posterior SCC, *13* anterior crus of the superior SCC

Considerations regarding the internal auditory canal:
1. Is it narrow/tapering/double/bulbous/absent?

Considerations regarding the posterior fossa and petromastoid:
1. Overall appearance, maintenance of symmetry, presence of mass.
2. Pneumatisation of petromastoid.

Normal MRI Anatomy

An example of the normal anatomy of the inner auditory meati on MRI imaging can be seen in Figs. 40.2 and 40.3.

Systematic Review of MRI Images

When systematically reviewing MRI images it is helpful to start peripherally and work centrally, and to include the petromastoid, middle ear cleft, membranous labyrinth, otic capsule, cranial nerves VII and VIII, the brainstem and the auditory pathway. Again, there are several questions to consider.

Consideration regarding the petromastoid/middle ear cleft:
1. Are the air cells aerated?

Considerations regarding the membranous labyrinth:
1. Assess the scala tympani and vestibuli (recent high-resolution MRI can visualise the macula).
2. Is there normal partitioning of the cochlea?

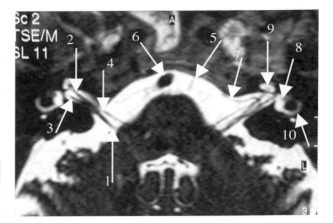

Fig. 40.2 Axial T2-weighted magnetic resonance image (MRI) through the internal auditory meati (IAMs): normal anatomy (see arrows). *1* Vestibulocochlear nerve (VIII), *2* cochlear nerve, *3* inferior vestibular nerve, *4* facial nerve (VII), *5* abducent nerve, *6* basilar artery, *7* vascular loop, *8* vestibule, *9* middle turn of cochlea, *10* lateral SCC. Note that the V-shaped division of the eighth nerve into the cochlear and inferior vestibular nerves occurs at the level of the inferior internal auditory canal (IAC)

3. Is there loss of the normal T2W high signal of the membranous labyrinth, implying obliteration?
4. Is the vestibular aqueduct +/− endolymphatic sac enlarged?

Considerations regarding the otic capsule
1. Although there is limited bony detail gross pathology is visible, so include in your review.

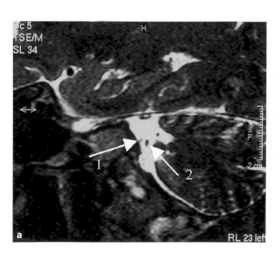

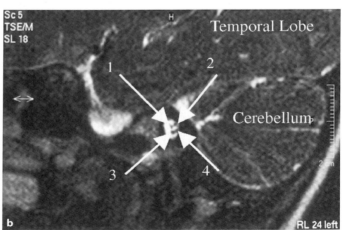

Fig. 40.3a,b Sagittal oblique T2-weighted MRI through the IAMs: normal anatomy (see arrows). **a** Through the cisternal space: *1* facial nerve, *2* vestibulocochlear nerve. Note the normal difference in size of the nerves VII and VIII before nerve VIII divides. **b** Through the lateral IAC: *1* facial nerve, *2* superior vestibular nerve, *3* cochlear nerve, *4* inferior vestibular nerve

Considerations regarding cranial nerves VII and VIII and the cisternal spaces:

1. Review the vestibular, cochlear and ampullary divisions; are they present and of normal size?
2. Is there a cerebellopontine angle mass? Is there a vascular loop indenting the root entry zone (REZ) of the eighth nerve?

Considerations regarding the brainstem and auditory pathways:

1. Assess from the REZ to the superior temporal gyrus.

Review the scout films in both imaging modalities for visible pathology such as cervical spinal pathology in Klippel-Feil and a postnasal space mass causing middle ear effusions.

When is Early Imaging Essential?

Early imaging is essential in the assessment of post-meningitis hearing loss, in order to evaluate the child's suitability for cochlear implantation (CI), as there is a limited time window before the possible onset of labyrinthitis ossificans. Ossification of the cochlea can render implantation technically more difficult or impossible. The presence of ossification in a recently deaf child is evidence that implantation should proceed on an urgent basis. The degree of ossification can influence the choice of ear for implantation, the surgical approach and the cochlear implant system used (Young et al. 2000).

Progressive hearing loss should be imaged early because of the increased risk of underlying radiologically detectable pathology.

Children under the age of 2 years gain maximum benefit following CI due to improved language skills, and should undergo early assessment by a CI team and referral for early imaging.

Imaging Algorithms for Conductive, Sensorineural and Mixed Hearing

Conductive Hearing Loss

CT is the modality of choice for imaging conductive hearing loss (CHL). Close inspection of the EAC, tympanic membrane (TM), middle ear cleft (in particular the ossicles and oval and round windows) and adjacent otic capsule is essential.

Sensorineural Hearing Loss

Historically, CT has been the preferred imaging modality for sensorineural hearing loss (SNHL) in children under 15 years of age. However, MRI is now the imaging modality of choice unless there is a suspicion of associated external or middle ear pathology. In SNHL, particular attention should be paid to the inner ear and central auditory pathway.

Mixed Hearing Loss

CT is the modality of choice. MRI may be required to demonstrate retrocochlear anatomy.

Part 2. Radiological Abnormalities Found in Children with Hearing Loss

Embryology of the Inner and Middle Ear and the EAC

Inner Ear

The radiographic appearance of some inner ear malformations correlates with arrest at a particular stage of embryonic development (Jackler et al. 1987). The development of the inner ear is complex, probably originates from three sources (neural crest, cephalic mesoderm and somatic mesoderm) and begins at around 3 weeks gestation, and reaches adult dimensions by 23 weeks of gestation (Couly et al. 1993).

1. Week 6: formation of SSCs, utricle and saccule begins.
2. Week 11: the 2.5 turns of the cochlea are formed.
3. Week 23: the otic capsule is ossified (Fisher and Curtin 1994).

Middle Ear

The middle ear space, including the mastoid air cells, the inner surface of the TM and the Eustachian tube arise from the endoderm of the first pharyngeal pouch. The ossicles and their attachments are derived from the first and second branchial arches during the 6th–38th weeks of gestation (Swartz and Harnsberger 1997). The first branchial arch gives rise to the head and neck of the malleus, and the body and short process of the incus. The second branchial arch forms the manubrium of the malleus, the long process of the incus and the stapes superstructure (with the exception of the footplate).

External Ear

The EAC develops from invagination of the ectoderm of the first branchial cleft, during the 4th week of gestation.

1. Week 4: the otic pit (invagination of ectoderm) is apparent.

2. Weeks 4–8: a solid core of epithelium, called the meatal plug, extends to the middle ear.
3. Week 26: The core canalises from a medial to lateral direction, giving rise to the EAC (Fisher and Curtin 1994).

Conductive Hearing Loss

This is the most common type of hearing loss; transmission of sound is impeded in the external and/or middle ear. CHL may be congenital or acquired. Otitis media (acute or chronic) is by far the most frequent aetiology. Impacted cerumen, foreign bodies and aural atresia are common causes of CHL. Less frequent aetiologies are isolated congenital middle ear anomalies and anomalies associated with an inherited syndrome (Bergstrom 1994). Various inherited syndromes are associated with middle ear anomalies; these include the craniofacial anomalies such as Treacher Collins, branchio-oto-renal (BOR) syndrome and CHARGE (acronym of Coloboma of the eyes, Heart defect, Atresia of the choanae, Retardation of growth and development, Genital hypoplasia, Ear anomalies) association.

Radiological Features of Congenital Aural Dysplasia

Congenital aural dysplasia describes a spectrum of disease ranging from complete atresia to various degrees of EAC stenosis (which may be due to bony or fibrous tissue), and is the result of abnormal development of the first branchial arch.

The incidence of aural atresia is approximately 1 in 10,000 live births (Swartz and Harnsberger 1997). Unilateral atresia is more common than bilateral, males are more commonly affected, and right EAC anomalies are more frequent than left (Anson and David 1980; Fig. 40.4). There is an association with malformations of the TM, ossicles and middle ear. However, inner ear development is usually normal, as it occurs at an earlier period of gestation. Aural atresia is observed in various syndromal abnormalities including Treacher-Collins, Goldenhars, Crouzon, Klippel-Feil and CHARGE association.

In bilateral EAC atresia, CT evaluation before surgical repair is mandatory in order to demonstrate normal oval and round windows and bony labyrinth and to exclude congenital cholesteatoma (Fisher and Curtin 1994; Fig. 40.5).

Congenital Middle Ear Anomalies

A range of ear abnormalities occurs in each of the syndromes associated with hearing loss; the characteristic radiological features of some syndromes are not defined, whilst others have normal imaging features. Hence, the role of imaging is to guide the management of the hearing loss rather than diagnosis of the syndrome.

Isolated middle ear anomalies are frequently bilateral (Swartz and Faeber 1985). The stapes is the most commonly involved ossicle, and the malleus is the least commonly involved (Fisher and Curtin 1994). The stapes may

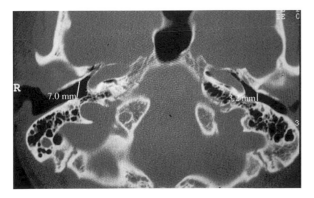

Fig. 40.4 Axial CT petrous temporal bone showing a unilateral bony stenosis of the left external auditory canal (EAC). Unilateral bony stenosis of the EAC is usually more common on the right side (4:1)

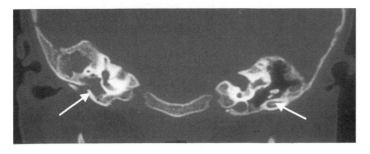

Fig. 40.5 Coronal CT in a patient with bilateral bony atresia with a pneumatised middle ear cleft on the left. Note the bony atretic plates (*arrows*)

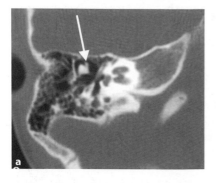

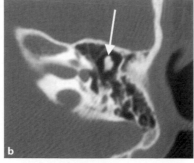

Fig. 40.6a,b Axial CT of the petrous temporal bone through the epitympanum (attic): compare the hypoplastic head of malleus in **a** with the normal sized head of malleus on the other side in **b** (*arrows*)

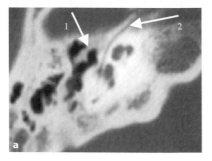

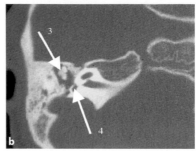

Fig. 40.7a,b Axial CT through the right petrous temporal bone. Note the bony web fixing the head of the malleus to the anterior wall of the epitympanum (*1*) and the abnormal facial nerve canal (*2*) in **a**, and the crudely shaped ossicles (*3*) and small oval window (*4*) in a patient with CHARGE syndrome in **b**

40

be absent, fixed to the oval window or demonstrate crural deformity (Eelkema and Curtin 1989). Congenital fixation of the stapes is secondary to ossification of the annular ligament and ankylosis of the stapes footplate. It may be associated with other ossicular anomalies, the most common of which is hypoplasia of the long process of the incus. The malleus may also be fixed to the anterior attic wall and there may be aplasia or dysplasia of the oval or round windows (Figs. 40.6 and 40.7).

Syndromes Associated with Congenital CHL

Otocraniofacial Syndromes

Craniofacial Microsomia

Underdevelopment of the face (hemifacial microsomia), is usually unilateral, but bilateral and asymmetrical disease is seen in 20% of cases (Phelps and Lloyd 1990). Possible radiological findings include:

1. Caudally situated pinna.
2. Microtia.
3. EAC atresia or stenosis.
4. The middle ear cavity is occasionally normal, but more frequently under- or non-pneumatised.
5. Absent or abnormal ossicles (fused or laterally placed).
6. Descent of the tegmen.
7. The bony labyrinth is usually normal.
8. The porus of the IAC is abnormally high and markedly higher than the lateral opening of the EAC (Phelps and Lloyd 1990).

Goldenhars Syndrome

Also known as occulo-auriculo-vertebral dysplasia, Goldenhars is a sporadic non-hereditary syndrome that is detected in infancy. It is considered a variant of hemifacial microsomia with additional features of epibulbar dermoids, and vertebral anomalies. Hearing loss may be conductive, sensorineural or mixed (Gorlin et al. 2001).

Treacher Collins Syndrome

Also known as mandibulofacial dysostosis, this is a disorder of craniofacial development with an autosomal dominant pattern of inheritance and variable expression. Around 60% of cases are due to new mutations (Gorlin et al. 2001). Possible radiological findings include:

1. Microtia.
2. Atresia of the EAM (around 50% of all patients).
3. Reduction in size of the attic and antrum (all patients).
4. Ossicular anomalies are common.
5. Altered course of facial nerve.
6. The lateral semicircular canal may be dysplastic with normal cochlear function (Phelps and Lloyd 1990; Fig. 40.8).

BOR Syndrome

Also known as ear pits deafness, this is an autosomal dominant disorder that consists of branchial-derived anomalies and otologic and renal malformations. The

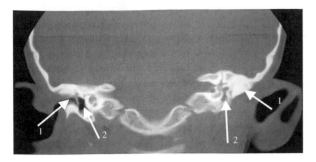

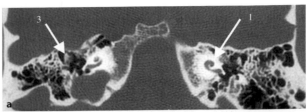

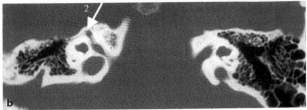

Fig. 40.8 Coronal CT petrous temporal bone in Treacher Collins syndrome. Note the deformed auricles, the bony atresia of the left and stenosis of the right EACs (1) and the slit-like Middle ear clefts (2); opacified on the left

Fig. 40.9a,b Axial CT petrous temporal bones: branchio-oto-renal (BOR) syndrome. Note the characteristic appearance of the cochlea. The distal turns are markedly hypoplastic and located anteriorly in relation to the normal axis of the modiolus (*1* in **a**). Note also the obtuse anterior genu of the facial nerve (*2* in **b**) and the crudely formed and laterally positioned ossicles (*3* in **a**)

hearing loss may be conductive, sensorineural or mixed. Ear pits are found in 80% of BOR syndrome cases, with associated deformities of the middle and/or inner ears, branchial cysts or fistulae (60%) and renal anomalies (15%; Phelps and Lloyd 1990). The radiological findings include:

1. Minor ossicular anomalies: the stapes is usually affected (and often has only one crus), crudely shaped malleus and incus (Figs. 40.9 and 40.10).
2. Obtuse angle of the anterior genu of the facial nerve canal.
3. Marked hypoplasia of the distal turns of the cochlea.
4. Short and bulbous IACs.
5. Short petrous pyramids that point upwards (Phelps and Lloyd 1990).

CHARGE Association

Possible radiological findings of CHARGE association include:

1. EAC atresia.
2. Atretic oval window.
3. Minor ossicular anomalies.
4. Absence of semicircular canals (most characteristic feature; Fig. 40.11).
5. Mondini deformity (Morimoto et al 2006).

X-Linked Deafness

The hearing loss is mixed. The conductive component is secondary to congenital fixation of the stapes footplate. The sensorineural component is progressive. The characteristic radiological features are:

1. Widening of the lateral end of the IAC.
2. Deficiency or absence of bone between the lateral end of the IAC and basal turn of the cochlea (Phelps and Lloyd 1990).

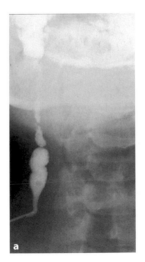

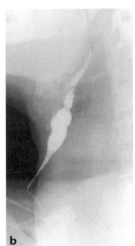

Fig. 40.10 Anteroposterior (**a**) and lateral (**b**) contrast radiographs demonstrating a branchial fistula in a patient with BOR syndrome. Contrast is injected via a sinus in the lower cervical region (anterior border of the sternocleidomastoid muscle) and exits in the oropharynx

Fig. 40.11 Axial CT showing the petrous temporal bone. Note the absence of SCCs that is pathognomonic and occurs in 50% of patients with CHARGE syndrome

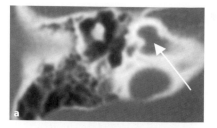
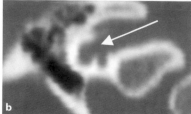

Fig. 40.12a,b Axial (**a**) and coronal (**b**) CT of the petrous temporal bone in a patient with X-linked deafness. Note the lack of a bony plate between the IAC and cochlea (*white arrow*)

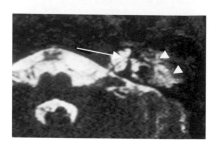

Fig. 40.13 X-linked deafness. Axial T2-weighted MRI through the IAMs. Note the absence of the bony plate between the IAC and cochlea (*arrows*) and the secretions in the middle ear cleft (*arrowheads*)

These features are bilateral and symmetrical and their recognition is particularly important as a cerebrospinal fluid gusher will develop if the stapes footplate is opened in an attempt to correct the CHL (Figs. 40.12 and 40.13).

Craniosynostoses

Crouzon Syndrome

Crouzon is the most common syndromal cause of craniosynostosis. Affected individuals have a characteristic facies with proptosis, hypertelorism, divergent strabismus and maxillary hypoplasia. CHL occurs in around half the cases and may be due to Eustachian tube dysfunction (Gorlin et al. 2001). Possible radiological findings include:
1. EAC atresia.
2. Ossicular anomalies.
3. Under-pneumatised petromastoid.
4. Upward tilting petrous pyramids.
5. Abnormalities of the bony labyrinth (large vestibule, dysplastic semicircular canal; Phelps and Lloyd 1990; Gorlin et al. 2001).

Otocervical Syndromes

Klippel-Feil Anomaly and Wildervanck Syndrome

Klippel-Feil anomaly consists of fusion of one or more cervical vertebrae (associated with various other vertebral abnormalities), webbed neck and low posterior hairline. An association with both CHL and more commonly SNHL is well recognised (Phelps and Lloyd 1990).

Wildervanck Syndrome is the association of Klippel-Feil anomaly with abducens paralysis and hearing loss. The hearing loss may be sensorinreural or conductive. Most of the reported cases are female (Gorlin et al. 2001). Possible radiological features include:
1. Abnormalities of the pinna.
2. EAC atresia.
3. Ossicular anomalies.
4. Abnormalities of the bony labyrinth (Mondini deformity, dysplastic semicircular canal; Gorlin et al. 2001).

Acquired CHL

Acquired causes of conductive hearing loss include:
1. Acute otitis media.
2. Otitis media with effusion.
3. Chronic otitis media.
4. Impacted wax/foreign body.
5. Trauma (e.g. ossicular disruption).
6. Tympanosclerosis.
7. Tuberculosis.

The first four aetiologies listed are by far the most common and are not routinely imaged.

Trauma: Ossicular Disruption

Ossicular disruption may occur at any age. The incus is most frequently involved. The most commonly involved joints are the incudostapedial followed by the malleo-incudal joints (Figs. 40.14–40.16).

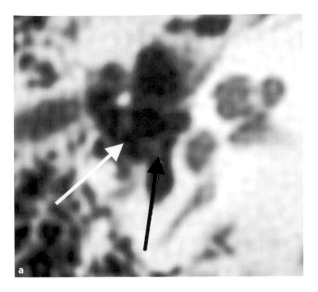
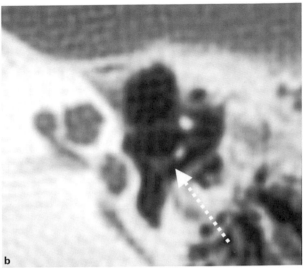

Fig. 40.14a,b Magnified axial CT images. Note the posterior angulation of the incudostapedial joint (ISJ; *white arrow*) in **a**, which is due to ISJ disruption rather than in keeping with (the stapes is indicated by the black arrow), and compare with the normal ISJ alignment (*dotted white arrow*) on the left side (**b**) in the same patient

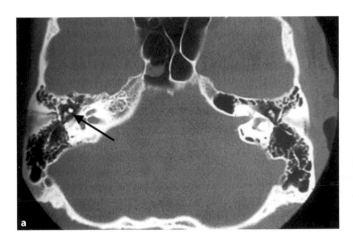
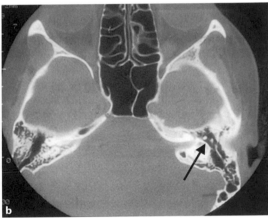

Fig. 40.15 a Widening (subluxation) of the malleoincudal joint on the right (*black arrow*); compare with the normal, left side. **b** The malleus is widely separate from the incus (*black arrow*), in keeping with malleoincudal dislocation

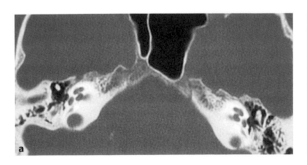
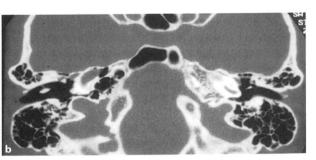

Fig. 40.16 a Note the absence of the incus in its normal location and compare to the normal, left side. **b** The dislocated incus is visible within the EAC

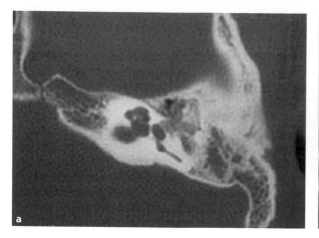
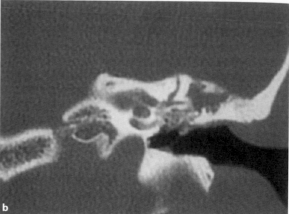

Fig. 40.17a,b Axial (**a**) and coronal (**b**) CT petrous temporal bone images. Note how difficult it is to clearly delineate the ossicles as they are surrounded by soft tissue containing multiple foci of calcification, in keeping with tympanosclerosis

Tympanosclerosis

Tympanosclerosis is a sequela of chronic otitis media where there are multiple punctate foci of calcification (hyalinised collagen) within the tympanic membrane or around the ossicles, with or without associated soft tissue (Fig. 40.17).

Sensorineural Hearing Loss

SNHL indicates dysfunction of the cochlea, cochlear nerve or auditory pathway. The prevalence of SNHL at the age of 6 years is estimated at 1.5–2 per 1000 children (Chan 1994).

Congenital SNHL

Congenital SNHL can be divided into the syndromal and the more common non-syndromal disorders. At least 80 loci have been identified in relation to non-syndromic hearing loss. The most common is connexin 26, a gap junction protein responsible for the intercellular transport of ions, which accounts for around 50% of non-syndromic SNHL – there are no associated imaging features (Kenneson et al. 2002). Although half of all SNHL is congenital (Fisher and Curtin 1994), the majority of these patients have no demonstrable radiological abnormality of the ears or auditory pathways.

Abnormal Development of the Inner Ear

The radiographic appearance of some inner ear malformations correlates with arrest at a given stage of embryonic development. This is particularly true of cochlear anoma-lies, which are traditionally divided into named deformities, but in reality represent a spectrum of abnormalities:
1. Michel deformity.
2. Common cavity.
3. Cystic cochleovestibular malformation.
4. Mondini deformity.
5. Widened vestibular aqueduct.
6. Dysplastic semicircular canals.
7. IAC anomaly.
8. Vestibulocochlear hypoplasia/aplasia.

Michel Deformity

In Michel's deformity, there is complete failure of inner ear development, resulting in labyrinthine aplasia and hypoplasia of the petrous pyramid. It correlates to arrest of development in the 3rd week of gestation. The external and middle ear may be normal and hearing loss may be unilateral or bilateral (Fig. 40.18).

Common Cavity

This results from a developmental arrest in the 4th week of gestation, leading to a primitive cochlear sac that is continuous with the vestibular cavity, with no bony separation from the arachnoid space, predisposing the child to meningitis (Fig. 40.19).

Cystic Cochleovestibular Malformation

A cystic cochleovestibular malformation consists of a dysplastic cochlea with a widened basal turn and incomplete partitioning of the distal turns, a dilated ductus reuniens and vestibule (Fig. 40.20).

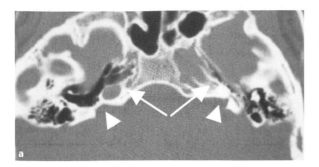
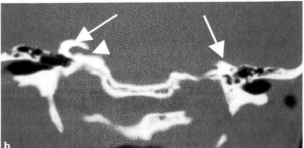

Fig. 40.18a,b Axial (**a**) and coronal (**b**) CT petrous temporal bone in a patient with Michel deformity. This is extremely rare, and more commonly a primitive otocyst is present. There is hypoplasia of the petrous pyramids (*arrows*) with no vestige of a labyrinth. Note also the tapered IACs (*arrowheads*). The middle ear clefts and ossicles are present, but abnormally formed

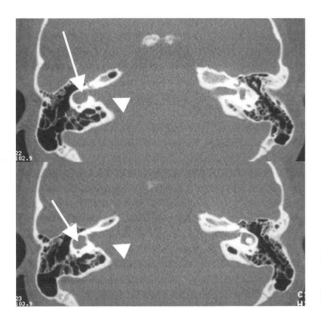

Fig. 40.19 Axial CT petrous temporal bone showing a common cavity deformity on the right (*arrows*) with hypoplastic petrous pyramid and widened IAC (*arrowheads*). Compare to the normal left side

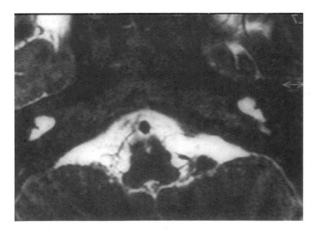
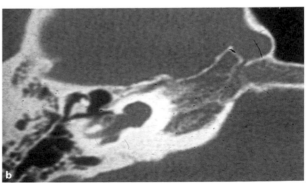

Fig. 40.20a,b Fine T2-weighted axial MRI (**a**) and axial CT (**b**) in two patients with cochleovestibular malformation. Note the dysmorphic cochlea in continuity with a dilated vestibule and deformed SCCs

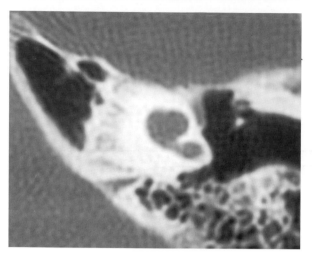

Fig. 40.21 Axial CT of the left petrous temporal bone in a patient with Mondini deformity. Note the normal size of the basal turn and incomplete partitioning of the distal turns

40

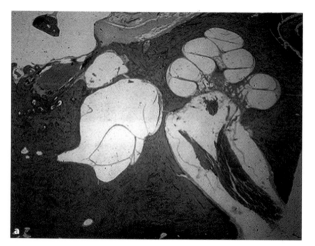

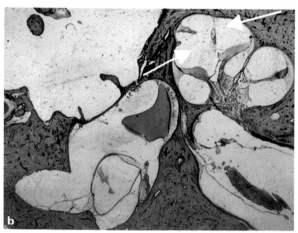

Fig. 40.22a,b Histopathology of the normal (**a**) versus the Mondini (**b**) cochlea. Note the incomplete partitioning of the distal turns in **b** (*white arrows*)

Widened Vestibular Aqueduct

The calibre of the normal vestibular aqueduct is equal to or smaller than that of the posterior semicircular canal (Eelkema and Curtin 1989). A widened vestibular aqueduct is defined as an increase in the anteroposterior diameter of the mid-portion of the descending limb, of greater than 1.5 mm. This is most clearly seen on the axial images (Fisher and Curtin 1994). Hearing loss is usually bilateral and progressive (Fig. 40.23).

Dysplastic Semicircular Canals

The semicircular canals may be entirely absent. The frequency of congenital anomalies of the semicircular canals is related to their chronology of development (Eelkema and Curtin 1989; Curtin 1988). The first to develop and least likely to be anomalous is the superior semicircular canal. The lateral semicircular canal, which appears last, is the most likely to be malformed (Jackler et al. 1987; Fig. 40.24).

Abnormalities of the IAC

The IAC may be enlarged or stenosed. A wide IAC may be normal but can be associated with neurofibromatosis (Fig. 40.25). A bulbous shape of the medial ends of the IACs is seen in X-linked deafness, which is characteristically associated with an absent bony plate between the cochlea and the IAC. The IACs are also short and bulbous in BOR syndrome.

Hypoplasia and Aplasia of the Vestibulocochlear Nerve

The vestibulocochlear nerve is clearly visualised on MRI and is normally considerably larger than the adjacent VII nerve. Hypoplasia or aplasia of the nerve is most frequently seen in conjunction with a narrow IAC. However, it is now recognised that VIII nerve hypoplasia can occur with an IAC of normal dimensions (Fig. 40.26).

Cochlear Nerve Aplasia and Hypoplasia

The cochlear division of the VIII nerve may be absent or hypoplastic in an otherwise radiologically normal VIII nerve trunk (Fig. 40.27).

Syndromes Associated with Congenital SNHL

These include: Pendred, Usher, Waardenberg, Alport, Jervel-Lange-Nielson and Stickler syndromes.

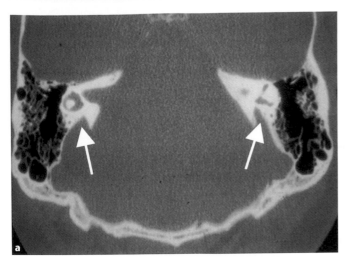
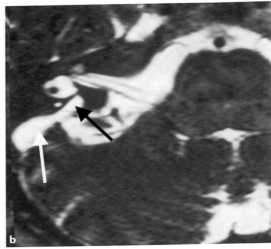

Fig. 40.23a,b Axial CT (**a**) and MRI (**b**) images in patients with widened vestibular aqueducts (*arrows*). Note that the MRI demonstrates both the enlarged vestibular aqueduct (*black arrow*) and endolymphatic duct (*white arrow*)

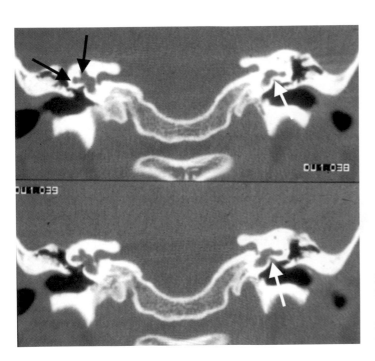

Fig. 40.24 Coronal CT of the petrous temporal bone. Note the dysplastic superior and lateral SCCs (*black arrows*). Isolated dysplasia of the lateral SCC may be associated with normal hearing. Note also the narrow oval windows (*white arrows*)

Pendred Syndrome

Pendred is the most common syndromal cause of deafness. The pattern of inheritance is autosomal recessive and the syndrome results in a triad of goitre, positive perchlorate test and SNHL. Possible radiological features are:

1. Mondini deformity.
2. Enlarged vestibule and deficient modiolus.
3. Widened vestibular aqueduct and wide endolymphatic sac (Phelps and Lloyd 1990; Fig. 40.28).

Ushers Syndrome

This syndrome accounts for 3–6% of the congenitally deaf (Chan 1994). Imaging is usually normal.

Waardenburgs Syndrome

The clinical features of this syndrome include dystopia canthorum (lateral displacement of the medial canthi but normal interpupillary distance), pigmentary abnormali-

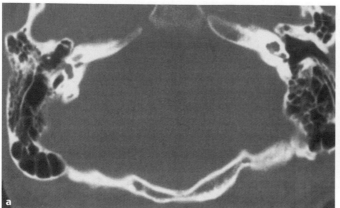

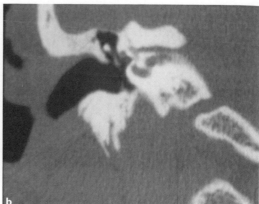

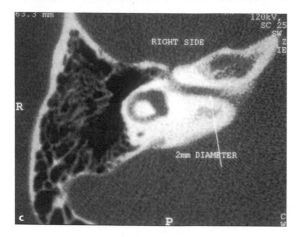

Fig. 40.25a–c CT petrous temporal bone imaging demonstrating a variety of IAC anomalies: bilaterally absent IACs in **a** (axial CT), double IAC in **b** (coronal CT right side) and narrow IAC (2 mm in diameter) in **c** (axial CT right side)

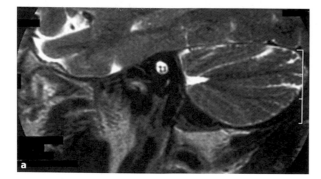

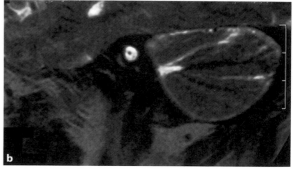

Fig. 40.26a,b Sagittal T2-weighted MRI through the IAC. Compare the normal side (**a**) where the three main divisions of the eighth nerve and the facial nerve are visible, with the hypoplastic eighth nerve in **b** where the facial nerve is readily visualised in the antero-superior IAC, but there is only a ghost of an outline of the three main divisions of the eighth nerve

ties of the skin, iris and hair (white forelock) and SNHL. Imaging is usually normal, although abnormalities of the vestibular system have been reported (Phelps and Lloyd 1990).

The Otoskeletal Syndromes (Bone dysplasias)

Osteogenesis Imperfecta

Osteogenesis imperfecta is an autosomal disorder of type I collagen synthesis, the features of which include osteoporosis, blue sclera, dentinogenesis imperfecta and

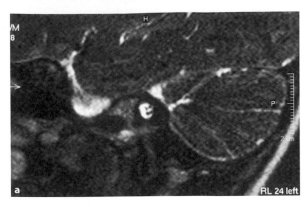
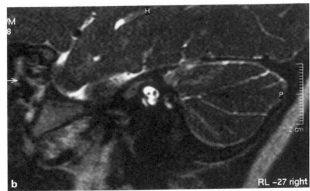

Fig. 40.27a,b Sagittal T2-weighted MRI through the IAC. Note the normal-sized cochlear division in **a** and compare with **b**, which demonstrates absence of the cochlear division in the anteroinferior IAC in a patient with profound unilateral hearing loss

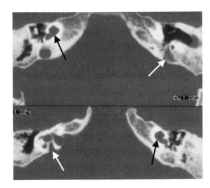
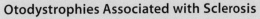

Fig. 40.28 Axial CT of the petrous temporal bone. Note the bilateral Mondini cochlea (*black arrows*) and widened vestibular aqueducts (*white arrows*)

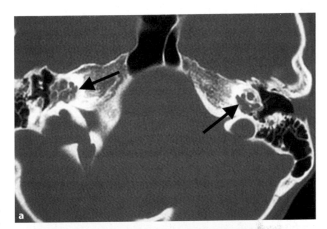
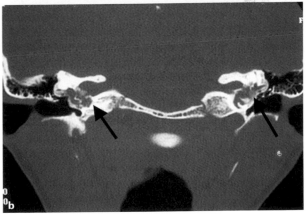

hearing loss. Hearing loss is most common in the type I disease, affecting up to 40% of cases, and may be conductive or sensorineural (Swartz and Harnsberger 1997). The changes are indistinguishable from severe pericochlear otospongiosis, with extensive demineralisation of the petrous bone encroaching on the otic capsule. Other possible features include thin ossicles, which together with fracture of the stapes contribute to the CHL (Fig. 40.29).

Otodystrophies Associated with Sclerosis

The otodystrophies, which are associated with an increase in bone density, cause a progressive mixed deafness. These include:
1. Osteopetrosis causing loss of the normal corticomedullary differentiation (Fig. 40.30).
2. Hyperostosis corticalis generalista (Von Buchem's disease; Fig. 40.31).
3. Craniometaphyseal dysplasia (Fig. 40.32).

Fig. 40.29a,b Axial (**a**) and coronal (**b**) CT of the petrous temporal bone in a patient with osteogenesis imperfecta. Note the extensive demineralisation encroaching on the otic capsule (*black arrows*)

4. Progressive diaphyseal dysplasia (Engelman's disease; Fig. 40.33).
5. X linked hypophosphataemia (Fig. 40.34).

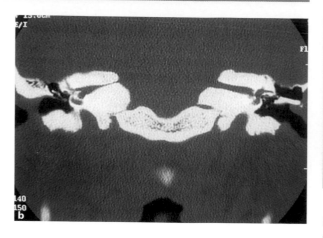

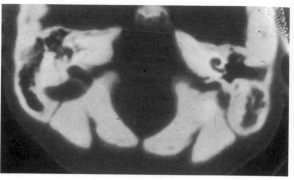

Fig. 40.30 Coronal CT of the petrous temporal bone in a patient with osteopetrosis, demonstrating diffusely sclerotic bone with loss of the normal corticomedullary differentiation. Note the evidence of previous canal wall-up mastoid surgery on the left

Fig. 40.31 Otodystrophies associated with sclerosis: in common with the dysplasias associated with increased bone density, there is involvement of the calvaria and skull base (see also Figs. 40.32–40.34). Cranial nerve palsies may occur due to encroachment on the skull base foramina. Axial CT petrous temporal bone in a patient with Von Buchem's disease

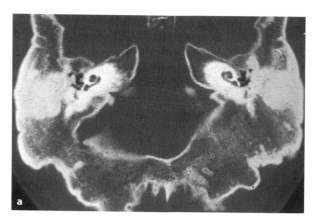

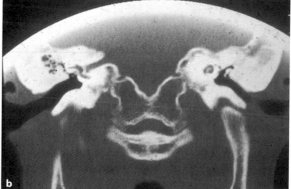

Fig. 40.32a,b Axial (a) and coronal (b) CT of the petrous temporal bone in a patient with craniometaphyseal dysplasia

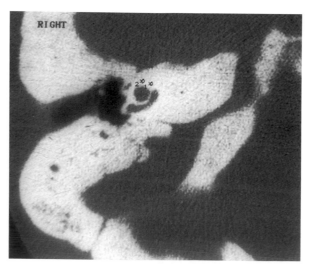

Fig. 40.33 Axial CT petrous temporal bone in a patient with progressive diaphyseal dysplasia

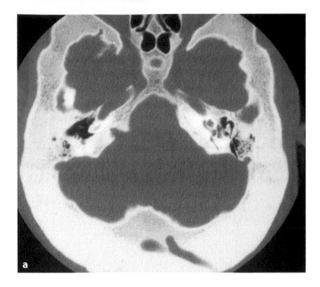

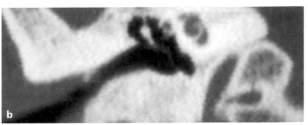

Fig. 40.34a,b Axial (a) and coronal (b) CT petrous bone in a patient with X-linked hypophosphataemia

The last four conditions cause expansion (as well as sclerosis), which encroaches on the neural foramina, middle ear cleft and IAC, as well as diffuse involvement of the calvaria and skull base.

Acquired SNHL

There are several causes of acquired SNHL. Prenatal causes include:

1. Drug exposure.
2. Prenatal infection with TORCH (toxoplasmosis, other agents, rubella, cytomegalovirus and herpes simplex).
3. Erythroblastosis fetalis.

Postnatal causes include:

1. Otoskeletal syndromes (see above).
2. Meningitis (labyrinthitis obliterans).
3. Other infections (adenovirus, influenza, mumps, chicken pox, Epstein-Barr virus).
4. Hyperbilirubinaemia.
5. Trauma (mechanical, noise exposure, barotraumas).

Post-Meningitic Labyrinthitis Obliterans

Labyrinthitis ossificans is the pathological ossification of the membranous labyrinth, in response to a destructive process (DeSouza et al. 1991). As early as 2 weeks after the onset of meningitis, fibrosis is present, followed by new bone formation, which is demonstrable radiologically in the 1st month. The most profound ossification occurs following meningitis (DeSouza et al. 1991). The rate of hearing loss increases when diagnosis is delayed by more than 3 days (Smith 1988).

There are two radiological patterns of response of the membranous labyrinth following meningitis:

1. Areas of marked signal loss on the T2W images, usually patchy, but occasionally involving the whole labyrinth, representing calcific or "fibrous" obliteration (Figs. 40.35 and 40.36).
2. A less common response is a generalised mild decrease in the normally observed T2W high signal intensity within the labyrinth. At cochleostomy, the labyrinthine fluid in the scala tympani has the consistency of paste, but insertion of a cochlear implant electrode may still be possible (Fig. 40.37).

The Future

The future for imaging of the deaf child undoubtedly includes the increasing use of MRI. Improvements in the technology may facilitate a more clear demonstration of the membranous labyrinth and shorter scan times. The role of functional MRI, which is an invaluable tool in the assessment pre-lingually deaf children, is also expanding.

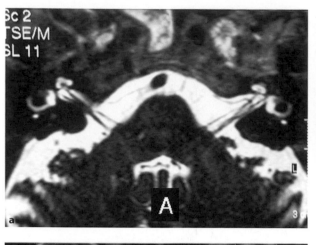

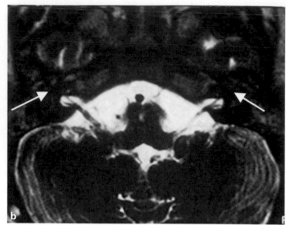

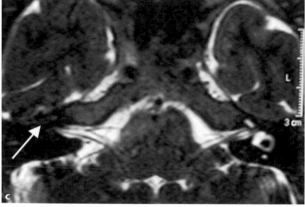

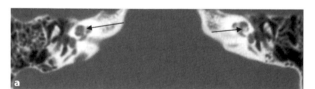

Fig. 40.35a–c Axial T2-weighted MRI images through the IACs. Compare the normal labyrinth in **a** with the total obliteration of the labyrinth in **b** (*white arrows*) and the obliteration of the right membranous labyrinth in **c** (*white arrow*)

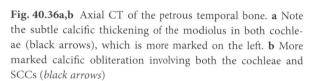

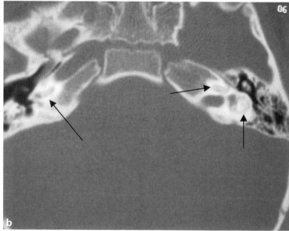

Fig. 40.36a,b Axial CT of the petrous temporal bone. **a** Note the subtle calcific thickening of the modiolus in both cochleae (black arrows), which is more marked on the left. **b** More marked calcific obliteration involving both the cochleae and SCCs (*black arrows*)

40

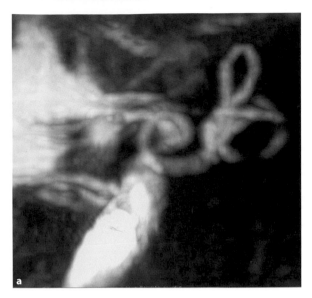
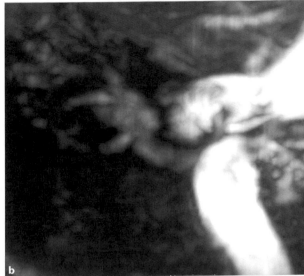

Fig. 40.37a,b Maximum-intensity projections of the membranous labyrinth. Compare the normal side in **a** with **b**, where there is a generalised decrease in the signal intensity

Summary for the Clinician

- CT is the imaging modality of choice in the investigation of CHL and mixed hearing loss, and provides excellent detail of bony and pneumatised structures. MRI is the first-line imaging modality for the investigation of SNHL unless there is a suspicion of associated external or middle-ear pathology. Impacted cerumen, foreign bodies and aural atresia are common causes of childhood CHL. The majority of patients with congenital SNHL have no demonstrable radiological abnormality. In congenital syndromic hearing loss, imaging of the temporal bone and auditory pathways is used to guide treatment (such as suitability for cochlear implantation) rather than to diagnose the syndrome. Early imaging is essential in children with progressive hearing loss (who are more likely to have a radiological abnormality) and post-meningitic hearing loss (as labyrinthitis obliterans may occur as early as 2 weeks after onset of infection).

References

1. Anson BJ, David J (1980) Developmental anatomy of the ear. In: Paparella MM, Shumrick DA (eds) Otolaryngology, Vol 1. Basic Sciences and Related Disciplines. Saunders, Philadelphia, pp 3–25
2. Bergstrom LB (1994) Anomalies of the ear. Otolaryngology 1:24–28
3. Casselman JW, Offeciers EF, De Foer B, et al (2001) CT and MR imaging of congenital abnormalities of the inner ear and internal auditory canal. Eur J Radiol 40:94–104
4. Chan KH (1994) Sensorineural hearing loss in children, classification and evaluation. Otolaryngol Clin North Am 27:473–486
5. Couly GF, Coltey PM, Le Douarin NM (1993) The triple origin of skull in higher vertebrates: a study in quail-chick chimeras. Development 17:409–429
6. Curtin HD (1988) Congenital malformations of the ear. Otolaryngol Clin North Am 21:317–336
7. DeSouza C, Paparella MM, Schacrern P, et al (1991) Pathology of labyrinthine ossification. J Laryngol Otol 105:621–624
8. Eelkema EA, Curtin HD (1989) Congenital anomalies of the temporal bone. Semin Ultrasound CT MR 10:195–212
9. Fisher NA, Curtin HD (1994) Radiology of congenital hearing loss. Otolaryngol Clin North Am 27:511–531
10. Gorlin R, Cohen M, Hennekam R (2001) Syndromes of the Head and Neck, 4th edn. Oxford University Press, New York

11. Jackler RK, Luxford WM, House WF (1987) Congenital malformation of the inner ear: a classification based on embryogenesis. Laryngoscope 97: 2–14

12. Kenneson A, Van Naarden Braun K, Boyle C (2002) GJB2 (connexin 26) variants and nonsyndromic sensorineural hearing loss: a HuGE review. Genet Med 4:258–274

13. Morimoto AK, Wiggins RH III, Hudgins PA, et al (2006) Absent semicircular canals in CHARGE syndrome: radiologic spectrum of findings. AJNR Am J Neuroradiol 27:1663–1171

14. Parker MJ, Fortnum H, Young ID, et al (1999) Variations in genetic assessment recurrence risks quoted for childhood deafness: a survey of clinical geneticists. J Med Genet 36:125–130

15. Phelps PD, Lloyd GAS (1990) Diagnostic Imaging of the Ear, 2nd edn. Springer-Verlag, London

16. Smith AL (1988) Neurologic sequelae of meningitis. N Engl J Med 319:1012–1013

17. Swartz JD, Faeber EN (1985) Congenital malformations of the external and middle ear: high-resolution CT findings of surgical import. AJR Am J Neuroradiol 144:501–506

18. Swartz JD, Harnsberger HR (1997) Imaging of the temporal bone, 3rd edn. Thieme, New York

19. Weissman JL (1996) Hearing loss. Radiology 199:593–611

20. William WML (1999) What is a 'Mondini' and what difference does a name make. AJNR Am J Neuroradiol 20:1442–1444

21. Young NM, Hughes CA, Byrd SE, et al (2000) Post meningitic ossification in paediatric cochlear implantation. Otolaryngol Head Neck Surg 122:183–188

Chapter 41

Acute Otitis Media in Children

Ingeborg Dhooge

41

Core Messages

- Acute otitis media (AOM) is one of the commonest paediatric infectious diseases. Its clinical spectrum may extend from a benign, self-limiting condition to a prolonged, complicated disease.
- A first episode before the age of 6 months is a strong and independent risk factor for recurrent AOM.
- AOM results from the interaction between microbial load (viral and bacterial), Eustachian tube dysfunction and an immature immune response.
- Most children recover well from AOM, even without antibacterial therapy.
- The clinician must bear in mind that if left untreated, the complications of otitis media may rapidly progress, with potentially life-threatening consequences.
- The presence of a normal tympanic membrane does not exclude the possibility of an otogenic complication of AOM.
- In most patients, the choice of treatment is empirical, and should be based on the available local epidemiological information on the commonest pathogens and their patterns of susceptibility

Contents

Introduction

Acute Otitis media (AOM) is one of the most common paediatric infectious diseases. The clinical spectrum may extend from a benign, self-limiting condition to a prolonged and sometimes complicated disease. Although in industrialised countries serious complications are rare, the burden of AOM is large, with impaired quality of life and high direct and indirect socio-economic costs. First described by Hippocrates in 450 BC, this disease continues to present one of the more troublesome medical problems of infancy and childhood.

Definitions

The following definitions are taken from Bluestone et al. (2002).

Otitis Media

This is an inflammation of the middle ear cleft, without reference to aetiology or pathogenesis.

Acute Otitis Media

In AOM, the presence of an infected effusion in the middle ear cleft occurs in conjunction with the rapid onset of one or more local or systemic signs and symptoms of acute infection. There is an advantage in grading the severity of AOM, since treatment guidelines should be graded according to the severity of the illness.

AOM Without Effusion (Myringitis)

This is characterised by erythema and opacification of the eardrum. Blisters or bullae may be present in cases of "bullous myringitis". In cases of myringitis, it may be difficult to establish, clinically, whether or not there is also a middle ear effusion.

Recurrent Otitis Media

Ten to twenty percent of children develop recurrent otitis media, with at least three episodes of AOM in 6 months or more than four episodes of AOM in 12 months, with evidence that the middle ear has returned to normal between episodes. These are called "otitis-prone" children.

Otorrhoea

This is a discharge from the ear. The acute onset of ear pain, fever and a purulent discharge through a perforation of the tympanic membrane (or tympanostomy tube) is evidence of AOM. This is called "AOM with perforation".

Epidemiology

AOM is mainly a disease of the young, occurring most commonly between the ages of 3 months and 3 years. The peak incidence is between ages 6 and 11 months. By 3 years of age, 50–85% of children have had AOM (Teele et al. 1989). The incidence decreases with age, and by 7 years of age relatively few children still experience episodes of AOM. Population-based studies from Finland and USA suggest an overall increase in AOM over the past 10–20 years, probably as a result of the increased attendance at day-care centres by younger children and infants. This trend should, however, be interpreted cautiously because changes in health-care systems, access to and use of care, and awareness of otitis media may have increased.

Predisposing Factors and Environmental Pressure

Host-Related Parameters

Age

The onset of a first episode before 6 months of age is a strong and independent risk factor for recurrent AOM. An early first acute suppurative otitis media episode may induce an inflammatory process in the middle ear, predisposing to recurrent attacks, and leading to the residual presence of otitis media with effusion or, alternatively, could reflect an innate predisposition for middle ear disease.

Gender

A small but significantly higher incidence in males has been reported (Teele et al. 2002).

Race

Native Americans, Canadian Inuits and Australian aboriginal children have a higher incidence of otitis media compared with similarly aged white children (Leach and Morris 2001). Although the difference in disease incidence for the different racial groups may be real, confounding factors like variability in socio-economic status, climate, access to medical care and diagnostic facilities of the health-care workers make this difference in prevalence of otitis media difficult to interpret.

Altered Host Defences and Underlying Diseases

Children with craniofacial defects or malformations (cleft palate, submucous cleft, craniofacial abnormality), altered physiologic defences (Eustachian tube dysfunction, barotraumas, cochlear implantation), congenital or acquired immunologic deficiencies (acquired immune deficiency syndrome, immunoglobulin deficiencies, chronic granulomatous disease, immunosuppressive drugs) are at risk for severe and recurrent AOM. Children with Down syndrome are at risk for recurrent AOM. Recent studies have implicated gastric reflux in the pathogenesis of otitis media; however, clear evidence is lacking (Heavner et al. 2001).

Genetic Predisposition

Twin studies have confirmed the role of heredity in recurrent otitis media (Kvaerner et al. 1996). Recurrent otitis media seems to be associated with genetically determined immunoglobulin markers, including allotype G2m(23) (Kelly 1993). However, it seems logical to suspect that many other genes are contributing. Knowledge of a child's genetic susceptibility could lead to individualised prevention and treatment strategies.

Prenatal and Perinatal Factors

Very low birth weight (<1500 g) or very preterm birth (<33 weeks of gestation) increases the risk of otitis media (Kvaerner et al. 1996). There is also a significant relationship between low levels of passively transferred maternal pneumococcal antibodies (measured in cord blood) and early otitis media (Becken et al. 2001). Finally, a meta-analysis of risk factor studies reported a 13% reduction in otitis media associated with exclusive breast-feeding lasting for 3–6 months (Uhari et al 1996).

Environmental Factors

Climate and Seasons

AOM is more common in the autumn and winter, along with the increase in viral respiratory infections, a common and well-recognised trigger. Birth in autumn is associated with higher otitis media recurrence (Daly et al. 1999).

Day Care/Home Care, Exposure to Other Children

Exposure to other children at home (siblings) or in a day-care setting increases the risk of otitis media, with the relative risk being proportionate to the number of children in a setting (Uhari et al. 1996). Centre care compared to home care produced the largest effect, with less difference in risk between family care and home care (Bennett and Haggard 1998). An infant who enters day care in the 1st year of life is at risk for early onset of otitis media.

Passive Smoking and Environmental Pollution

Meta-analyses confirm the increased incidence of otitis media associated with exposure to passive cigarette smoke (Uhari et al. 1996). High concentrations of sulphur dioxide in air samples, from atmospheric pollution, are significantly associated with an increased incidence of pneumococcal disease and middle ear disease.

Socio-Economic Status/Poverty

Crowded living conditions, poor sanitation and inadequate medical care have been associated with otitis media. However, the importance varies among studies.

Use of Dummies (Pacifiers)

Studies from Finland have shown that use of a dummy is a risk factor for otitis media (Niemelä et al. 2000).

Pathogenesis of otitis media

Several reasons (anatomical, physiological and immunological) account for the high incidence of otitis media in young children (Fig. 41.1). AOM is an infectious disease, resulting from the interaction between microbial load (viral and bacterial), Eustachian tube dysfunction and an immature immune response. In general, the following events can be envisaged: (1) pathogens must adhere to the nasopharyngeal epithelium; (2) pathogens must be able to enter the middle ear cavity through the Eustachian tube; (3) pathogens must be able to overcome the defensive mechanisms of the middle ear.

Eustachian Tube Dysfunction

The Eustachian tube has three important functions with respect to the middle ear: ventilation (equalising the pressure between the middle ear and ambient air), protection of the middle ear from ascending nasopharyngeal secretions or pathogens, sounds and pressure variations and clearance of secretions towards the nasopharynx. Clearance of the middle ear is achieved by mucociliary transport in the Eustachian tube directed towards the nasopharynx, and the pumping action of the Eustachian tube during closing.

The infant Eustachian tube is anatomically different from the adult tube, contributing to the increased incidence of otitis media in early childhood. In infants and young children, the Eustachian tube is short, lacks stiffness and is horizontally orientated. In cleft palate children, anatomical and functional disturbances of the Eustachian tube explain the high incidence of middle ear pathology. Dysfunction of the Eustachian tube can be enhanced by inflammation within the tube, but the tube can also be obstructed from external pressure such as from adenoids. A viral infection of the nasopharynx facilitates nasopharyngeal bacterial adherence and colonisation, and subsequent entry into the Eustachian tube, due to viral destructive interference in the mucociliary system.

Immature Immune Response

The nasopharynx is a natural reservoir for potential middle ear pathogens. Nasopharyngeal colonisation by potential middle ear pathogens is usually not followed by disease, since this is prevented by an active mucociliary clearance and powerful innate and adaptive immune systems.

Various secreted antimicrobial components of the innate immune system such as lysozyme, lactoferrin and defensins are found on the epithelium lining of the upper airway. These microbicidal proteins and peptides can selectively disrupt bacterial cell walls and membranes, sequester microbial nutrients or act as decoys for microbial attachment.

The primary adaptive immune defence against pathogens at the port of entry of the upper respiratory tract takes place in the organised mucosa-associated lymphoid

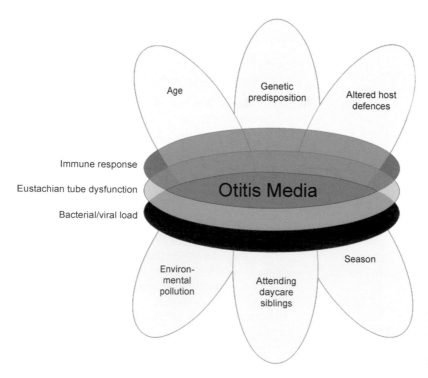

Fig. 41.1 Important factors involved in the pathogenesis of otitis media (adapted from Rosenfeld and Bluestone 2003)

tissue of Waldeyer's ring. Lymphoid cells of the adenoid can recognise and destroy nasopharyngeal pathogens. In addition, effector and memory lymphocytes are produced that migrate to neighbouring mucosal sites to reinforce the local immune response. Furthermore, locally produced secretory antibodies (sIgA and IgM) in nasopharyngeal secretions inhibit pathogen adherence (viral and bacterial) and reduce nasopharyngeal bacterial colonisation.

Serum antibodies protect the middle ear cavity from disease (Karma et al. 1995). High IgG2 concentrations are found in cord blood and in serum from newborns. The peak incidence of AOM is between ages 6 and 11 months. This coincides with a decline of maternally derived serum antibody levels, before the capacity to mount an antibody response to capsular polysaccharides has developed. The decrease in incidence of AOM after 18–24 months parallels the development of antibodies against the capsular polysaccharides of *Streptococcus pneumoniae*. Children with recurrent otitis media may lack secretory IgA or specific IgG2 antibodies (Dhooge et al. 2002). Finally, mucociliary deficiencies are evident in all children with amotile ciliary (Kartagener's) syndrome. Otitis media is therefore seen in those children from birth.

Microbial Infection

Respiratory viral infections usually precede or coincide with AOM in children. Viruses appear to reduce the protective and clearance capacity of the Eustachian tube and hence facilitate the entry of bacteria into the middle ear cavity. They also enhance or prolong the inflammation in the middle ear, and may significantly impair otitis media resolution. Respiratory syncytial virus is the most common virus isolated from middle ear fluid in children with AOM, followed by parainfluenza, rhinovirus, influenza, enteroviruses and adenovirus. In 5–20% of AOM cases, the cause is viral infection alone (Heikkinen et al. 1999), while co-infection with bacterial pathogens is much more common, occurring in 65% of cases. *S. pneumoniae* and non-typable *Haemophilus influenzae* are the two main bacterial pathogens. *S. pneumoniae* is isolated in 30–50% of cases, and *H. influenzae* in 20–30% of cases. *Moraxella catarrhalis* is the third most common bacteria, and is isolated in 3–20% of cases. *S. pyogenes* and *Staphylococcus aureus* is encountered in 1–5% of the cases (Bluestone et al. 1992). Most cases of AOM in infants under 2 months of age are caused by pathogens similar to those causing AOM in older children (Turner et al. 2002). Of the three major bacterial pathogens, *S. pneumoniae* has been associated with the greatest virulence and the most severe findings in AOM. It is also commonly associated with complications of otitis media. There is some evidence that the microbiology of AOM may be changing as a result of routine use of the conjugated pneumococcal vaccine.

In approximately 20% of cases of AOM, neither bacterial nor viral pathogens can be detected in the middle ear effusion (Heikkinen et al. 1999).

Natural History and Complications

The majority of children with AOM experience clinical resolution within 4–7 days of diagnosis with symptomatic treatment only (Glasziou et al. 2004). Complications are rare. Takata et al. (2001) made a pooled random effects estimate of the incidence of mastoiditis of 1 per 1000 in children with AOM not treated with antibiotics. Infants and children less than 2 years of age, those with recurrent AOM, or those with severe clinical symptoms are subgroups of children who are more prone to develop complications and should be evaluated with extra care. Children with predisposing factors (immune deficiencies, cleft palate, craniofacial abnormalities) also need particular care.

Acute Perforation

During an episode of AOM, the tympanic membrane can rupture due to pressure from pus accumulating in the middle ear space. Many clinicians consider such perforations a part of the disease process rather than a complication, especially because the majority heal uneventfully within 1–2 weeks.

Suppurative Complications

Early complications of otitis media result from spread of infection beyond the middle ear space. The effectiveness of antibiotic therapy and the low incidence of complications have resulted in an atmosphere of complacency in the treatment of otitis media in developed countries, as well as a lack of familiarity with the manifestations of impending complications among treating clinicians. The clinician must bear in mind that complications of otitis media, if left untreated, may rapidly progress with potentially life-threatening consequences.

The complications of otitis media are divided clinically into intratemporal (extracranial) and intracranial. Spread of infection through the osseous boundaries of the middle ear may occur by direct extension by bone erosion, through anatomic or preformed pathways, or by haematogenous or thrombophlebitic spread.

Computed tomography (CT) scanning with intravenous contrast is the imaging modality of choice in screening for complications of otitis media. Magnetic resonance imaging with gadolinium and angiography are useful when intracranial involvement is suspected.

Intratemporal (Extracranial) Complications of Otitis Media

Intratemporal complications are more common than intracranial complications, with acute mastoiditis accounting for the majority of cases. Facial paralysis and subperiosteal abscess are the most common second-stage complications.

Palva et al. (1985) reported an annual acute mastoiditis incidence of 0.3/100,000 for a Finnish population of one million. In The Netherlands, where the antibiotic prescription rate for AOM is at present low, the incidence of acute mastoiditis (3.8/100,000) is markedly higher. Mastoiditis is characterised by erythema, tenderness and swelling of the mastoid region associated with anterior displacement of the auricle (Fig. 41.2), posterior canal wall protrusion, otalgia, and a dull tympanic membrane. Post-auricular fluctuance is associated with subperiosteal abscess and confirms the presence of coalescence within the mastoid cavity. Patients previously treated with antibiotics can present with "masked mastoiditis" characterised by a prolonged course of mild symptoms, low-grade fever, a variable degree of otalgia and subtle neurological signs. The presence of a normal tympanic membrane does not exclude the possibility of an otogenic complication. A previous antibiotic course can clear the middle ear, but obstruction of the aditus ad antrum can trigger osteitis, which can spread, causing complications.

CT scanning allows the differentiation between mere opacification of the mastoid system, which is common in acute purulent otitis media, and disruption of the cellular system or demineralisation of the bone by osteoclastic activity, indicative of acute mastoiditis. Resorption of the bony septae in the mastoid will cause coalescence of the mastoid air cells. Finally, mastoiditis can extend medi-

ally to the mastoid apex (Gradenigo syndrome) or to the neck, via an infected, thrombosed sigmoid sinus (Bezold's abscess).

In the absence of coalescence, approximately 75–90% of cases can be effectively treated with intravenous antibiotics and myringotomy or tympanostomy tube insertion to ensure the drainage of the middle ear and to harvest a specimen for bacterial culture. Close to 20% of these patients will continue to be symptomatic despite antibiotic therapy and require an urgent cortical mastoidectomy. If the CT scan shows coalescence or bone erosion, initial management should be a myringotomy, mastoidectomy and appropriate antibiotic coverage.

Subperiosteal Abscess

Subperiosteal abscess of the mastoid can be defined as a purulent collection lateral to the mastoid cortex. Treatment varies from simple post-auricular aspiration, incision and drainage of the abscess, or incision and drainage with mastoidectomy.

Facial Palsy

As a complication of AOM, facial palsy is rarely encountered today, with an estimated incidence of 0.005%. It can occur in children during an episode of AOM or it can occur as a complication of acute mastoiditis. Management consists of myringotomy or tympanostomy tube insertion, and intravenous antibiotic therapy while awaiting culture results. Mastoid surgery is only performed in the presence of coalescent disease or other associated complications seen on CT scan (Popovtzer et al. 2005). Complete facial nerve recovery can be expected in >95% of patients with AOM.

Labyrinthitis

This results when infection spreads from the middle ear or mastoid air cells, or both, into the inner ear. Labyrinthitis may also be caused by meningitis, which may or may not be a complication of OM. Clinically, during the course of AOM, the patient presents with a severe sensorineural hearing loss and vertigo.

Intracranial Complications of Otitis Media

Among the intracranial complications, meningitis is the most frequently encountered, followed by lateral sinus thrombosis, brain abscess and otogenic hydrocephalus. These are life-threatening diseases associated with high mortality and serious residual symptoms.

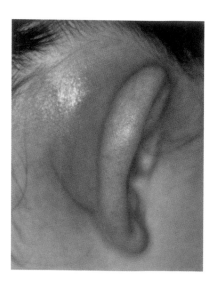

Fig. 41.2 Acute mastoiditis (by permission, from Becker 1984)

Assessment and Diagnosis

Symptoms and Signs

Children with AOM usually present with a history of rapid onset of signs and symptoms of an ear infection, irritability and sleep disturbances in an infant or toddler, otorrhoea and/or fever. However, most of these signs overlap with those of a common cold and almost any other acute infection. Earache has the highest predictive value for AOM, but the absence of earache does not exclude AOM (Kontiokari et al. 1998).

Infection with *S. pneumoniae* is associated with higher fever and more severe earache than other pathogens, while *H. influenzae* is commonly associated with conjunctivitis.

Clinical history alone is poorly predictive of the presence of AOM, especially in younger children. To establish the diagnosis with certainty, the presence of middle ear fluid must be confirmed by examination of the ear.

Otoscopy

Adequate illumination of the tympanic membrane requires proper lighting and an open ear canal. For pneumatic otoscopy, a speculum of proper shape and diameter must be selected to permit a seal in the external auditory canal. In small children, the otoscopic diagnosis can be difficult because of a small ear canal and the presence of wax. Appropriate restraint of the child to permit adequate examination is necessary.

The tympanic membrane is bulging and opaque (Fig. 41.3) and has limited or no mobility on pneumatic otoscopy. Fullness or bulging of the tympanic membrane combined with abnormal colour and absent mobility has the highest predictive value for AOM (Karma et al. 1993). Redness of the tympanic membrane caused by inflammation may be present and must be distinguished from the pink flush evoked by crying or high fever. In bullous myr-

ingitis, blisters may be seen on the tympanic membrane. The presence of purulent secretions in the external auditory canal (otorrhoea) as a result of tympanic membrane perforation is an obvious sign.

Ultimately, the gold standard for diagnosing AOM continues to be tympanocentesis with subsequent middle ear fluid culture for the identification of causative pathogens. However, tympanocentesis is not, now, a routine measure in the management of AOM.

Conventional Tympanometry

Tympanometry is an objective, quantitative method of assessing tympanic membrane mobility and the presence or absence of middle ear fluid. Most studies have used Jerger type B (absent impedance peak) or C^2 (peak pressure <-200 mmH$_2$O) tympanograms to diagnose middle ear effusion (Feldman 1976). The sensitivity and specificity of tympanometry are high (sensitivity 94%, specificity 50–70%). Because tympanometry is unable to distinguish a serous from a purulent effusion, the results must be combined with the history and clinical examination of the patient.

Conventional Audiometry

Pure tone audiometry or visual reinforcement audiometry can be used to diagnose the conductive hearing loss associated with AOM in young children.

Other Diagnostic Procedures

In evaluating a child with recurrent AOM, other diagnostic procedures can be helpful in determining predisposing factors: for example, X-rays of the nasopharynx or nasopharyngeal fibroscopy to assess adenoid size (Fig. 41.4), and immunologic evaluation.

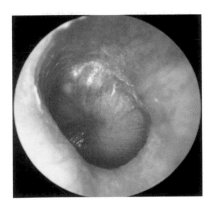

Fig. 41.3 The typical appearance of the tympanic membrane in acute otitis media

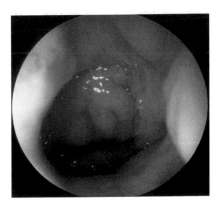

Fig. 41.4 Nasendoscopic view of the nasopharynx, showing adenoid hypertrophy

Imaging

In the routine evaluation of a child with an uncomplicated AOM, imaging of the temporal bone is not warranted.

Treatment

Medical

Symptomatic Treatment

Pain and fever are common features of AOM, and management of the pain associated with AOM is an essential part of care. Paracetamol and non-steroidal anti-inflammatory drugs are effective analgesics and therefore the mainstay of pain management for AOM. Adequate dosage is necessary: paracetamol (rectally or orally administered) at 60 mg/kg/day in four to six divided doses; ibuprofen (oral administration) at 20–30 mg/kg/day in three to four divided doses.

Ear drops contain analgesic and antibacterial agents or both. Some beneficial effects of ear drops in AOM-associated otalgia have been reported. However, some substances in ear drops can induce allergy (neomycin) or are potentially ototoxic (aminoglycosides, with continued use) when the tympanic membrane is not intact. Ototopic agents such as ofloxacin and ciprofloxacin with or without steroids are effective and safe in the treatment of acute otorrhoea occurring in case of a perforated ear drum or through a tympanostomy tube.

Although often prescribed, there is no proven benefit from oral decongestants and antihistamines in the management of AOM (Flynn et al. 2004). These agents may relieve accompanying nasal symptoms.

Antibacterial Treatment

Immediate Antibacterial Treatment Versus Watchful Waiting

Concerns about the rising rates of bacterial resistance and the significant costs of antibacterial prescriptions have focussed the attention of the medical community on the need for judicious use of antibiotics. The strategy of "watchful waiting" in selected children is based on results of randomised controlled trials performed over the last 30 years demonstrating that most children recover well from AOM even without antibacterial therapy (Rosenfeld and Kay 2003). The decision to observe or to treat (with antibiotics) is based on the child's age, the diagnostic certainty and the severity of the disease (Table 41.1). As only few data are available on the youngest age groups, and as younger age has been demonstrated to be associated with poorer outcomes for AOM, a more aggressive approach is recommended for these children. Obviously in children with underlying medical conditions that may alter the natural course of AOM (Down syndrome, cleft palate, immunodeficiency or presence of a cochlear implant) a more aggressive approach is recommended. If the "observation option" is used, the clinician should share with parents or caregivers the degree of diagnostic certainty and consider their preference. Observation is only an option when there is ready access to adequate follow-up care. If watchful waiting results in clinical failure after 48–72 h, the start of antibacterial therapy should be considered.

Choice, Dosage and Duration of Antibacterial Treatment in AOM

The choice of treatment is empirical in most of the patients and should be based on the available local epide-

Table 41.1 Management of acute otitis media (AOM) according to age, diagnostic certainty and severity of disease

Age	Certain diagnosis[a]	Uncertain diagnosis
<6 months	Antibacterial therapy	Antibacterial therapy
6 months to 2 years	Antibacterial therapy	Antibacterial therapy if severe[b] illness; observation if non-severe illness
≥2 years	Antibacterial therapy if severe[b] illness; observation if non-severe illness	Observation

[a] A certain diagnosis of acute otitis media meets all three criteria: (1) rapid onset, (2) signs of middle ear effusion and (3) signs and symptoms of middle ear inflammation.

[b] In case of severe AOM, the child presenting with moderate-to-severe otalgia, fever equal to or higher than 39°C orally (39.5°C rectally), while in non-severe AOM, there is mild otalgia and fever less than 39°C orally (39.5°C rectally), or no fever

miological information on the most common pathogens and their susceptibility patterns. Differences in antibiotic consumption and factors promoting the carriage and spread of antimicrobial resistant organisms, such as the organisation of childcare in day-care centres contribute to national differences in resistance profiles.

Between 10 and 50% of upper respiratory *S. pneumoniae* isolates are estimated to be penicillin resistant, the majority being of intermediate resistance (MIC between 0.1 and 1.0 µg/ml). Approximately 20–30% of isolates of *H. influenzae* and up to 100% of *M. catarrhalis* derived from the upper respiratory tract are estimated to be β-lactamase-positive worldwide.

Amoxicillin remains the drug of choice in the treatment of uncomplicated AOM because of its efficacy against *S. pneumoniae* and a favourable pharmacodynamic profile, as well as safety, low cost, acceptable taste, and narrow microbiological spectrum. All intermediately resistant *S. pneumoniae* strains and many highly resistant *S. pneumoniae* strains can be effectively eradicated using a high amoxicillin dose (80–90 mg/kg/day) (Piglansky et al. 2003). High-dose amoxicillin-clavulanate (40 mg/kg/day amoxicillin component in three divided doses) is recommended as second-line empirical treatment for non-responding patients treated initially with other antibacterial agents or in patients for whom additional coverage

for ß-lactamase-producing *H. influenzae* and *M. catarrhalis* is desired. Risk factors for the presence of bacterial species likely to be resistant to amoxicillin include recent receipt (less than 30 days) of antibacterial treatment, and day-care attendance (Brook and Gober 2005; Table 41.2).

In case of non-IgE-mediated penicillin allergy, cefuroxime 50 mg/kg/day in two divided doses may be used. In the patient who is vomiting or cannot otherwise tolerate oral medication, a single intramuscular dose of parenteral ceftriaxone (50 mg/kg) has been shown to be effective for the initial treatment of AOM (Leibovitz et al. 2000). In selected cases, macrolides (azithromycin 10 mg/kg per day on day 1 followed by 5 mg/kg/day for 4 days as a single daily dose, or clarithromycin (15 mg/kg/day in two divided doses) can be an option. However, the two main common pathogens involved in AOM, *S. pneumonia* and *H. influenzae*, display a major resistance to macrolide antibiotics.

The optimal duration of antibiotic treatment for AOM remains uncertain. A course of 10 days is justified in the case of otorrhoea, in children <2 years of age, in day-care attendants and in case of history of chronic or recurrent AOM. In other cases a 5- to 7-day course is recommended.

Risks of antibiotics include allergic reactions, gastric intolerance, accelerated bacterial resistance and unfavourable changes in nasopharyngeal bacterial flora.

Table 41.2 Choice of antibiotic in the management of acute otitis media (adapted from Segal et al. 2005)

I. First-line therapy
(1) Amoxicillin (50 mg/kg/day in three divided doses, for 5–7 days): Empirical treatment of first episode of AOM Empirical treatment of AOM in areas with low prevalence of pneumococcal penicillin resistance
(2) Amoxicillin (80–90 mg/kg/day in three divided doses for 5–7 days): Empirical treatment of AOM in children having received antibiotics during previous months; in otitis prone children; in day-care attendants Empirical treatment of AOM in areas with high prevalence of pneumococcal penicillin resistance
(3) Amoxicillin/clavulanate (40 mg/kg/day amoxicillin component) + amoxicillin 40 mg/kg/day in three divided doses for 5–7 days): Empirical treatment of AOM in neonates Empirical treatment of AOM in immunocompromised patients Empirical treatment of AOM in areas with high prevalence of β-lactamase-producing organisms Empirical treatment of AOM in patients who received antibiotics for AOM during preceding month
II. Second-line therapy[a]
(1) Amoxicillin/clavulanate (40 mg/kg/day amoxicillin component in three divided doses) for 5–7 days
(2) Intramuscular ceftriaxone (50 mg/kg/day) for 3 days

[a] Therapeutic failure is not considered before 72 h of first-line therapy.

Treatment failure with Initial Antibacterial Treatment for AOM

When antibacterial agents are prescribed for AOM, the time course of clinical response should be 48–72 h. If initially febrile, the patient's temperature is expected to return to normal within 48–72 h. Irritability should diminish, and sleeping and eating patterns should begin to normalise. If the patient does not improve by 48–72 h, reassessment of the patient is necessary. A patient who fails to respond to a second, different oral antibiotic should be treated with a 3-day course of parenteral ceftriaxone (50 mg/kg/day once daily) because of its superior efficacy against *S. pneumoniae*, compared with alternative oral antibacterials (Leibovitz et al. 2000).

If the patient still does not improve, admission to hospital and tympanocentesis with Gram-stain, culture, and antibacterial-agent sensitivity studies of the fluid is essential to guide additional therapy.

"Alternative" Medical Treatments

None of these modalities (homeopathy, osteopathic and chiropractic manipulation, acupuncture, nutritional supplements) has been subjected to a published, peer-reviewed, clinical trial. A general concern about herbal products is the lack of any oversight into product quality and purity.

Surgical Therapy

Myringotomy

Tympanocentesis or myringotomy, the incision of the tympanic membrane, used to be part of the routine treatment of AOM in some countries. Five randomised studies compared antibiotics with a combination of myringotomy and antibiotics. All of these studies showed that the surgical procedures did not improve symptoms or resolution.

Table 41.3 Indications for myringotomy

Severe otalgia or high fever
Confirmed or potential suppurative complication
Unsatisfactory response to antibiotic therapy
Onset of AOM during antibiotic treatment
AOM in newborns
AOM in patient with primary or secondary immunodeficiency

Tympanocentesis and myringotomy should therefore be reserved for children suffering from severe illness, failure to respond to antibiotics or impending complications, to provide adequate drainage of the middle ear and for microbiological diagnosis (Table 41.3).

Tympanocentesis can be performed under general anaesthesia, or after local anaesthesia of the ear drum, using a myringotomy knife or an intramuscular needle attached to a 2-cm^3 syringe. The anteroinferior or posteroinferior quadrant of the ear drum is incised.

Tympanostomy Tube Insertion

With the growing evidence that long-term antimicrobial prophylaxis for recurrent AOM is associated with the emergence of resistant *Pneumococcus*, a possible alternative is tympanostomy tube placement. Children with recurrent AOM who receive tympanostomy tubes have 67% fewer episodes of AOM than controls (Rosenfeld and Bluestone 2003). Transient otorrhoea occurs in 16% of patients in the post-operative period, and later in 26%, but is infrequently chronic, recurrent or requires tube removal. Risk factors for early post-tympanostomy tube otorrhoea are the presence of purulent middle ear fluid, bacteria in culture of middle ear fluid, young age, and marked mastoid cloudiness on radiographs.

Several controlled trials of prophylactic ear drop use after tube insertion show conflicting results and limited clinical benefits. Silastic tubes impregnated with silver oxide yielded a lower post-intubation otorrhoea rate (5.1% versus 9.8%) when compared with non-impregnated identical tubes (Chole and Hubbell 1995). Middle ear discharge in a child with tubes can be treated initially with ototopic agents such as ofloxacin and ciprofloxacin or a short course of aminoglycoside and steroid drops. If the middle ear discharge continues for longer than 1 week despite appropriate topical antibiotics, re-examination of the child is necessary. If the persistence of otorrhoea is not attributable to poor compliance to the treatment, more intensive therapy is necessary, including daily cleansing of the ear canal in combination with oral antibiotics. Sometimes the reason for the persistent discharge is biofilm formation on the tube or cholesteatoma. In selected cases, removal of the tube may even be necessary to stop the discharge.

Adenoidectomy

Adenoidectomy reduces the incidence of AOM by 0–3 episodes per child-year. This procedure also significantly reduces the chance of future tube insertions for children aged 2 years or older who have recurrent otitis media after tube extrusion (relative decrease of 52%; Rosenfeld and Bluestone 2003). Recently, Coyte et al. (2001) showed that the benefit of adenoidectomy is already apparent at age 2 years and is the greatest for children aged 3 years or older irrespective of adenoid size. Adenoidectomy has a 0.2–0.5% incidence of haemorrhage and a 2% incidence of transient velopharyngeal insufficiency.

Follow-Up

Once the patient has shown clinical improvement, follow-up is based on the usual clinical course of AOM. Persistent middle ear fluid after resolution of acute symptoms is common and should not be viewed as a need for active therapy. Two weeks after an episode of AOM, 60–70% of children have middle ear fluid, decreasing to 40% at 1 month and 10% to 25% after 3 months (Rosenfeld and Kay 2003). It is important to establish that otitis media with effusion resolves. Evaluation of the hearing is particularly important for children with cognitive or developmental problems.

Prevention of AOM

To prevent the onset of AOM episodes and to reduce the incidence of recurrent AOM, several environmental control measures are recommended. Prolonged breastfeeding, limiting dummy (pacifier) use and eliminating exposure to tobacco smoke have been postulated as reducing the incidence of AOM. These recommendations, however, are mainly based on non-randomised controlled epidemiological trials.

The efficacy of antibiotic prophylaxis on the prevention of recurrent otitis media has been evaluated in a meta-analysis (Williams et al. 1993). The small benefit on episodes per month must be balanced against the risk of drug-induced side effects and the disadvantage of promoting antibiotic resistance.

The use of xylitol, a polyol sugar-alcohol that inhibits the growth of S. Pneumoniae, was shown to significantly reduce AOM incidence. But compliance with this treatment is very poor, mainly due to the unpractical dosing schedule (chewing gum or syrup five times daily). The use of xylitol only during upper-respiratory infections showed no effect in preventing AOM (Uhari et al. 1998).

In more than 75% of cases, an episode of AOM is preceded by a viral upper respiratory tract infection. Consequently, the reduction of upper airway infections by altering child-care attendance patterns, by limiting large-group day-care, avoiding full-time day-care attendance or by postponing day care until the age of 6 months, is often recommended. Intranasal fluticasone propionate administered during viral upper-respiratory infections has no effect and might even increase AOM incidence.

Immunoprophylaxis with killed (Clements et al. 1995) and live-attenuated intranasal influenza vaccines (Belshe and Gruber 2000) has demonstrated more than 30% efficacy in the prevention of AOM during the influenza season in children older than 2 years. In younger children, the efficacy of killed influenza vaccine in the prevention of AOM could not be demonstrated (Hoberman et al. 2003).

Vaccines for respiratory syncytial virus, parainfluenza virus and adenovirus, currently under development, hold additional promise.

The 23-valent polysaccharide vaccine against *S. pneumoniae* covers 90% of all known pneumococcal infections in developed countries and has marginal benefit for children older than 2 years, favouring those with previous AOM episodes (Straetemans et al. 2002). The pneumococcal conjugate vaccines are shown to be immunogenic in children younger than 2 years and are highly effective against invasive pneumococcal infections. Although the pneumoccocal conjugate vaccine decreases the proportion of AOM due to vaccine-related *S. pneumoniae* serotypes by 56–67%, this effect is counteracted by an increase in AOM caused by other bacterial pathogens of the upper airway (*H. Influenzae* and *Moraxella*) or by non-vaccine pneumococcal serotypes (van Kempen et al. 2006).

Sequelae

The sequelae of AOM in children include:

1. Hearing loss (conductive/sensorineural).
2. Perforation of the tympanic membrane without otitis media.
3. Chronic suppurative otitis media with/without cholesteatoma.
4. Atelectasis of the middle ear/adhesive otitis media.
5. Ossicular discontinuity/ossicular fixation.

Summary for the Clinician

- AOM refers to an acute infection or inflammation in the middle ear with local or systemic signs and symptoms and the presence of an effusion in the middle ear. AOM is usually a self-limiting disease. The use of the delayed antibiotic-prescription strategy is appropriate in the majority of cases. Only a small percentage of children with AOM will benefit from antibiotic therapy. However, the clinician must bear in mind that complications of AOM, if left untreated, may rapidly progress with potentially life-threatening consequences.

41

References

1. Becken ET, Daly KA, Lindgren BR, Meland MH, Giebink GS (2001) Low cord blood pneumococcal antibody concentrations predict more episodes of otitis media. Arch Otolaryngol Head Neck Surg 127:517–522

2. Becker W (1984) Atlas of Ear, Nose and Throat Diseases, 2nd edn. Georg Thieme Verlag, Stuttgart

3. Belshe RB, Gruber WC (2000) Prevention of otitis media in children with live attenuated influenza vaccine given intranasally. Pediatr Infect Dis J 19:S66–71

4. Bennett KE, Haggard MP (1998) Accumulation of factors influencing children's middle ear disease: risk factor modelling on a large population cohort. J Epidemiol Community Health 52:786–793

5. Bluestone CD, Gates GA, Klein JO, Lim DJ, et al (2002) Recent advances in otitis media, 1: definitions, terminology, and classification of otitis media. Ann Otol Rhinol Laryngol 111:8–18

6. Bluestone CD, Stephenson JS, Martin LM (1992) Ten-year review of acute otitis media pathogens. Pediatr Infect Dis J 11:S7–11

7. Brook I, Gober AE (2005) Antimicrobial resistance in the nasopharyngeal flora of children with acute otitis media and otitis media recurring after amoxicillin therapy. J Med Microbiol 54:83–85

8. Chole RA, Hubbell R (1995) Antimicrobial activity of Silastic tympanostomy tubes impregnated with silver oxide. Arch Otolaryngol Head Neck Surg 121:562–565

9. Clements DA, Langdon L, Bland C, Walter E (1995) Influenza A vaccine decreases the incidence of otitis media in 6- to 30-month-old children in day care. Arch Pediatr Adolesc Med 149:1113–1117

10. Coyte PC, Croxford R, McIsaac W, Feldman W, Friedberg J (2001) The role of adjuvant adenoidectomy and tonsillectomy in the outcome of the insertion of tympanostomy tubes. N Engl J Med 344:1188–1195

11. Daly KA, Brown JE, Lindgren BR, Meland MH, Le CT, Giebink GS (1999) Epidemiology of otitis media onset by six months of age. Pediatrics 103:1158–1166

12. Dhooge I, van Kempen M, Sanders L, Rijkers G (2002) Deficient IgA and IgG2 anti-pneumococcal antibody levels and response to vaccination in otitis prone children. Int J Pediatr Otorhinolaryngol 64:133–141

13. Feldman AS (1976) Tympanometry – procedures, interpretation and variables. In: Feldman AS, Wilber LA (eds) Acoustic Impedance and Admittance – The Measurements of Middle Ear Function. Williams and Wilkins, Baltimore, pp 103–155

14. Flynn CA, Griffin GH, Schultz JK (2004) Decongestants and antihistamines for acute otitis media in children. Cochrane Database Syst Rev (3):CD001727

15. Glasziou PP, Del Mar CB, Sanders SL, Hayem M (2004) Antibiotics for acute otitis media in children. Cochrane Database Syst Rev (1):CD000219

16. Heavner SB, Hardy SM, White DR (2001) Transient inflammation and dysfunction of the Eustachian tube secondary to multiple exposures of simulated gastro oesophageal refluxant. Ann Otol Rhinol Laryngol 110:928–934

17. Heikkinen T, Thin MT, Chonmaitree T (1999) Prevalence of various respiratory viruses in the middle ear during acute otitis media. N Engl J Med 340:260–264

18. Hoberman A, Greenberg DP, Paradise JL, et al (2003) Effectiveness of inactivated influenza vaccine in preventing acute otitis media in young children: a randomized controlled trial. JAMA 290:1608–1616

19. Karma PH, Bakaletz LO, Giebink GS, Mogi G, Rynnel-Dagoo B (1995) Immunological aspects of otitis media: present views on possibilities of immunoprophylaxis of acute otitis media in infants and children. Int J Pediatr Otorhinolaryngol 32:S127–134

20. Karma PH, Sipilia MM, Kataja MJ, Penttilia MA (1993) Pneumatic otoscopy and otitis media. II. Value of different tympanic membrane findings and their combinations. In: Lim DJ, Bluestone CD, Klein JO, Nelson JD, Ogra PL (eds) Recent Advances in Otitis Media: Proceedings of the Fifth International Symposium. Decker Periodicals, Burlington, Ontario, pp 41–45

21. Kelly KM (1993) Recurrent otitis media: genetic immunoglobulin markers in children and their parents. Int J Pediatr Otorhinolaryngol 25:279–280

22. Kontiokari T, Koivunen P, Niemelä M, Pokka T, Uhari M (1998) Symptoms of acute otitis media. Pediatr Infect Dis J 17:676–679

23. Kvaerner KJ, Tambs IC, Harris JR, Magnus P (1996) The relationship between otitis media and intrauterine growth: a co-twin study. Int J Pediatr Otorhinolaryngol 37:217–225

24. Leach AL, Morris PS (2001) Perspectives on infective ear disease in indigenous Australian children. J Paediatr Child Health 37:529–530

25. Leibovitz E, Piglansky L, Raiz S, Press J, Leiberman A, Dagan R (2000) Bacteriologic and clinical efficacy of one day vs. three day intramuscular ceftriaxone for treatment of nonresponsive acute otitis media in children. Pediatr Infect Dis J 19:1040–1045

26. Niemelä M, Pihakari O, Pokka T, Uhari M (2000) Pacifier as a risk factor for acute otitis media: a randomized, controlled trial of parental counseling. Pediatrics 106:483–488

27. Palva T, Virtanen H, Mäkinen J (1985) Acute and latent mastoiditis in children. J Laryngol Otol 99:127–136

28. Piglansky L, Leibovitz E, Raiz S, Greenberg D, Press J, Leiberman A, Dagan R (2003) The bacteriologic and clinical efficacy of high-dose amoxicillin as first-line therapy for acute otitis media in children. Pediatr Infect Dis J 22:405–412

29. Popovtzer A, Raveh E, Bahar G, Oestreicher-Kedem Y, Feinmesser R, Nageris B (2005) Facial palsy associated with acute otitis media. Otolaryngol Head Neck Surg 132:327–329

30. Rosenfeld RM, CD Bluestone CD (2003) Clinical efficacy of surgical therapy. In: Rosenfeld RM, Bluestone CD (eds) Evidence-Based Otitis Media (2nd edn). BC Decker, Hamilton, ON, pp 227–240

31. Rosenfeld RM, Kay D (2003) Natural history of untreated otitis media. In: Rosenfeld RM, Bluestone CD (eds) Evidence-Based Otitis Media (2nd edn). BC Decker, Hamilton, ON, pp 180–198

32. Segal N, Leibovitz E, Dagan R, Leiberman A (2005) Acute otitis media – diagnosis and treatment in the era of antibiotic resistant organisms: updated clinical practice guidelines. Int J Pediatr Otorhinolaryngol 69:1311–1319

33. Straetemans M, Sanders EAM, Veenhoven RH, Schilder AGM, Damoiseaux RAMJ, Zielhuis GA (2002) Pneumococcal vaccines for preventing otitis media. Cochrane Database Syst Rev 2:CD001480

34. Takata GS, Chan LS, Shekelle P, Morton SC, Mason W, Marcy SM (2001) Evidence assessment of management of acute otitis media: I. The role of antibiotics in treatment of uncomplicated acute otitis media. Pediatrics 108:239–247

35. Teele DW, Klein JO, Rosner B (1989) Epidemiology of otitis media during first seven years of life in children in greater Boston: a prospective, cohort study. J Infect Dis 160:83–94

36. Turner D, Leibovitz E, Aran A, Piglansky L, Raiz S, Leiberman A, Dagan R (2002) Acute otitis media in infants younger than two months of age: microbiology, clinical presentation and therapeutic approach. Pediatr Infect Dis 21:669–674

37. Uhari M, Kontiokari T, Niemelä M (1998) A novel use of xylitol sugar in preventing acute otitis media. Pediatrics 102:879–884

38. Uhari M, Mäntysaari K, Niemelä M (1996) A meta-analytic review of the risk factors for acute otitis media. Clin Infect Dis 22:1079–1083

39. van Kempen MJ, Vermeiren JS, Vaneechoutte M, Claeys G, Veenhoven RH, Rijkers GT, Sanders EA, Dhooge IJ (2006) Pneumococcal conjugate vaccination in children with recurrent acute otitis media: a therapeutic alternative? Int J Pediatr Otorhinolaryngol 70:275–285

40. Williams RL, Chalmers TC, Stange KC, Chalmers FT, Bowlin SJ (1993) Use of antibiotics in preventing recurrent otitis media and in treating otitis media with effusion: a meta-analytic attempt to resolve the brouhaha. JAMA 270:1344–1351

Otitis Media With Effusion

Peter J. Robb

42

Core Messages

1. The initial management of otitis media with effusion is watchful waiting and the monitoring of hearing.
2. Medical treatments have not been proven to be effective in the management of otitis media with effusion. Treatment of associated rhinitis is helpful. Nasal autoinflation may produce benefit if used regularly.
3. Complementary and alternative treatments have not been proven to be effective in the management of otitis media with effusion.
4. Insertion of ventilation tubes for children over 3 years of age with a bilateral hearing impairment associated with otitis media with effusion, who have failed watchful waiting, is effective in restoring hearing thresholds. The measurable benefits are short-lived and modest.
5. The large benefits reported by parents are at odds with the modest short-term benefits measured in well-designed scientific studies over a more appropriate period.
6. The combination of ventilation tubes and adenoidectomy in children over 3 years of age is beneficial in terms of hearing, general health and development. The benefit is sustained over 2 years after intervention and is cost-effective.
7. The benefit from surgery for bilateral otitis media with effusion in children under the age of 3 years is no better than with watchful waiting.
8. At present there is no evidence to support the surgical management of unilateral otitis media with effusion.

Contents

Introduction

Otitis media with effusion (OME or "glue ear") is the most common cause of hearing impairment in childhood. The condition is generally self-limiting, but may occur during a period when poor hearing will impede speech and language development. The effects are mostly short term, but in children in whom the condition recurs throughout childhood, some effects on behaviour and cognition are detectable up to the age of 10 years and beyond (Bennett and Haggard 1999).

There is evidence that untreated OME may produce lasting effects on behaviour and development, particularly attention and hyperactivity (Silva et al. 1982). However, in a longitudinal study, Bennett and Haggard (1998) showed that continuation of such a developmental impact into the teens was restricted to those few whose middle ear disease had lasted through late childhood.

OME is characterised by an inflammation of the middle ear accompanied by the accumulation of serous or mucoid fluid in the middle ear (Zeilhuis 1998). Inflammation of the middle ear results in metaplasia of the middle ear mucosa, with proliferation of mucus glands and goblet cells. Vascular proliferation precedes the production of a lymphocyte and plasma cell infiltrate (Ishii et al. 1980; Sadé 1966). Signs of acute inflammation are typically absent, although emerging evidence supports a covert biofilm infection as a major contributing cause of the inflammatory changes in the middle ear cleft (Fergie et al. 2004).

The prevalence of OME has a bimodal distribution rising from birth to a first peak around the age of 2 years, falling away via a subsidiary second peak around 5 years of age (Zeilhuis 1998). These peaks coincide with initial attendance at day-care and primary school, reflecting corresponding peaks in the exposure to infective pathogens. The prevalence of OME in children of 7.5–8.0 years of age is approximately 8%, although this is subject to wide variation, dependent on season. During the months of November to April, in the northern hemisphere, the prevalence may be double that during other seasons (Schilder et al. 1993). About 80% of children aged 10 years will have been affected by an episode of otitis media with effusion during childhood, mostly in the first 3 years of their life (Williamson 2002). Over half of cases of OME follow episodes of acute otitis media (AOM), and children with OME typically experience up to five times more episodes of AOM than those without OME (Zeilhuis et al. 1989).

Epidemiology

There are many aetiological risk factors, and only recently has a coherent picture emerged of their relative significance.

Birth Order

Having an older sibling is a risk factor for OME (Sassen et al. 1997).

Gender

Male sex is a weak, but consistent factor for cumulative incidence and prevalence of OME (Teele et al. 1989).

Breast-Feeding

In numerous studies, breast-feeding has been reported as reducing the risk of ear and respiratory infections, and hence, of OME (Duffy et al. 1997; Paradise et al. 1997) Maternal immunity has been proposed as the mechanism underlying this protective effect. Breast-fed infants carry reduced numbers of bacteria in their nasopharynx. A two-fold increase in risk of first episodes of AOM or OME was found in infants exclusively formula-fed as opposed to those breast-fed for 6 months. However, a large longitudinal birth cohort study of over 12,000 children born in 1970, whilst confirming other established risk factors, found the protective effect of breast-feeding to be weak (Bennett and Haggard 1998). This illustrates that depending on the nature of the population, the strength of the risk factors is variable.

Day-Care

Attending day-care imparts a risk of OME up to three times that for children cared for at home or by a child-minder in a small group. The risk is also higher in families with a large number of siblings at home (Paradise et al. 1997).

The influences of season, day-care attendance and family size are likely to be inter-related variables, the common element being increased exposure to both viral and bacterial respiratory pathogens. The day-care environment can furthermore be a forcing ground for bacterial resistance due to heavy antibiotic prescribing and re-circulating infections (Barnes et al. 1995).

Parental Smoking

Maternal, but not paternal smoking was shown to be associated with presence of middle ear effusion in the children (8–18 years) of British servicemen (Green and Cooper 1991). In a large, longitudinal cohort study, a similar dependence on parent gender was found, suggesting a direct relation to dose (Bennett and Haggard 1998). Controlling statistically for further influential factors, a systematic quantitative review from the UK (Strachan and Cook 1998) concluded that there is likely to be a causal relationship between parental smoking and both acute and chronic middle ear disease in children.

Infection

In a study of 1679 children, Karma proposed that OME was the end state of an infectious cascade initiated by an episode of AOM. While the acute phase may respond to antibiotic treatment, the chronic stage of effusion was unlikely to do so (Karma 1988).

Infective pathogens stimulate an immune response, with release of cytokines (Kubba et al. 2000). Respiratory viruses may predispose to bacterial infection, or may stimulate an immune response themselves. The release of inflammatory mediators upregulates the mucin genes expressed in the middle ear, leading to the secretion of mucin-rich fluid, recognised clinically as the middle ear effusion seen at myringotomy.

In a small study of middle ear effusions that produced "sterile" cultures, polymerase chain reaction (PCR) confirmed the presence of bacteria (typically *Haemophilus influenzae, Streptococcus pneumoniae* and *Moraxella catarrhalis*), in apparently sterile middle ear fluid (Fergie et al. 2004).

Confocal laser scanning microscopy and vital dye examination of middle ear tissue biopsy samples taken at the time of ventilation tube insertion have demonstrated biofilm colonies in 80% of ears (Kerschner et al. 2005).

In the context of a biofilm infection, the fulfilment of Koch's postulates, using traditional methods of culturing bacteria as proof of infectious aetiology, is no longer a tenable approach to the confirmation of bacterial infection. More recent studies of culture-negative middle ear effusions found that PCR techniques could demonstrate bacterial mRNA as a marker for metabolically active organisms in culture-sterile middle ear effusions (Rayner et al. 1998). The inference is that bacteria, in a form that could not be previously demonstrated, are present even in "sterile" effusions, cultured by traditional techniques. Much current evidence points to bacterial biofilm colonies as a major cause of middle ear inflammation and of persistence of middle ear effusion. Rosenfeld concluded that the benefits from antibiotic treatment in the OME phase are so slight that, in the face of drug resistance from widespread low-dose use, the prescribing of antibiotics is a poor clinical policy (Rosenfeld and Post 1992).

As evidence gathers that persistent OME is likely to be largely due to a biofilm infection, there will be many implications for the future management of OME. The use of biofilm-resistant surfaces, probiotic treatment, chemical or mechanical disruption of the protective glycocalyx of the biofilm and, ultimately, modulation of the biofilm phenotype are all modalities of treatment for OME that have been proposed (Goessler 2005).

Immune Deficiency and Allergy

This topic is discussed in Chapters 10 and 34.

Reflux of Gastric Acid

There is accumulating evidence that gastric acid may act as an inflammatory co-factor in the development of low-grade inflammation of the Eustachian tube and middle ear mucosa. In a study of middle ear effusions at the time of myringotomy in 54 children aged 2–8 years, 83% of the effusions contained pepsin/pepsinogen at concentrations up to 1000-fold greater than those in serum (Tasker et al. 2002). One direct causal hypothesis is that inflammation caused by the acid reflux improves the conditions for bacterial colonisation. This could also facilitate chronic biofilm infection. As yet, no trial of anti-reflux treatment for the management of OME has been reported, perhaps because there are many other contributing risk factors, none of which is likely to have a dominant influence. The common factor of inflammation suggests that diverse types of insult can influence different stages of the immune cascade that allows the establishment of a biofilm colony, resulting in persistence of the middle ear effusion (Fig. 42.1).

Symptoms and Signs of OME

OME may be asymptomatic. Discomfort from the presence of the middle ear effusion does occur, but is hard to measure, and clinical reports from older children suggest that it is not always an important symptom. In younger children, poor articulation, language delay and poor balance may be observed (Golz et al. 1998). In older children, nursery teachers or schoolteachers often draw attention to the hearing loss when inattention in a group setting is noted. Poor social interaction and disengagement from class activities that require good "signal in noise" hearing are frequently reported. Frequently, a hearing loss is noted at a routine hearing screening assessment, before which there was little parental concern about the child's hearing.

Diagnosis

Clinical diagnosis following a full history is made by examination of the ears and age-appropriate audiological testing. The tympanic membrane is best assessed with otomicroscopy, but in general clinical practice, a bright halogen otoscope provides clear illumination. Loss of the light reflex, dullness, amber-gold colouration of the tympanic membrane due to middle ear effusion, and an air-fluid meniscus are all common findings in cases of confirmed middle ear effusion. The apparently more horizontal appearance of the malleus that is often seen results from negative middle ear pressure drawing the long process of the malleus medially. Attic retraction or retraction of the posterior pars tensa of the tympanic membrane may be visible. These findings do not necessarily indicate a more severe or persistent type of OME, and are not absolute indications for urgent surgical intervention. Otoscopy alone is poorly predictive of the hearing loss associated with the presence of middle ear fluid, and while pneumatic otoscopy may aid diagnosis, audiometry is es-

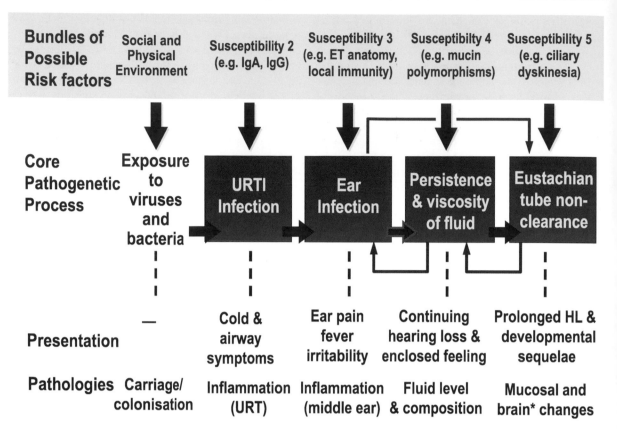

Fig. 42.1 The cascade leading to the development and persistence of otitis media with effusion (with permission after Haggard MP, Medical Research Council OME study group). *ET* Eustachian tube, *HL* hearing loss, *URT* upper respiratory tract

sential to assess the degree of hearing loss, as a marker for the wider impact and likelihood of resolution.

There is an important difference between making the simple diagnosis of middle ear effusion and the more complex assessment of the persistence and effects of OME in the individual child.

The clinical findings on otoscopy described above supported by a B or C2 tympanogram, indicate that a middle ear effusion happens to be present on the day of the examination. Hearing thresholds and systematic questioning about possible developmental effects are practical clinical tools to assess the medium-term persistence of the disease, and hence provide some pointers to the need for intervention.

Audiology

In younger children, below the age of 2 years, visual reinforcement audiometry, using sound field testing or delivering the sound to each ear separately with "inserts", and bone-conduction testing, produce reliable thresholds.

Older children are conditioned using play audiometry in sound field or with headphones and can also cooperate with speech testing using the toy identification test. Tympanometry alone is a useful screening tool, and if used as a first routine test will reduce the audiometric workload to 69%, but still identify 95% of hearing-impaired children (MRC Multi-Centre Otitis Media Study Group 1999). It will however, fail to detect the sensorineural hearing loss that will be present in 0.1–1.0% of children.

Natural History

Without treatment, the natural history of OME in childhood is predominantly one of spontaneous resolution. Watchful waiting with monitoring of hearing over a 6-month period will result in spontaneous resolution of the OME in over 90% of children (Browning 2001). This strategy does, however, assume that early specialist referral and prompt surgical intervention will be available when required.

42

Complications

There is no evidence that treating OME surgically reduces the risk of cholesteatoma formation or permanent damage to the tympanic membrane. Retraction of the pars tensa and tympanosclerosis are frequently seen following OME, although the incidence of these is higher in those who have had a ventilation tube insertion. This makes the evaluation of side effects of treatment very difficult (Rakover et al. 2000).

Treatment

Medical

There is no evidence that medical treatments produce lasting resolution of OME. Several systematic reviews have been undertaken assessing the benefits of antibiotics or a combination of antibiotics with oral corticosteroids. None of these reviews have found a material or lasting benefit from these treatments (Rosenfeld and the Post 1992). The unwanted side effects of medical treatment, though not common, vary from the troublesome (e.g. gastric irritation) to the potentially life-threatening (e.g. anaphylactic shock), and these treatments have a minimal role in contemporary practice.

The role of intranasal corticosteroids is under investigation. There is a high association between rhinitis and OME (personal communication, Umapathy D, University of London MSc thesis). Intranasal corticosteroids reduce the need for grommet insertion (Scadding et al. 2000). Fluticasone and mometasone are minimally systemically absorbed, are free from major side effects (Allen et al. 2002) and are helpful in treating any associated rhinitis in children over 4 years of age. Younger children with allergic rhinitis may be treated with intranasal sodium cromoglycate. Those with recurrent infection should be screened for immunocompetence (see also Chapter 10).

Despite repeated claims by their protagonists, and that of parents and patients, there is no convincing evidence to support the efficacy of "complementary medicine", such as cranial osteopathy, homeopathy or aromatherapy, for OME. In studies of other conditions in adults there is now strong evidence that, with very few exceptions, such treatments act as placebos.

Nasal auto-inflation of the Eustachian tubes (for example using Otovent® balloons) may produce benefit if used regularly (Blanshard et al. 1993). The drawbacks of this simple, attractive treatment are the inability of 12% of children aged 3–10 years to use such a nasal balloon and poor compliance with the need to use the balloons three or more times a day. The costs of this treatment must be borne by the parents. An automated, battery-operated version of this treatment (the Earpopper®) is also available, but as yet of unproven additional benefit.

The initial management involves reassuring parents of the self-limiting nature of OME and the likelihood that surgical treatment will not be required. Monitoring the child's hearing over a 3- to 6-month period will identify those children with persistent OME who may benefit from surgical treatment. These numbers are much smaller than the numbers of children in whom OME is known to be present at some stage in their lives.

Hearing Aids

There have been no randomised trials of the provision of hearing aid versus other treatments for OME, and there are no published indications or guidelines for the prescription of hearing aids in the management of OME. In a small UK study of 48 children with OME (Flanagan et al. 1996), compliance by the children issued with a hearing aid was high. However, 13% of children continued to use the hearing aid in the affected ear after the OME had resolved, suggesting the possibility of learned dependency as an undesired side effect. Although providing a child with hearing aids avoids the cost and possible risks of ventilation tube insertion, there is still a need to establish whether OME is sufficiently persistent, and its effects severe enough, to justify this measure.

Surgical

Grommet Surgery (Ventilation Tubes)

Surgical intervention improves the hearing thresholds of children over the age of 3 years, where watchful waiting has confirmed failure of resolution of OME, and where a bilateral hearing loss of 20 dBHL or worse persists. Insertion of grommets produces considerable immediate improvement in hearing. However, over the period of 1 year following surgery, this averages out as providing only a modest improvement in hearing. This benefit also depends on grommet design and the time lapse before extrusion of the grommets begins. The measurable improvement in hearing is definite, but the wider and longer-term benefit is, perhaps, disappointing when compared to parental reports of improvement immediately after surgical intervention. In children over the age of 3 years, the UK MRC TARGET trial has shown very small benefits in developmental variables, including speech and language, behaviour and child quality of life, in the 2-year period after surgery. There are considerable benefits to hearing level and to physical health including sleep pattern, especially if the adenoids are removed at the time of grommet insertion. It would be helpful to have an evidence base for selective targeting of these latter benefits (Haggard 2005, personal communication).

These benefits depend on whether adjuvant adenoidectomy is carried out at the time of ventilation tube insertion. In children under the age of 3 years, spontaneous resolution of OME is more likely; for this reason and because of the difficulty of getting reliable information over time about the child, it is hard to define particular children of this age who might benefit from intervention. In younger and mildly affected children, evidence consistently shows that watchful waiting is as effective as early surgical management for OME (Paradise et al. 2005; Rovers et al. 2001). Accessible and high-quality audiological services would be needed in primary care to define subgroups of these younger children who would benefit from intervention.

In some circumstances (e.g. cleft palate), where chronicity of the OME is anticipated, surgical intervention has traditionally been recommended. A recent long-term review of the sequelae of OME in this group concludes that a more conservative approach is likely to be beneficial in the long term (Sheahan et al. 2002).

Adenoidectomy

Including adenoidectomy at the time of grommet insertion provides clear additional benefits, compared with grommet insertion alone (Maw and Bawden 1994). In the TARGET randomised trial of children aged 3.25–7 years old, additional benefits were measured in terms of hearing level and physical, particularly respiratory, health. The hearing benefits had not disappeared 2 years following the intervention (Haggard 2005, personal communication). The extra benefits in these two fields provided by adenoidectomy are small yet reliable during the first 6 months when grommets are in place. The benefit of adenoidectomy assumes greater importance when the grommets extrude.

The traditional technique for adenoidectomy is blind curettage of the nasopharynx. This is a technically unsatisfactory procedure, risking trauma to the Eustachian tube cushions and even the anterior cervical spine, while inadequately clearing adenoidal tissue from the choanae. Adenoidectomy under direct vision is the recommended technique. The suction coagulation and Coblation® techniques enable bloodless adenoidectomy under direct vision, and day-case discharge from hospital where appropriate. The higher risk of post-operative haemorrhage found after tonsillectomy with monopolar diathermy has not been identified after adenoidectomy using monopolar suction coagulation (Hartley et al. 1998; Walker 2001).

There are technical difficulties in achieving surgical clearance of the nasopharynx using a microdebrider (Yanagisawa and Weaver 1997) and suction coagulation is usually necessary to achieve haemostasis. Nasopharyngeal stenosis has been reported as a significant risk following KTP (potassium titanyl phosphate) laser adenoidectomy (Giannoni et al. 1998).

Whether all children having surgical treatment for OME should also have their adenoids removed depends on whether a group that do not receive extra benefits can be clearly defined. It is possible to define such a group, but not in terms of improvement in hearing.

The American Academy of Pediatrics 2004 Guidelines recommended against adenoidectomy in children undergoing ventilation tube surgery for the first time for OME (American Academy of Family Physicians et al. 2004). This was for medicolegal reasons rather than reasons of effectiveness. In contrast, the TARGET results show that in the OME child over 3 years of age, the combined operation of grommets plus adenoidectomy delivers, over a 2-year period, benefits roughly three times greater than those provided by short-stay grommets alone, so some further modification to guidelines may be anticipated.

Complications of Surgical Management

Premature Extrusion of the Grommets and Perforation

Standard ventilation tubes will normally extrude between 6 and 9 months after insertion. The permanent perforation rate is less than 2–3%. While the insertion of a long-stay (>18 months) tympanostomy tube on a single occasion seems attractive, the complication rate and the permanent perforation rate are unacceptably high at about 20% (Golz et al. 1999). There is no well-controlled evidence on the clinical and cost-effectiveness of short-stay versus medium-stay (12–18 months) ventilation tubes, although there may be a clinical argument in favour of short-stay tubes for those children undergoing adjuvant adenoidectomy.

Otorrhoea

Post-operative otorrhoea occurs in about 15% of children after grommet surgery, and is persistent or recurrent in about 5% of children 1 year after the operation. Studies have shown no association between swimming and otorrhoea in children with ventilated ears.

The instillation of antibiotic ear drops at the time of surgery reduces otorrhoea in the immediate post-operative period; further evidence suggests that a single instillation of antibiotic ear-drops at the time of surgery is as effective as a 5-day course post-operatively, if the middle ear fluid is not infected at the time of operation.

Given the concerns of ototoxicity surrounding the use of aminoglycoside ear-drops, quinolone drops are recommended.

Myringosclerosis (Tympanosclerosis)

While tympanosclerosis of the tympanic membrane (myringosclerosis) is reported to occur in 39–65% of ears after grommet surgery, the associated average hearing loss is typically less than 5 dBHL. There may be effects on the acoustic reflex and on hearing speech in noise, but the noted ambiguity between disease sequelae and treatment side effect applies here also. Myringosclerosis also occurs naturally in ears after untreated recurrent AOM and persistent OME.

Atelectasis

Atelectasis (collapse of the pars tensa of the tympanic membrane), also discussed in Chapter 43, and attic retraction have been reported in up to 20% of untreated ears, as opposed to 37% of ears following grommet surgery. Retraction pockets have been reported in up to 52% of ears following grommets and 40% of untreated ears with OME, making it difficult to attribute a causal relationship with either the disease or the intervention, as intervention may itself be more likely in OME of longer duration. However, the TARGET study has suggested that atelectasis and tympanic membrane perforation are less common long-term complications than was previously thought (Browning 2001).

Post-adenoidectomy Haemorrhage

The post-operative primary haemorrhage rate after adenoidectomy is approximately 0.6% (Lowe 2005, personal communication, UK National Prospective Tonsillectomy Audit data). There are no mortality figures for adenoidectomy alone, as published data invariably include those having simultaneous tonsillectomy. The mortality rate of approximately 1:50,000 for adenotonsillectomies is due almost entirely to tonsillectomy or to non-surgical causes.

Summary for the Clinician ↓

- For most children with OME, particularly younger children under the age of 3 years, watchful waiting and monitoring of hearing, usually over 3 months is effective (Rovers et al. 2005). To some extent, this allows a further period of possible spontaneous resolution, increasing the per capita cost-effectiveness of surgical intervention by concentrating it on those in whom the effusion does not resolve. The ability to deliver appropriate watchful waiting depends on the availability of audiology support. At the time of writing, the waiting time for a children's ENT outpatient appointment in England and Wales currently varies between 7 and 20 weeks. The range of waiting times after listing for grommet surgery is 4–22 weeks. It is desirable to have shorter waiting times for ENT outpatient appointments and for day-case surgery; where these times are short, there is special need to have the watchful waiting process clearly defined. In the absence of such desirable rapid access, by the time many children with OME are seen in an ENT clinic, they will have in effect completed a period of watchful waiting. To then make them wait longer for surgery (where indicated) seems perverse. Two possible solutions are: a shortened waiting period between listing and admission for surgery, or listing for surgery at their first ENT visit of those that meet criteria, but with rigorous preoperative tympanometry and audiometry to confirm that there is still the need for surgical intervention. Diagnosis and monitoring in the primary care setting, with direct listing and confirmation of planned surgery in a pre-admission clinic is another model that could provide a patient pathway for the surgical management of OME.

References

1. American Academy of Family Physicians; American Academy of Otolaryngology–Head and Neck Surgery; American Academy of Pediatrics Subcommittee on Otitis Media With Effusion (2004) Otitis media with effusion. Pediatrics 113:1412–1429

2. Allen DB, Meltzer EO, Lemanske RF, et al (2002) No growth suppression in children treated with the maximum recommended dose of fluticasone proprionate aqueous nasal spray for one year. Allergy Asthma Proc 23:407–413

3. Barnes DM, Whittier S, Gilligan PH, et al (1995) Transmission of multiple drug resistant *Streptococcus pneumoniae* in group day care: evidence suggesting capsular transformation of the resistant strain in vivo. J Infect Dis 171:890–896

4. Bennett KE, Haggard MP (1998) Accumulation of factors influencing children's middle ear disease: risk factor modelling on a large population cohort. J Epidemiol Community Health 52:786–793

5. Bennett KE, Haggard MP (1999) Behaviour and cognitive outcomes in middle ear disease. Arch Dis Childhood 80:28–35

6. Blanshard JD, Maw AR, Bawden R (1993) Conservative treatment of otitis media with effusion by autoinflation of the middle ear. Clin Otolaryngol Allied Sci 18:188–192

7. Browning GG (2001) Watchful waiting in childhood otitis media with effusion. Editorial. Clin Otolaryngol 26:263–264

8. Duffy LC, Faden H, Wasielewski R, et al (1997) Exclusive breastfeeding protects against bacterial colonization and day care exposure to otitis media. Pediatrics 100:E7

9. Fergie N, Bayston R, Pearson JP (2004) Is otitis media with effusion a biofilm infection? Clin Otolaryngol 29:38–46

10. Flanagan PM, Knight LC, Thomas A (1996) Hearing aids and glue ear. Clin Otolaryngol 21:297–300

11. Giannoni C, Sulek M, Friedmann EM, et al (1998) Acquired nasopharyngeal stenosis: a warning and review. Arch Otolaryngol Head Neck Surg 124:163–167

12. Goessler MC (2005) OME as a biofilm disorder: clinical implications. Abstracts of the 5th Extraordinary International Symposium on Recent Advances in Otitis Media, 26 April 2005, Amsterdam

13. Golz A, Angel-Yeger B, Parush S (1998) Evaluation of balance disturbances in children with middle ear effusion. Int J Pediatr Otorhinolaryngol 43:21–26

14. Golz A, Netzer A, Joachims HZ, et al (1999) Ventilation tubes and persisting tympanic membrane perforations. Otolaryngol Head Neck Surg 120:524–527

15. Green RE, Cooper NK (1991) Passive smoking and middle ear effusions in children of British servicemen in West Germany – a point prevalence survey by clinics of outpatient attendance. J R Army Med Corps 137:31–33

16. Hartley BEJ, Papsin BC, Albert DM (1998) Suction diathermy adenoidectomy. Clin Otolaryngol 23:308–309

17. Ishii T, Toriyama M, Suzuki JI (1980) Histopathological study of otitis media with effusion. Ann Otol Laryngol Rhinol 89:83–86

18. Karma P (1988) Secretory otitis media – infectious background and its implication for treatment. Acta Otolayngol (Stockh) 449:47–48

19. Kerschner KE, Link TR, Burrows A, et al (2005) Otitis media as a biofilm disease in humans. Abstracts of the 5th Extraordinary International Symposium on Recent Advances in Otitis Media, 26 April 2005, Amsterdam

20. Kubba H, Pearson JP, Birchall JP (2000) The aetiology of otitis media with effusion: a review. Clin Otolaryngol 25:181–194

21. Maw AR, Bawden R (1994) Does adenoidectomy have an adjuvant effect on ventilation tube insertion and thus reduce the need for re-treatment? Clin Otolaryngol 19:340–343

22. MRC Multi-Centre Otitis Media Study Group (1999) Sensitivity, specificity and predictive value of tympanometry in predicting a hearing impairment in otitis media with effusion. Clin Otolaryngol 24:294–300

23. Paradise JL, Rockette HE, Colborn DK, et al (1997) Otitis media in 2253 Pittsburgh infants: prevalence and risk factors during the first two years of life. Pediatrics 99:318–333

24. Paradise JL, Campbell TF, Dollaghan CA, et al (2005) Developmental outcomes after early or delayed insertion of tympanostomy tubes. N Engl J Med 353:576–586

25. Rakover Y, Keywan K, Rosen G (2000) Comparison of the incidence of cholesteatoma surgery before and after using ventilation tubes for secretory otitis media. Int J Pediatr Otorhinolaryngol 56:41–44

26. Rayner MG, Zhang Y, Gorry M, et al (1998) Evidence of bacterial metabolic activity in culture-negative otitis media with effusion. JAMA 279:296–299

27. Rosenfeld RM, Post JC (1992) Meta-analysis of antibiotics for the treatment of otitis media with effusion. Otolaryngol Head Neck Surg 1016:378–386

28. Rovers MM, Ingels K, van der Wilt GJ, et al (2001) Otitis media with effusion in infants: is screening and treatment with ventilation tubes necessary? CMAJ 165:1055–1056

29. Rovers MM, Black N, Browning GG, et al (2005) Grommets in otitis media with effusion: an individual patient data meta-analysis. Arch Dis Child 90:480–485

30. Sadé J (1966) Middle ear mucosa Arch Otolaryngol 84:137–143

31. Sassen ML, Brand R, Grote J (1997) Risk factors for otitis media with effusion in children 0 to 2 years of age. Am J Otolaryngol 18:324–330

32. Scadding GK, Parikh A, Alles R, et al (2000) Treatment of allergic rhinitis and its impact in children with chronic otitis media with effusion. J Audiol Med 9:104–117

33. Schilder AGM, Zeilhuis GA, van den Broek P (1993) The otological profile of a cohort of Dutch 7.5–8-year olds. Clin Otolaryngol 18:48–54

34. Sheahan P, Blayney AW, Sheahan JN, et al (2002) Sequelae of otitis media with effusion among children with cleft lip and/or palate. Clin Otolaryngol 27:494–500

35. Silva PA, Kirkland C, Simpson A, et al (1982) Some developmental and behavioural problems associated with bilateral otitis media with effusion. J Learn Disabil 15:417–421

36. Strachan DP, Cook DG (1998) Parental smoking, middle ear disease and adenotonsillectomy in children. Thorax 53:50–56

37. Tasker A, Dettmar PW, Panetti M, et al (2002) Reflux of gastric juice and glue ear in children. Lancet 359:493

38. Teele DW, Klein JO, Rosner B, the Greater Boston Study Group (1989) Epidemiology of otitis media during the first seven years of life in children in Greater Boston. A prospective cohort study J Infect Dis 160:83–94

39. Walker P (2001) Pediatric adenoidectomy under vision using suction-diathermy ablation. Laryngoscope 111:2173–2177

40. Williamson I (2002) Otitis media with effusion. Clin Evid 7:469–476

41. Yanagisawa E, Weaver EM (1997) Endoscopic adenoidectomy with the microdebrider. Ear Nose Throat J 76:72–74

42. Zeilhuis GA, Heuvelmans-Heinen EW, Rach GH, et al (1989) Environmental risk factors for otitis media with effusion in preschool children. Scand J Prim Health Care 7:33–38

Chronic Otitis Media

43

John Hamilton

Core Messages

- The data concerning chronic suppurative otitis media in aboriginal communities, progressive tympanic membrane retraction and cholesteatoma show that these are all more prevalent in children than in adults.

- The rates of persistent middle ear inflammation after tympanic membrane repair, failure of tympanic membrane repair and recurrence of cholesteatoma after intact canal wall mastoidectomy are also higher in children.

- The patterns of cholesteatoma development are different in children and may also reflect the higher prevalence of pars tensa atrophy in this population. The pattern of cholesteatoma spread is also different in children.

- When dealing with cholesteatoma in a child, the surgeon may choose to use a different surgical technique to that employed in adults. This is because the problems of removing the cholesteatoma, obtaining a dry ear and preventing the recurrence of disease are all greater in a child.

- In disease that has a tendency to recur, it is important to follow the patient up until the disease is unlikely to recur. This is particularly true of cholesteatoma in children and may also be true of retraction pockets and tympanic membrane perforations in children. Healthcare providers as well as surgeons should take this into consideration so that adequate follow-up after treatment is not neglected. Parents must also have this fact carefully explained to them.

- When dealing with a child who presents with a chronic tympanic membrane perforation at a very young age, the surgeon needs to consider carefully the optimum age at which to undertake tympanoplasty. This reflects of the impact of early age on the success of tympanic membrane repair.

- The surgeon managing a child with an advanced pars tensa retraction pocket faces a difficult decision whether to intervene or not. There is no high-quality evidence to guide the decision.

- The more forceful nature of otitis media in children is a common factor that may link all of these features through the medium of chronic otitis media. It is suggested that pathological changes in the tympanic membrane and ossicles are often secondary to generalised chronic middle ear inflammation.

- Children form a special population, with more aggressive and persistent otitis media and a higher rate of complications of this disease. The surgeon entrusted to manage this disorder in a child faces a more difficult task than the surgeon dealing only with adult chronic otitis media.

Contents

43

Introduction

Chronic otitis media is defined as chronic inflammation of the mucosa and submucosa of the middle ear. Chronic otitis media is recognised to be part of a continuum of inflammatory middle ear disease that also includes acute otitis media and otitis media with effusion.

Prolonged inflammation of the mucosa of the middle ear results in changes not only to the mucosa and submucosa, but also to the tympanic membrane and ossicles. As the middle ear cleft is a region of great anatomical complexity, the consequences of this inflammation are remarkably varied. Table 43.1 classifies the effects of chronic otitis media on the anatomical elements of the temporal bone.

The aim of this chapter is to identify the pathological consequences of this inflammation on the tissues of the temporal bone, detail the most common symptoms

Table 43.1 Classification of chronic otitis media: temporal bone complications

Underlying disease process	Target organ	Complication
Chronic otitis media		
	Mucosa	Granulation tissue
		Glandular metaplasia
		Squamous metaplasia
		Sclerosis
	Temporal bone	Bone erosion
		Osteoneogenesis
	Tympanic membrane	Perforation
		Atrophy
		Sclerosis
		Myringitis
		Cholesteatoma
	Ossicles	Bone erosion
		Sclerosis
	Facial Nerve	Neuritis
	Labyrinth	Labyrinthitis

caused by these changes in children and discuss their management. In-depth description of surgical techniques will not be covered and the reader is directed towards the many operative texts available.

Histology of Chronic Inflammation of the Middle Ear Mucosa

The histological features of chronic inflammation of the middle ear lining are well established (Friedmann 1956). Otitis media is characterised by submucosal inflammatory infiltrates and mucosal metaplasia, with the development of glandular structures, mucus-producing cells and ciliated cells.

As chronic inflammation results in tissue destruction and attempts at healing, the histological features of chronic otitis media include mononuclear cell infiltrates and submucosal fibrosis, osteitis, new bone formation and the formation of highly vascular granulation tissue.

The aetiology of acute and chronic inflammation of the middle ear is covered in Chapters 41 and 42 on acute otitis media and otitis media with effusion, respectively.

Perforation of the Tympanic Membrane and Chronic Suppurative Otitis Media

The response of the tympanic membrane to chronic inflammation of its mucosal surface is complex. The changes in the tympanic membrane echo the battle between tissue destruction and healing seen throughout the middle ear mucosa. They are, however, not confined to the mucosal layer alone.

Perforated tympanic membranes resected for histological analysis bear evidence of inflammation, excessive fibrosis, tympanosclerosis, epithelial hyperplasia, rete ridges, epithelial ingrowth and epithelial inclusion (Somers et al. 1997). A perforated tympanic membrane, therefore, is not simply a defect in an otherwise normal eardrum; it is a feature of a structure in which chronic inflammation has prevented the defect from healing.

Chronic suppurative otitis media (CSOM) was defined in 1996 by a World Health Organisation (WHO) workshop as "a stage of ear disease in which there is chronic infection of the middle ear cleft ... in which a non-intact tympanic membrane ... and discharge (otorrhoea) are present." The same report qualifies this definition by stating that the otorrhoea should be present for 2 weeks or longer (WHO 1996).

According to the panel reporting to the Seventh Post-Symposium Research Conference of the International Symposium on Recent Advances in Otitis Media, CSOM is defined by otorrhoea of at least 6 weeks duration in the presence of a chronic tympanic membrane perforation.

Furthermore, a perforation of the tympanic membrane is deemed to be chronic if present for 3 months (Bluestone et al. 2002).

It is important to note that this term, CSOM, has a quite different meaning from "chronic otitis media", which was defined in the introduction to mean chronic inflammation of the middle ear cleft. Unfortunately, the similarity of the two terms often causes confusion.

Older textbooks use confusing, and outdated terminology to describe tympanic membrane perforations, such as: central, "tubo-tympanic" and "safe" perforations, and marginal, attico-antral and "unsafe" perforations. This division was used to indicate the increased possibility of cholesteatoma in the latter group. The underlying chronic mucosal changes are the same in either group and it is the presence of the ingrowth of keratinsing epithelium into the middle ear cleft that defines cholesteatoma, rather than its site of origin. However, this classification is obsolete in the era of microscopic examination. It is better to carefully examine and describe the pathology, be it a perforation, a retraction pocket or cholesteatoma.

Epidemiology

This topic is also discussed in Chapters 41 and 42. The WHO recognises that a high prevalence of CSOM in children represents a significant health burden (see Table 43.2):

1. The populations with the highest prevalence of CSOM in childhood are the Inuit and Australian Aboriginals, who frequently have prevalence percentage rates in double figures.
2. Apache and Navaho Indians, rural Maori and Solomon Islanders as well as some rural Indian and African populations have been found to have a point prevalence of CSOM of over 5% in children.

Table 43.2 World Health Organisation's (WHO) classification of the prevalence of chronic suppurative otitis media (CSOM)

Prevalence of CSOM in children (%)	WHO grade	WHO suggested response
1–4	"an avoidable burden"	Manage in the "general health care context"
>4	"a massive public health problem"	Requires "urgent" attention

3. By contrast, a well-planned national study in South Korea found a rate of less than 1% in the paediatric population.

4. No recent general screening of large paediatric populations has been performed recently in Europe or the United States; however, audiometric screening studies of small populations suggest a point prevalence of less than 1% in these countries.

5. In South Korea, a rising prevalence of tympanic membrane perforation with age is found, a phenomenon that continues into later life (Kim et al. 1993). Findings in the UK, although less systematically researched, appear more similar to the Korean pattern. For instance, the UK National Study of Hearing found a high rate (4.1%) of tympanic membrane perforation in the British adult population (Browning and Gatehouse 1992).

6. By contrast, data from aboriginal populations indicate a high prevalence of tympanic membrane perforation in very young children, with a somewhat lower prevalence in adulthood (Fig. 43.1; Gilchrist and Hills 1991; Kim et al. 1993).

In populations provided with modern medical care, a further cause of paediatric tympanic membrane perforation is surgical insertion of tympanostomy tubes (see Table 43.3). A detailed meta-analysis from eight studies providing separate outcomes for both long-term and short-term tubes indicated that long-term tubes increased the relative risk of chronic perforation by 3.5 (95% confidence interval: 1.5–7.1) compared with short-term tubes (Kay et al. 2001).

Symptoms

The key symptoms of CSOM are otorrhoea and hearing loss. The otorrhoea is generally intermittent, but profuse when present. In mild cases there may be almost no discharge; in severe cases the discharge may be continuous. The hearing loss is generally slight unless associated with other complications of chronic otitis media, such as ossicular erosion. Profuse ear discharge filling the external ear canal will also impair hearing. Other otological symptoms are rare in children with CSOM.

43

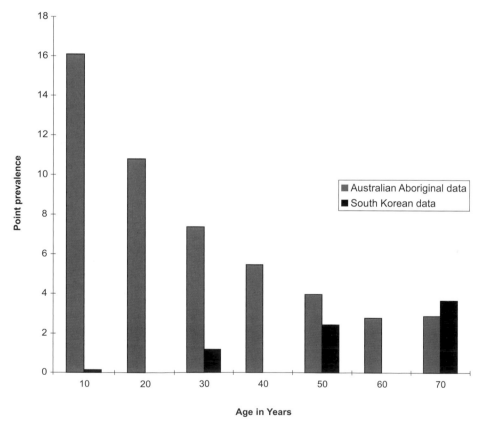

Fig. 43.1 Age-related point prevalence of ear discharge in Australian Aboriginal and South Korean populations. These data are intended to contrast the distribution of chronic suppurative otitis media in the two populations. Data adapted from Gilchrist and Hills (1991) and Kim et al. (1993)

Table 43.3 Prevalence of chronic perforation of the tympanic membrane in children after ventilation tube insertion

Type of ventilation tubes used in study group	Number of ears in study group	Number of ears with chronic perforation in study group	Percentage of ears with chronic perforation in study group (%)
All tubes	20,222	964	4.8
Short-term tubes	8,107	175	2.2
Long-term tubes	3356	556	16.6

Signs

The symptoms of CSOM are shared by cholesteatoma and tympanic membrane atrophy. The most important objective of the physical examination, therefore, is to determine the status of the tympanic membrane. Mucopurulent discharge, however, may obscure the child's tympanic membrane. This is best cleared by mopping, which is usually well tolerated, and the administration of topical steroid/antibiotic ear drops. It is important to obtain a clear view of the tympanic membrane to establish the presence of any pathology. If it proves impossible to obtain a clear and full view of the affected tympanic membrane, the child's ear should be examined under anaesthetic.

The perforated tympanic membrane may be also affected by sclerosis, atrophy, retraction and myringitis. If the myringitis is exuberant, the granulation tissue may become pedunculated, in which case it is termed an "aural polyp". The polyp may obscure the tympanic membrane; in children, they are usually friable and easily removed with microsuction.

If the polyp is more fibrous, it cannot be removed easily. In this circumstance, the removal should be performed by sharp dissection to prevent injury to underlying structures. If an aural polyp is not associated with any mucopurulent discharge, the possibility of neoplasia should be considered and the polyp removed for histological examination.

Investigation

The diagnosis is based on the inspection of the ear. The factors that influence the treatment are the patient's symptoms and signs and, importantly, the patient's age. In most cases, the only investigation required is a pure-tone audiogram with masked bone conduction in the affected ear, when the ear is dry. This should reflect the patient's reported hearing disability and provides the surgeon with data upon which to base the likelihood of associated ossicular pathology. In general, a perforation alone causes little hearing loss (<20 dBHL). The audiogram is also evidence of the hearing status prior to any intervention.

Treatment

Treatment is aimed both at controlling symptoms and restoring the integrity of the tympanic membrane. Good control of ear discharge can result in almost complete loss of symptoms so that it is not always necessary to proceed to early closure of the tympanic membrane defect, particularly in very young children.

Prophylaxis

Despite the identification of risk factors and the introduction of guidelines for the community management of otitis media in severely affected indigenous populations, there has been no change in prevalence of CSOM in the most affected Australian Aboriginal and Inuit communities over the past 20 years. Even the introduction of improved housing and better access to healthcare has not provided a consistent decrease in the prevalence of CSOM in these communities in the past 15 years.

The ideal treatment of otorrhoea through a chronic tympanic membrane perforation in high-risk communities should include improvements in nutritional status and living environment and education about the disease, as well as more overtly medical strategies.

The introduction of well-managed salt-water swimming pools to remote Aboriginal communities where children were previously swimming in stagnant water holes established a benefit in a community with a high prevalence of paediatric tympanic membrane perforation (Lehmann et al. 2003).

By contrast, in the developed world the most useful patient advice to eliminate ear discharge is to ensure that the ear is kept scrupulously dry both when washing and when swimming. With the diligent use of ear plugs or the avoidance of swimming altogether, it is often possible to prevent otorrhoea in the presence of a tympanic membrane perforation. This often results in a symptom-free child. However, it can be taxing to keep a child's ear completely dry and despite the lack of symptoms, the majority of parents will accept the offer of tympanic membrane closure.

Medical Treatment

Medical treatment aims to clear any infection in the ear and reduce the chronic mucosal inflammation. It does not, however, treat the structural changes to the tympanic membrane or middle ear. It offers what may only be a temporary improvement of the symptoms of CSOM, as symptoms often recur. The two main bacteria isolated in CSOM, with or without cholesteatoma, are *Staphylococcus aureus* and *Pseudomonas aeruginosa*. In uncomplicated CSOM, topical medication in the form of ear drops is the treatment of choice. Drops contain an antibiotic, commonly an aminoglycoside, or more recently a quinolone, to combat infection, and a corticosteroid to reduce the inflammatory response. Oral antibiotics are usually reserved for patients with other bacterial infections, systemic symptoms or complications.

It must be remembered that mycobacteria, including atypical variants, can be found infecting the middle ear and mastoid and must be considered, especially in cases that seem unresponsive to normal treatment.

A variety of systematic reviews of medical treatment of CSOM have been published. The Cochrane Database intends to publish seven reviews on this topic. Many trials on this topic are of low quality and not all of these studies included children.

Two large and well-designed studies co-ordinated by the Liverpool School of Tropical Medicine offer high-quality guidance. Smith et al. (1996) demonstrated that topical and systemic antibiotics after ear mopping resulted in better resolution of otorrhoea than mopping alone. The result of mopping alone was the same as no treatment.

McFadyen et al. (2005) demonstrated that topical antiseptics are less effective at drying discharging ears than topical quinolones.

The following statements offer a guide to the evidence-based treatment of ear discharge in CSOM in children:

1. It seems probable that topical treatment with antibiotics after mopping is more effective than systemic treatment with antibiotics. The importance of adequately cleaning the ear prior to instilling the drops cannot be over-emphasised.
2. It is not clear whether topical quinolones are more effective than other topical antibiotics for the control of CSOM. However, topical quinolones do not carry the potential for ototoxicity associated with aminoglycosides.
3. Caution should be exercised when using topical aminoglycosides for children with discharging, perforated ears. The use of aminoglycoside ear drops should be for short periods, never more than 2 weeks at a time, and only used in the presence of active CSOM, where the risk of ototoxicity from pus in the middle ear cleft

probably outweighs that from aminoglycoside drops. Ototoxicity from aminoglycoside drops appears to be dose-related and to occur following prolonged courses. The child's parents should be counselled about the risks. Microbiology guidance should be sought, especially if there is failure to respond after an initial course of treatment.

Surgical Closure of Tympanic Membrane Perforations in Children with CSOM (Tympanoplasty)

Surgical intervention is the treatment of choice to close the perforation. Spontaneous healing of chronic tympanic membrane perforations is uncommon and medical interventions are not curative. The medical literature provides ample evidence that a high rate of closure is possible in adults when surgery is performed in an adept manner. In children, however, there is a higher failure rate.

The conclusions of many individual studies that suggest that the age of the child makes no difference to success rate are compromised by small sample sizes, leading to insufficient power. A meta-analysis of paediatric tympanoplasty (Vrabec et al. 1999) provided an authoritative analysis of parameters that correlate with closure of the tympanic membrane. The following conclusions were drawn:

1. There is a significant association of greater success of surgical repair with advancing age, from age 6 years to age 13 years.
2. No other parameter correlates with success, despite the findings of smaller individual studies.

The presence of an open perforation carries an ongoing risk of acute bacterial infection. Choosing when to repair a young child's perforated ear is thus a balance between the morbidity caused by leaving the perforation open and the decreasing risk of surgical failure as the child grows older. In the developed world, scrupulous attention to keeping the child's ear dry can minimise any morbidity while awaiting an appropriate age for surgery. As a child matures, he or she also becomes more able to understand and prepared to undergo the surgical procedure. This is often more important in the post-operative period, when young children find it hard to tolerate removal of dressings from the ear and suction toilet of the ear canal.

It is important to realise that chronic otitis media, with middle ear inflammation, may persist despite closure of the perforation, as witnessed by the identification of otitis media with effusion behind the intact repaired tympanic membrane in children in 10.6% of cases.

For descriptions of surgical techniques for closing tympanic membrane perforations, the reader is referred to general ENT surgical textbooks.

43

Tympanic Membrane Atrophy and Retraction Pockets: Pars Tensa

Atrophy of the tympanic membrane, with associated development of a retraction pocket, especially in the posterior-superior quadrant of the pars tensa (Figs. 43.2–43.5), has a clear role in the subsequent development of a cholesteatoma.

In histological studies of human temporal bones, tympanic membrane atrophy is clearly associated with chronic middle ear inflammatory changes. Some animal model studies have demonstrated that tympanic membrane atrophy can result from intense middle ear inflammation. Other studies have failed to produce atrophy despite intense middle ear inflammation. It is fair to state that, in general, the factors that promote atrophy are not yet known.

Pathology

Atrophy of the pars tensa of the tympanic membrane occurs through loss of the collagenous fibrous layer. Following the loss of this stiff structural element, the thinned area of tympanic membrane can be more easily displaced by any pressure difference across it. The relative negative middle ear pressure found in association with chronic otitis media results in medial displacement, "retraction", of the weakened area.

Tympanic membrane atrophy with retraction may focally affect any segment of the tympanic membrane, and the affected area is described as a "retraction pocket". In the pars tensa it most commonly affects the posterior and superior quadrants, but it can affect the entire tympanic membrane. An atrophic area of the tympanic membrane may become complicated by adhesion of the retracted area to underlying structures, the ossicles or promontory.

In a small proportion of cases, pars tensa retraction may become associated with erosion of the ossicles, most commonly starting with the lenticular process of the incus. This erosion may stabilise without damaging the ossicles enough to cause a significant conductive deafness. More severe tympanic membrane retraction pockets erode the long process of the incus and the stapes superstructure and can progress to become cholesteatoma.

An important aim in the management of tympanic membrane atrophy is to distinguish retraction pockets that develop these complications from those that do not. Often, this can only be done by repeated observation over months or years ("watchful waiting").

Epidemiology

Population-based surveys have been conducted in a number of countries. The point prevalence of tympanic membrane retraction was determined as 1.9% in Navajo

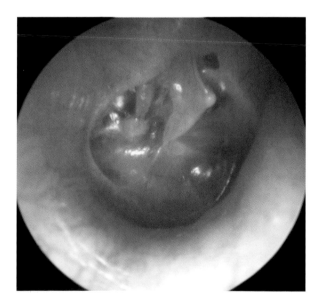

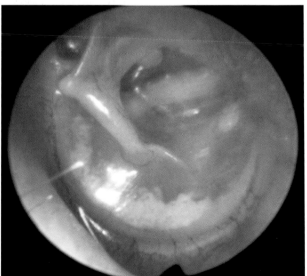

Fig. 43.2 Early retraction pocket. Although the extent and depth of this retraction pocket are both limited, the lenticular process of the incus is absent and the incus no longer articulates with the stapes. The retraction pocket is adherent to the head of the stapes; this arrangement is rarely associated with more than 15 dB conductive hearing loss

Fig. 43.3 Late retraction pocket. This retraction pocket has eroded the long process of the incus and the stapes superstructure. The pocket is adherent to the clearly visible facial nerve. Nonetheless, the middle ear is ventilated and the pocket is clean. This arrangement is usually associated with 30 dB conductive hearing loss or more

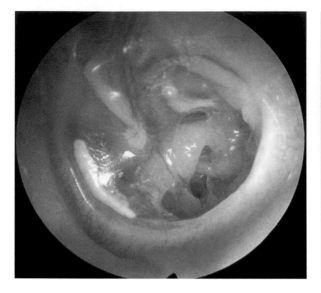

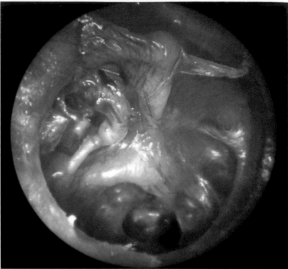

Fig. 43.4 End-stage atelectatic ear. The atrophic part of this tympanic membrane has retracted onto the promontorium and has perforated. The margins of the retracted area are draped around the margins of the posterior mesotympanum and may be left in place, resulting in residual cholesteatoma if the surgeon repairing this perforation does not recognise its origins

Fig. 43.5 Pars tensa cholesteatoma. This retraction pocket has started to accumulate keratin not only in the sinus tympani, but also in the hypotympanum. Despite this, the ossicular chain is intact

43

children, 1.3% in a cohort of 15-year-old children in the Dunedin area of New Zealand, and a study of Danish children found that 5.4% of 684 5-year-old children had tympanic membrane atrophy, of whom 0.3% had retraction and adherence to the ossicles. Prospective follow-up of English children with persistent otitis media with effusion has confirmed an increase in the prevalence of tympanic membrane retraction with increasing duration of follow-up: 15% developed some degree of retraction and 2% were found to have advanced pars tensa retraction (Maw and Bawden 1994).

Data collected from Gloucestershire Royal Hospital between 1993 and 1996 on patients undergoing surgery for pars tensa retraction confirms that this condition is commonly found in children, with a peak prevalence of surgery for retraction pockets at the age of 10 years (Fig. 43.6).

Classification

Since a menacing minority of retraction pockets progressively deteriorate to form cholesteatomas, terminology and classifications have been devised to facilitate the surveillance of the deterioration of the retracted area. The earliest and best known of these is Sadé's classification (Sadé et al. 1981a). Sadé defined the following:

1. Atelectasis: "diffuse retraction of the tympanic membrane towards the promontorium", with four grades

of atelectasis classified on an ordinal scale (see Table 43.4).
2. Retraction pocket: "focal retraction of the pars tensa towards or into the antrum and attic.

Numerous other authors have defined classifications of retracted tympanic membranes. No evidence has been presented so far that any of these other classifications provides a more precise prediction of disease progression than the original Sadé classifications.

Table 43.4 Sadé classification (1981a) of atelectasis of the tympanic membrane. A fifth stage of perforation of the retracted area was also recognised. Focal posterosuperior atelectasis was also termed "retraction pocket"

Grade	Description
Grade 1	The "retracted drum"
Grade 2	The drum is touching or adhering to the incus or stapes
Grade 3	The drum is touching the promontory
Grade 4	The drum adheres to the promontory

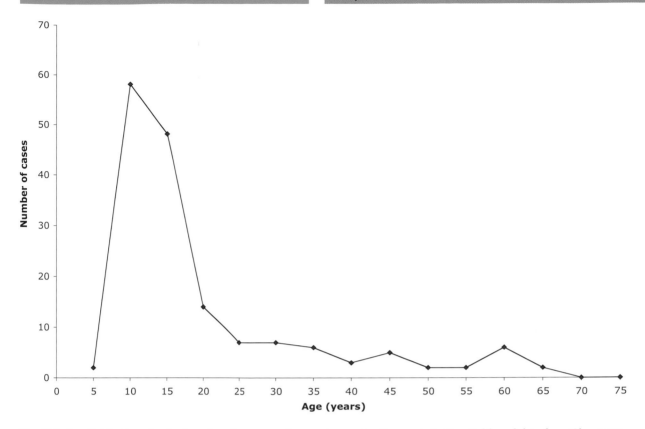

Fig. 43.6 Age distribution of patients undergoing surgery for pars tensa retraction pockets. Hospital-based data from Gloucestershire Royal Hospital, UK. At the time of data collection, retraction pocket excision was aggressively pursued for all ears with Sadé grade III or IV atelectasis

Natural History

Surveillance of patients with tympanic membrane retraction over a mean of 3–5 years has established that:

1. Retraction without atrophy (grade I atelectasis; see Table 43.4) is usually a transitory condition. It rarely progresses to more advanced stages and frequently reverts to a normal tympanic membrane. This behaviour is clearly different from that found in more advanced stages of this disease.
2. Grades II and III of the disease are quite dynamic, having the ability to improve, deteriorate or remain the same; 16% may be expected to deteriorate over 3–5 years.
3. Grade IV atelectasis, on the other hand, does not spontaneously revert back earlier stages of the disease. This is significantly different from to the behaviour of grades I–III.
4. Of grade IV retractions towards the promontory, 16% will progress to perforation, within 3–5 years.
5. A large number of pars tensa retraction pockets (PTRPs) that progress towards the facial recess and antrum present for the first time at a late stage. Ten percent

of clean pockets retracting in this direction will begin to the accumulate keratin debris within 3–5 years.

On the basis of this data, it is clear that the majority of cases of pars tensa atrophy are incidental and present no risk to the child's health. However, a definite percentage will progress to perforation or cholesteatoma, particularly those pockets retracting towards the antrum and attic.

Symptoms

Patients with pars tensa atrophy and retraction may suffer symptoms because of the retraction itself, the underlying otitis media or complications arising from the retracted tympanic membrane. However many children develop asymptomatic atrophic tympanic membranes, at least initially, which may only be discovered at otoscopy.

The otitis media may cause pain if acute, hearing loss if associated with effusion, and discharge if the inflammation results in acute perforation of the tympanic membrane. The retracted segment may collect keratin debris. If this becomes infected it may lead to hearing loss and discharge.

The mobility of the atrophic segment may also result in symptoms. Many children with pars tensa atrophy avoid performing Valsalva's manoeuvre, as this causes pain. A proportion also note distorted hearing if the atrophic area is distended by auto-inflation or swallowing. Some children develop techniques to drop their middle ear pressure to protect against this. These include sniffing and Toynbee manoeuvres.

Erosion of the incus and stapes may occur and result in conductive hearing loss.

Principles of Surgical Intervention for Tympanic Membrane Atrophy and Retraction Pockets

The surgeon may be prompted to treat the atrophic PTRP either for symptomatic or pathological reasons. There is little controversy about treatment for established problems.

The surgeon also may be prompted to treat PTRP to prevent pathological complications. Such prophylactic intervention is controversial. This is because there is no test that is sufficiently accurate for identifying those pockets that are at high risk for progression of disease. Without an accurate test, any effective policy of prophylaxis will necessarily result in the surgical treatment of some ears that are not unstable. Accordingly, many surgeons prefer to delay surgery with the aim of minimising surgery on asymptomatic, possibly stable PTRPs. However, this approach will inevitably result in some ears developing complications before intervention. It is necessary to involve the parents in the decision-making processes and help them to understand the options.

Partial resolution of this dilemma is possible if the prophylactic treatment is simpler and less taxing for the patient than the treatment for established complications. Although this hope has been offered in the management of PTRP by the introduction of retraction pocket excision, lack of evidence for or against this treatment has limited its impact.

Surgical Treatment of Tympanic Membrane Atrophy

Grommet Insertion

The best available evidence suggests that this may not affect the progression of tympanic membrane retraction. Insertion of multiple ventilation tubes can also results in further generalised tympanic membrane scarring as well as atrophy at the site of tube insertion (Maw and Bawden 1994). At best, this treatment offers temporary ventilation of the middle ear with stabilisation of hearing.

Reinforcement Tympanoplasty

Excision of the retraction pocket with grafting of the tympanic membrane remains a widely performed procedure. Once the retraction pocket has been excised, the tympanic membrane is repaired as for a chronic tympanic membrane perforation. The graft material is usually cartilage, perichondrium or temporalis fascia, designed to reinforce the intact posterior tympanic membrane and prevent recurrence of the pocket. If the pocket is removed intact, there need be no concern about residual disease. If the pocket is adherent to the middle ear walls and tears during removal, a second-look procedure may be necessary since in children, the risk of residual disease is as high as with cholesteatoma surgery (Roger et al. 1997).

Retraction Pocket Excision

In the 1980s, Iain Stewart (Stewart et al. 1988) serendipitously noted that simple excision of a retraction pocket is usually associated with spontaneous healing of the tympanic membrane. This novel procedure is of interest because it is specific for retraction pockets and it is significantly less invasive than combined excision and repair. As it can be performed via a permeatal approach as a day-case procedure, it has been suggested as more appropriate than excision with grafting for prophylaxis against cholesteatoma (Marquet 1989).

Up to the present, no high-quality evidence has been presented to support the use of any of these prophylactic treatments compared with watching and waiting. The complication rates and effect on hearing, compared with an untreated group, are not documented and the long-term results, particularly the disease relapse rate, are not well defined. On the other hand, watching and waiting is not without its complications and may later result in the child undergoing a major procedure to remove cholesteatomas.

In summary, the treatment of atrophy and retraction of the pars tensa of the tympanic membrane remains a difficult and controversial area. It is important to involve the child's parents in the decision-making process, and to help them to understand that retraction pocket disease is not a static process, but may dynamically change for better or worse. Surgery at an early stage may not be appropriate, but may be the option of choice 1 year later if progression has occurred. In all cases, watchful waiting is needed, with regular observation of an at-risk child.

Attic Retraction Pockets

(see Figures 43.7–10) It is important to separate Attic retraction pockets from the posterosuperior quadrant pockets described in the previous section. Attic retractions arise in the pars flaccida. In Sadé's own series (Sadé et al. 1981a), 28% of cholesteatomas were congenital and 7% were related to central perforations. Of the remaining 58%, one-third were in the attic, while two-thirds were posterior marginal cholesteatomas. Tos et al. (1987) described four stages of attic retraction (see Table 43.5 and Figs. 43.7–43.10).

It is important to be aware that a large cholesteatoma may be found behind the smallest defect in the scutum (Fig. 43.8). Accordingly, this classification does not reflect the progression from retraction to attic cholesteatoma in children in the same way that the Sadé classification reflects the development of a PTRP into cholesteatoma. Any defect of the lateral attic wall must be treated with suspicion, and erosion of the attic wall is only one sign that might heighten the possibility of underlying cholesteatoma. Others include mucus, an attic polyp or keratin, whether dry ("wax") or moist keratin covering the scutum.

These signs can sometimes be difficult to identify in a child who is reluctant to permit close examination. If the history suggests the possibility of cholesteatoma and the pars tensa is normal, then meticulous examination of the attic is required. In small children this is likely to require examination under anaesthetic so that cleaning of the scutum can be performed and an unhurried, detailed examination of the attic region can be performed.

Table 43.5 Tos classification of attic retraction pockets (Tos et al. 1987). In this series, type I was found in 9–11% of children between 5 and 10 years, type II in 7–13%, type III in 1.1–4% and type IV in only 0.4–0.9%

Stage I	Mild retraction, with air still present between the pocket and malleus neck
Stage II	Pocket touches malleus neck +/− erosion of neck
Stage III	Pocket begins to expand: limited erosion of outer attic wall
Stage IV	More severe erosion of outer attic wall, pocket attached to malleus head and incus

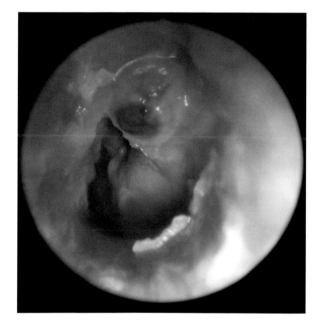

Fig. 43.7 Attic polyp. If the examining doctor encounters the presence of a red polyp that obscures the lateral attic wall and is surrounded by mucopus in a patient with ear discharge, it is almost certain that there is an attic cholesteatoma hidden behind the polyp. It is usually an easy matter to remove the polyp, which is generally very friable, with microsuction. Children are frightened by the noise of this procedure so it is important to place the sucker on the polyp before the suction is turned on. If the sucker is slowly withdrawn it will avulse the polyp without pain and without disquiet

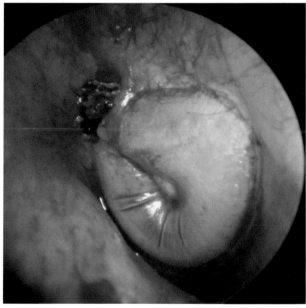

Fig. 43.8 Attic crust. Dry keratin is brown and forms the main component of wax. The examiner should enquire why this wax is localised over the attic. There is often an attic cholesteatoma full of moist keratin deep to this dry crust. It simply requires removal of the crust to confirm the diagnosis, although in most children this procedure will require examination under anaesthetic

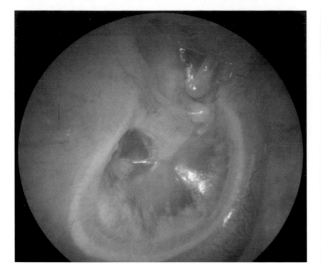

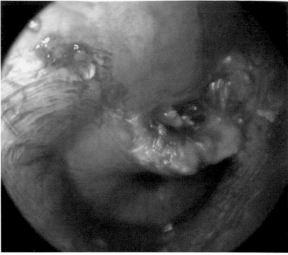

Fig. 43.9 Attic retraction pocket. This retraction pocket is extensive but shallow. Although the malleus head can be seen, the pocket is not accumulating keratin. If the margins of the pocket are hidden, a high-definition computed tomography scan will determine if there is keratin accumulating out of sight

Fig. 43.10 Attic cholesteatoma. Once the polyps, mucopus or crusts have been removed, the underlying cause for these signs can be identified

Cholesteatoma

Cholesteatoma is the accumulation of keratin after keratinising epithelium invades the middle ear space, usually from the tympanic membrane. This intriguing behaviour is inherited from the foetal organ that forms the external ear canal; this structure invades the mesenchyme of the future temporal bone and generates the keratinising epithelium of the canal and tympanic membrane.

Table 43.6 Diagnosis of congenital cholesteatoma: criteria of Derlacki and Clemis (1965)

1	White mass medial to an intact tympanic membrane
2	Normal pars tensa and flaccida
3	No previous history of ear discharge, perforation or previous otological procedure

Pathogenesis and Classification

Congenital Cholesteatoma

Epidermal cysts are found medial to an intact tympanic membrane in children and in adults, usually attached to the promontory anterior to the malleus handle (Fig. 43.11 and 43.12). These are considered to be "congenital" if they fulfil the criteria of Derlaki and Clemis (1965; see Table 43.6). However, it has been proposed that prior bouts of acute otitis media are not grounds for excluding congenital cholesteatoma, since it is unusual for a child to have no episodes of otitis media in its first 5 years.

A vestigial structure that separates from the foetal ear canal, the "epidermoid formation", has been identified medial to the tympanic membrane. It is probable that most congenital cholesteatomas may originate from this organelle.

It should be noted that some epidermal cysts that fulfil the criteria of Derlacki and Clemis (1965) do not present until the fourth or fifth decade of life. These may result

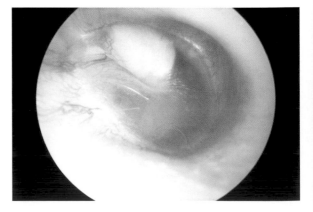

Fig. 43.11 Congenital cholesteatoma viewed through the tympanic membrane of the right ear (reproduced with permission of Professor Leslie Michaels)

43

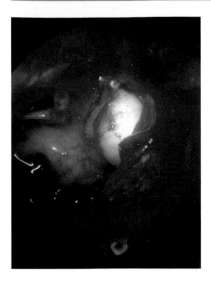

Fig. 43.12 The same congenital cholesteatoma as shown in Fig. 43.11: operative view (reproduced with permission of Professor Leslie Michaels)

brane. Animal models have confirmed that squamous epithelial proliferation is promoted by chronic middle ear inflammation.

4. Metaplasia: epithelial transformation from the columnar endothelium of the middle ear cleft into keratinising epithelium in response to chronic middle ear inflammation. This acquired cholesteatoma may give rise to epithelial cysts. It has also been debated whether some apparently acquired cholesteatomas may be due to late perforation of congenital epithelial cysts through the tympanic membrane.
5. Trauma: massive blunt trauma, with a temporal bone fracture involving the external auditory canal and tympanic membrane, may implant keratinising squamous epithelium within the middle ear complex.
6. Iatrogenic causes of middle ear epithelial cysts include implantation of squamous epithelium as a result of surgery to the tympanic membrane. The otologist must always be aware of this possibility when operating on the tympanic membrane.

A combination of retraction and proliferation is probably responsible for most acquired cholesteatomas.

from metaplasia rather than a congenital focus. The reported incidence of congenital cholesteatoma in the literature has risen from 2% in 1977 to 28% in 1989. This increase probably largely represents better identification of congenital cholesteatoma.

Congenital cholesteatomas are usually slow growing at first, behaving like "pearls" of keratin, with intact matrices. Once the matrix has been breached, for example by infection, after the cholesteatoma has broken through the tympanic membrane, congenital cholesteatomas behave in a more aggressive way, typical of paediatric cholesteatoma.

Acquired Cholesteatoma

More commonly, keratin accumulates within a diverticulum of tympanic membrane squamous epithelium that extends into the middle ear. Recognised mechanisms leading to such "acquired" cholesteatomas include:

1. Immigration: the ingrowth of squamous epithelium into the middle ear through a defect in the tympanic membrane. While this mechanism continues to be recognised, it is responsible for only a very small proportion of cholesteatomas.
2. Retraction: progressive retraction of the bilaminar tympanic membrane, either in the pars flaccida or associated with atrophy of the pars tensa.
3. Papillary proliferation: proliferation of the basal layers of the keratinising epithelium of the tympanic mem-

Epidemiology

Estimates based on retrospective analysis of hospital operation data and the population served have demonstrated an incidence of 0.3–1.6/10,000 per year in Europe and North America. Extremes of 0.04/10,000 per year in Gothenburg and 6.6/10,000 per year in Israel have also been reported. Congenital cholesteatoma may make up 9.2–28% of children's cholesteatoma, with 3% occurring bilaterally. The age at presentation differs, with congenital cholesteatoma tending to present around 5 years of age (5.6±2.8) and acquired cholesteatoma later in childhood, at around 10 years of age (9.7±3.3; Nelson et al. 2002). The age distribution of the patients undergoing cholesteatoma surgery in a population-based study from Iowa in 1976 showed a peak incidence in the second decade of life. Less rigorous collection of data from Gloucester Royal Hospital (author's own series) shows a comparable picture (Fig. 43.13).

Anatomy of Paediatric Cholesteatoma

Paediatric cholesteatoma differs from adult disease in its origin, its pattern of spread and its pattern of erosion. Children's middle ear clefts are also in a state of continuing development when compared to the adult. Persisting immaturity of the middle ear and Eustachian tube leads to continuing chronic otitis media and negative middle ear pressure, which can predispose to recurrent disease formation. The surgeon has to treat disease mindful that

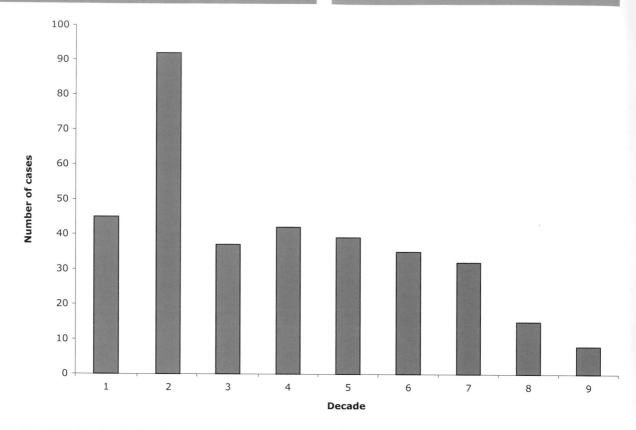

Fig. 43.13 Age distribution of patients undergoing primary surgery for cholesteatoma. Hospital based data from Gloucestershire Royal Hospital (UK), 1997–2006. These data indicate that the disease reaches peak prevalence in the second decade

43

the underlying causes may or may not be only rectified by growth.

In children, there is a significantly higher rate of pars tensa cholesteatoma (Fig. 43.5) than in adults.

Paediatric cholesteatoma more frequently involves the extremes of the middle ear space (the Eustachian tube, the anterior mesotympanum, the retrolabyrinthine area and the mastoid tip) than cholesteatoma in adults. This leads to more technically challenging surgery and an increased risk of residual disease post-operatively. Paediatric cholesteatoma erodes the lateral semicircular canal, the bone over the facial nerve and the ossicles less frequently than cholesteatoma in adults.

It has been suggested that paediatric cholesteatoma is more aggressive than adult disease. Some studies have suggested an increased epithelial growth rate, but the greater spread of paediatric disease is possibly a result of the more pneumatised mastoid in the child and a more open architecture of the air cells, allowing easier spread of the squamous epithelium.

Treatment

Medical

Once the diagnosis of cholesteatoma has been established in a child that can tolerate a general anaesthetic, there is no justification for withholding the surgical removal of the keratin matrix. Antibiotic/steroid ear drops and oral antibiotics may be used to try to control the infection while the child is waiting for surgery.

Imaging

Computed tomography imaging of the temporal bone can be very helpful in paediatric cholesteatoma. Images allow for visualisation of the extent of mastoid pneumatisation, which can assist in planning the surgical approach. It can help with estimation of disease extent, which is often greater in children than that seen in adult disease, and for extension in to the petrous apex (see Chapter 40).

Surgical

The aims of cholesteatoma surgery are:

1. Removal of all cholesteatomas.
2. Prevention of the development of further cholesteatomas.
3. Obtaining a "robust" ear, which remains dry, self-cleaning and free of infection after exposure to water.
4. Restoration of hearing.

Removal of cholesteatomas is more likely after radical resection of the pneumatised temporal bone and bony ear canal to obtain good exposure of the disease. By contrast, the acquisition of a dry, hearing ear, requires a more conservative technique, with the preservation or reconstruction of important functional elements. These antagonistic principles ensure that the successful treatment of cholesteatoma is particularly challenging.

Surgical Approaches for the Removal of Cholesteatoma and Restoration of a Stable, Dry Ear

There are many surgical approaches that can be utilised for the removal of cholesteatomas. The choice of approach depends on a number of factors, including the extent of disease, pneumatisation of the temporal bone, complications (if present), parental choice and the ability to maintain long-term follow up. Each approach has pros and cons and these need to be examined with the specific case in mind. In paediatric cholesteatoma, the surgeon should have the ability to fit the surgical approach to the patient's needs, using a repertoire of techniques rather than a single approach for all cases.

Small or localised cholesteatomas can often be managed by limited local surgery. For instance, cholesteatoma of the posterosuperior pars tensa can be treated by local excision, with repair and reinforcement of the tympanic membrane with cartilage or fascia. Localised cholesteatoma of the lateral epitympanum can be managed by atticotomy with or without repair of the scutum using cartilage or bone pâté.

More extensive cholesteatoma, which extends into the mastoid air cell system, requires a surgical procedure that involves the removal of mastoid bone. This can present problems with subsequent healing. Several procedures that are intended to provide good exposure of disease and high rates of stable healing have been designed. All of these require meticulous surgery to fulfil these aims.

Mastoid Cavity Surgery

The surgically created space within the mastoid is known as the mastoid cavity. It might be envisaged that incorporation of this space into the ear canal would merely result in an enlarged but otherwise normal canal. However, this is not necessarily the case, as the mechanism that maintains the stability of the external ear canal, the migration of the keratinising epithelium from the tympanic membrane towards the cartilaginous part of the ear canal, tolerates distortion of the canal only up to certain limits. If the surgically created canal/cavity is irregular, the self-cleaning mechanism fails and the new canal either collects keratin or fails to maintain a keratinising epithelium, or both. Only if this bowl is smooth and free of recesses will the new canal tolerate exposure to the external environment.

The most important factor influencing the outcome of a dry ear in mastoid cavity surgery is adequate lowering of the facial ridge (Wormald and Nilssen 1998). Other techniques that can help include exenterating the mastoid air cells, removing the mastoid tip and widening the cartilaginous meatus to match the cavity. The advantages of this approach include good exposure of the middle ear cleft with good access to areas of the ear such as the epitympanum. Following surgery, the areas explored remain exposed and can easily be examined in an outpatient setting. Moreover, if the surgery has been performed well, the patient is treated in a single operation. It is a big "if", however, and even a dry mastoid cavity often needs occasional aural toilet, especially in the immediate post-operative period. With a child, aural toilet is often not tolerated, especially in the younger age group. This can lead to significant problems and the need for recurrent examinations under general anaesthesia to keep the ear under control. The term "mastoid misery" has been coined for this situation (Males and Gray 1991). This grades discharge, smell, wax, vertigo and discomfort from 0 to 3 each. 0 is "never" and 3 is "always". A total score of 8 or more is an indication for revision surgery. The mastoid in cases of paediatric cholesteatoma is often well pneumatised, especially in congenital cases. In a highly pneumatised temporal bone, a mastoid cavity resulting from cholesteatoma surgery is large and will often fail to heal. It is better to anticipate these problems, and the following strategies can be employed to improve the likelihood of obtaining a healthy cavity:

1. Minimising the size of the new canal in temporal bones with a large mastoid air cell system by obliterating the mastoid cavity. There are many techniques for achieving this, including local soft-tissue flaps and use of drilled bone (bone pâté) or hydroxyapatite granules. The same outcome can also be achieved by reconstruction of the ear canal wall with bone, cartilage, fascia or artificial prostheses.
2. Incorporating the mastoid cavity without obliteration into the canal. This should only be performed in temporal bones with a small mastoid air cell system.

The surgeon who chooses to construct a mastoid cavity must not only construct the shape of the mastoid cavity with care, but must also ensure that the size of the cavity be minimised to obtain a robust, dry ear.

Combined Approach Tympanoplasty

An alternative to removal and reconstruction of the canal wall is to leave it in place and work around it whilst removing the cholesteatoma. By retaining the normal bony canal, the normal keratinising epithelial lining of the canal is also to be expected to have reformed once healing is complete. Healing can be expected to be faster, the need for aural toilet (hated by children) minimised and the return to activities loved by children, such as swimming, more likely.

One important disadvantage of this approach is the restriction imposed by the canal wall on the field of view. The field of view is improved by creating a posterior tympanotomy. This entails removing bone between the facial nerve and posterior wall of the ear canal and chorda tympani in order to link the mesotympanic and mastoid spaces. This posterior approach provides a view of the facial recess, posterior middle ear and hypotympanum, spaces which may not be directly visible down the ear canal. It also gives rise to the name by which the procedure is best known: "combined approach tympanoplasty".

Even so, in a well-pneumatised temporal bone, cholesteatoma may be hidden in these areas and further improvements in inspection for concealed cholesteatoma have come from the introduction of angled mirrors and endoscopes.

After surgery, the mastoid bowl cannot be inspected from the ear canal and a further procedure is required to determine whether or not this space has been completely cleared of cholesteatoma. In general, this "second-look" procedure requires formal re-exploration of the ear to inspect the mastoid space. This should be undertaken when the middle ear cleft has healed and the cholesteatoma has had time to grow large enough that it will not be missed. The procedure should not be delayed so long that the cholesteatoma is difficult to remove. The optimum interval from the first procedure to the second is 9–18 months.

It would be desirable to avoid a full exploration at the "second look" if the ear could be determined to be healthy. As yet, radiological investigations are not sufficiently accurate to identify small cholesteatomas, although progress is being made in this field with diffusion magnetic resonance scanning. Some surgeons advocate introducing endoscopes through a tiny stab wound as a diagnostic procedure, with progression to full surgery only once cholesteatoma has been identified. However, the tendency in children of the mastoid cortex to regrow has limited the role of this technique outside the adult population.

In the past, the combined approach tympanoplasty has colloquially been described as "canal wall up" surgery to distinguish it from mastoid cavity surgery, which has been termed "canal wall down". These approaches have also been loosely described as "closed" and "open", respectively, in respect of the state of the mastoid at the end of surgery. Over the past 40 years there has been much controversy concerning the merits of these approaches on the outcomes of cholesteatoma surgery. With the introduction of smaller cavity surgery and the many obliteration techniques mentioned above, the distinction between canal wall up and canal wall down surgery has become blurred. It has also become clearer that the outcomes of cholesteatoma surgery are highly operator dependent; all of the techniques described above are capable of providing very good outcomes if appropriately chosen and carefully performed.

Residual and Recurrent Cholesteatoma

Residual Cholesteatoma

Residual cholesteatoma is cholesteatoma left in the middle ear by the surgeon at the end of a surgical procedure. Studies examining the location of residual cholesteatoma indicate that the commonest site is the sinus tympani. The anterior epitympanum and the retained ossicular chain provide other sites associated with high rates of residual cholesteatoma. That this happens is testimony to the difficulty of removing cholesteatoma. Retrospective analyses of risk factors for residual cholesteatoma in children using multivariate analysis indicate that the presence of the factors shown in Table 43.7 independently heighten the risk of residual disease.

Reported rates of residual cholesteatoma in children range from 23 to 44% after combined approach tympanoplasty (Glasscock et al. 198; Kinney 19881; Sanna et al. 1988), and from 6 to 38 % in mastoid cavity surgery (Charachon 1988; Mills and Padgham 1991; Sivola and Palva 1999).

Rates of residual disease after surgery are decreasing, partly as a consequence of improving visualisation techniques. Significant advances in this respect have come from the introduction of endoscopes and angled mirrors. However, the single most significant improvement

Table 43.7 Risk factors for residual cholesteatoma in children

| Erosion of the ossicular chain |
| Presence of posterior mesotympanic cholesteatoma, especially if adherent |
| Presence of inflamed middle ear mucosa |
| Operator ability |

43

has come from the introduction of the fibre-guided laser as a tool for removing cholesteatoma safely from around the ossicles, the middle ear and mastoid. A prospective trial of cholesteatoma surgery with and without a potassium titanyl phosphate laser has confirmed that the rate of residual disease is lower by a whole order of magnitude when the laser is used (Hamilton 2005).

Recurrent Cholesteatoma

Recurrent cholesteatoma is cholesteatoma that results from new ingrowth of squamous epithelium into the middle ear cleft from the repaired tympanic membrane. In most cases this represents a repeat of the process that led to the original cholesteatoma. Recurrent cholesteatoma in children may be caused by middle ear adhesions and persistent chronic otitis media. Recurrent cholesteatoma can develop over a long period of time, which means that a child who has been treated for cholesteatoma will need careful long-term follow up. In the past, combined approach tympanoplasty has had a notorious reputation for recurrent cholesteatoma. Studies using life table analysis have confirmed a higher rate of recurrent disease after combined approach tympanoplasty (Austin 1989), and that children have a higher risk of developing recurrent cholesteatoma than adults.

Other series have also examined recurrence rates in children. After combined approach tympanoplasty, Kinney (1988) noted a 25% recurrence rate at 5 years, Sanna et al. (1988) an 11% recurrence rate over 2–10 years and Charachon (1988) a 20% retraction pocket rate at 5 years. The risk of retraction after combined approach tympanoplasty has been reduced by completely obliterating the mastoid and epitympanum.

After mastoid cavity surgery, Silvola and Palva (1999) found that 25% of cases developed further retraction pockets, with 42% of these becoming retraction cholesteatomas after as much as 13 years.

Careful attention to reinforcing the weaker areas of the tympanic membrane is necessary in combined approach tympanoplasty to try and prevent further retraction. Tragal or conchal cartilage is generally used for this purpose. Some surgeons feel that a period of middle ear ventilation with a tympanostomy tube can also be beneficial.

Children with cholesteatoma present a more difficult group to treat when compared to adults. An adult understands the reasons for treatment and the need for often long and extensive follow up, frequently with microsuction of the ear. Children, by contrast, may not be able to appreciate the reasons behind what may be painful surgery and potentially uncomfortable sessions in the outpatient clinic. They may not allow the use of ear drops, ear suction, or even good visualisation of the tympanic membrane. This makes management of a difficult disease process even more challenging, and these factors should be borne in mind when considering the surgical options.

Changes in the Ossicles Secondary to Chronic Middle Ear Inflammation

Epidemiology

Chronic otitis media is often complicated by erosion of the ossicles. The ossicular chain was intact in just 37% of cases in a survey of 1100 ears with chronic otitis media (Tos 1979; Fig. 43.14). Involvement of the ossicles was highest when retraction pockets or cholesteatoma involved the ossicular chain. A similar large survey identified a lower rate of ossicular involvement in patients with perforated ears that were not discharging (Sadé et al. 1981b). This study also included an age-related analysis and demonstrated that the rate of ossicular involvement was lower in the ears of younger patients.

Pathology

Loss of ossicular integrity secondary to chronic otitis media has been termed resorptive osteitis and is mediated by osteoclasts. Bone damage is ultimately due to the chronic inflammatory process. The commonest defect is erosion of the long process of the incus, but erosion of any of the ossicles can occur. Other pathological processes that contribute to hearing loss include tympanosclerosis, fibrocystic sclerosis, sclerosing osteitis and fibrosis of the tympanic membrane, as well as tympanic membrane perforation.

Symptoms

The possibility of ossicular involvement should be entertained in any child with hearing loss associated with chronic otitis media, especially if the hearing loss persists when the ear canal is clean and the presence of a middle ear effusion has been excluded.

Signs

In addition to the signs of the tympanic membrane involvement of chronic otitis media, it may be possible to see a defect in the long process of the incus or stapes superstructure through a posterior perforation. Much less frequently, the manubrium of the malleus may be noted to be shortened or absent. In other cases, ossicular pathology may be inferred from the presence of a conductive hearing loss of over 20 dBHL in the presence of a tympanic membrane perforation, a retraction pocket or cholesteatoma.

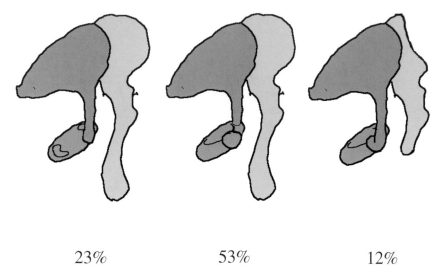

23%   53%   12%

Fig. 43.14 Prevalence of erosion of the ossicular chain in chronic otitis media. Pooled data for chronic otitis media associated with cholesteatoma, tympanic membrane atrophy and tympanic membrane perforation (Tos 1979)

43

Diagnosis

Confirmation of the presence of ossicular defects is possible by computed tomography scanning. If the child has cholesteatoma, the state of the ossicular chain can be defined as part of the wider investigation of the child's diseased ear. Tympanotomy remains the gold standard investigation for hearing loss caused by stiffening of the ossicular chain, although experimental attempts to define this condition prior to surgery using laser Doppler interferometry have proven successful.

Treatment

The decision on whether to offer treatment to restore hearing after ossicular erosion depends on whether the middle ear environment is likely to provide a stable result and whether the intervention is likely to influence auditory perception. The presence of continuing chronic otitis media mitigates against ossicular reconstruction, and this should only be considered in a stable, dry, chronic-otitis-media-free ear.

It is possible to reconstruct the ossicular chain by interposing rigid prostheses, including the patient's own ossicular remnants. The geometry of the ossicular defect does not always lend itself to stability of the prosthesis, so some reconstructions are more favoured than others. Reconstruction is usually performed between the tympanic membrane, manubrium or long process of incus on the one hand and the capitulum, stapes footplate or vestibule on the other.

Amplification, using hearing aids must always be borne in mind as a risk-free alternative to surgery.

Outcome Measures

Surgeons usually measure the success of ossicular reconstruction by assessment of the reduction of the conductive hearing loss: the difference between the air-conduction threshold and the bone-conduction threshold. Although this measure is of technical value when comparing surgical techniques, it is not a good guide to the patient's perception of success.

Other parameters influence auditory perception: the operated ear may contribute little to auditory perception if it is also impaired by sensorineural hearing loss; it may also contribute little if the hearing in the opposite ear remains very much better. Accordingly, the single most reliable indicator of patient's judgement of the benefit of ossicular surgery is the post-operative air-conduction threshold in the operated ear (Smyth and Patterson 1985), as this reflects the function of the entire ear on the operated side. This measure and the role of the other ear are neatly summarised by the Belfast Rule of Thumb: the patient can be expected to derive benefit from surgery if, after the operation, the air-conduction threshold in the operated ear is either less than 30 dBHL, or is greater than the air-conduction threshold in the opposite ear by no more then 15 dBHL.

Factors that Influence the Success of Ossicular Reconstruction

While a patient with symptomatic chronic otitis media can be offered high rates of success of disease removal and post-operative dry ear, as well as low rates of disease recurrence, the outcome of surgical reconstruction of the ossicular chain remains more variable. The presence of even mild sensorineural hearing loss limits the benefit to the patient of any ossicular reconstruction. In children there is a higher rate of useful hearing after ossicular reconstruction simply because children usually have better cochlear function.

One factor that is likely to influence outcomes in children is the presence of a middle ear effusion. It may be prudent to treat or allow any middle ear effusion to settle prior to performing an ossiculoplasty in a child's ear.

It is well established that the status of the ossicular chain prior to surgery is an important influence on surgical outcome. In essence, the greater the disruption of the chain prior to surgery, the less successful the surgery. In particular, the prior presence of the stapes superstructure has been repeatedly highlighted as the most important independent predictor of technically successful ossicular surgery (Modugno et al. 2000). Other middle ear factors that have been shown to independently influence the post-operative air–bone gap in ossicular surgery in adults include mucosal fibrosis, drainage and whether the procedure is revision surgery (Dornhoffer and Gardner 2001)

Studies using laser Doppler vibrometry have demonstrated that the outcome of ossicular surgery is sensitive to the density and stiffness of the prosthesis. The tension in the reconstructed chain should be kept to a minimum and the prosthesis should be positioned to minimise any rotation forces within the reconstructed chain.

The outcome of ossicular surgery is dependent on several variables including those factors discussed above, as well as the otologist him- or herself. One prospective randomised controlled trial of ossicular reconstruction has identified the operator as the most important variable influencing surgical outcome (Mangham and Lindeman 1990).

Complications of CSOM in Children

Intra- and extracranial complications of CSOM seem relatively uncommon in children in developed countries. When they occur, they are the same as those that occur in adults. Ludman (1996) separates complications into those within the cranial cavity (extradural abscess, subdural abscess, sigmoid sinus thrombosis, otitic hydrocephalus, meningitis and brain abscess) and those within the temporal bone (facial palsy and labyrinthine infection). Treatment consists of antibiotic therapy, with neurosurgical intervention when required and surgical management of problems in the temporal bone itself.

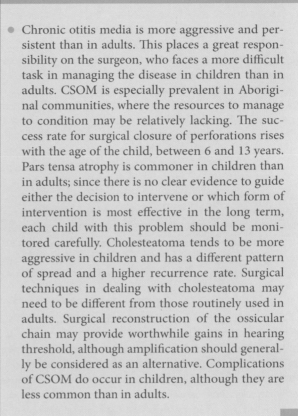

Summary for the Clinician

- Chronic otitis media is more aggressive and persistent than in adults. This places a great responsibility on the surgeon, who faces a more difficult task in managing the disease in children than in adults. CSOM is especially prevalent in Aboriginal communities, where the resources to manage to condition may be relatively lacking. The success rate for surgical closure of perforations rises with the age of the child, between 6 and 13 years. Pars tensa atrophy is commoner in children than in adults; since there is no clear evidence to guide either the decision to intervene or which form of intervention is most effective in the long term, each child with this problem should be monitored carefully. Cholesteatoma tends to be more aggressive in children and has a different pattern of spread and a higher recurrence rate. Surgical techniques in dealing with cholesteatoma may need to be different from those routinely used in adults. Surgical reconstruction of the ossicular chain may provide worthwhile gains in hearing threshold, although amplification should generally be considered as an alternative. Complications of CSOM do occur in children, although they are less common than in adults.

References

1. Austin DF (1989) Single-stage surgery for cholesteatoma: an actuarial analysis. Am J Otol 10:419–425
2. Bluestone CD, Gates GA, Klein JO et al (2002) Definitions, terminology and classification of otitis media. Ann Otol Rhinol Laryngol 111:8–18
3. Browning GG, Gatehouse S (1992) The prevalence of middle ear disease in the adult British population. Clin Otolaryngol 17:317–321
4. Charachon R (1988) Surgery of cholesteatoma in children. J Laryngol Otol 102:680–684
5. Derlacki EL, Clemis JD (1965) Congenital cholesteatoma of the middle ear and mastoid. Ann Otol Rhinol Laryngol 74:706–727
6. Dornhoffer JL, Gardner E (2001) Prognostic factors in ossiculoplasty: a statistical staging system. Otol Neurotol 22:299–304
7. Friedmann I (1956) The pathology of otitis media. J Clin Pathol 9:229–236
8. Gilchrist CA, Hills LJ (1991) A semi-Markov model for ear infection. Aust J Stat 33:5–16
9. Glasscock ME, Dickins JRE, Wiet R (1981) Cholesteatoma in children. Laryngoscope 91:1743–1753

10. Hamilton JW (2005) The efficacy of the KTP Laser in cholesteatoma surgery. Otol Neurotol 26:135–139

11. Kay DJ, Nelson M, Rosenfeld RM (2001) Meta-analysis of tympanostomy tube sequelae. Otolaryngol Head Neck Surg 124:374–380

12. Kim CS, Jung HW, Yoo KY (1993) Prevalence and risk factors of chronic otitis media in Korea: results of a nationwide survey. Acta Otolaryngol 113:369–375

13. Kinney SE (1988) Intact canal wall tympanoplasty with mastoidectomy for cholesteatoma: long term follow up. Laryngoscope 98:1190–1194

14. Lehmann D, Tennant MT, Silva DT, et al (2003) Benefits of swimming pools in two remote Aboriginal communities in Western Australia: an intervention study. BMJ 327:415–419

15. Ludman H (1996) Complications of suppurative otitis media. In: Kerr AG, Booth JB (eds) Scott Brown's Otolaryngology, 6th edn. Butterworth-Heinemann, London, pp 1–29

16. Males AG, Gray RF (1991) Mastoid misery: quantifying the distress in a radical cavity. Clin Otolaryngol Allied Sci 16:12–14

17. Mangham CA, Lindeman RC (1990) Ceravital versus plastipore in tympanoplasty: a randomized prospective trial. Ann Otol Rhinol Laryngol 99:112–116

18. Marquet J (1989) My current cholesteatoma techniques. Am J Otol 10:124–130

19. Maw AR, Bawden R (1994) Tympanic membrane atrophy, scarring, atelectasis and attic retraction in persistent, untreated otitis media with effusion and following ventilation tube insertion. Int J Pediatr Otorhinolaryngol 30:189–204

20. McFadyen C, Gamble C, Garner P, et al (2005) Topical quinolone vs. antiseptic for treating chronic suppurative otitis media: a randomised controlled trial. Trop Med Int Health 10:190–197

21. Mills RP, Padgham ND (1991) Management of childhood cholesteatoma. J Laryngol Otol 105:343–345

22. Modugno GC, Pirodda A, Saggese D, et al (2001) Multivariate analysis in predicting functional results in tympanoplasty. In: Magnan J, Chays A (eds) Proceedings of the Sixth International Conference on Cholesteatoma and Ear Surgery. Label Production, Marseille, pp 973–976

23. Nelson M, Roger G, Koltai PJ (2002) Congenital cholesteatoma. Arch Otolaryngol Head Neck Surg 128 810–814

24. Roger G, Denoyelle F, Chauvin P, et al (1997) Predictive risk factors of residual cholesteatoma in children: a study of 256 cases. Am J Otol 18:550–558

25. Sadé J (1993) Treatment of cholesteatoma and retraction pockets. Eur Arch Otorhinolaryngol 250:193–199

26. Sadé J, Avraham S, Brown M (1981a) Atelectasis, retraction pockets and cholesteatoma. Acta Otolaryngol 92:501–512

27. Sadé J, Berco E, Buyanover D, et al (1981b) Ossicular damage in chronic middle ear inflammation. Acta Otolaryngol 92:273–283

28. Sanna M, Zini C, Gamoletti R, et al (1988) Surgery for congenital and acquired cholesteatoma. Adv Otorhinolaryngol 40:124–130

29. Silvola J, Palva T (1999) Paediatric one-stage cholesteatoma surgery: long term results. Int J Paediatr Otorhinolaryngol 49:S87–90

30. Smith AW, Hatcher J, Mackenzie IJ, et al (1996) Randomised controlled trial of chronic suppurative otitis media in Kenyan schoolchildren. Lancet 348:1128–1133

31. Smyth GD, Patterson CC (1985) Results of middle ear reconstruction: do patients and surgeons agree? Am J Otol 6:276–279

32. Somers T, Houben V, Goovaerts G, et al (1997) Histology of the perforated tympanic membrane and its muco-epithelial junction. Clin Otolaryngol 22:162–166

33. Stewart IA, Silva PA, Said S, et al (1989) Surgical treatment of retraction pockets. In: Tos M, Thomsen J, Pietersen E (eds) Cholesteatoma and Middle Ear Surgery. Proceedings of the Third International Conference on Cholesteatoma and Mastoid Surgery. Kugler and Ghedini, Amsterdam, pp 443–448

34. Tos M (1979) Pathology of the ossicular chain in various chronic middle ear diseases. J. Laryngol Otol 93:769–780

35. Tos M, Stangerup SE, Larsen P (1987) Dynamics of eardrum changes following secretory otitis media. Arch Otolaryngol Head Neck Surg 113:380–385

36. Vrabec JT, Deskin RW, Grady JJ (1999) Meta-analysis of pediatric tympanoplasty. Arch Otolaryngol Head Neck Surg 125:530–534

37. WHO/CIBA Foundation Workshop (1996) Prevention of Hearing Impairment from Chronic Otitis Media. WHO/PDH/98.4. CIBA Foundation, London

38. Wormald PJ, Nilssen EL (1998) The facial ridge and the discharging mastoid cavity. Laryngoscope 108:92–96

43

Chapter 44

Bone-Anchored Hearing Aid (BAHA) and Softband

44

David W. Proops

Core Messages

- Children with congenital conductive hearing loss need long-term solutions.
- Conventional surgery for congenital conductive hearing loss has provided uncertain and generally poor results.
- The bone-anchored hearing aid (BAHA) offers a safe, robust and reliable solution.
- The Softband BAHA device is a short-term option that requires further evaluation for all conductive hearing losses.
- Acquired conductive hearing loss is a very common problem and speech and language development and behaviour and bone conduction devices may have a part to play in its management.
- Prosthetic osseointegrated pinnae are an effective alternative to autologous reconstruction of the pinna in microtia.

Contents

Introduction

This chapter will deal with the use of bone-anchored hearing aids (BAHAs) and will also cover Softband, a non-surgical application of the hearing aid part of BAHA in certain situations.

The main application of BAHA is to congenital conductive hearing loss. This includes various forms of microtia, when osseointegrated titanium bone screws may also be used as an attachment for artificial pinnae, if required. BAHA is also used in cases of congenital conductive hearing loss. This can occur in isolation or as a feature of various syndromes (see Chapter 8).

Conventional otosurgery is notoriously unsuccessful in congenital conductive deafness and the results of surgery in ears damaged by chronic suppurative otitis media can be disappointing in younger children. Air conduction aids are not always suitable, because they cannot be fitted if there is an absent or severely deformed pinna or ear canal. Bone-conducting hearing aids are the best medical option and would be used more often were they more comfortable.

The discovery of osseointegration has offered both secure, sensation free fixation and direct bone conduction amplification. The BAHA and Softband in children offer predictable benefits with minimal risk. Exciting opportunities may lie ahead to utilize bone conduction to benefit those with temporary as well as permanent conductive hearing loss.

Conductive Hearing Loss in Children

Conductive hearing loss is the result of failure of sound energy to be transmitted to the inner ear. This might be due to fluid in the middle ear space, abnormalities of the eardrum or ossicular chain, or to absence of the ear canal and drum.

Short-lasting conductive hearing loss in childhood probably gives no long-term sequelae, but in those children with persistent otitis media or with bilateral congenitally malformed ears then the effects on speech and language, attentiveness and behaviour, and hence educational performance, can be devastating. It is thus vital to identify these children early and have options to alleviate the conductive hearing loss.

Management of Congenital Conductive Hearing Loss

The management of congenital conductive hearing loss requires a brief understanding of the embryology of the ear. The middle ear and ossicular chain originate from the mesenchyme of the first two branchial arches, whereas the cochlea is an out-pouching of the central nervous system. This means that most people with a congenital ear abnormality have normal cochlear anatomy and function. Congenital ear malformations are often sporadic forms of the first and second arch. Some are sporadic and some are syndromal; however, there is a group of syndromes that have congenital ear abnormalities as one of their features (Table 44.1). A fuller description of syndromes that include hearing loss can be found in Chapter 8.

Classification of Congenital Ear Disorders

This topic is also discussed in Chapter 39. The management of congenital ear disorders requires a classification of the congenitally abnormal ear. There have been many, and these have usually been based on the presumed association between external and middle ear deformities as the basis of decision making about the benefits of surgical intervention. The most useful is Cremers et al. (1987). which represents three types:

1. Type 1: Mild, with a reduced-sized middle ear and a narrow or stenotic ear canal. This rare type is the only one suitable for surgical reconstruction.
2. Type 2: Medium – the commonest. The auricle is rudimentary, the canal atretic, the ossicles malformed and the facial nerve aberrant.
3. Type 3: Severe – not only is the external and middle ear severely affected, but the inner ear may be as well.

Investigations of Congenital Middle and External Ear Malformations

In some centres, much reliance is placed upon radiological investigations. Although this helps classification, it rarely affects management. The audiological evaluation must be undertaken as early as possible. The question to be asked is simple: "Is the deafness conductive, sensorineural or mixed?". In bilateral cases, the case for intervention is overwhelming. Until recently, the benefit of intervening in unilateral cases early, or ever, was questioned because of the "Belfast rule of thumb". Smyth (1980) showed that

Table 44.1 Syndromes that have congenital ear abnormalities as one of their features

Eponym	Pathological name
Treacher Collins syndrome	Mandibulofacial dysostosis
Apert's syndrome	Acrocephalosyndactyly
Crouzon's syndrome	Craniofacial dysostosis
Klippel Feil syndrome	Otocervical syndrome
Goldenhar's syndrome	Oculoauriculovertebral dysplasia
Turner's syndrome	Gonadal aplasia
Patau syndrome	Trisomy 13/15 syndrome
Edwards' syndrome	Trisomy 18 syndrome
Down's syndrome	Trisomy 21 syndrome
Pierre Robin syndrome	Cleft Palate, micrognathia and glossoptosis
Di George syndrome	Third and fourth pharyngeal pouch syndrome

unless the affected ear could be brought to within 15 dB of the normal ear, the patient perceived no benefit. Because the benefits of conventional otosurgery were so poor and unpredictable, and because children with monaural hearing seemed to fare well without hearing aids, it became a "tenet" that children with a unilateral congenital conductive hearing loss had a handicap that was not worthy of address, because the risks outweighed the benefits.

As the extent of the handicap of being monaural, especially in terms of hearing speech in the presence of background noise and in directional hearing has been revealed, the effect of BAHA in reducing both these handicaps safely and predictably has been demonstrated. There may now be a case for applying BAHA to unilateral congenital deafness.

So what audiological investigations are needed? This depends on age: in older cooperative children, air- and bone-conduction audiometry, with masking can be used, with aided thresholds and speech audiometry, using a conventional bone conductor. This is much more difficult in very young children, but visual reinforcement audiometry supplemented by air- and bone-conduction auditory brainstem audiometry can be undertaken.

Aiding Options for Congenital Conductive Hearing Loss

If there is an external ear of reasonable shape and a meatus, then a conventional aid can by tried. Conventional hearing aids, however, are often disliked by parents and are uncomfortable for children. The natural response of young children is to pull out the aid from their ears and parents need to be very patient if a regular pattern of wearing is to be achieved.

If it is not possible to fit such an aid, then a bone-conducting device must be employed. The principles of bone conduction have been known for many years: Tonndorf (1966) identified that on reaching the cochlea, vibratory energy causes alternate compression and expansion of the cochlear shell. Compression of the cochlea would not produce inner ear fluid displacement if the cochlear scalae were of equal size and shape. However, the total volume of the scala vestibuli is smaller than that of the scala tympani. The oval window is also less compliant than the round window, so the cochlear partition is forced downwards as a result of the forces produced by vibration of the skull.

Conventionally, bone-conduction hearing aids were kept in place on the skull with a sprung metal band. Although effective, this is uncomfortable and, to some, unsightly, and has been superseded by the "Softband". This is an elasticated head band to which a bone-conducting device is held. Surprisingly, less pressure than was anticipated was required to gain benefit.

Surgical Management of Congenital Conductive Hearing Loss

Reconstructive Surgery of the External and Middle Ear

This topic is also discussed in Chapter 39. When the only management option was surgical, then poor results were seen as an acceptable cost for the occasional, but relatively rare, good results. The purpose of this type of surgery is to create a socially useful level of hearing, but in the reported series, which are likely to be the better ones, social levels of hearing were only achieved in between 31 and 71% of cases. Rates of re-stenosis and otorrhoea were reported as 33% by Fenner et al. (1981), 24% stenosis and 18% otorrhoea by Colman (1976) and 10% by Cremers et al. (1988).

Selection of cases has been stressed by Jahrsdoerfer et al (1992), who devised the grading system, which, in his reported cases, only demonstrated 25% to be suitable for surgery to give a 70% chance of getting within 25 dB of the contralateral ear. The level of complexity and complication of the surgery makes justification very difficult in unilateral cases.

The Bone-Anchored Hearing Aid

Branemark et al. (1977) discovered that commercially pure titanium, when placed in bone, becomes firmly attached without an intermediate connective tissue layer. The principle of osseointegration applied to the concept of direct bone conduction with hearing aids was introduced by Tjellström (1989).

The BAHA is a semi-implantable bone-conducting hearing device that is secured to the skull by an osseointegrated titanium fixture. This direct coupling of mechanical vibration of the skull provides high-quality transmission of sound.

BAHA Surgical Procedure

In children, surgery is performed as a two-staged procedure under a general anaesthetic. At the first stage, the titanium implant is installed and 3 months later, the skin-penetrating abutment is placed and the skin flap thinned. When the soft tissue has healed, the hearing aid can then be fitted to the abutment (Tjellström et al. 1983).

This technique requires greater surgical expertise in children because of the reduced thickness of bone and the different composition of the skull bone. This means that surgery should not be attempted much before the second birthday and until that age, the hearing aid part of the device can be employed using a Softband.

Results in Bilateral Congenital Conductive Hearing Loss

BAHA has been shown to be safe in children (Stevenson et al 1997; Tietze and Papsin 2001; Tjellström et al. 2001).

Several studies have shown that in audiological terms, the BAHA out-performs conventional bone conductors (Snik et al. 1995b). The sound field thresholds were better and, consequently, significant improvements have been reported in speech perception scores in quiet. The reason for the better aided thresholds and speech perception with the BAHA system is that the sound quality remains acceptable even at higher volume settings. Significant improvements in speech-in-noise test scores have been reported (Snik et al. 1995a, b). Apart from audiometric measurements, disease- and handicap-specific questionnaires show that the BAHA system affords greater benefit than conventional devices (Dutt et al 2002a, b; Snik et al. 1995a, b).

Long-term results have also been studied by questionnaires, which showed that 5 and 10 years after fitting, most patients are still using their BAHA systems on a daily basis and were satisfied with the results (Ganström 2000).

Some of the children with bilateral congenital conductive hearing loss have gone on to have a sequential second-side BAHA and as this is becoming standard practice with adults, and as the evidence that two are better than one accumulates (Dutt et al. 2002a, b), it is likely that bilateral provision in children with bilateral conductive loss may become the norm, as it is using conventional aids.

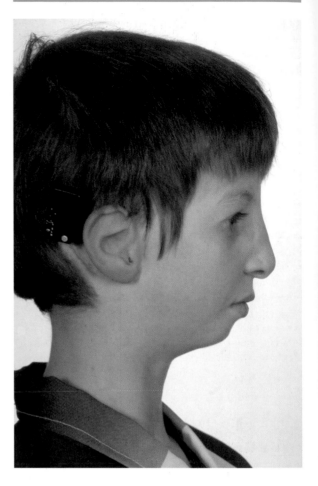

Fig. 44.1 Boy with Treacher Collins syndrome. Artificial pinna and bone-anchored hearing aid (reproduced with permission)

Unilateral Congenital Conductive Hearing Loss

Single-sided deafness has become of much greater interest lately as it has become increasingly recognised that it does pose a greater handicap and disability than previously recognised. Great effort is expended in chronic ear surgery addressing unilateral hearing loss. BAHA is now being used for rehabilitating acquired single-sided sensorineural loss in adults (Snik et al. 2002). The question needs to be asked and answered whether single-sided conductive hearing loss in children should not receive the same attention.

ing follow up. Clinical results show a high degree of safety and a limited number of complications. If a fixture is lost, re-operation is relatively simple to perform (Zeitoun et al. 2002).

For those with anotia or microtia, osseointegrated retained prostheses can be employed (Fig. 44.1). These have the advantage of requiring simple and safe surgery, and the cosmetic results are assured if good technical skills are available from prosthetists. Autologous reconstruction, while favoured by some parents, is a more difficult technique with significant donor site morbidity, and requires several long operations with much more uncertain outcome.

Fixture Survival and Skin Care

Percutaneous implantation of the titanium screws is achieved in 90–98% of cases and osseointegration seems to be as successful in children as adults. However, children are more susceptible to trauma. Approximately 90% of implants remain free from serious skin reactions dur-

Providing a Service for Children with Congenital Conductive Deafness

These children require a dedicated multidisciplinary team who can assess and support the complex need of each child and the impact that any intervention may have. The

BAHA service must work closely with the child and their parents and involve them in every step of the procedure. The long-term commitment both in healthcare needs, graduation to an adult service and funding must be carefully organized.

The British National Deaf Children's Society (NDSC 2003) have written a quality standard on BAHAs for children and young people, which sets out the requirements for such a service and quality standards that should be achieved (www.ndcs.org.uk). In school children, it may be beneficial to couple a personal FM system to the BAHA system.

Softband

The BAHA can now be used in the transcutaneous way by connecting the device to a special plastic disc held in place by an elastic band around the head, called the BAHA Softband. By this method, bone conduction vibrations are transmitted transcutaneously, which although less effective, is nevertheless a good temporary solution for children under 2 years, and those awaiting implantation. Lately, interest has been expressed at using the Softband in the management of otitis media with effusion (Medical Research Council Multicentre Otitis Media Study Group 2001). This is an engaging prospect and further studies are awaited.

Summary for the Clinician

- The results of conventional surgery for congenital conductive hearing loss have been variable and often disappointing. BAHA offers a safe and robust solution, and is as successful in children as it is in adults, although the skin-penetrating abutment is more likely to suffer trauma in children. It should not be considered until after the child's second birthday and the surgical technique requires greater surgical expertise in children. The Softband BAHA device seems to be a reliable short-term option, especially for infants and children too young to receive prosthetic BAHA. Osseointegrated prostheses are also available for children with microtia and can provide good cosmetic results.

References

1. Branemark PI, Hansson BO, Adell R, et al (1977) Osseointegrated implants in the treatment of the edentulous jaw. Scand J Plast Reconstr Surg 11:S11–16
2. Colman BH (1976) Congenital Deformities of the ear. The International Otology Workshop, Chicago
3. Cremers CWR, Oudenhoven JMTM, Marres EHM (1987) Congenital aural atresia: a subclassification and superficial management. Clin Otolaryngol 9:119–127
4. Cremers CWR, Temissen E, Marres EHM (1988) Classification of congenital aural atresia and results of reconstructive surgery. Adv Otorhinolaryngol 40:9–14
5. Dutt SN, McDermott AL, Burrell SP, et al (2002a) Patient satisfaction with bilateral bone anchored hearing aids, the Birmingham experience. J Laryngol Otolaryngol 28:37–46
6. Dutt SN, McDermott AL, Jelbert A, et al (2002b) The Glasgow Benefit Inventory in the evaluation of patient satisfaction with the bone anchored hearing aid: quality of life issues. J Laryngol Otolaryngol 28:7–14
7. Gantström G (2000) Osseointegrated implants in children. Acta Otolaryngol 543:118–121
8. Jahrsdoerfer RA, Yeakley JW, Aguilar EA, et al (1992) Grading system for the selection of patients with congenital auricular atresia. Am J Otol 13:6–12
9. Medical Research Council Multicentre Otitis Media Study Group (2001) Surgery for persistent otitis media with effusion, generalizability of results for the UK trial (TARGET). Trial of Alternative Regimens in Glue Ear Treatment. Clin Otolaryngol Allied Sci 26:417–424
10. NDSC (National Deaf Children's Society) (2203) Quality Standards in Bone Anchored Hearing Aids for Children and Young People. NDSC, London UK
11. Smyth GDL (1980) Ossiculoplasty in chronic ear disease. In: Smyth GDL (ed) Monographs in Clinical Otolaryngology. Churchill Livingstone, Edinburgh, pp 146–174
12. Snik AFM, Mylanus EAM, Cremers CWRJ (1995a) Bone anchored hearing aids in patients with sensorineural hearing loss and persistent otitis media. Clin Otolaryngol 20:31–35
13. Snik AFM, Mylanus EAM, Cremers CWRJ (1995b) The bone-anchored hearing aid compared with conventional aids. Otolaryngol Clin N Am 28:78–83
14. Snik AFM, Mylanus EAM, Cremers CWRJ (2002) The bone anchored hearing aid in patients with a unilateral air–bone gap. Otol Neurotol 23:61–66
15. Stevenson DA, Proops DW, Wake MB, et al (1997) Osseointegrated implants in the management of childhood ear abnormalities: the initial Birmingham experience. J Laryngol Otol 107:502–509
16. Tietze L, Papsin B (2001) Utilization of bone anchored hearing aids in children. Int J Pediatr Otorhinolaryngol 58:75–80
17. Tjellström A, Rosenhall U, Lindström J, et al (1983) Five year experience with skin penetrating bone anchored implants in the temporal bone. Acta Otolaryngol 95:568–575

18. Tjellström A, Håkansson B, Granström G (2001) Bone anchored hearing aids. Current status in adults and children. Otolaryngol Clin N Am 34:337–364

19. Tjellström A (1989) Osseointegrated appliances and their application in the head and neck. Adv Otorhinolaryngol 3:39–70

20. Tonndorf J (1966) Bone conduction. Studies in experimental animals. Acta Otolaryngol 213:1

21. Zeitoun H, De R, Thompson SD, Proops DW (2002) Osseointegrated implants in the management of childhood ear abnormalities: with particular emphasis on complications. J Laryngol Otol 116:87–91

Cochlear Implantation in Children

45

Mary Beth Brinson and John Graham

Core Messages

- Children identified with profound deafness at birth should be referred before the age of 6 months to cochlear implant programmes.
- Children deafened by meningitis, regardless of degree of hearing loss, should be referred without delay to a cochlear implant programme and should also be considered for bilateral implants.
- Unaided thresholds of hearing are the only valid threshold measurements; aided thresholds are no indicator of suitability for implantation.
- Congenitally deaf children suitable for implantation should receive their implants before their first birthday. Outcomes are significantly worse for those implanted after the age of 2 years.
- Although there is a place for implanting older children, and those with other disabilities, they should be assessed by an experienced paediatric cochlear implant team; if offered an implant, there should be realistic counselling of the family regarding potential outcomes.

Contents

Introduction

Cochlear implantation is now a mainstream option for the management of children with severe-to-profound hearing loss. Worldwide, approximately 65,000 people have cochlear implants, of whom approximately 25,000 are children. Cochlear implants are suitable for children from the 1st year of life onwards. Current research indicates that among congenitally deafened children, those who are implanted at a very young age seem to have the best outcomes from cochlear implantation. With the implementation of universal neonatal hearing screening (UNHS) in many developed countries and with the ability to obtain objective, frequency-specific and ear-specific hearing thresholds using auditory brainstem responses (ABR) and auditory steady state responses (ASSR) at, or shortly following birth, it is no longer necessary to delay intervention until the child is able to perform conventional behavioural tests. Yoshinaga-Itano et al. (1998) published seminal research that demonstrated that children who were identified with hearing loss early, and provided with amplification or implantation soon afterwards, were able to achieve much better outcomes in speech and language development than children whose hearing loss was identified later or who had delayed intervention.

A cochlear implant is a surgically implanted prosthetic device. All cochlear implants consist of five basic parts (Fig. 45.1): a microphone, speech processor, transmitting coil, internal receiver/stimulator, and an electrode array.

The microphone captures the speech signal or environmental sounds. The speech processor selects the important parts of the signal and converts these to an electronic format that can best be used to stimulate the cochlear nerve. This is known as the programme, or map. The transmitting coil uses radio frequencies to send the information to the internal device. The internal receiver–stimulator changes the signal to electrical impulses and also contains an internal magnet. The electrode array receives the electrical signal and sends it to the spiral ganglion cells of the cochlear nerve, which lie in the modiolus, the central core of the cochlea. A photograph of a cochlear implant in situ is shown in Fig. 45.2.

A cochlear implant bypasses the damaged hair cells in the cochlea, and directly stimulates the remaining spiral ganglion cells. With a few exceptions, it is the cochlear hair cells, rather than the cochlear nerve fibres, that are absent or damaged in both congenital and acquired profound sensorineural deafness. Currently available cochlear implants have arrays that have between 12 and 24 separate electrodes. Each electrode encodes a frequency band. Several speech-processing strategies are available. Following surgery to place the receiver–stimulator and the electrode array, the incision is allowed to heal for approximately 4 weeks. Then the patient attends a series of appointments with the audiologist to programme the external speech processor. A programme is created using a combination of patient input and objective measures. This programme shapes the input from the speech processor.

45

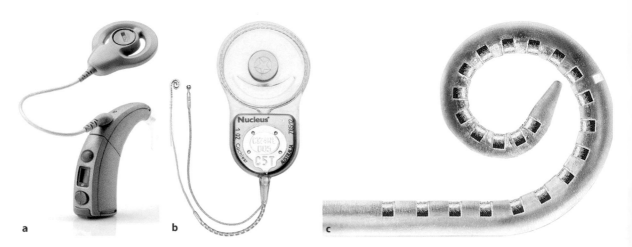

Fig. 45.1a–c Example of a cochlear implant. **a** External parts: speech processor, which contains the microphone, battery, and electronics to receive the electrical signal from the microphone, manipulate it, and change to a radio signal, for transmission across the scalp. The cable leads to the transmitting aerial, with a central magnet to couple with the implanted magnet and hold the aerial in place on the scalp. **b** The implanted part of a typical cochlear implant. The receiving aerial, with a central magnet (to couple with the external magnet shown in **a**). This leads the signal into the main implant package, which decodes the radio signal, converts it back into an electrical signal and sends it down the main cable, terminating in 22 active electrodes. There is also a single, ball-shaped, indifferent electrode, which is placed deep to the temporalis muscle. **c** An enlarged view of an intracochlear electrode array. There are 22 active electrodes, which lie in the scala tympani and the shape of the array holds it coiled close to the modiolus

For a description of speech-processing strategies and implants currently commercially available, the reader is referred to the manufacturers' literature and websites and to texts such as Cooper and Cradock's "Cochlear Implants, A Practical Guide, 2nd edition (Cooper and Cradock 2006). The websites of four commonly used cochlear implant manufacturers are:

1. www.cochlear.com
2. www.bionicear-europe.com
3. www.medel.com
4. www.neurelec.com

www.bcig.org (the website of the British Cochlear Implant Group) also has useful information.

A cochlear implant has the potential to restore "near normal" hearing sensitivity, with hearing thresholds around 30 dBHL, or better, across the frequency range. In most previously hearing but deafened adults and children,

a cochlear implant will be expected to restore the ability to discriminate speech. In congenitally deaf children, implanted before their second birthday, even though there will have been a period of auditory deprivation before implantation, a cochlear implant will usually be expected to allow that child's central auditory pathways to mature and enables a cortical "template" for language and speech to be laid down while the plasticity of the brain still allows this; as a result, many such children are provided with the opportunity to understand speech and language, to produce spoken language and to attend mainstream schools.

Team Approach

Successful cochlear implantation requires a multidisciplinary team. Each team member is responsible for a crucial part of the evaluation and habilitation or rehabilitation.

Referral Guidelines

It is imperative to have clear referral guidelines to ensure timely management of the hearing loss. The implementation of newborn hearing screening (UNHS) has enabled accurate identification of hearing loss from birth. This should allow very early identification of children with severe or profound hearing loss, which is most important, since it is now well established that children should ideally receive an implant at no later than 2 years of age for optimum benefit (Waltzman and Cohen 1998; Yoshinago-Itano 1999).

The authors make no excuse for introducing, near the beginning of this chapter, a list of referral guidelines for those who are responsible for the care of newly diagnosed deaf children. We hope that this will make it easier for those not actively involved in cochlear implant work to select those children who may benefit from a cochlear implant and to refer such children to cochlear implant teams at an early stage and with the minimum of delay. Most general paediatric audiology clinics, and those responsible for funding children for implantation, will not have the relevant equipment, time or multidisciplinary expertise to make the special judgments that a well-founded implant team is accustomed to making on a daily basis. It is therefore better to have relatively generous criteria for onward referral of potentially suitable children. Cochlear implant teams would prefer to take the responsibility of rejecting several unsuitable children, after proper counselling of the parents, than to be presented, too late, with one potentially suitable child for whom the window of opportunity of gaining access to spoken language and the ability to learn to speak has now closed.

Referral guidelines are often based mainly on audiometric data. It should be noted that teams now use un-

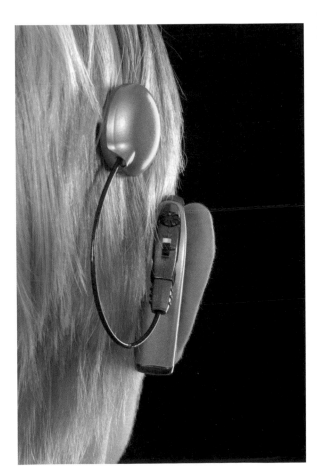

Fig. 45.2 Photograph of a typical multichannel cochlear implant in place. The speech processor is hooked behind the pinna. The external transmitting aerial is held magnetically against the scalp and exactly over the internal receiving aerial

aided thresholds, rather than aided ones, in their selection criteria for implantation: with the widespread use of digital hearing aids, aided audiograms are no longer considered valid criteria for excluding a child for implantation. Also, aided thresholds do not provide accurate information about the ability to discriminate sounds. They only provide information regarding sound detection levels.

The following four categories of referral criteria are generally recommended by cochlear implant programs.

Group I: Congenital Profound Hearing Loss

Children who are identified with a bilateral profound (>90 dBHL) hearing loss at birth (Fig. 45.3) should be referred to a cochlear implant centre by 6 months of age, since they otherwise face an insurmountable hurdle to oral language development. It is appropriate to refer these children for cochlear implant assessment in the first 6 months of life. With appropriate intervention, management and family counselling, these children can often receive a cochlear implant by their first birthday. Children who receive a diagnosis of profound hearing loss after the age of 1 year should also be referred immediately to a cochlear implant centre for evaluation.

Group II: Progressive Hearing Loss

This group encompasses children with bilateral hearing loss that is not initially profound enough to need a co-

chlear implant, but which on careful follow-up becomes progressively or suddenly worse. This can happen in children with congenital rubella and cytomegalovirus infection and also in those who have wide vestibular aqueducts (WVA) (see below, and Chapters 7, 8 and 40). These children may already have developed good speech and language, but are then found to have deteriorating hearing sensitivity on pure tone and speech perception audiometry, and may also be noted to have worsening speech production. Other children, for example those with autoimmune disease causing deafness, may have fluctuating hearing loss that may slowly deteriorate, bringing them within the criteria for an implant.

Group III: Severe-to-Profound Bilateral Hearing Loss

Children 2 years or older with a bilateral severe-to-profound hearing loss should be referred for cochlear implant evaluation (Fig. 45.4). Some children in this group make excellent progress with conventional hearing aids. Others, often with the same auditory thresholds, do not, and may benefit more from a cochlear implant. This group will need in-depth analysis of oral speech and language development to establish whether adequate progress is being made using conventional hearing aids. A careful analysis of the method of language learning and school placement needs to be made. Children older than about 5 years of age who have been using sign language as the primary method of language acquisition and are

45

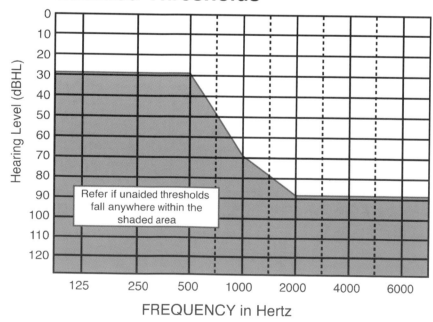

Fig. 45.3 The lower, shaded part of this audiogram chart shows the unaided levels of hearing that are recommended for referral to a cochlear implant team (courtesy of the Royal National Throat, Nose and Ear Hospital cochlear implant department)

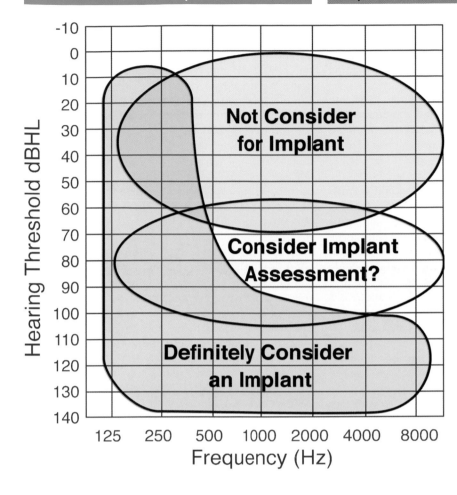

Fig. 45.4 This figure (by courtesy of the Ear Foundation) shows both the levels of profound hearing loss that should be referred to a cochlear implant team and the levels of severe hearing loss that may also benefit from a cochlear implant, together with those levels of hearing not suitable for a cochlear implant

placed in a signing-only educational environment need very careful assessment, as these children often will not benefit substantially from cochlear implantation.

Group IV: Sudden Hearing Loss

Sudden hearing loss can result from, for example, meningitis, autoimmune disease, chemotherapy, ototoxicity or head injuries. A child deafened by meningitis should be referred to a cochlear implant programme immediately, if possible as soon as the deafness has been identified. An early magnetic resonance imaging (MRI) scan is also imperative in these children, since with rapidly progressive ossification, the period during which it is possible to insert implants before the cochlea becomes ossified may be a matter of only a few weeks. Ossification may also occur in some cases of autoimmune deafness.

Children who are not making the expected progress with proper hearing aids, no matter what their hearing thresholds are, should be considered for referral. Some of these may have auditory neuropathy (AN) and may benefit

from cochlear implantation (see Chapter 7: OTOF gene). Some patients with AN who are not developing speech and language at a normal rate should also be referred to an experienced paediatric cochlear implant team (Berlin et al. 2001; Mason et al. 2003; Shallop et al. 2001).

It cannot be emphasised strongly enough that delaying the referral of a suitable child to a cochlear implant programme, for whatever reason, will inevitably lead to loss of potential long-term benefit in terms of oral speech and language development. There is no disputing that "early is better". In the past, it was suggested that a decision about implantation should be delayed until a child is "old enough to make up his or her own mind". This view has been proved to be entirely incorrect. Early referral has the potential to change the course of a child's life.

Assessment

Children referred for cochlear implantation assessment will usually been seen in an initial clinic. This is an opportunity for the child and parents to be introduced to the concept of the cochlear implant and for the team to determine if further assessment is warranted. Following the initial clinic, the child may be referred on to full assessment, discharged back to the referrer or occasionally reviewed after an interval if it appears that the hearing loss is progressive.

Once a child has been seen in the initial clinic and accepted as a possible cochlear implant candidate, it is essential that the team works quickly but thoroughly to establish whether or not that child will be expected to benefit from a cochlear implant. Each team member has a rôle in this assessment, and usually it is possible for the different team members to work in tandem, rather than sequentially, to speed up the assessment.

The full assessment entails thorough measurement not only of hearing thresholds, but also of the child's ability to discriminate speech and of his or her speech and language development. There is discussion of the child's present and future educational placement, psychological evaluation, particularly with regard to the child's family, and consideration of other medical or surgical aspects of the individual child. There should be documentation of every step in assessing the child's progress before, during and after implantation. Cochlear implant teams will have formal methods of using the information acquired during assessment to reach a decision. An example is the Children's Implant Profile, devised by the Nottingham programme in the UK (Nikolopoulos et al. 2004).

The team members include audiological scientists, teachers of the deaf, speech and language therapists, psychologists, medical members (otologists and audiological physicians) and the parents and family of the child. There should also be access to scientists/engineers, to sign language interpreters and to efficient secretarial and administrative support. The rôles of all team members tend to overlap, and most teams have a coordinator, to provide overall monitoring and direction for the team.

Audiological Scientist

The compilation of a complete audiological profile is crucial. An experienced paediatric audiological scientist will be responsible for completing the comprehensive objective and subjective audiological testing needed for assessment. The audiologist must be experienced and knowledgeable about hearing aids, able to make judgments about candidacy, and later to "map" the speech processor following surgery.

Unaided thresholds of hearing are the only valid threshold measurements. Aided thresholds from children using hearing aids are not a reliable guide to candidacy. Aided thresholds only predict the quiet levels of sound that the child has access to and do not take into account distortion of these sounds or predict the child's ability to discriminate speech and develop spoken language using these amplified sounds. In the extreme case

of dead regions of the cochlea, a child may respond to all tones presented, but is unable to discriminate between pure tones an octave or more apart. However, it is essential that a child being assessed for implantation should be using hearing aids and that these aids are optimised for the individual child. Occasionally, this may mean that the audiologist will provide different aids from those in use at the time of the initial referral.

Speech and Language Therapist

This topic is discussed further in Chapter 5. The speech and language therapist will be responsible for assessing the child's overall communication and listening skills. This may involve parent questionnaires, constructing vocal profiles and video analysis of early interaction and communication. They will also monitor the child's progress in terms of speech and language and may provide support and recommendations for local professionals. This will be particularly important if an implanted child is not making the expected progress.

Teacher of the Deaf

The role of an experienced teacher of the deaf overlaps with that of other team members in several fields, as well as focusing on educational aspects. They advise on eventual school placement and monitor educational progress. They also monitor hearing aid use, provide counselling for families, check the child's functional use of hearing and liaise with the child's local teachers of the deaf, helping with any problems that are found.

Psychologist

There are often unresolved problems within the family of a deaf child at the time of referral to the cochlear implant team. It will greatly help, both during the assessment process, at the time of admission for surgery and after implantation if the team's paediatric psychologist can be closely involved from the time of assessment onwards. In some cases no active intervention is necessary, but in many cases there are unresolved problems related to the parents' acceptance of deafness and their "mourning" for a child with deafness. They may also need to deal with parents who think implant is a "cure" for deafness and refuse to consider the long-term implications of having a deaf child. The psychologist will also have the training to identify additional developmental delay, and behavioural problems, both in the child and in the parents, that might prevent successful mapping or habilitation.

At the time of writing, relatively few members of the "deaf community", congenitally deaf adult couples who have a congenitally deaf child, will present their child for implantation, but when this does occur such parents need particular care and the expertise of a psychologist accustomed to communicating with congenitally deaf, signing adults. Similarly, when the family has one congenitally deaf parent, the role of the psychologist will be important, both in counselling before implantation and in the family dynamics during the long-term habilitation of the child.

Medical Team Members

Medical members of the team include otologists and audiological physicians. As well as taking overall clinical responsibility, and in the case of otologists, performing the surgery, they will undertake whatever diagnostic tests are required to establish the aetiology of the deafness. It is also helpful for the team to have a close relationship with a clinical geneticist and a radiologist experienced in the field of otological imaging in children. It is very helpful for the implant team to have a close relationship with a paediatrician accustomed to dealing with children with hearing loss and with various forms of developmental delay. For surgery, a paediatric anaesthetist is essential.

Parents

It must be remembered that, compared to team members, the child's close family are, if anything, even more closely involved in the decision to offer an implant to a child. In some families, siblings and grandparents may have rôles equal to those of the parents. There may also be differences in language and culture to be taken into account. Any implant team will have encountered parents who themselves have social and communication problems quite separate from those associated with having a deaf child. The responsibility of the team is to recognise these, but to remember that their primary duty is to the care of the child and of that child's future. Most parents, however, are highly supportive of the implant team and devote all of their energy towards a successful outcome from the implant process. Useful websites, providing support for parents include www.deafnessatbirth.org.uk
The decision to offer an implant is taken as a joint decision on the part of the multidisciplinary team, the parents and possibly others outside the team such as teachers and local paediatricians.

Implantation Criteria

These are the main criteria that a paediatric cochlear implant team will use during the assessment process to decide whether or not to offer an individual child a cochlear implant.

The Child

1. Children with bilateral profound sensorineural hearing loss. These children should be implanted before 18 months of age if at all possible for the best outcomes (Osberger et al. 2002). Many centres routinely implant at 9–10 months of age.
2. Children deafened by meningitis need to be fast-tracked through the assessment process. The invasion of the cochlea by bacteria during an episode of meningitis carries a high risk that both cochleae will be rapidly obliterated by new bone. This can begin less than 1 month after meningitis and can progress rapidly, making normal insertion of the electrodes into the scala tympani difficult or impossible.
3. Children with bilateral severe-to-profound sensorineural hearing loss not receiving sufficient benefit from hearing aids should be implanted by the age of 2 years.
4. Older children who are receiving inadequate benefit from their hearing aids, as demonstrated on speech perception tests in the auditory-only condition (severe-to-profound hearing loss). These children receive marginal or minimal benefit from traditional amplification.
5. Children with progressive sensorineural hearing loss resulting in severe-to-profound to profound hearing thresholds.

The Child's Environment

1. There should be appropriate motivation and expectations from the family and child, if possible.
2. There should be appropriate educational placement, to enhance development of auditory skills.

These are guidelines for cochlear implant candidacy. The actual cochlear implant assessment is tailored for each individual child, and other factors may be involved in the decision of the team. As the design of cochlear implants has developed, and outcomes improved, children with less profound degrees of hearing loss have been found to progress better with implants than with hearing aids.

Factors Affecting the Outcome of Cochlear Implantation

Many factors influence the outcome of cochlear implantation. Some of these factors are known and are good predictors of how the recipient will perform. However, with all patients, there are unknown and immeasurable factors that may affect success. These factors include spiral ganglion cell survival, additional learning difficulties and speech and language disorders. This is particularly true with very young children, as some problems only become apparent over time. Factors that are known to affect outcome are:

1. Age at implantation: generally younger is better.
2. Duration of deafness. In congenital deafness this means implanting early, in acquired deafness it implies implanting as soon as possible after the deafness occurs.
3. Age of onset of severe-to-profound acquired deafness.
4. Parental expectations: realistic parental expectations are essential. Parents who have unreasonable hopes for the progress of their child can experience great disappointment when these expectations are not met.
5. Available appropriate education options: children who receive a cochlear implant need intensive oral and aural habilitation. It is essential that these services are available. It is not unheard of for families to move house to be near appropriate educational and rehabilitation services.
6. The child's cognitive function: in terms of speech and language development, it has been shown that deaf children who suffer from severe cognitive impairment do not make any greater progress with cochlear implants than they would if their hearing were normal. If the decision is made to implant a child with a lesser degree of cognitive impairment, it is essential to ensure that the parents understand that the implant will not change any other disability that the child may have.
7. Aetiology of deafness: certain causes of deafness can have generally poorer outcomes. An example is post-meningitic deafness in which there is also some neurological damage.

The ideal candidate for cochlear implantation will have deafness identified by UNHS at birth, will have had the deafness quantified early using ABR and ASSR and will have been fitted with hearing aids soon afterwards. He or she will have no other developmental problems. He or she will have been referred to a cochlear implant programme by the age of 6 months and will have received an implant by his first birthday. After implantation, he will respond to sound, and mapping of the speech processor will take place with no problems. If the date of implantation is considered his "birth date", progress made in terms of speech and language development would be expected to be roughly parallel with that of a normal hearing child, but delayed by the number of months equivalent to his age at implantation.

Surgery

Once an implant has been offered and the choice of device agreed, the child will be admitted to a children's facility for the implant operation to take place. Normally implants are performed with the child admitted to a paediatric ENT ward, with paediatric- and ENT-trained nursing staff. To allow continuity, one team member may be allocated to the child and family over the period of surgery, post-operative course and initial device programming.

Approach

Most implant surgeons use the standard approach, with a short post-aural incision, 3–4 mm behind the post-aural crease, and minimal shaving of hair. The perichondrium and temporalis muscle are incised 2 cm posterior to the line of the skin incision. A "pocket" of pericranium is raised posterior to the incision to accommodate the implant package. A transmastoid approach is usually preferred by experienced otologists, with facial nerve monitoring. The size of the cortical mastoid cavity created will depend on the existing anatomy, and can be a little cramped in children younger than 1 year of age; however, there is seldom any major problem of access; many small children have a relatively deep facial recess, making the creation of a posterior tympanotomy easier than in an adult. Although damage to the facial nerve has been described during this part of the procedure, it should occur rarely, if ever, at the hands of an experienced otologist.

The cochleostomy is performed in the same way as in an adult, drilling with a diamond burr to flatten the promontory anterior to the round window niche and about the width of two stapes heads inferior to the incudostapedial joint. A disc-shaped white area of endosteum is eventually exposed and followed inferiorly and anteriorly for 1 or 2 mm, then carefully lifted from the anterior-inferior wall of the scala tympani, avoiding any damage to the basilar membrane.

Preparation of the Bed for the Receiver–Stimulator Package

The skull of a young child is relatively thin and it is often necessary to expose the dura, which must not be damaged. Some surgeons place sutures in the skull to stabilise the implant package, others rely on the small pocket of elevated pericranium to do this.

Insertion of the Electrode Array

This is performed in exactly the same way as in adults using the appropriate technique for the type and make of implant used.

45

Special Medical and Surgical Situations

Jervell and Lange-Nielsen Syndrome

This should be detected during the diagnostic phase of implant assessment. It is a hereditary potassium channel disorder that affects both the cochlea and the myocardium. The myocardial lesion causes a prolonged QTc interval. This electrocardiographic abnormality can produce a particular form of ventricular tachycardia called "torsade des pointes", which can lead to ventricular fibrillation when the myocardium is challenged by sympathetic activity, for example during exercise or anaesthesia. It does not preclude general anaesthesia, as long as the anaesthetist is aware of the problem and administers beta-blockers. Long term, some children with the syndrome may require beta-blocker treatment or a cardiac pacemaker or pacemaker-defibrillator.

Meningitis

Otologists recommend that children receiving cochlear implants should begin a course of vaccine against common strains of *Pneumococcus* before implantation. This is because there is a potential risk of bacterial middle ear infections passing through the cochleostomy and reaching the cerebrospinal fluid (CSF), to cause meningitis. The most likely organism that could cause this is *Pneumococcus*. Manufacturers now recommend antibiotic cover for cochlear implant surgery. The risk of meningitis is greater when there is a surgical "gusher" at operation, and steps must be taken to seal the cochleostomy effectively.

Prematurity

Some children referred for implantation have become deaf during a complicated post-natal period in the neonatal intensive care unit. Such children may have other problems related to their initial low birth weight and prematurity, and a close liaison with the neonatal unit is important.

Otitis Media

Middle ear effusion (otitis media with effusion, OME) is common in young children. During the assessment of a child for implantation, it is important to eliminate the conductive element of the hearing loss during threshold estimation. There is no clear guidance on the best way of dealing with OME either when it has been identified before implant surgery or if it is identified for the first time during the implant operation. Clinically, it is a question of balancing the risk of low-grade infection being present at surgery, perhaps involving biofilms, and the risk to an implant if a ventilation tube is left in place. Acute otitis media, on the other hand, will mean postponing the operation while antibiotics are administered. Some surgeons have advocated adenoidectomy and ventilation tube insertion before implant surgery. There seems to be evidence that this is more effective than simply ignoring the presence of OME.

Ossified Cochleae

As stated above, a child deafened by meningitis should be referred immediately and then fast-tracked through the assessment process. There is the strongest possible case for offering children deafened by meningitis bilateral implants; otherwise the non-implanted ear may not be available for later implantation using normal electrodes. Both computed tomography and MRI are useful in determining the extent of ossification; however, MRI is essential and can demonstrate a slight fading of the signal from the perilymph on T2-weighted imaging as the earliest sign of ossification. This process is dynamic and may be very rapid, and a further MRI may need to be performed as close as possible to the time of surgery. Several strategies have been described to deal with ossifying and already ossified cochleae. At an early stage the cochlea may simply contain fluid of a stiff, paste-like consistency, allowing full insertion of the electrode, especially those that have a central stilette, producing some rigidity (the Nucleus Freedom), or introduced from an external rigid tube (the Clarion HiRes). Later in the process of ossification, with the early laying down of new bone, this may be relatively soft, allowing disobliteration of the cochlea. In some cases, only the basal half of the basal turn is ossified and, once this part has been cleared, the rest of the basal and second turn are found to be patent. Since the meningitis bacteria gain entry to the cochlea through the cochlear aqueduct and initially reach the scala tympani, the scala vestibuli may, at first, not be affected and the implant may be introduced into it. Once the new bone is mature and hard, some form of tunnel needs to be drilled into the promontory to allow electrodes to be placed close to the modiolus, to allow stimulation of whatever remains of the spiral ganglion. The technique described by Bredberg et al. (1997) allows the maximum number of electrodes to be placed on each side of the spiral ganglion, using a pair of tunnels, one drilled to follow the normal path of the first part of the basal turn, the second, parallel to the first, following the path of the upper basal turn. Temporal bone practice is advised before undertaking this procedure. "Split" electrode arrays are available from two manufacturers; these consist of two arrays, each pair containing 12 or 20 electrodes, depending on the manufacturer. One electrode array is inserted into each of the two tunnels.

Congenital Malformation of the Cochlea

See Chapter 40 for a fuller description of this topic. Jackler et al. (1987) produced a classification of congenital dysplasias of the cochlea based on the stage of in utero development at which the cochlea stopped growing. At worst, there is no cochlea (Michel deformity), then a small cochlear bud or common cavity, a larger common cavity, and finally, the Mondini deformity, and about 1.5 turns of the cochlea, instead of the normal 2.5 turns, and an incomplete partition separating the turns. In any of the situations where the cochlea is present but malformed, there may or may not be an abnormal, direct communication between the vestibule and the internal auditory canal (IAC), allowing CSF to flow through the cochlea once the cochleostomy has been performed: a so-called surgical gusher. An abnormally WVA may be present, especially in Pendred syndrome, with or without a Mondini deformity. WVA may also so associated with a surgical gusher, suggesting that it may in some cases be associated with the abnormal communication between vestibule and IAC mentioned above.

Children with Mondini deformity can commonly be implanted in the usual way, with the reasonable confidence that spiral ganglion cells will be present in a modiolus. There are no clear guidelines on which electrode arrays may be best to use in a common cavity; however, it seems logical to choose an array more likely to lie against the wall of the cavity, since this is where any neural tissue will be found.

Two other technical problems may be associated with placing implants in common cavities: (1) it may not be possible to drill into the cavity through the promontory in the usual way, via a posterior tympanotomy, when the promontory itself is relatively concave, rather than convex, and cannot be seen through the tympanotomy; (2) a wide connection between vestibule and IAC may allow the electrode to pass directly into the IAC. It may be possible to obtain a better access to the promontory by removing the posterior canal wall. However, an easier strategy (McElveen et al. 1997) is to "blue line" the lateral semicircular canal and make a slot-shaped opening into the canal. This allows the electrode to be bent back on itself as a loop, the apex of which can be introduced through the slot and the loop then fed towards the common cavity, avoiding the risk of insertion into the IAC. One manufacturer, MedEl, has provided a special electrode for this purpose.

Some congenitally deaf children have abnormally narrow vestibulocochlear or cochlear nerves. There may be suspicion that this is the case when the IAC is found to be abnormally narrow on imaging; however, abnormality of the cochlear nerves may also be present with IACs of normal dimensions (see Chapter 40). There have been case reports of children in this situation in whom an implant failed to provide any sensation of sound. In others, good hearing levels were obtained, although in a series of 6 cases (J Bell M, Beale T et al. 2007) personal communication) long-term results showed disappointing outcomes in terms of speech discrimination and spoken language, suggesting that the quality of information transmitted through these abnormal nerves can be relatively poor.

Surgical "Gusher"

In this situation, as described above, CSF at relatively high pressure emerges from the cochleostomy and floods into the middle ear. Some control of the speed of flow can be obtained by tilting the head of the operating table upwards. A muscle plug can be inserted into the cochleostomy to control the flow while the implant is prepared for insertion. If the tip of an appropriate fine sucker end is placed just at the rim of the cochleostomy, this keeps the middle ear clear of fluid, gives the surgeon a better view and helps the insertion. There is clearly a risk of post-operative meningitis in this situation and a stable and solid seal to the cochleostomy is mandatory.

When the cochlear nerve is absent, or the cochlea itself is not present, an auditory brainstem implant (ABI) may be possible (Colletti et al. 2002); more information is needed on the long-term results of ABI in congenital deafness.

Chronic Suppurative Otitis Media

It is uncommon for chronic suppurative otitis media to be the cause of bilateral profound sensorineural deafness in children; however, there are rare cases when either surgery for cholesteatoma or the disease process itself leads to bilateral profound deafness. Cochlear implantation can usually be performed once complete eradication of the disease has been achieved.

Complications After Implantation

(See also Bhatia et al. 2004)

Device Failure

All devices currently on the market have a failure rate, although this is very small (Conboy et al. 2004). In an adult or an older child, significant failure of the device is obvious. In a small child such failure may be less evident. Signs of failure or malfunction of the implant include non-responsiveness to sound or a change in responsiveness, facial twitching and or pain in response to sound. Some children who have developed some language may indicate a change in the quality of sound or new additional sounds, like pinging or popping. Sometimes, parents notice a change in the quality of the child's speech or his level of responsiveness. Some of these signs are also indications that a remapping is necessary. Although device failure can be very traumatic for the patient, it is relatively simple to reopen the original incision and replace the device. Once the device is replaced, performance usually returns to prefailure levels rather quickly.

Infection

This is less common than might have been expected. The fact that middle ear infections are more common in children and the middle ear may contain biofilms might have resulted in such infections being a common problem in implanted children; however, this does not seem to be the case. Acute middle ear infections do occur, however, and need robust management with substantial courses of antibiotics. If there is not a rapid response to this treatment, the child should be admitted to hospital, if necessary for intravenous antibiotic therapy.

Skin Breakdown

This may occur for no obvious reason, or may be the result of a blow over the implant or friction, for example from a helmet. This situation can be remedied either by moving the implant package away from the skin defect, excising non-viable skin and closing the defect in a straight line (the second author's preference) or by rotating scalp flaps to provide cover for the exposed implant.

Facial Nerve Stimulation

This can be a problem in implanted patients. It can accompany intracochlear infection, incomplete implant failure or occur for no particular reason. The electrodes that are producing the stimulation should be "switched off", but after a period may be reintroduced, gradually using levels of current well below those that originally caused the problem. If it is necessary to leave a few electrodes switched off, this is not a problem, as in all modern implants there is a built-in redundancy in the total number of electrodes. These electrodes can remain off with no worsening of performance.

Further Considerations

Bilateral Cochlear Implantation in Children

Bilateral implantation has been shown to improve a deaf child's ability to localise sound and to discriminate

speech in the presence of background noise (Litovsky et al. 2006). This has general advantages, but especially in the classroom. For children or adults deafened by meningitis, in whom the cochleae are ossifying, bilateral implantation is strongly advisable, since for both ears there may be a very small window of opportunity for placing an electrode in a non-obstructed cochlea. There are also strong indications for bilaterally implanting children with visual problems, including those with Usher's syndrome. Such children will need to rely particularly on their hearing in the future, for communication and for awareness of their environment.

As evidence continues to accumulate regarding the benefits of bilateral cochlear implantation, the practice is becoming a more mainstream option for all children. An unresolved question is whether, in a congenitally deaf child with a unilateral cochlear implant, the second side will still be able to benefit from an implant after an interval of, say. 20 or 40 years or more. It is possible that after such an interval the cochlear nucleus on the contralateral side may not be capable of adequate onward transmission of signals arriving from the auditory nerve.

Future Prospects

Experimental work is taking place in the fields of hair cell regrowth and of neurotropic agents, designed to persuade the hair cells to regrow or the dendrites serving the spiral ganglion to grow towards the implant electrodes. Implants are being designed that will contain a central hollow core to allow delivery of these agents.

Hybrid devices are already available to be used in cases when low-frequency hearing is relatively well preserved. These have short electrode arrays, introduced into the basal few millimetres of the basal turn, with minimal damage. They allow electrical stimulation of the high-frequency, basal part of the spiral ganglion, but are linked to a conventional hearing aid, to amplify the lower frequencies.

A totally implantable device, with no external parts, is another desirable future development.

The greatest need for cochlear implantation, in terms of numbers, is in the developing world (see Chapter 13), where the rates of profound deafness are highest and the availability of all kinds of health services is lowest. Effective but affordable cochlear implants would allow some increase in the number of children receiving implants in these countries.

Finally, although cochlear implants have revolutionised the outlook for profoundly deaf children, it is important to realistic about the likely benefits, especially in children implanted late and those who may have other problems. In the 1940s to 1960s the introduction of electrical hearing aids made a huge impact on children with moderate-to-severe deafness, enabling them to acquire spoken language and communicate orally. It was confidently predicted that these benefits would also extend to profoundly deaf children. Sadly, for the majority this did not happen. Many of these children were deprived of access to signing during their education. As adults, many of them resent the way they were treated. An optimistic approach to the benefits of cochlear implantation for suitable children is entirely appropriate for the majority, diagnosed and implanted early. We do, however, need to be vigilant in identifying those who, for whatever reason, fail to develop speech and language understanding and production at the expected rate, and to be prepared to tailor their overall management to match their perception of sound.

Summary for the Clinician

- Cochlear implantation has been shown to be an effective treatment for some types of deafness for adults and children. Much progress has been made since the advent of cochlear implants, with most recipients achieving some degree of open-set speech recognition. The degree of success of cochlear implantation is largely dependent on having an experienced cochlear implant team involved from the beginning of the assessment.
- Current trends in cochlear implantation include bilateral implantation for adults and children and cochlear implants for patients with less profound degrees of hearing loss. Research is now focusing on obtaining better speech understanding in noisy environments (i.e. classrooms, workplace) and better perception of music.

References

1. Berlin C, Hood L, Rose K (2001) On renaming auditory neuropathy as auditory dys-synchrony. Audiol Today 13:15–17
2. Bhatia K, Gibbin KP, Nikolopoulos TP, O'Donoghue GM (2004) Surgical complications and their management in a series of 300 consecutive pediatric cochlear implantations. Otol Neurotol 25:730–739
3. Bradley J, Bell M, Beale T, et al. (2007) Variable long term outcomes from cochlear implantation in children with hypoplastic auditory nerves. Cochlear Implants International 8: In press
4. Bredberg G, Lindstrom B, Lopponen H, et al (1997) Electrodes for ossified cochleas. Am J Otol 18:42–43
5. Colletti V, Carner M, Fiorino F, Sacchetto L, Miorelli V, Orsi A, Cilurzo F, Pacini L (2002) Hearing restoration with auditory brainstem implant in three children with cochlear nerve aplasia. Otol Neurotol 23:682–693
6. Conboy PJ, Gibbin KP (2004) Paediatric cochlear implant durability, the Nottingham experience. Cochlear Implants Int 5:131–137
7. Cooper HR, Cradock LC (eds) (2006) Cochlear Implants: A Practical Guide. Whurr, London
8. Jackler RK, Luxford WM, House WF (1987) Congenital malformations of the inner ear: a classification based on embryogenesis. Laryngoscope 97:2–14
9. Litovsky RY, Johnstone PM, Godar SP (2006) Benefits of bilateral cochlear implants and/or hearing aids in children. Int J Audiol 45:S78–S91
10. McElveen JT, Carrasco VN, Miyamoto RT, et al (1997) Cochlear implantation in common cavity malformations using a transmastoid labyrinthotomy approach. Laryngoscope 107:1032–1036
11. Mason JC, De Michele A, Stevens C, et al (2003) Cochlear implantation in patients with auditory neuropathy of varied aetiologies. Laryngoscope 113:45–49
12. Nikolopoulos TP, Dyar D, Gibbin KP (2004) Assessing candidate children for cochlear implantation with the Nottingham Children's Implant Profile (NchIP): the first 200 children. Int J Pediatr Otorhinolaryngol 68:127–135
13. Osberger MJ, Zimmerman-Phillips S, Koch DB (2002) Cochlear implant candidacy and performance trends in children. Ann Otol Rhinol Laryngol Suppl 185:62–65
14. Shallop JK, Peterson A, Facer GW, et al (2001) Cochlear implants in five cases of auditory neuropathy: postoperative findings and progress. Laryngoscope 111:555–562
15. Waltzman S, Cohen N (1998) Cochlear implantation in children younger than 2 years old. Am J Otol 19:158–162
16. Yoshinago-Itano C (1999) Benefits of early intervention for children with hearing loss. Otolaryngol Clin N Am 32:1089–1102
17. Yoshinago-Itano C, Sedey AL, Couloter D, et al (1998) Language of early- and later-identified children with hearing Loss. Pediatrics 102:1161–1171

45

Chapter 46

The Dizzy Child

46

Linda Luxon and Waheeda Pagarkar

Core Messages

- Dizziness is a non-specific term, whereas the term "vertigo" implies an illusion of movement due to lesions in the vestibular system, but children are often unable to make the distinction.
- Dizziness in children is most commonly due to migraine and its equivalents, otitis media with effusion, and vestibular neuritis.
- A detailed history is invaluable in arriving at a diagnosis in a dizzy child.
- Clinical examination of a dizzy child must include observation of play and normal activities, together with examination of eye movements, gait and posture, Dix Hallpike test and the central nervous system.
- Vestibular testing includes rotational chair tests, bithermal caloric tests, posturography, vestibular evoked myogenic potentials and subjective visual vertical.
- Vestibular rehabilitation therapy is useful in the management of vestibular dysfunction in children.

Contents

Introduction

Dizziness is a lay term used to describe many different sensations, including unsteadiness, imbalance, clumsiness, light-headedness and vertigo. However, vertigo is a medical term referring to an illusion of movement, which may be subjective (personal perception of motion) or objective (observation of motion of the environment), and is characteristically associated with disorders of the vestibular system. Young children are often unable to describe these different perceptions, and thus any complaint of dizziness, instability or vertigo should be considered in the broad context of the "dizzy child" for diagnostic purposes.

Balance depends upon sensory input from the visual, vestibular and somatosensory systems (Fig. 46.1). The development of these systems occurs at different rates, with the somatosensory system maturing first, followed by vision and lastly by the vestibular system. Children under the age of 1–2 years perform poorly under conflicting sensory conditions such as in a moving car, although they may perform well under conditions of sensory deprivation, such as visual loss. This suggests that although the vestibular system is developed, the adaptive and integration mechanisms mature later. Postural sway in children improves with increasing age and children do not exhibit the sensory integration seen in adults until the age of 14 years.

The incidence of vertigo as a primary complaint in children, as judged from hospital records, has been reported to be less than 1%, whereas population-based surveys have reported a childhood prevalence of between 8%

(aged 1–15 years) and 18% (school children 5–15 years; Niemensivu et al. 2006). Prevalence studies may be influenced by the fact that children may find it difficult to describe dizziness, associated signs may be absent and medical advice may not be sought, as peripheral disorders in children are frequently associated with early compensation.

Pathology in many different systems may give rise to dizziness, ranging from self-limiting inner ear disorders to life-threatening neurological disease (Table 46.1). The prevalence of different conditions depends on the population studied: otolaryngology clinics report a predominance of otological causes, while paediatric neurology clinics report a higher incidence of neurological pathology. Nonetheless, certain conditions occur frequently in all studies; specifically, migraine-associated vertigo, otitis-media-related dizziness, benign paroxysmal vertigo, trauma and vestibular neuritis together account for more than half of children with dizziness (Niemensivu et al. 2006).

In attempting to establish a diagnosis in a dizzy child and to differentiate vestibular vertigo, from neurological and paediatric conditions giving rise to dizziness/vertigo, the clinician needs to be armed with four clinical tools:

1. A working knowledge of the causes of balance disorders in children.
2. An appropriate diagnostic strategy including key points in the history.
3. A good knowledge of eye movement examination and interpretation.
4. An understanding of appropriate investigations and their interpretation.

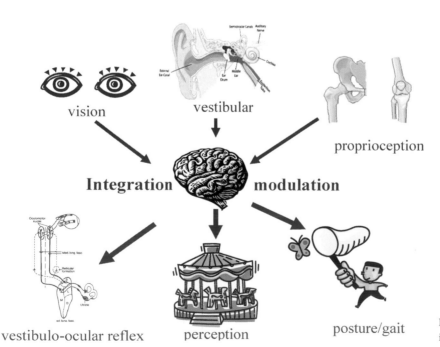

Fig. 46.1 Mechanisms of balance in children

Table 46.1 Causes of dizziness/vertigo/imbalance in children. *CHARGE* Acronym of: coloboma, heart defects, atresia of the choanae, retardation of growth and development, genital and ear anomalies, *BPPV* benign paroxysmal positional vertigo, *BOR* branchio-oto-renal syndrome, *CP* angle cerebellopontine angle, *BPT* benign paroxysmal torticollis

Causes		Conditions
1. Congenital	a) Malformations	Enlarged vestibular aqueduct Vestibular dysplasia Semicircular canal malformation Arnold Chiari malformation
	b) Syndromes associated with hearing loss	CHARGE, Usher, BOR, Pendred, Alstrom, Alport
2. Otologic	a) Inflammatory/infective	Otitis media with effusion, chronic suppurative otitis media, cholesteatoma, vestibular neuritis, labyrinthitis, meningitis
	b) Traumatic	Concussion, perilymphatic fistula, cochlear implant surgery
	c) Degenerative disorders	Menière's disease, BPPV
	d) Ototoxic medications	Gentamicin, cisplatin, diuretics
3. Neurological	a) Migraine and migraine precursors	Basilar migraine, migraine without aura, BPT, BPV, cyclical vomiting, abdominal migraine
	b) Neoplasia (CP angle, posterior fossa, brainstem)	Vestibular schwannoma, neurofibromatosis 2, medulloblastoma, glioma, ependymomas
	c) Other neurological causes	Episodic ataxia, epilepsy
4. Cardiovascular		Long QT syndrome, orthostatic hypotension
5. Metabolic disturbances		Diabetes, electrolyte disturbances
6. Ocular disorders		Refractive errors, strabismus
7. Psychological causes		Anxiety, panic

This knowledge enables the clinical consultation to lead to appropriate other referrals and the differentiation of labyrinthine from neurological vertigo (Table 46.2).

This chapter will first describe the features that a clinician should look for in taking the history and in the general examination of the child with dizziness. A repertoire of relevant investigations will be described, with the likely findings in different pathologies. The different disorders that may cause dizziness in a child will be described and the chapter ends with a description of management strategies for the dizzy child.

Clinical Evaluation

An accurate history, an eyewitness account of episodes, opportunistic observation of play and detailed clinical examination prove invaluable in making a diagnosis. A diary of symptoms may give valuable insight into the frequency, duration, triggers and associated symptoms.

History

In addition to a general systemic review of all systems to identify conditions with vestibular manifestations or those that will compound the presentation or treatment strategy for vestibular pathology, it is essential to take a detailed otological history to raise the suspicion of otitis media, neurofibromatosis or other otological pathology.

The specific history should include information about:
1. Quality of symptoms, such as light-headedness, rotation, fatigue and inattention.
2. Duration of individual attacks: a brief episode suggests benign paroxysmal positional vertigo (BPPV) or

epilepsy; one lasting hours is more suggestive of migraine; days: of vestibular neuritis.

3. Duration of overall complaint.
4. Severity of symptoms over time (reducing with vestibular compensation, fluctuating but not reducing with migraine).
5. Triggers.
6. Associated symptoms.

In children with congenital or severe/profound acquired hearing loss or delayed motor milestones, questions related to absent vestibular function are pertinent: difficulty walking in the dark or on uneven surfaces, difficulty learning to ride a bicycle or skate, general clumsiness, absence of motion sickness and absence of dizziness on fairground rides, all of which point to loss of vestibular input. In a child with absent vestibular function, motor milestones are frequently delayed, with walking age later than 18 months. The possibility of vestibular failure or hypofunction should always be considered in a child who has had meningitis or treatment with cytotoxic drugs.

A history of recurrent acute vertigo or cyclical vomiting should raise the suspicion of migraine and prompt questions about motion sickness, which is common in this condition, abdominal pains, headaches and a family history of migraine. A history of head trauma or, for example, a recent viral infection will raise the suspicion of

labyrinthine concussion or of benign paroxysmal vertigo or vestibular neuritis in a dizzy child.

Triggers for, and symptoms associated with, the dizziness should always be sought: body position (cardiovascular causes), head movement (vestibular dysfunction), motion sickness (migraine), visual stimuli (visuo-vestibular mismatch associated with vestibular dysfunction), stressful environment (psychological element, e.g. bullying), eating certain foods or exercise (migraine), loss of awareness (epilepsy).

General Examination

Observation of gait and play may reveal unsteadiness and clumsiness. Home video recordings are useful both to assess children, who are shy in hospital, and to monitor progress. Examination of the ears is vital in all children with dizziness, but particularly in seriously ill, malnourished or immigrant children who may have undiagnosed chronic middle ear disease with labyrinthine erosion. All children should be examined for dysmorphic features to define syndromes with vestibular involvement (e.g. CHARGE and branchio-oto-renal, BOR, syndrome). A general paediatric and developmental examination should be undertaken to exclude non-vestibular diseases that may give rise to imbalance or dizziness: cardiovascular pathology, endocrine disease, autoimmune pathology.

Table 46.2 Differentiation between peripheral and central vertigo. *ENG* Electronystagmography, *VNG* Videonystagmography, *OKN* optokinetic nystagmus, *VOR* vestibulo-ocular reflex

Signs and symptoms	Peripheral vertigo	Central vertigo
Symptoms	Severe rotatory vertigo, improves over a short time (days)	Gradual, moderate, persistent
Eye movements	Normal, conjugate	Low gain broken pursuit, dysconjugate eye movements, dysmetric or slow saccades
Cranial nerve palsy	Absent	Present
Spontaneous nystagmus	Horizontal, unidirectional	Vertical, gaze-induced, dysconjugate, bidirectional,
Positional nystagmus	Latent period, rotational geotropic, adapts and fatigues, marked nausea, pallor and sweating	Vertical, dysconjugate, bidirectional, ageotropic, persistent, non-fatiguable, often asymptomatic or projectile vomiting
Cerebellar signs	Absent	Present
ENG/VNG recording	VOR suppression normal, normal OKN, pursuit and saccades	Poor VOR suppression/abnormal OKN, deranged pursuit and/or saccades
Caloric testing	Nystagmus enhanced in absence of fixation	No enhancement of nystagmus in absence of fixation

46

Specific neuro-otological examination requires a detailed neurological examination to exclude motor, sensory and cerebellar loss. There should be an assessment of stance and gait, which provides input about the severity of the disability, but little site of lesion information. Oculomotor examination provides diagnostic information about site and side of vestibular dysfunction (Table 46.2).

Eye Movement Examination

This is the key to identification of the site of vestibular pathology and includes examination for overt or latent strabismus, horizontal and vertical eye movements, horizontal and vertical gaze tests, smooth pursuit, saccades and optokinetic nystagmus. A small flashing toy for pursuit and saccadic testing and an optokinetic drum with interesting images, for example cartoon characters or animals, can be used to maintain the child's interest during assessment. Nystagmus due to a peripheral lesion is best seen in the absence of optic fixation, using Frenzel's glasses (10+ diopter lenses that prevent fixation), during fundoscopic examination in the dark or with a videonystagmoscope.

Doll's head eye movements may be used to assess the vestibulo-ocular reflex (VOR) in younger children.

Other signs should be routinely sought to assess vestibular dysfunction:

Dix-Hallpike Positional Test

This test may be the only abnormal clinical sign in a dizzy child and is, therefore, essential (Fig. 46.2). Importantly, it differentiates labyrinthine from central positional nystagmus. In BPPV (most commonly affecting the posterior semicircular canal), severe vertigo associated with horizontal, rotatory, geotropic nystagmus occurs after a short latent period and fatigues on repeated testing. Any positional nystagmus that does not conform to these criteria or is vertical, dysconjugate, rotational in an unexpected direction (e.g. non-geotropic), not preceded by a latent period or is associated with profuse or projectile vomiting must be further investigated with magnetic resonance imaging (MRI) and a neurological opinion to exclude central positional nystagmus, most commonly secondary to a posterior fossa lesion.

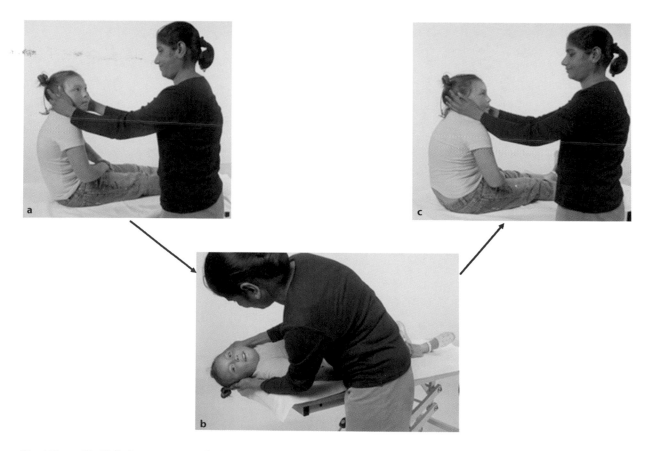

Fig. 46.2a–c The Hallpike manoeuvre. The head is turned to 45° towards the examiner with the child seated on the couch (**a**). The examiner then rapidly reclines the child, with the head hanging over the edge of the couch, and the eyes are observed for nystagmus (**b**). The latency, direction and duration of nystagmus are observed. The child is then brought back to the original position, and the eyes observed for reversal of nystagmus (**c**)

Halmagyi Head Thrust Sign

This test is a simple clinical manoeuvre that enables the detection of total unilateral or bilateral vestibular loss (Fig. 46.3). The child fixes gaze on the nose of the examiner, who holds the child's head between his or her hands and then makes a very rapid (high-acceleration) 30° rotational movement to right or left ("head thrust"), asking the child to keep the gaze fixed on the examiner's nose. When the head is rapidly turned toward the side of absent vestibular function, one or more "catch up" saccades are observed.

Head-Shaking Nystagmus

This test elicits an asymmetry in the vestibular inputs to the VOR and, if such an abnormality exists, generates a nystagmic response. An asymmetry may be due to labyrinthine or more central pathology and thus the test points to vestibular dysfunction, but is not site specific. The head is vigorously rotated right and left with eyes closed for about 30 seconds. Upon stopping, the eyes are opened and (preferably using Frenzel lenses) nystagmus, usually beating away from the side of the lesion, is observed in children with vestibular asymmetry.

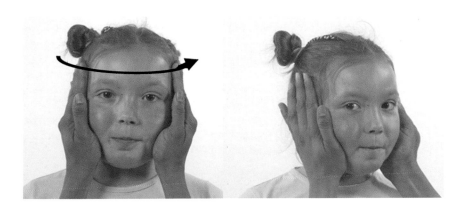

Fig. 46.3a,b The Halmagyi head thrust test. The child is asked to fixate on the examiner's nose (**a**) while the examiner passively moves the child's head rapidly in the yaw plane to one side in the direction of the arrow to the position shown in **b**. The examiner looks for a movement of the eyes during the head thrust and a refixation saccade back to the target. A normal response is that the eyes remain fixed on the target by virtue of the vestibulo-ocular reflex. A positive head thrust is a sign of reduced vestibular function on the side of head movement. The eye travels with the head during the high-velocity movement, and a refixation saccade is necessary to view the target. The test is similarly done in the opposite direction after bringing the head in the centre. Bilateral refixation movements are seen with bilateral vestibular failure (e.g. ototoxicity)

46

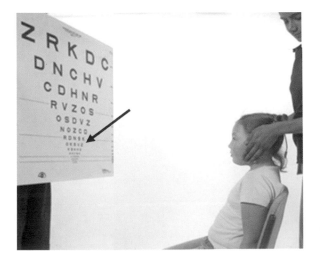
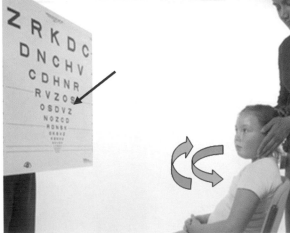

Fig. 46.4a,b The dynamic visual acuity test. The child is asked to read the lowest possible line on a LOGMAR eye chart (**a**) with best corrected vision (i.e. glasses). The manoeuvre is repeated while passively shaking the child's head at approximately 2 Hz in the yaw plane (**b**), and the number of lines of acuity "lost" during the headshake is recorded. A drop of more than two lines is a sign of bilateral vestibular hypofunction. For younger children the "E" chart or a picture chart may be used

Dynamic Visual Acuity

This test assesses the ability of the VOR to maintain gaze on an object during head motion (Fig. 46.4). The child is asked to read a visual acuity chart from a distance of 1.5 m with the head stationary and then repeat the task while moving the head from right to left at approx 2–4 Hz in time with a metronome. The test can also be done by passive movement of the head as shown in Fig. 46.4. A worsening of visual acuity by at least three lines on a visual acuity chart is abnormal and is found in bilateral vestibular loss. Younger children may require a picture chart of familiar objects such as animals decreasing in size down the chart.

Tests for Posture Control and Gait

Various tests are used, including the Romberg test, Unterberger test (marching on the spot with the hands outstreched in front of the body; Fig. 46.5), standing on foam test with and without vision, standing on one leg and tandem gait (Fig. 46.6). The principle is to reduce the visual and proprioceptive contribution to balance, which may bring out instability from an underlying vestibular dysfunction. The limitations include: no published, standardised, age-related, normative data for children, lack of specificity for vestibular dysfunction and lack of studies comparing clinical tests with quantitative vestibular testing. In infants, examination of the Moro reflex and neck-righting reflexes are useful indicators of vestibular function.

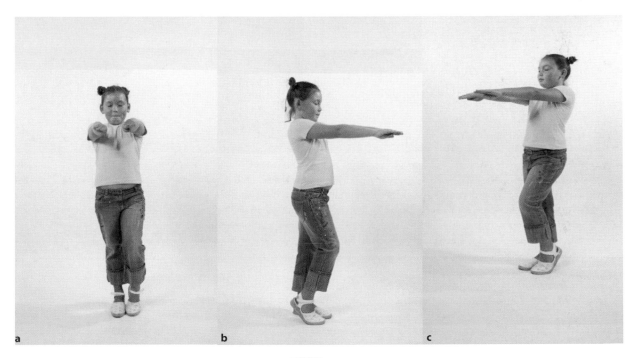

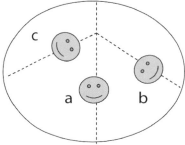

Fig. 46.5a–c The Unterberger test. The child is asked to march on the spot with arms extended and eyes closed, for 1 min (**a**). The degree of rotation and linear movement at the end of the manoeuvre is noted. Some children with uncompensated unilateral vestibular dysfunction deviate toward the affected side (**b**) or move forward/backwards as well as deviate (**c**). Positions **a, b** and **c** are shown diagrammatically as positions **a, b** and **c**, respectively, in the circle below. In **b** the child deviates in the anticlockwise direction, whereas in position **c**, she moves backwards and in the clockwise direction. The *dotted lines* in the circular diagram represent the direction of the face and hands

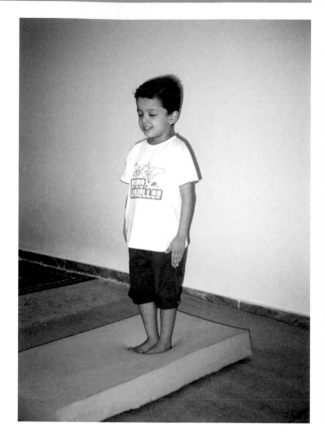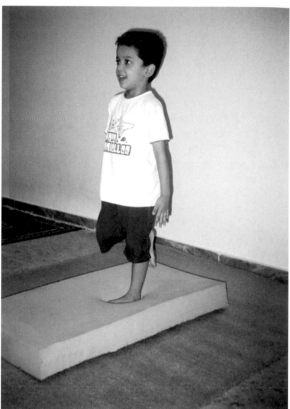

Fig. 46.6 The foam test. The child is asked to stand on a foam mat with both feet together with eyes open (*left*) and then eyes closed. The test is then repeated standing on each leg (*right*). Normal children can stand with both feet steadily, while older children (>8 years) will stand on one leg with no difficulty. Vestibular dysfunction will lead to instability, with a tendency to fall to the affected side. In vestibular failure, children will find it extremely difficult to stay upright, even on both legs, with eye closure

46

Neurological Examination

Examination of the cranial nerves, motor (especially cerebellar function) and sensory systems are essential to exclude neurological disease with vestibular involvement.

Investigations for the Dizzy Child

The vestibular system is anatomically developed and functionally responsive by birth. VOR responses in neonates are poor, but the majority of normal children demonstrate vestibular responses to caloric and rotational stimuli by the age of 2 months. By 10 months, absence of VOR responses may be considered abnormal. Optokinetic nystagmus to a rotating drum is evident from 3 to 6 months of age, and is similar to adults by 3–6 years of age. Smooth pursuit should be similar to adults by the age of 5 years. Speed, appropriate selection of tests and skill in performing test optimally are the key to obtaining valuable data from vestibular tests in children, as they rapidly become bored or tired and do not tend to tolerate repetition of tests.

Eye Movement Recordings

These are used to evaluate the presence of nystagmus with and without optic fixation, smooth pursuit, saccades, optokinetic nystagmus, the VOR and VOR suppression with optic fixation. Measurement of the VOR in children is generally limited to responses from the horizontal semicircular canals, which are stimulated by caloric irrigation or by rotational chair tests. Horizontal and vertical eye movements can be recorded using electro-oculography (EOG) or video-oculography (VOG). Particular difficulties encountered with children are that EOG may be difficult to calibrate for those under 3 years of age, due to inattention and developmental immaturity of the oculomotor system, while young children tend to pull off the goggles required for VOG. Results must be compared with age-matched controls.

Rotational Chair Tests

These are more helpful than caloric testing if the goal is primarily to assess the presence or absence of vestibular function; as small children are able to sit in their mother's lap during the testing, vertigo is less intense than during caloric tests, multiple frequencies of rotational stimuli can be applied and there is no dependence on the thermal energy transfer to the inner ear. However, the disadvantage is that bilateral stimulation makes the detection of mild unilateral lesions impossible without sophisticated analysis software.

Bithermal Caloric Test

These use the maximum slow-phase velocity or duration of nystagmus from each ear to calculate canal paresis and directional preponderance, using the Jongkees formula:

$$\frac{(LC + LW) - (RC + RW)}{(LC + LW + RC + RW)} \times 100 = \% \text{ caloric paresis;}$$

$$\frac{(LC + RW) - (RC + LW)}{(LC + LW + RC + RW),} \times 100 = \% \text{ directional preponderance}$$

where RC, RW, LC and LW indicate the peak slow-component velocity or the duration of nystagmus from right cool, right warm, left cool and left warm irrigations, respectively.

Although normative data differ between laboratories, a rule of the thumb is that a canal paresis of greater than 22–25% indicates unilateral peripheral vestibular loss, and a directional preponderance of greater than 26–30% indicates a significant asymmetry. Each laboratory should, however, obtain their own normative data. Studies of ice-cold caloric responses in infants indicate that nystagmus is well observed by the age of 6 months in full-term and 9 months in preterm infants (Eviatar et al. 1979). However, ice-cold water should not be used as a routine, because of the intense strength of response in normal vestibular function and the discomfort associated with such a cold temperature. If standard caloric testing fails to yield a vestibular response, then irrigation for 1 min with water at 20°C is adequate to confirm the absence of a caloric response.

Posturography

This technique has very limited diagnostic value, but the sensory organisation test of dynamic posturography provides information about the contribution of different sensory inputs involved in balance. This information can be used to design appropriate motor and sensory rehabilitation strategies. Its use is limited to cooperative children 3 years or older. The greatest development of sensory integration occurs between the ages of 4 and 6 years, with the response to altered sensory conditions becoming similar to that exhibited by adults when the child is 7–10 years of age.

Vestibular Evoked Myogenic Potentials

Vestibular evoked myogenic potentials (VEMPs) are reproducible, short-latency alternations in neck-muscle activity (measured in the sternocleidomastoid) induced by intense sound stimuli (80–90 dBnHL) in subjects regardless of their hearing status (Sheykholeslami et al. 2005). The reflex pathway is postulated to originate in the saccule with transmission through the inferior vestibular nerve. VEMPs may be absent in tumours of the eighth nerve, vestibular neuritis and trauma to the eighth nerve. VEMPs can be evoked in very young children and are a useful measure of otolith function, which is otherwise difficult to measure in clinical settings. They may also provide an indication of vestibular function in a child who has visual disturbance impeding measurement of the VOR or in a child who will not cooperate with caloric or rotational testing. Difficulties in recording VEMPs in children may arise in maintaining sternocleidomastoid muscle tension at the desired level, making recording sessions much longer.

Subjective Visual Vertical

The subjective visual vertical (SVV) test requires the child to align a luminous bar to the true vertical in a totally darkened room (i.e. in the absence of any visual clues). The test is a simple way of assessing otolith function and, to a lesser extent, function of the vertical semicircular canals, but is limited in use to older children. SVV is deviated towards the side of the peripheral vestibular lesion, and this improves with time, although it may persist even after compensation.

Other Tests

Audiological tests including pure-tone audiometry, impedance studies, speech audiometry, otoacoustic emissions with and without suppression and auditory brainstem responses are useful in identifying combined auditory and vestibular pathology and in indicating the presence of a retrocochlear lesion, allowing prioritisation of children for imaging.

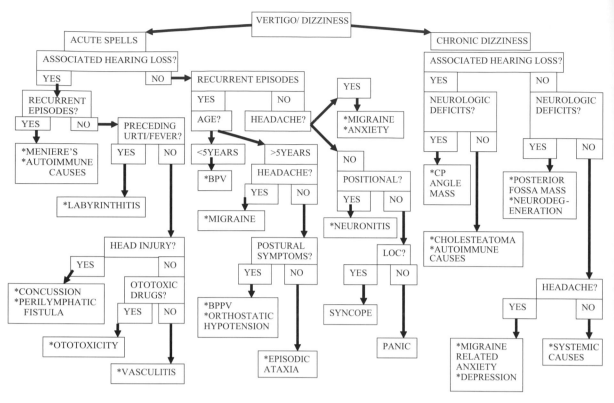

Fig. 46.7 A diagnostic approach to dizziness in children (adapted from Ravid et al. 2003)

Table 46.3 Genetic causes of hearing loss associated with vestibular symptoms. *EVAS* Enlarged vestibular aqueduct syndrome

Cause of deafness	Gene mutation	Clinical features
Syndromic		
Usher syndrome type 1	MYO7A	Vestibular areflexia
Usher syndrome type 3	CDH23	Variable vestibular function
Pendred syndrome	SLC26A4	EVAS, vertigo, 30% bilateral vestibular failure, 30% normal vestibular function
CHARGE syndrome	Gene CDH7	Absent semicircular canals, vestibular dysplasia, vestibular hypofunction
BOR syndrome	EYA1	EVAS, vertigo
Jervell and Lange Nielsen syndrome	KCNQ1	Vestibular hypofunction
Neurofibromatosis 2	NF2	Bilateral vestibular schwannomas, café-au-lait spots, vestibular dysfunction
Non-syndromic		
DFNA9/DFNA11	COCH	Progressive hearing loss, vertigo
DFNB2	MYO7A	Severe to profound loss
DFNB4	SLC 26A4	Severe to profound loss
DFNB12	CDH 23	Severe to profound loss

Other tests depend on clinical manifestations. Imaging with MRI and computed tomography (CT) are useful to rule out intracranial space-occupying lesions, traumatic fractures and congenital anomalies. Electrocardiogram (ECG), electroencephalogram (EEG) and genetic and blood testing may be useful in selected children, depending on clinical indications.

By adopting a structured history, examination and investigation, as outlined above, it is possible to come to a diagnosis in the majority of children presenting with dizziness and/or vertigo or imbalance (Fig. 46.7).

Causes of Vertigo/Dizziness/Imbalance in Children

Congenital Disorders

Both syndromic and non-syndromic causes of hearing loss may also be associated with vestibular symptoms (Table 46.3; see also Chapters 8 and 40).

Syndromic Hearing Loss and Vestibular Dysfunction

Usher's Syndrome

Type l is characterised by profound hearing loss, retinitis pigmentosa and absent vestibular function; some cases of type III may also have vestibular hypofunction. Type II generally has less marked hearing loss and has normal vestibular function. The diagnosis of type 1 has important prognostic and rehabilitative implications because of the dual sensory impairment: loss of vision and congenital profound hearing loss.

Pendred Syndrome

This refers to sensorineural hearing loss (SNHL) with goitre, and is a recessively inherited disorder. It is commonly characterised by the Mondini malformation and enlarged vestibular aqueduct, with vestibular loss in one-third of cases.

Enlarged Vestibular Aqueduct Syndrome

The vestibular aqueduct is a J-shaped bony canal that extends from the medial wall of the vestibule to the posterior surface of the petrous temporal bone. It is normally < 1.5 mm in diameter when measured at the midpoint of the long limb of the "J". When enlarged (Fig. 46.8), it is associated with fluctuating or progressive SNHL and vestibular symptoms. The latter are reported in less than one-third of cases and range from episodic vertigo to incoordination and imbalance (Berrettini et al. 2005), and reduced caloric responses are frequently found. Transmission of intracranial pressure fluctuations into the membranous labyrinth, either across the widened vestibular aqueduct or through abnormal communication between the internal auditory canal and the vestibule, has been thought to result in cochlear damage and stimulation of vestibular sensory receptors. Enlarged vestibular aqueduct syndrome can be an isolated abnormality or can occur as part of Pendred's and BOR syndrome.

Congenital Long-QT Syndrome

Long-QT syndrome (LQT) is an inherited ion channel disease caused by mutations in the genes encoding for the transmembrane sodium or potassium ion channel proteins. It usually manifests in childhood and adolescence, with the clinical presentations range from dizziness to syncope and sudden death. Such individuals are at risk from drugs that affect potassium repolarisation channels and further prolong the QTc, interval allowing ventricular arrhythmias, such as some antihistamines (terfenadine, astemizole, high doses of ebastine, mizolastine, loratadine), ketaconazole and macrolide antibiotics. One type – Jervell-Lange-Nielsen syndrome (autosomal-recessive) – is associated with profound SNHL and vestibular hypofunction. The diagnosis rests on clinical and electrocardiographic features (abnormally long QTc interval) and family history.

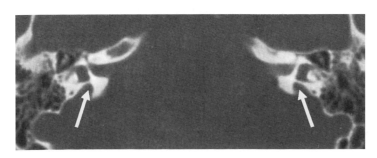

Fig. 46.8 Computed tomography (CT) scan showing enlarged vestibular aqueducts (indicated by *arrows*)

CHARGE Syndrome

This is a condition characterised by an association of defects: coloboma, heart defects, atresia of the choanae, retardation of growth and development, genital and ear anomalies. The characteristic inner ear abnormalities seen in are shown in Fig. 46.9.

Nonsyndromic Hearing Loss and Vestibular Dysfunction

Vestibular abnormalities are commonly associated with isolated genetic deafness of all patterns of inheritance; the documented mutations leading to this combination of findings are shown in Table 46.3.

Mutations in the DFNA9 locus cause an autosomal-dominant progressive SNHL and Menière-like vertigo symptoms with progressive impairment of vestibular function, and are an example of non-syndromic hearing loss with vestibular involvement. The mutations cause a disruption in the function of cochlin protein, an important component of the extracellular matrix of the inner ear (Cremers et al. 2005).

Otological

Inner Ear Infection or Inflammation

Otitis Media with Effusion

The aetiology of the balance disturbance in otitis media with effusion (OME) remains ill defined, but two theories predominate:

1. A change of pressure inside the middle ear influences the flow of inner ear fluids.
2. Toxins in the middle ear fluid leak into the inner ear and affect the vestibular receptors (Waldron et al. 2004).

Although children with OME rarely complain of dizziness or vertigo, they can present with frequent falls, impaired balance, clumsiness and delay in motor develop-

ment. Abnormal findings on electronystagmography and motor proficiency tests have been reported in a significant number (58%) of children with OME as compared to controls (Golz et al. 1998). Similarly, fixed and moving platform posturography and sway magnetometry have shown balance disorders in children with OME. Tympanostomy tubes have been reported to result in significant improvement in balance (Casselbrant et al. 1995; Waldron et al. 2004).

Chronic Suppurative Otitis Media and Cholesteatoma

See also Chapter 43. Cholesteatoma is a skin cyst that behaves like a localised tumour. Both chronic suppurative otitis media and cholesteatoma can be associated with dizziness and vertigo, by causing bone destruction and perilymphatic fistulae, or by causing serous labyrinthitis. There is invasion of bacterial toxins and inflammatory cells into the inner ear as the round window membrane permeability changes due to infection (Mehta and Stakiw 2004). The lateral semicircular canal may be involved in bony destruction by the cholesteatoma.

Vestibular Neuritis

Vestibular neuritis in children, as in adults, is characterised by sudden onset of severe rotatory vertigo, spontaneous horizontal nystagmus without neurological signs and unilateral loss of vestibular function on the affected side, as a result of a viral infection of Scarpa's ganglion. Vertigo is made worse with head movement, but recovery is usually very rapid. In a series of 21 children with vestibular neuronitis (Taborelli et al. 2000), nearly 50% had a preceding upper respiratory infection. Acute symptoms completely subsided within 3 months in 66% and within 2 years in 100% of children. A floating sensation and unsteadiness were present after 1 year in 30% of children. The incidence of unilateral canal paresis reduced from 100% in the 1st week, to 66% after 3 months, 14% after 2 years, and there was complete recovery of vestibular function at 5 years (Taborelli et al. 2000).

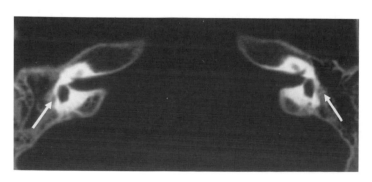

Fig. 46.9 Axial CT showing absent semicircular canals in CHARGE syndrome. The vestibule is slightly enlarged (*arrows*). The top of the basal cochlear turn is seen in this section (Satar et al. 2003)

46

Labyrinthitis

This is an infection or inflammation of the labyrinth. Symptoms are similar to vestibular neuritis, but may additionally include SNHL and tinnitus. Three types are described: serous labyrinthitis, otogenic suppurative labyrinthitis and meningogenic suppurative labyrinthitis.

Serous labyrinthitis represents an irritation of the inner ear without bacterial or viral invasion. As a result of otitis media or surgical opening of the labyrinth, toxins may spread from the middle ear into the inner ear through the round or oval window. Otogenic suppurative labyrinthitis involves bacterial invasion of the inner ear from contiguous areas within the temporal bone. Meningogenic suppurative labyrinthitis occurs when bacteria spread from the subarachnoid space into the inner ear during meningitis. Specific viral illnesses causing labyrinthitis include mumps, measles, influenza and infectious mononucleosis. The hearing loss resolves completely or partially in about 50% of cases (Mehta and Stakiw 2004).

Meningitis

Vestibular loss as result of labyrinthine or eighth nerve pathology occurs more commonly (in 40–80%) than deafness, following bacterial meningitis. This manifests itself clinically as regression in motor milestones in younger children and poor balance in the older ones. MRI scan may indicate labyrinthitis ossificans of the lateral semicircular canal (Fig. 46.10). Long-term follow up into adulthood of these children indicates that vestibular symptoms compensate very well, but residual symptoms of imbalance when walking in the dark may remain (Hugosson et al. 1997).

Traumatic

Head Injury

Of children with closed-head trauma and whiplash injury, 50–60% suffer labyrinthine concussion (Mehta and Stakiw 2004), which may occur with or without temporal bone fractures. Symptoms include dysequilibrium, vertigo and dizziness. Post-traumatic dizziness may be accompanied by headache, insomnia and personality changes (Nečajauskaitė et al. 2005) and vestibular symptoms, which may result from BPPV, post-traumatic migraine, intracranial hypertension and emotional stress. Temporal bone fractures occur in approximately 10% of cases of paediatric blunt-head trauma, with conductive or SNHL and facial nerve paralysis in addition to dizziness. Conductive hearing loss is more common, although SNHL is associated with a poorer prognosis. In the vestibular system, there may be caloric hyporeflexia, spontaneous or positional nystagmus (46%) and central ENG disturbances (43%) immediately after head trauma, but at 2 years follow up, these abnormalities are reduced to 18% and 12%, respectively (Vartianen et al. 1985).

Benign Paroxysmal Positional Vertigo

BPPV in children is believed to be due to a displacement of otoconia, originating from the utricle, and most commonly migrating into the posterior semicircular canal (Marcelli et al. 2006). The condition is rare in children as compared to adults, but similar deposits of otoconia have been detected in the paediatric labyrinth on temporal bone examinations. Very young children may have deposits on the lateral cupula, in keeping with their recumbent posture. Aetiology is most commonly post-traumatic or may follow vestibular neuritis. Characteris-

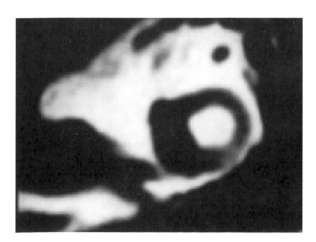 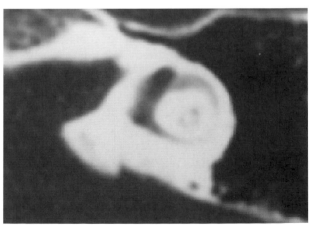

Fig. 46.10 Post-meningitis labyrinthitis ossificans. The figure on the *left* shows a normal lateral semicircular canal, whereas the figure on the *right* shows that the lumen of the lateral semicircular canal is obliterated

tic symptoms of positional vertigo on neck extension are seen, and the diagnosis is confirmed by the typical nystagmus on the Dix-Hallpike test. The symptoms usually subside spontaneously without treatment within 1 year, or may resolve immediately after canalith-repositioning manoeuvres.

Perilymphatic Fistula

This condition results from an abnormal communication between the middle and inner ears, which allows the escape of perilymphatic fluid. Symptoms include sudden, fluctuating or progressive hearing loss, positional vertigo, tinnitus, positional nystagmus and a positive fistula test. Perilymphatic fistula (PLF) may be congenital or acquired and occurs following head trauma, barotrauma, surgical trauma, meningitis, chronic ear infections or may occur spontaneously (Mehta and Stakiw 2004). Congenital PLF is thought to arise from a deformity or weakness of the temporal bone, rendering the ear unusually susceptible to pressure changes. Diagnosis rests on a high index of suspicion, audiometry indicating a conductive or SNHL and findings on the CT scan, but, in some cases, the diagnosis is defined only on exploratory surgery. Conservative treatment, such as maintaining the upright head position and avoiding heavy lifting, can be tried, but if ineffective, surgical sealing of the leak should be attempted.

Cochlear Implant Surgery

Cochlear electrode implantation may alter normal inner ear fluid homeostasis, induce direct trauma to the vestibular sensory structures, cause inflammation and resultant fibrosis or hair cell loss, or may result in electrical stimulation of the vestibular system (Buchman et al. 2004). Dizziness is reported in 3% of children postoperatively and compensation occurs with time. In addition, electrical stimulation may cause vertigo on device activation, but although reported, this is uncommon with more modern electrodes.

Studies have reported a reduction in the caloric response in the implanted ear in up to 40% of cases, with similar findings on rotational testing. One study has also identified a further deterioration in the caloric response at 2 years follow up, and an accompanying reduction in the caloric response of the unimplanted ear to a lesser extent (Buchman et al. 2004), although no clear explanation for this latter finding has been proposed. Posturography findings are variously reported to have improved, worsened or remained the same.

Limited data on pathologic analysis of temporal bones in patients with cochlear implants have indicated the presence of fibrosis and hydrops in the vestibule; this latter finding may explain the cases of children with delayed vertigo. Perilymphatic fistula has anecdotally been reported after cochlear implantation.

Idiopathic

Menière's Disease

Menière's disease is an idiopathic condition of the membranous labyrinth associated with the pathologic finding of endolymphatic hydrops, but the pathophysiology remains poorly understood and genetic, metabolic and autoimmune mechanisms have all been implicated. The condition is rare in childhood but may account for up to 4 % of children with dizziness (Akagi et al. 2001; Niemensivu et al. 2005), while 3–5% of patients with Menière's disease experience the onset of symptoms during childhood. Symptoms in children are similar to those in adults: fluctuating hearing loss, episodic vertigo and tinnitus. More importantly, children with congenital SNHL may develop secondary hydrops, with episodic vertigo and worsening of hearing loss (Huygen and Admiraal 1996).

Ototoxicity

Aminoglycoside antibiotics (gentamicin is particularly vestibulotoxic), loop diuretics (e.g. frusemide), salicylates (i.e. aspirin) and chemotherapeutic agents (e.g. cisplatin) may cause ototoxicity. The risk increases in very young children (<3 years) treated with multiple ototoxic medications, prolonged treatment, prematurity and preexisting kidney and inner ear disorders. With aminoglycosides, prevalence rates of 2–15% have been reported for ototoxicity (Mehta and Stakiw 2004) and may occur with both local and systemic administration. Symptoms include a bilateral high-frequency SNHL, tinnitus and dizziness, although bilateral vestibulopathy may occur, especially with gentamicin. Management is geared towards prevention, with monitoring of drug levels, but vestibular hypofunction responds well to vestibular rehabilitation in children, who compensate rapidly.

Neurological

Migraine and Migraine Precursors

Migraine and its precursors are the commonest causes of dizziness in the paediatric population. The prevalence of migraine in children is about 5%, and its equivalents may be considered as age-dependent expressions of an inherited migrainous disposition. The prevalence is higher in the teenage population (21.7%) with girls being affected three times as commonly as boys in this age group (Split and Neuman 1999). The association of vertigo with migraine has long been recognised in adults, but less so in children. Approximately 38% of teenage girls and 21% of teenage boys with migraine complained of dizziness (Split and Neuman 1999). At present, the International Classification of Headache Disorders (ICHD) does not include a specific category for migrainous vertigo. However, as in adults, vertigo or dizziness may occur in children with a history of migraine.

Migrainous vertigo may occur without headache, but with abdominal pain, and may be the first presentation of migraine in children. It may be rotatory or associated with a constant feeling of unsteadiness. There may be a delay of several years between the onset of migraine and vertigo. The vertigo may have no temporal relation to the headache and its duration may be shorter or longer than the migraine aura. Motion sickness has been reported in 60% of patients with migraine, whereas the incidence in the normal population is only 20% (Kayan and Hood 1984). Vestibular function tests may identify canal paresis as well as abnormalities on rotational chair testing and visual fixation (Choung et al. 2003), but often there may be few definitive abnormalities despite severe symptoms. Table 46.4 lists the types of migraine associated with dizziness.

Basilar Migraine

The age of onset is usually less than 7 years, the majority of sufferers being girls. A family history of migraine is frequent. The key features are vertigo, nausea or vomiting, ataxia, visual field defects, diplopia, tinnitus, weakness (hemiplegia, diplegia, quadriplegia) and loss of consciousness. These early transient features last for up to 1 h and are followed by headache. Unlike other types of migraine, headache may be occipital in origin, with the presence of additional neurological abnormalities. Children may require neuroimaging to rule out a posterior fossa lesion.

The criteria for diagnosis of basilar migraine are clinical and are given in Table 46.5. Vestibular test results vary, but may merely show a directional preponderance on caloric irrigation (Mehta and Stakiw 2004). The differential diagnosis includes episodic ataxia, complex partial seizures, stroke and familial hemiplegic migraine (FHM) with cerebellar signs. Children may develop classic migraine on follow up.

Familial Hemiplegic Migraine

FHM is a dominantly inherited disorder resulting from mutations in the calcium channel gene *CACNA1A*, in which migraine headaches are heralded by an aura of hemiparesis. Patients with FHM may also have additional basilar-type symptoms during the aura, but some degree of hemiparesis is always present. Overlap of clinical fea-

Table 46.4 Migraine types associated with dizziness in children (Lewis and Pearlman 2005)

Migraine without aura
Migraine with aura
■ Typical aura with migraine headache
■ Basilar-type migraine
Childhood periodic syndromes, commonly precursors of migraine
■ Cyclical vomiting
■ Abdominal migraine
■ Benign paroxysmal vertigo of childhood
■ Benign paroxysmal torticollis

Table 46.5 International Classification of Headache Disorders Criteria for Basilar-type Migraine

A	At least two attacks fulfilling criteria B–D
B	Aura consisting of at least two of the following fully reversible symptoms, but no motor weakness: dysarthria, vertigo, tinnitus, diplopia, visual symptoms, ataxia, decreased level of consciousness, decreased hearing, bilateral paraesthesias
C	At least one of the following:
	[i] At least one aura symptom develops gradually over ≥5 min and/or different aura symptoms occur in succession over ≥5 min
	[ii] Each aura symptom lasts ≥5 and up to 60 min
D	Headache fulfilling criteria *for migraine without aura* begins during the aura or follows aura within 60 min
E	Not attributed to another disorder

tures with episodic ataxia and FHM have led to the hypothesis that migraine may be a manifestation of a form of channelopathy.

Benign Paroxysmal Vertigo

This a common, but unrecognised condition that was first described by Basser in 1964 and is characterised by paroxysmal, nonepileptic recurrent episodes of vertigo (Drigo et al. 2001). The age of onset is commonly 2–4 years, and sex distribution is equal. Attacks occur when the child is awake and are sudden in onset. The child appears anxious, pale, fearful and sweaty, grasps for support, may sway and remain immobile. Younger children may cry, while older ones describe a "falling" or "spinning" sensation. Episodes typically last for a few seconds to minutes, but rarely may continue for hours and be associated with nausea, vomiting, unusual head postures and visible spontaneous nystagmus. Frequency varies between several times a day to once every 1–3 months and decreases with increasing age, often abating within 2 years of onset or after the age of 5 years. There is no loss of consciousness and there is complete recovery after the attack. Absence of attacks for 6 months is usually a sign of recovery.

Neurological examination is normal. The EEG between, as well as during, episodes is normal, as are CT scan findings. Caloric tests and audiometry in most studies have been reported as normal (Mira et al. 1984).

The diagnosis of BPV is clinical, and one of exclusion. A recent study indicated raised levels of CPK-MB of muscular origin in children with BPV, and suggested further studies to evaluate this as a diagnostic marker (Rodoo and Hellberg 2005). The differential diagnoses to be considered include epilepsy, posterior fossa or cerebellopontine angle tumours, vestibular neuritis, otologic pathology, Ménière's disease, basilar migraine and BPPV.

BPV is considered as a precursor of migraine. There is a greater incidence of migraine among BPV sufferers than controls (24% vs 10.6%) and there is a greater incidence of BPV among migraine sufferers than controls (8.8% vs 2.6%). There is a family history of migraine in 36% of children affected by BPV, and most children suffer from motion sickness. In a long-term follow-up study of 19 children with BPV, 21% developed migraine, which was more likely to be of basilar type (Lindskog et al. 1999).

The pathogenesis of BPV is not known, but it has been variously considered as a manifestation of peripheral vestibular dysfunction, central vestibular dysfunction or a dysfunction of the vestibulocerebellar pathways. Treatment includes reassurance regarding the benign nature of the condition, anti-emetics and a trial of cyproheptadine 2–4 mg nightly for a brief duration of 4–6 weeks for children with frequent episodes (Lewis and Pearlman 2005).

Benign Paroxysmal Torticollis

This paroxysmal dyskinesia typically begins in infancy (2–8 months) and presents with episodic torticollis to the right or left, with or without associated pallor, vomiting, ataxia, behavioural changes and dystonic features, including truncal or pelvic posturing (Lewis and Pearlman 2005). Episodes last between 4 hours and 4 days, decline as the child gets older, and usually disappear in entirely by mid-childhood. Although not included in the recent ICHD classification, benign paroxysmal torticollis (BPT) is thought to be a variant of basilar migraine. There is often a family history of migraine and, more recently, children with BPT were shown to have muta-

tions in the *CACNA1A* gene (similar mutations are also present in familial hemiplegic migraine and episodic ataxia). This raises questions regarding the varying phenotypic expression of calcium channelopathies at different stages of development. Neurological findings in children are normal. The diagnosis is clinical and some studies have suggested an underlying vestibular disorder such as labyrinthitis or involvement of vestibulocerebellar connections (Drigo et al. 2000). After disappearance of BPT, 27% of children may present with BPV, cyclic vomiting, recurrent abdominal pain or migraine (Drigo et al. 2000). Differential diagnoses include Sandifer syndrome (gastro-oesophageal reflux), idiopathic torsion dystonia, complex partial seizures and congenital or acquired lesions of the craniocervical junction. Management consists of reassurance, but cyproheptadine may be tried for disabling episodes.

Cyclical Vomiting

This may have a migrainous basis and the clinical features include recurrent spells of severe vomiting. The mean age of onset is 5 years; boys and girls are equally affected and most children outgrow their symptoms by the age of 10 years. Attacks occur every 2–4 weeks and last for 24–40 h, typically commencing in the early hours of the morning; there are no interval symptoms. Treatment should focus on maintaining hydration, using anti-emetics and sedation (Lewis and Pearlman 2005). There is a much higher prevalence of migraine in children with cyclical vomiting compared to controls (82% vs 14% controls). Investigations should be directed to rule out neurological and gastrointestinal pathology, but if these are absent, migraine prophylaxis should be advocated.

Abdominal Migraine

Episodes begin at 4–10 years of age and are characterised by crampy, moderate to severe periumbilical abdominal pain, nausea and vomiting with associated pallor. They typically last 1–72 h. Symptoms resolve completely between episodes and frequency of episodes declines within 2 years after onset. Of children with abdominal migraine, 90% have a family history of migraine in a first-degree relative and 70% will develop classical migraine headache later in life (Lewis and Neuman 2005).

Episodic Ataxia Type 2

This is an inherited disorder, with mutations in the *CACNA1A* gene, characterised by spontaneous episodes of ataxia lasting 10 min to several hours or days, usually triggered by stress and exertion and often dramatically relieved by treatment with acetazolamide (Jen et al. 2004). Vertigo, fluctuating generalised weakness, seizures and a history of migraine may be associated. Onset is before the age of 20 years and a positive family history may be obtained, although de novo mutations are known. Children may have ataxia and gaze-evoked or downbeating nystagmus between episodes. Ataxia is mild and slowly progressive over many years. Cerebellar atrophy can be detected in children with long-standing symptoms. It may be worthwhile considering this diagnosis in a child not responding to antimigrainous treatment.

Neoplasia

Infratentorial tumours account for 60–70 % of intrinsic brain tumours in children, who present with gait abnormalities, ataxia, dizziness, cranial nerve palsies, symptoms of increased intracranial pressure, irritability and decline in school performance. Dizziness alone is rarely a presenting feature. Vestibular symptoms are produced due to involvement of the central vestibular pathways in the cerebellum and brainstem. A careful eye movement and cranial nerve examination is often a pointer to the diagnosis. Common intracranial tumours include medulloblastoma, astrocytoma, ependymoma, craniopharyngiomas and metastatic lesions.

Vestibular schwannomas are uncommon in children compared to adults, and often present as large tumours, because symptoms are dismissed or overlooked. Care should be taken to identify rare cases of neurofibromatosis type 2. Symptoms are produced by pressure on the vestibulocochlear nerve and adjoining cerebellum and brainstem. The audiogram may indicate an asymmetric SNHL, and auditory-evoked responses are commonly abnormal. Vestibular tests (eye movement recording and caloric testing), may indicate an ipsilateral peripheral abnormality and/or central vestibular lesion. MRI imaging of the brainstem and posterior fossa is diagnostic.

Cardiovascular Causes

Routine examination should include blood pressure measurement in the supine and upright position as well as an ECG and a referral to a cardiologist if required.

Orthostatic Hypotension

This is defined as a persistent decrease in systolic blood pressure of more than 20 mmHg or a decrease in diastolic blood pressure of more than 10 mmHg within 3 min of assuming the upright position. This can be detected in many otherwise healthy asymptomatic adolescents and may occur with vasovagal syncope. It may occur in ill-

nesses involving primary or secondary autonomic disturbances, such as familial dysautonomia, diabetes and peripheral neuropathies such as Guillian Barré syndrome. Postural tachycardia syndrome may present with orthostatic intolerance. Clinical features include lightheadedness during orthostatic stress and occasionally syncope. Head-up tilt testing helps in a diagnosis and can be performed in children from the age of 6 years. Treatment is largely supportive and palliative, but in some cases mineralocorticoids and vasoactive agents may be useful.

Miscellaneous Causes

Ocular Disorders

Failures in binocular vision or in convergence can be responsible for inadequate gaze stabilisation during movement and blurred vision during fixation, which may generate a sensation of imbalance and dizziness.

Psychological Causes

Vertigo of Psychogenic Origin

In children with unexplained vertigo, dizziness, headache and fainting, a psychiatric diagnosis should be considered, but underlying primary vestibular pathology should always be excluded before this diagnosis is made. Remarkably little work has been conducted on the psychological correlates of vestibular disease in children, although this is a well-recognised association of symptoms in adults, and anecdotally there seems to be a similar presentation in children. In contrast, depression, anxiety, panic attacks and avoidance behaviour, in association with vestibular symptoms, should particularly prompt the careful exclusion of underlying vestibular pathology.

Management of Dizziness

A dizzy child frequently needs input from a multidisciplinary team, including audiovestibular physician, otolaryngologist, paediatrician, neurologist, physiotherapist, audiologist, play therapist and child psychiatrist. Having made a diagnosis, a management plan comprising of several components should be established:

1. Explanation of diagnosis to child and family.
2. Treatment of primary pathology where appropriate.
3. Treatment of acute vestibular symptoms.
4. Treatment of BPPV with particle-repositioning manoeuvres.
5. Correction of any factors that may delay or preclude compensation, such as visual impairment or psychological factors.

6. Vestibular rehabilitation physiotherapy for chronic symptoms of peripheral vestibular disorder.
7. Re-introduction of exercise activity (e.g. school games, swimming, dance classes).
8. Monitor, reassurance and discharge.

Accurate diagnosis is essential to treat the pathology underlying a vestibular disorder.

Treatment of Paediatric Migraine

Avoiding alterations of sleep patterns and meal times, dietary avoidance of chocolates, caffeine, citrus fruits and dairy products, with stepwise re-introduction may be useful. Ibuprofen and acetaminophen are effective in the acute treatment of headaches in younger children, while sumatriptan nasal spray is effective for adolescents (>12 years of age). For preventive therapy, flunarizine is probably effective, but is not universally available. Although other medications are widely used (propranolol, pizotifen, amitryptiline and valproate), there is insufficient data to recommend them for the preventive therapy of migraine (Lewis and Neuman 2004), but on an empirical basis in children who are suffering frequent symptoms, a therapeutic trial may be of value.

Vestibular Management

Acute vestibular symptoms may require vestibular sedatives and anti-emetics, together with strong reassurance of the benign nature of the condition in cases of peripheral pathology. However, in these cases, vestibular sedatives and anti-emetics should be discontinued as soon as possible, as they impair vestibular compensation. Generic treatment of peripheral vestibular abnormalities by a specialist vestibular rehabilitation physiotherapist should then be started. Thought should be given to the need for any specific psychological treatment, and any other disorder that may impact on compensation should be treated, if possible.

Vestibular rehabilitation therapy (VRT) consists of a series of physical exercises that include eye, head and body movements performed with the objective of accelerating compensation mechanisms. VRT is a safe and efficacious therapeutic option in children with peripheral vestibular disturbances and should be combined with everyday physical activities and sport. Children with bilateral vestibular loss are better trained to use substitutive sensory and motor strategies and are counselled to avoid situations in which both the visual and proprioceptive systems are rendered unreliable (e.g. such as swimming in the dark or underwater). Deficits in vision are corrected and sensory input is optimised to enhance compensation.

Central vestibular pathology is particularly difficult to treat. There is now some evidence to suggest that central vestibular disorders may also benefit from VRT, but vestibular sedative drugs and anti-emetics may be essential (e.g. cinnarizine, flunarizine, prochlorperazine, metoclopramide). Other drugs that have been found of empirical value include clonazepam, carbamazepine, sodium valproate and domperidone.

Summary for the Clinician

● Balance disorders in childhood are less common than in adults and until recently have often been overlooked in the paediatric age group. Frequently, it may be felt that vestibular investigations are not helpful in diagnosis in this age group, with the result that no diagnosis has been established and no treatment has been instituted. However, such disorders may manifest with disabling and frightening symptoms for both the child and family. A rational structured approach to assessment will commonly allow a diagnosis to be established and appropriate management to be started, with good outcomes.

References

1. Akagi H, Yuen K, Maeda Y, et al (2001) Meniere's disease in childhood. Int J Pediatr Otorhinolaryngol 61:259–264
2. Basser LS (1964) Benign paroxysmal vertigo of childhood (a variety of vestibular neuronitis). Brain 87:141–152
3. Berrettini S, Forli F, Bogazzi F, et al (2005) Large vestibular aqueduct syndrome: audiological, radiological, clinical and genetic features. Am J Otolaryngol 26:363–371
4. Buchman C, Joy J, Hodges A, et al (2004) Vestibular effects of cochlear implantation. Laryngoscope 114:1–22
5. Casselbrant M, Furman J, Rubenstein E, et al (1995) The effect of otitis media on the vestibular system in children. Ann Otol Rhinol Laryngol 104:620–624
6. Choung Y, Park K, Moon S, et al (2003) Various causes and clinical characteristics in vertigo in children with normal eardrums. Int J Pediatr Otorhinolaryngol 67:889–894
7. Cremers C, Kemperman M, Bom S, et al (2005) From gene to disease: a progressive cochlear–vestibular dysfunction with onset in middle age (DFNA9). Ned Tijdschr Geneeskd 149:2619–2621
8. Drigo P, Carli G, Laverda A (2000) Benign paroxysmal torticollis of infancy. Brain Dev 22:169–172
9. Drigo P, Carli G, Laverda A (2001) Benign paroxysmal vertigo of childhood. Brain Dev 23:38–41

46

10. Eviatar L, Miranda S, Eviatar A, et al (1979) Development of nystagmus in response to vestibular stimulation in infants. Ann Neurol 5:508–514

11. Golz A, Netzer A, Angel-Yeger B, et al (1998) Effects of middle ear effusion on the vestibular system in children. Otolaryngol Head Neck Surg 119:695–699

12. Hugosson S, Carlsson E, Borg E, et al (1997) Audiovestibular and neuropsychological outcome of adults who had recovered from childhood bacterial meningitis. Int J Pediatr Otorhinolaryngol 42:149–167

13. Huygen P, Admiraal R (1996) Audiovestibular sequelae of congenital cytomegalovirus infection in 3 children presumably representing 3 symptomatically different types of delayed endolymphatic hydrops. Int J Pediatr Otorhinolaryngol 35:143–154

14. Jen J, Kim G, Baloh R (2004) Clinical spectrum of episodic ataxia type 2. Neurology 62:17–22

15. Kayan A, Hood JD (1984) Neuro-otological manifestations of migraine. Brain 107:1123–47

16. Lewis D, Pearlman E (2005) The migraine variants. Pediatr Ann 34:486–497

17. Lindskog U, Odkvist L, Noaksson L, et al (1999) Benign paroxysmal vertigo in childhood: a long-term follow-up. Headache 39:33–37

18. Marcelli V, Piazza F, Pisani F, et al (2006) Neuro-otological features of benign paroxysmal vertigo and benign paroxysmal positioning vertigo in children: a follow-up study. Brain Dev 28:80–84

19. Mehta Z, Stakiw D (2004) Childhood vestibular disorders. Comm Disorders Qtr 26:5–16

20. Mira E, Piacentino G, Lanzi G, et al (1984) Benign paroxysmal vertigo in childhood. Diagnostic significance of vestibular examination and headache provocation tests. Acta Otolaryngol Suppl 406:271–274

21. Nečajauskaitė O, Endzinienė M, Jurėienienė K (2005) Prevalence, clinical features and accompanying signs of post traumatic headache in children. Medicina (Kaunas) 41:100–108

22. Niemensivu R, Pyykko I, Kentala E (2005) Vertigo and imbalance in children: a retrospective study in a Helsinki University Otorhinolaryngology Clinic. Arch Otolaryngol Head Neck Surg 131:996–1000

23. Niemensivu R, Pyykko I, Weiner-Vacher S, et al (2006) Vertigo and balance problems in children – an epidemiologic study in Finland. Int J Pediatr Otorhinolaryngol 70:259–265

24. Ravid S, Bienkowski R, Eviatar L (2003) A simplified diagnostic approach to dizziness in children. Pediatr Neurol 29:317–320

25. Rodoo P, Hellberg D (2005) Creatine kinase MB (CK-MB) in benign paroxysmal vertigo of childhood: a new diagnostic marker. J Pediatr 146:548–551

26. Satar B, Yetiser S, Ozkaptan Y (2003) Congenital aplasia of the semicircular canals. Otol Neurotol 24:437–446

27. Sheykholeslami K, Megerian C, Arnold J, et al (2005) Vestibular-evoked myogenic potentials in infancy and early childhood. Laryngoscope 115:1440–1444

28. Split W, Neuman W (1999) Epidemiology of migraine among students from randomly selected schools in Lodz. Headache 39:494–501

29. Taborelli G, Melagrana A, D'Agostino R, et al (2000) Vestibular neuronitis in children: study of medium and long term follow-up. Int J Pediatr Otorhinolaryngol 54:117–121

30. Vartiainen E, Karjalainen S, Karja J (1985) Vestibular disorders following head injury in children. Int J Pediatr Otorhinolaryngol 9:135–141

31. Waldron M, Matthews J, Johnson I (2004) The effect of otitis media with effusions on balance in children. Clin Otolaryngol Allied Sci 29:318–320

Chapter 47

The Facial Nerve

47

Chris Rittey

Core Messages

- Disorders of the facial nerve present to the otolaryngologist as well as to the neurologist.
- This chapter explains the relevant anatomy and outlines conditions that may result in nerve malfunction.

Contents

Anatomy

The facial nerve contains a variety of different types of fibres including somatic sensory fibres, which carry sensation from the skin of the outer ear and its immediate vicinity, visceral sensory fibres, which carry taste from the anterior two-thirds of the tongue and from the palate, visceral motor fibres, which supply secretomotor function in the submandibular and sub-lingual salivary glands, and branchial motor fibres, which innervate the muscles of facial expression and the stapedius (Fig. 47.1). These latter fibres comprise the vast majority of the facial nerve fibres.

The cutaneous sensation from the ear is provided by the Vth, IXth and Xth nerves and the fibres from all are carried with the vagus nerve. These fibres all enter the spinal trigeminal tract and then behave like trigeminal afferents.

The taste fibres from the anterior two-thirds of the tongue are conveyed in the chorda tympani and taste fibres from the palate in the nerve of the pterygoid canal. These sensory fibres are contained in a separate trunk, the nervus intermedius. This nerve trunk runs with the VIIIth nerve rather than the VIIth nerve through the subarachnoid space. It also contains the preganglionic parasympathetic fibres to the submandibular and sublingual salivary glands.

The visceral sensory fibres from the VIIth, IXth and Xth nerves all enter the solitary tract and terminate in the solitary nucleus. This extends from the rostral medulla to the caudal medulla and caudal pons.

The motor fibres that innervate the muscles of facial expression and the stapedius arise from the facial motor nucleus, which lies in the ventrolateral part of the caudal pons at about the same level as the VIth nerve nucleus. The fibres then project in a dorsomedial direction to wrap around the VIth nerve nucleus (the internal genu of the facial nerve) before turning back to leave the brainstem ventrolaterally.

The motor fibres of the facial nerve supply the frontalis muscle, all the muscles of facial expression including platysma and the stapedius muscle. The stapedius is responsible (with the tensor tympani) for damping down movement of the tympanic membrane and stapes which occurs in response to loud noises. Thus complete facial nerve paresis will lead to a failure of this process and hence hyperacusis.

Upper Motor Neurone Input

The facial motor nucleus is supplied by pyramidal upper motor neurones arising in the precentral gyrus and nearby areas of the frontal cortex. These upper motor neurones project bilaterally to the upper part of the face (presumably because of the requirement for bilateral motor activity in these areas such as blinking both eyes and wrinkling both sides of the forehead). However, the upper motor neurones to facial muscles below the eyes are predominantly crossed. The lower motor neurones of the facial nerve nucleus project to ipsilateral muscles. Thus, damage to the upper motor neurones will lead to contra-

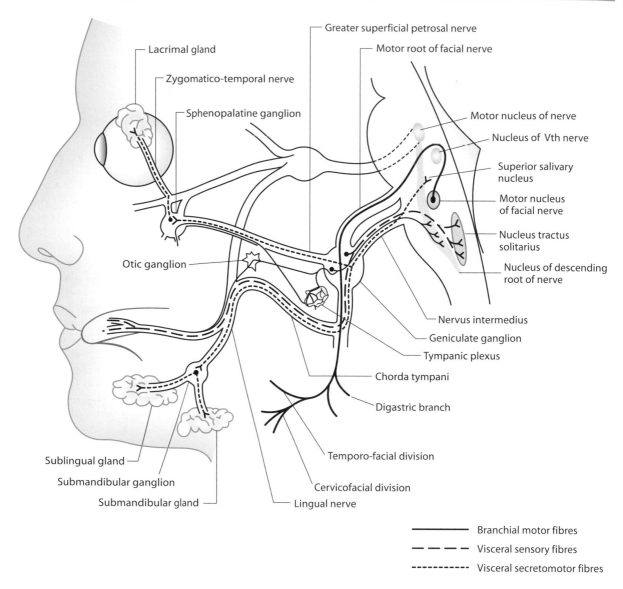

Fig. 47.1 Course of the facial nerve

47

lateral weakness of the lower part of the face, while damage to the lower motor neurones will lead to weakness of the ipsilateral facial muscles.

Clinical Assessment

As with all neurological assessment in children, the clinical examination must be tailored to the child. Thus, assessment of the older child will be similar to that of an adult, while assessment of the baby or infant will largely depend on observation of spontaneous facial movement and behaviour. It is often difficult to assess formally the function of the frontalis muscle (the muscle that results

in wrinkling of the forehead) in young children, and close observation of the child while playing and laughing is important. If the child becomes upset, then close observation of the facial expression during crying can be very helpful.

Formal assessment should include assessment of:

1. Ability to wrinkle the forehead.
2. Ability to forcibly close the eyes. In a lower motor neurone lesion, the eye closure is usually incomplete and the eye can be seen rolling up as the attempt is made (Bell's phenomenon). In an upper motor lesion, the weakness of eye closure is usually only evident as an inability to bury the eyelashes. It should be noted that ptosis is not a feature of facial palsy.

3. Ability to smile, show the teeth and blow out the cheeks.
4. Taste sensation.
5. Blink response – if this is impaired it is important to assess whether corneal sensation is intact. If corneal sensation is impaired, then the patient clearly has involvement of more than just the VIIth nerve.

In theory, impaired taste sensation should be helpful in localising a lesion within the facial nerve as the chorda tympani joins the facial nerve in the middle ear. However, this is often not the case, as taste fibres are frequently spared even when the lesion lies proximal to the middle ear. However, if there is impaired taste then the lesion must lie proximal to or within the petrous bone.

Examination of the facial nerve must be accompanied by a detailed assessment of the remainder of the cranial nerves as well as a good general neurological examination and a thorough general clinical examination (including examination of the ears, nose and throat). Clearly, the differential diagnosis of an isolated facial palsy is very different from that of a facial palsy accompanied by other neurological dysfunction.

Isolated Facial Weakness

Bell's Palsy

Bell's palsy is an acute unilateral weakness or paralysis of the face caused by facial nerve dysfunction for which no identifiable cause can be found. It is the commonest cause of unilateral facial weakness, accounting for up to 80% of all cases of lower motor neurone facial palsy (Bleicher et al. 1996). In the paediatric population, the annual incidence is approximately 3:100,000 in the first decade and approximately 10:100,000 in the second decade. It occurs equally in boys and girls and shows no particular racial predilection. It affects the left and right sides of the face approximately equally.

The cause of Bell's palsy is unclear. Various mechanisms including direct viral infection, post-infectious allergic or immune-mediated inflammatory neuritis, ischaemia and hereditary factors have been suggested. Pathological studies performed in nerves within a week of the diagnosis have shown inflammation, myelin breakdown, axonal damage and oedema. The oedema causes compression of the nerve within the facial canal and this may lead to further damage to the nerve, with axonal loss. Where there has been axonal loss as well as demyelination, then prognosis for complete recovery is poor.

The diagnosis is made when there is acute onset of complete unilateral facial weakness causing difficulty in closing the eye, slurring of speech and difficulties with eating and drinking. There is often a history of aching or pain in and around the ipsilateral ear for 24–48 h before the onset of the facial weakness. Involvement of taste, lacrimation and salivation is often seen and hyperacusis may also occur. Thorough neurological examination may reveal minimal involvement of adjacent cranial nerves, although significant involvement of other cranial nerves should raise doubts about the diagnosis. No abnormality is found on examination of the ear or the parotid gland.

In cases with isolated facial palsy, further investigation is unnecessary. However, the presence of other neurological signs or systemic abnormalities such as fever and otorrhoea, mandate further investigation including magnetic resonance imaging (MRI) and lumbar puncture (Alaani et al. 2005). In Bell's palsy, MRI may show enhancement of the facial nerve, and cerebrospinal fluid may show a mild elevation of protein with some pleocytosis.

The prognosis for recovery in Bell's palsy is excellent. More than 95% of children will experience complete recovery, although the facial muscles may remain weak for a few weeks to months. Occasionally, the process of recovery leads to aberrant innervation of the lacrimal glands by axons destined for the salivary glands and this may result in patients having excessive lacrimation before and during eating (so-called "crocodile tears"). Some information about prognosis may be obtained from neurophysiological studies, although these are not routinely used.

The most important component of treatment is protection of the cornea, which is at risk of drying due to incomplete eye closure and impaired blink reflex. This means the use of artificial tears during the day and artificial eye closure at night. There is no benefit from approaches such as electrical stimulation, massage or facial exercises. There is no clear evidence that steroids are of benefit in altering the prognosis of Bell's palsy and I do not recommend their use. One study has suggested that acyclovir with prednisone may be more effective than prednisone alone (Adour et al. 1996), but further studies are required before acyclovir can be recommended for children with Bell's palsy. Surgical decompression of the facial nerve has not been shown to have consistent benefit.

Rare Causes of Isolated Unilateral Facial Palsy

Acute facial palsies rarely present as a consequence of identifiable inflammatory conditions. Facial palsy is one of the commonest neurological features of Lyme disease (borreliosis). In this condition, the attacks of facial palsy may be recurrent and bilateral. In a review from Poland, 4 of 24 children with borreliosis presented with facial palsy. In all cases the facial palsy was initially unilateral, but within a few weeks the paresis appeared on the opposite side (Mlodzikowska-Albrecht et al. 1995).

Facial palsy has also been rarely reported in Kawasaki disease (Biezeveld et al. 2002) and as a complication of dental disorders (Friedman 1996). Isolated facial palsy has been reported with posterior fossa arachnoid cysts

(Pirotte et al. 2005), and as a rare complication of treatment with sumatriptan for migraine (Rothner et al. 2000). Rarely, muscle disorders may present with facial weakness, which simulates the pattern of facial nerve damage (Kazakov 1994).

Recurrent facial palsy also occurs in the Melkersson-Rosenthal syndrome. This condition is characterised by facial palsy, facial oedema and a furrowed tongue. The facial oedema is usually perioral, although periorbital oedema is also reported. The oedema and facial palsy may occur in isolation or simultaneously. With repeated attacks, there is often incomplete recovery of the facial palsy eventually leading to severe impairment in some cases. The cause of this syndrome is unknown, although biopsy sampling shows a non-caseating granulomatous abnormality. In many cases the complete triad of features is not present and the condition should be considered in patients with recurrent facial palsy (Greene and Rogers 1989).

Recurrent facial palsy is also associated with diabetes, hypertension and familial Bell's palsy (Hageman et al. 1990)

Congenital Facial Palsy

Congenital facial palsy should be distinguished from hypoplasia or paralysis of the depressor anguli oris muscle, in which the corner of the mouth fails to move downward on crying (Nelson and Eng 1972).

Congenital facial palsy may occur as a consequence of birth trauma or prenatal compression. It is seen in approximately 2.1 per 1000 live births (Falcon and Ericson 1990) and probably occurs as a result of pressure on the nerve distal to its emergence from the stylomastoid foramen against the sacral prominence of the mother's pelvis. It is rare for congenital facial palsy to occur as a result of birth trauma (Laing et al. 1996).

Congenital facial palsy is seen in several associated syndromes including Möebius syndrome, Poland syndrome and Goldenhar's syndrome (see also Chapter 8). Facial palsy is also seen in children with abnormalities of the external ear or mastoid. The pathology in these syndromes is different from that seen in isolated congenital facial palsy where abnormalities in the facial motor nucleus (Jemec et al. 2000) and agenesis of the facial nerve itself (Jervis and Bull 2001) have been described. Congenital tuberculosis presenting with congenital facial palsy and otorrhoea has also been described (Pejham et al. 2002). Familial congenital facial palsy has recently been described with abnormal neuroimaging (Kondev et al. 2004).

Facial weakness may be prominent in some infants with congenital muscle disorders, such as nemaline myopathy, congenital myotonic dystrophy or congenital or neonatal myasthenia. In most cases of congenital facial palsy, the cause remains obscure.

Facial Palsy as Part of Other Cranial Nerve Palsies

Facial weakness may co-exist with other neurological signs including other cranial nerve palsies. In this case, the differential diagnosis is much wider and includes inflammatory conditions, neoplasia, trauma, cerebral malformations, endocrine disorders and vascular abnormalities.

Inflammatory conditions such as Lyme disease, sarcoidosis, brucellosis, Sjögren syndrome and Miller Fisher syndrome may all present with facial palsy as part of a more diffuse neurological dysfunction. Local infection due to acute otitis media or mastoiditis may cause facial palsy, particularly if the bony canal containing the horizontal segment of the facial nerve is dehiscent, or if there is extension of infection into the petrous temporal bone. Basal meningitis, especially due to tuberculosis, may also lead to involvement of lower cranial nerves including the facial nerve. Brainstem abscesses most commonly occur in the pons, and involvement of the VIth and VIIth nerves is common (Suzer et al. 1996).

Ramsay Hunt Syndrome

In this condition, the herpes zoster virus causes damage to the facial nerve. This results in a very characteristic clinical picture. There is severe pain in the ear, which is followed by eruption of vesicles in or around the external auditory meatus. There may be extensive oedema, redness and tenderness of the ear; facial weakness develops 24–72 h thereafter. Other cranial nerves may be involved, particularly the Vth, VIIIth or IXth nerves, leading to sensory loss over the face or palate or sensorineural deafness. Although most patients recover, the rate of recovery is slightly less than that from Bell's palsy.

Trauma leading to fracture of the petrous bone may cause damage to the facial nerve. Compression of the nerve due to lesions of the cerebellopontine angle commonly leads to facial palsy. Careful assessment will reveal the presence of co-existent palsies of adjacent cranial nerves. Lesions such as cholesteatoma, meningioma, lymphoma as well as neuromas on the Vth, VIIth or IXth nerves can all present with a similar clinical picture. Neuroepithelial cysts may present in the posterior fossa, especially in the cerebellopontine angle. These lesions occur relatively commonly in childhood (Shuangshoti and Shuangshoti 1998). Acoustic neuroma rarely presents in childhood – facial palsy in this condition tends to be a late feature.

Pontine glioma is a rare tumour of the brainstem and usually occurs in young boys. The glioma expands the pons and produces a series of projecting exophytic lesions, which may project into the cerebellopontine angle and give the clinical picture of an extrinsic tumour in that area.

Some children with systemic malignancy may present with neurological features including facial nerve palsy. Of these, leukaemia and neuroblastoma are the commonest childhood systemic malignancies that present with neurological features. Intraparotid facial plexiform neurofibroma is extremely rare and has been described in childhood (Souaid et al. 2003).

Other compressive lesions that may lead to facial palsy include bone dysplasias such as osteopetrosis or osteopathia striata with cranial sclerosis (Kornreich et al. 1988).

Hemifacial Spasms

Hemifacial spasm consists of continual twitching movements, which are usually maximal around the mouth and eye. It is thought to be due to minor anatomical variation in the blood vessels running along the nerve. It is extremely rare in childhood, but in those patients affected the cause seems to be the same as in adults. Surgical microvascular decompression in childhood appears to have a similar outcome to that in adults (Chang et al. 2001). Hemifacial spasms in infancy are much more likely to be associated with serious intracranial pathology such as brainstem and cerebellar tumours or venous sinus thrombosis (Flüeler et al. 1990).

Other movement disorders may affect the face but are not the consequence of facial nerve pathology. These include common disorders such as tics and rare disorders such as familial dyskinesia and facial myokymia, which is characterised by limb movements that appear choreiform and perioral and periorbital myokymia (Fernandez et al. 2001).

Summary for the Clinician

- Facial nerve disorders in children are often complex and require careful assessment to ensure that there is no other underlying disease. It is important to remember that facial nerve palsy may form part of a more serious condition and appropriate steps should be taken to ascertain whether that is the case. The need for surgical treatment of traumatic facial weakness is rare, but may need to be done.

References

1. Adour KK, Ruboyianes IM, von Doersten PG, et al (1996) Bells palsy treatment with acyclovir and prednisone compared with prednisone alone; a double blind, randomized, controlled trial. Ann Otol Rhinol Laryngol 105:371–378

2. Alaani A, Hogg R, Saravanappa N, et al (2005) An analysis of diagnostic delay in unilateral facial paralysis. J Laryngol Otol 119:184–188

3. Biezeveld MH, Voorbrood S, Clur SB, et al (2002) Facial nerve palsy in a thirteen-year-old male youth with Kawasaki disease. Pediatr Infect Dis J 21:442–443

4. Bleicher JN, Hamiel BS, Gengler JS (1996) A survey of facial paralysis: etiology and incidence. Ear Nose Throat J 75:355–358

5. Chang JW, Chang JH, Park YG, et al (2001) Microvascular decompression of the facial nerve for hemifacial spasm in youth. Childs Nerv Syst 17:309–312

6. Falcon A, Ericson E (1990) Facial nerve palsy in the newborn: incidence and outcome. Plast Reconstr Surg 85:1–4

7. Fernandez M, Raskind W, Wolff J, et al (2001) Familial dyskinesia and facial myokymia (FDFM): a novel movement disorder. Ann Neurol 49:486–492

8. Flüeler U, Taylor D, Hing S, et al (1990) Hemifacial spasm in infancy. Arch Ophthalmol 108:812–815

9. Friedman G (1996) Facial nerve paralysis of dental origin in children. Pediatr Neurol 14:342–344

10. Greene RM, Rogers RS III (1989) Melkersson-Rosenthal syndrome: a review of 36 patients. J Am Acad Dermatol 21:1263–1270

11. Hageman G, Ippel PF, Jansen ENH, et al (1990) Familial, alternating Bells palsy with dominant inheritance. Eur Neurol 30:310–313

12. Jemec B, Grobbelaar AO, Harrison DH (2000) The abnormal nucleus as a cause of congenital facial palsy. Arch Dis Child 83:256–258

13. Jervis PN, Bull PD (2001) Congenital facial nerve agenesis. J Laryngol Otol 11:53–54

14. Kazakov VM (1994) Affection of mimic muscles, simulating damage of the facial nerve in patients with facioscapulohumeral muscular dystrophy. Eur Arch Otorhinolaryngol S96–101

15. Kondev L, Bhadelia RA, Douglass LM (2004) Familial congenital facial palsy. Pediatr Neurol 30:367–370

16. Kornreich L, Grunebaum M, Ziv N, et al (1988) Osteopathia striata, cranial sclerosis with cleft palate and facial nerve palsy. Eur J Pediatr 147:101–103

17. Laing JHE, Harrison DH, Jones BM, et al (1996) Is permanent congenital facial palsy caused by birth trauma? Arch Dis Child 74:56–58

18. Mlodzikowska-Albrecht J, Zarowski M, Steinborn B, et al (1995) Bilateral facial nerve palsy in the course of neuroborreliosis in children – dynamics, laboratory tests and treatment. Rocz Akad Med Bialymst 50:64–69

19. Nelson KB, Eng CD (1972) Congenital hypoplasia of the depressor anguli oris muscle: differentiation from congenital facial palsy. J Pediatr 81:16–20

20. Pejham S, Altman R, Li KI, et al (2002) Congenital tuberculosis with facial nerve palsy. Paediatr Infect Dis J 21:1085–1086

21. Pirotte B, Morelli D, Alessi G, et al (2005) Facial nerve palsy in posterior fossa arachnoid cysts: report of two cases. Childs Nerv Syst 21:587–590

22. Rothner AD, Winner P, Nett R, et al (2000) One-year toler-
    ability and efficacy of sumatriptan nasal spray in adoles-
    cents with migraine: results of a multicenter, open-label
    study. Clin Ther 22:1533–1546
23. Shuangshoti S, Shuangshoti S (1998) Neuroepithelial cyst
    of the cerebellopontine angle: a case report with a review of
    the literature. Neuropathology 18:328–335
24. Souaid JP, Nguyen VH, Zeitouni AG, et al (2003) Intra-
    parotid facial nerve solitary plexiform neurofibroma: a
    first paediatric case report. Int J Pediatr Otorhinolaryngol
    67:1113–1115
25. Suzer T, Coskun E, Cirak B, et al (2005) Brain stem ab-
    scesses in childhood. Childs Nerv Syst 21:27–31

47

Appendix

Robert J. Ruben

Developmental Data

Some of these data are replicated in individual chapters, but set out here as well.

Airway

Table 1 Siberry and Iannone (2005), The Harriet Lane Handbook. *ET* Endotracheal tube, *ID* internal diameter

Age	Premature	Newborn	Infant	1 year	3 year	6 year	10 year	Adolescent	Adult
Weight (kg)	1.5	3	5	10	15	20	30	50	70
ET size[a]	2.5–3.0 uncuffed	3.0–3.5 uncuffed	3.5–4.0 uncuffed	4.0–4.5 uncuffed	4.5–5.0 uncuffed	5.0–5.5 uncuffed	6.0–6.5 cuffed	>6.5 cuffed	>6.5 cuffed

[a]ET size (mm) = 116 + age (years)/4; approximate distance of insertion = ID × 3

Table 2 Casselbrant and Alper (2003). Storz bronchoscope sizes. *OD* outside diameter

Age	Premature	Premature–newborn	Newborn–6 months	6 months–1 year	1–2 years	3–4 years	5–7 years	Adult
Size	2.5	3.0	3.5	3.7	4.0	5.0	6.0	6.5
Length	20	20, 26	20, 26, 30	26, 30	36, 30	30	30, 40	43
ID (mm)	3.5	4.3	5.0	5.7	6.0	7.1	7.5	8.5
OD (mm)	4.2	5.0	5.7	6.4	6.7	7.8	8.2	9.2

Table 3 Wetmore 2003. Approximate size of tracheostomy tubes

Age	Premature <1000 g	Premature 1000–2500 g	Neonate–6 months	6 months–1 year	1–2 years	>2 years
ID (mm)	2.5	3.0	3.0–3.5	3.5–4.0	4.0–5.0	$\dfrac{\text{Age in years} + 16}{4}$

Sinuses

Table 4 Ónodi (1911). Development sinuses. All dimension are in mm. *h* Height, *l* length, *w* width, *DOS* diameter of sphenoid ostium I, *ND* no data

Age	0–1 year	1–2 years	3 years	3.5 years	6 years	7.5 years
Frontal	h 3.5–8	h 4.5–9	h 14–18	h 6.5	h 17–18	h 14–17
	l 3–9	l 4–5.5	l 11–16	l 6	l 10–13	l 4–11
	w 2–6	w 3–4	w 5–6	w 5	w 11–12	w 7–9
Maxillary antrum	h 3–9	h 8–9	h 13	h 13	h ND	h 23
	l 5–19	l 10–12	l 22	l 26	l ND	l 38
	w 2.5–8	w 3–7	w 13	w 20	w ND	w 20
Ethmoid anterior	h 1–8	h 4–10	h 6–7	h 3.5–11	h 8–10	h 8–13
	l 1–9	l 2.5–4.5	l 6–7	l 3–8	l 8–10	l 5–6
	w 1–6	w 1.5–4	w 3–4	w 3–6	w 6–7	w 7
Ethmoid posterior	h 2–8	h 5	h 6–7	h 3.5–10	h ND	h 10
	l 2–6	l 4	l 6–7	l 3.5–11	l ND	l 11–17
	w 1.5–8	w 3	w 3–4	w 3–11	w ND	w 6–9
Sphenoid	h 1–6	h 2–6	h 6	h 4.5–6	h 10	h 8–12
	l 1–5	l 3–5	l 6	l 3.5–5	l 6–7	l 12–13
	w 1–6	w 2–7	w 9	w 7	w 12	w 11
	DOS 0.5–2	DOS 1–1.5	DOS 2	DOS 1.5	DOS 1.5	DOS 4

The Adenoid

The adenoid is first identified as an accumulation of lymphocytes in the pharyngeal vault at 3 months gestation (100 mm crown–rump) and germinal centers are not seen until postpartum (Snook 1934). Magnetic resonance imaging has been used to observe adenoidal development. The adenoid was identified in 2/11(18%) of children less than 3 months of age, in 6/8 (75%) at 4 months of age and in all children at 5 months of age (Jaw et al. 1999). The adenoid increases in absolute size to 10 years of age and then diminishes, reaching minimum size at age 20 years (Vogler et al. 2000). The growth of the adenoid, in normal children age 1–11 years, remains in constant proportional to the size of the nasopharyngeal airway (Arens et al. 2002).

Language and Speech

For a full description of speech and language development see Chapter 5. See also the NICDC website cited in the reference list below.

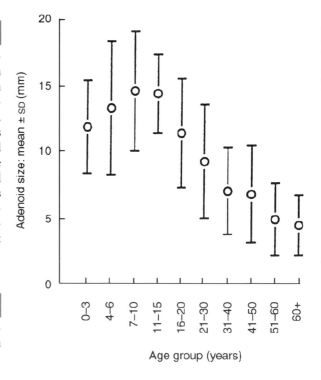

Fig. 1 The development and regression of the adenoid (Vogler et al. 2000)

References

1. Arens R, McDonough JM, Corbin AM, et al (2002) Linear dimensions of the upper airway structure during development: assessment by magnetic resonance imaging. Am J Respir Crit Care Med 165:117–122

2. Casselbrant ML, Alper CM (2003) Methods of examination. In: Bluestone CD, Stool SE, Alper CM, et al (eds) Pediatric Otolaryngology. Saunders/Elsevier, Philadelphia, pp 1379–1394

3. Jaw TS, Sheu RS, Liu GC, Lin WC (1999) Development of adenoids: a study by measurement with MR images. Kaohsiung J Med Sci 15:12–18

4. NICDC: Speech and Language: Developmental Milestones. http://www.nidcd.nih.gov/health/voice/speechandlanguage.asp#mychild. 10–21–2005

5. Ónodi A (1911) The accessory sinuses of the nose in children: 102 specimens reproduced in natural size from photographs. William Wood, New York

6. Siberry GK, Iannone R (eds) (2005) The Harriet Lane Handbook: A Manual for Pediatric House Officers, 17th edn. Elsevier Mosby, Philadelphia

7. Snook T (1934) The development of the human pharyngeal tonsil. Am J Anat 55:323–341

8. Vogler RC, Ii FJ, Pilgram TK (2000) Age-specific size of the normal adenoid pad on magnetic resonance imaging. Clin Otolaryngol 25:392–395

9. Wetmore RF (2003) Tracheotomy. In: Bluestone CD, Stool SE, Alper CM, et al (eds) Pediatric Otolaryngology. Saunders/Elsevier, Philadelphia, pp 1583–1598

Subject Index

Printing: Ten Brink, Meppel, The Netherlands
Binding: Ten Brink, Meppel, The Netherlands